ATLAS OF HISTOLOGY

with Functional Correlations

Thirteenth Edition

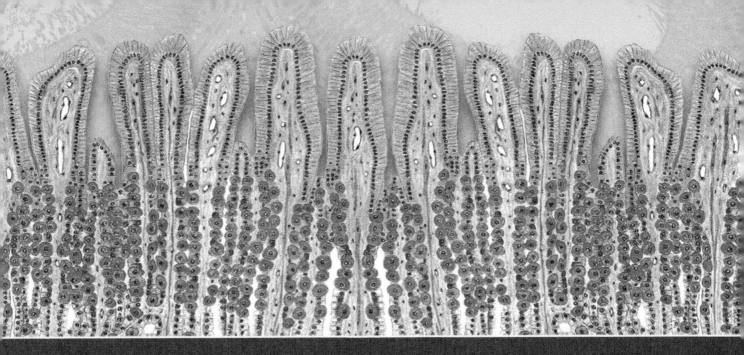

ATLAS OF HISTOLOGY

with Functional Correlations

Thirteenth Edition

Victor P. Eroschenko, PhD

Professor Emeritus of Anatomy
WWAMI Medical Program University of Idaho
Moscow, Idaho

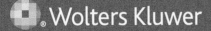 Wolters Kluwer

Philadelphia · Baltimore · New York · London
Buenos Aires · Hong Kong · Sydney · Tokyo

Not authorised for sale in United States, Canada, Australia, New Zealand, Puerto Rico, and U.S. Virgin Islands.

Acquisitions Editor: Crystal Taylor
Product Development Editor: Andrea Vosburgh
Editorial Coordinator: Annette Ferran
Marketing Manager: Michael McMahon
Designer: Terry Mallon
Production Project Manager: David Orzechowski
Compositor: SPi Global

Thirteenth Edition

Library of Congress Cataloging-in-Publication Data
Names: Eroschenko, Victor P., author.
Title: Atlas of histology with functional correlations / Victor P. Eroschenko.
Other titles: DiFiore's atlas of histology with functional correlations
Description: 13th edition. | Philadelphia : Wolters Kluwer, [2017] | Preceded by DiFiore's atlas of histology with functional correlations / Victor P. Eroschenko. c2013.
Identifiers: LCCN 2016046552 | ISBN 9781496316769
Subjects: | MESH: Histology | Atlases
Classification: LCC QM557 | NLM QS 517 | DDC 611/.018—dc23 LC record available at https://lccn.loc.gov/2016046552

Dedicated

To those who matter so much

Cassidy

Declan

Beckett

Ian

McKenzie

Sarah

Shannon

      and

      Diane

      Kathryn

      Tatiana

      Sharon

            and

            Todd

            Joshua

            Chadwick

                  and most especially and always

                  Elke

PREFACE TO THE THIRTEENTH EDITION

The thirteenth edition of *Atlas of Histology with Functional Correlations* (formerly *diFiore's Atlas of Histology with Functional Correlations*) continues to provide a colorful and expanded atlas of histologic images for medical, veterinary, dentistry, and pathology as well as students of the biological sciences.

As in previous editions, numerous comments from reviewers were helpful in suggesting improvement to the text and images of the atlas. Keeping these suggestions in mind, the composite and colorful illustrations of cells, tissues, and organs that made this atlas popular are maintained in the thirteenth edition. In addition, numerous photomicrographs were added throughout. While most of the images were prepared with light microscopy, other images with transmission and scanning microscopy are also included where it was necessary to show more precise and detailed morphology of different structures not visible with light microscopy.

The rapid advance in scientific research continues to produce volumes of new information that further our understanding of fundamental biological functions of cells as well as their subcellular and molecular components. Thus, in our contemporary era, the study of histology requires more than the recognition and identification of structural characteristics in different organs but also learning and understanding their diverse dynamics and functional correlations that maintain the homeostasis of living organisms.

CHANGES IN THE THIRTEENTH EDITION

- Descriptive text material has been carefully rewritten and updated for more concise presentation and easier understanding.
- Empty spaces have been condensed and replaced by text material and/or images.
- At least eight labeled Additional Histologic Images have been added to Chapters 2 and 3 through 22 to supplement the color illustrations and other histologic images.
- Chapters 2 through 22 now include five End-of-Chapter Review Questions with explanations for correct answers.
- The most important and latest functional correlations concerning the structure and function of various cells, tissues, and organs have been provided in a summarized format for easier reading and better comprehension of the new information.
- Composite lead-in art pages from previous editions have been dispersed throughout chapters to better correspond to their relevant topics.

LEARNING RESOURCES

The following Student and Instructor Resources are offered at Wolters Kluwer's learning resource center thePoint*.

Student Resources:

- Interactive Question Bank of more than 250 additional multiple-choice questions not included in the book, with explanations for correct answers

Instructor Resources:

- Interactive Image Bank including all images from the book with labels and leaders on, labels and leaders off, and labels off with leaders on options

- Supplemental Image Bank including more than 1,000 additional unlabeled photomicrographs not included in the book, organized by chapter; multiple images of similar structures are included
- Syllabus Conversion Guide indicating changes and additions between the twelfth and thirteenth editions.

For more information about accessing and licensing Instructor Resources, please contact your sales representative or visit thepoint.lww.com.

ACKNOWLEDGMENTS

I acknowledge the numerous colleagues who have graciously contributed their images to my previous editions of this atlas. In this edition, the donated images are credited with their names and their affiliated institutions. I shall always be grateful to these professionals for their generosity and assistance in improving this atlas.

The cooperation and assistance provided by the staff of the publishing company of Wolters Kluwer is sincerely appreciated. As with numerous past editions, I acknowledge the assistance of Crystal Taylor, my long-time acquisitions editor. I also was given the high privilege of working for the third time in preparing this edition with the most professional freelance editor, Kelly Horvath. Her hard work and dedication to accuracy and the best possible production of this atlas is sincerely appreciated. To all other professional individuals who assisted or were involved in production of this latest version of my atlas I express my sincere appreciation.

IN MEMORIAM

Since assuming the authorship of this atlas approximately 30 years ago, I have had the pleasure of collaborating with Dr. E. Roland Brown, the medical illustrator who ensured the accurate composition of each histological illustration for this atlas during all of this time. These beautiful color illustrations of numerous cells and tissues made this atlas unique and popular with histology students. As I was preparing the atlas for the thirteenth edition, I was informed that Roland passed away. With Roland's death, the field of medical illustration has lost a very talented artist, and I have lost a close and wonderful friend. The beautiful histologic illustrations that he prepared for all previous editions of the atlas will be enjoyed and appreciated by many students worldwide for many years. His talent will be sorely missed.

Victor P. Eroschenko, PhD
Professor Emeritus of Anatomy
Eagle, Idaho
November 2016

REVIEWERS

FACULTY

Rebecca Brown
LeMoyne College
Syracuse, New York

Raymond Coleman
Cornell University
Ithaca, New York

John Kmetz
University of Texas at San Antonio
San Antonio, Texas

Regina Munro
Chandler-Gilbert Community College
Chandler, Arizona

Holly Ressetar
West Virginia University School of Medicine
Morgantown, West Virginia

STUDENTS

Josh Agranat
Boston University School of Medicine
Boston, Massachusetts

Cheri Dijamco
University of Texas Health Science Center at San Antonio
San Antonio, Texas

Reza Khorasanee
University of Oxford
Oxford, United Kingdom

Jason Lipof
George Washington University Medical School
Washington, District of Columbia

Tina Lu
University of California San Diego School of Medicine
San Diego, California

Andrew Mendelson
Lake Erie College of Osteopathic Medicine
Erie, Pennsylvania

Nicholas Pettit
American Association of Colleges of Osteopathic Medicine
Chevy Chase, Maryland

Hope Taitt
SUNY Downstate Medical Center
Brooklyn, New York

Jennifer Townsend
University of California San Francisco
San Francisco, California

Samuel Windham
University of Missouri School of Medicine
Columbia, Missouri

CONTENTS

CHAPTER 3 CELLS AND THE CELL CYCLE 38

PART III Tissues

CHAPTER 4 EPITHELIAL TISSUE 44

SECTION 1   Classification of Epithelial Tissue 44

SECTION 2   Classification of Glandular Tissue 60

CHAPTER 5 **CONNECTIVE TISSUE 73**

CHAPTER 7   SKELETAL TISSUE: CARTILAGE AND BONE   118

CHAPTER 8 MUSCLE TISSUE 154

CHAPTER 9 NERVOUS TISSUE 179

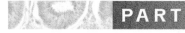

PART IV Systems

CHAPTER 10 CIRCULATORY SYSTEM 224

CHAPTER 14 DIGESTIVE SYSTEM PART II: ESOPHAGUS AND STOMACH 325

CHAPTER 16 DIGESTIVE SYSTEM PART IV: ACCESSORY DIGESTIVE ORGANS (LIVER, PANCREAS, AND GALLBLADDER)

CHAPTER 17 RESPIRATORY SYSTEM 402

CHAPTER 18   URINARY SYSTEM   428

PART I

Introduction

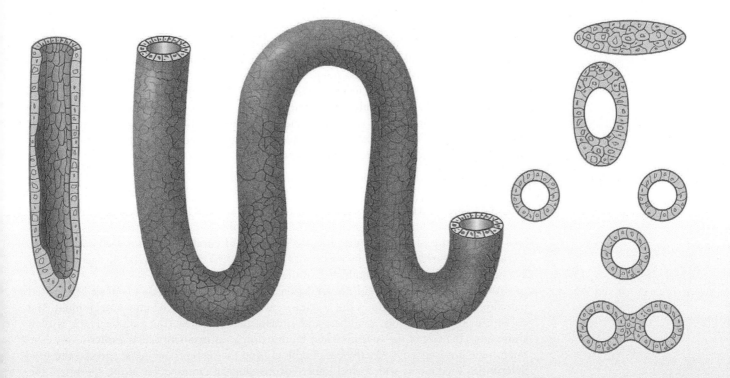

Histologic Methods

SECTION 1 Tissue Preparation and Staining of Sections

TISSUE PREPARATION: LIGHT MICROSCOPY

Histology is a visual as well as a very colorful science, which is studied with the aid of a light microscope. This chapter briefly describes the methodology used in preparing tissues for examination with microscopes and the different stains that were used to photograph the images. Most of the illustrations in this atlas are photographed from slides that have been prepared by the different methods described below.

Fixation

To preserve a section of tissue or organ for histological examination, the tissue specimen first undergoes **fixation** with different chemicals. Fixation permanently preserves the structural and molecular composition of the specimen. For light microscopy use, small pieces of the tissue specimen are immersed in the fixative, which hardens the specimen for sectioning and causes **cross-linkage** of **macromolecules** within the cells. This process reduces the cellular degeneration, preserves the integrity of cells and tissues, and increases their affinity to take up different stains that will show the composition of the specimen. The most commonly used fixative for light microcopy is the neutral-buffered **formaldehyde**.

Postfixation

After the tissue is fixed, usually overnight, water is first removed from the fixed specimen (dehydration) and passed through a series of ascending **alcohol** (ethanol) concentrations, usually from 50% to 100% ethanol. Before embedding the specimen in **paraffin** (wax) for slicing it into thin sections, it is cleared of alcohol by passing it through several changes of clearing agents such as **xylene**, which is miscible with both alcohol and paraffin.

After alcohol clearance and impregnation with xylene, the specimen is placed in melted paraffin. Paraffin then infiltrates the specimen, after which it is placed into a metal mold. The paraffin in the mold cools, solidifies, and encases the specimen. The paraffin block is then trimmed to the size of the specimen and mounted in an instrument called a **microtome**. The microtome precisely advances the paraffin block, and the sections are cut at specific and predetermined increments with a steel knife. For histological examination of the specimen, the sections are normally cut at 5 to 10 μm thick. The thin paraffin section is then collected and floated in a warm water bath to flatten and remove any wrinkles from the sections and placed onto a glass slide that has been covered with a thin layer of mounting medium, which adheres the specimen to the glass slide or the slides are dried in an oven so that the specimen attaches to the glass.

Staining of Sections

There are numerous stain-specific cell organelles, different cell types, fibers, tissues, and organs. The thin paraffin sections that are placed on the glass slide are colorless. To see the structural details in a given specimen, the sections must be stained. To stain the specimen in the section, paraffin must first be dissolved with solvents such as **xylene** and the sections rehydrated with a series of decreasing **alcohol** concentrations. The hydrated sections can then be stained with a variety of water-soluble stains, which selectively stain various components of the specimen and allow visual differentiation between the different cellular and tissue components. After completion of staining, the specimen is again dehydrated and immersed in xylene, after which a suitable mounting medium is put on the specimen and a thin protective glass coverslip placed over the specimen on the slide. The coverslip allows for viewing of the stained specimen on the glass slide with the light microscope via a light beam that passes through the specimen attached to the glass slide.

Most of the stains used for histological slide preparations act like the acidic or basic compounds. Structures in the specimen that stain with basic stains are called **basophilic** and those that stain with acidic stains are called **acidophilic**. The most common stains that are used for histological sections are **hematoxylin** and **eosin** stains.

TISSUE PREPARATION: OTHER METHODS

Frozen Section Procedures

Besides paraffin sections, there are also procedures in which the tissues are first frozen for rapid microscopic examination of a specimen that may be taken during surgery. This type of procedure is called cryosection; however, frozen sections are of lesser quality than those fixed in formalin and embedded in paraffin. The instrument for cryosectioning is the **cryostat**, which is a microtome inside a freezer. The tissue is removed from an organism, placed onto a metal stub, embedded in a gellike medium, and frozen to about −20°C to −30°C; such low temperatures are required for fat or lipid-rich tissue. The specimen is secured in a chuck and is cut frozen on the microtome 5 to 10 μm thick. Individual or single frozen sections are cut at low temperature, picked up and put on a glass slide, and then stained. The freezing of tissue eliminates the need for chemical fixation, is faster, and maintains most enzyme and immunological functions. It also can be used to examine temperature-sensitive or lipid-soluble molecules or where rapid analysis of the tissue is needed. Sectioning with the cryostat is similar to that of paraffin sectioning; both methods use a rotary type of microtome.

In addition to rotary microtomes, there are nonrotary or sliding or sledge microtomes. In these units, the tissue sample is put into a holder, which then is moved back and forth across the knife. The sledge or sliding microtome is primarily used for cutting large samples of tissues or organs embedded in paraffin, such as sections of the brain, kidneys, and other biological structures for histological examinations. Typical section thickness produced by a sledge microtome is between 1 and 60 μm. After sectioning, the samples undergo routine preparation for staining with different type of stains.

Transmission and Scanning Electron Microscopy

Examining the tissue sections with a **transmission electron microscope (TEM)** allows for much higher magnification and greater resolution. The fixatives and procedures are different from those of tissue preparation for histological slide examination. The specimen that is to be collected is either previously perfused with the fixative in the body or removed from the organism, cut into small pieces, and directly immersed in the fixative for rapid fixation. In addition, the primary fixative for TEM specimens is cold-buffered **glutaraldehyde** in which the specimens are first immersed. Following glutaraldehyde fixation, the specimens are rinsed in several buffers and then postfixed in cold **osmium tetroxide**, which reacts with phospholipids. Osmium tetroxide imparts an electron density to the cells and tissues because of its heavy metal. This allows for image formations for viewing with TEM. Following fixation and postfixation, the tissues are embedded in epoxy resin, which then polymerizes and forms a hard plastic tissue block. The plastic blocks are trimmed, and ultrathin sections are cut from them with a special instrument called an ultramicrotome, using either a diamond knife or special glass knives. The thin sections are then collected on small copper grids and stained with **uranyl acetate** and **lead citrate**. Using the TEM, the electron beams pass through the ultrathin stained specimen, resulting in high-resolution, high-contrast black-and-white images on the screen for recording.

In contrast to TEM with thin sections, the **scanning electron microscope (SEM)** uses larger, solid pieces of tissue to view a three-dimensional image of the surface of the specimens. The collected tissue samples are fixed in the same fixative as that used for TEM, namely, cold-buffered glutaraldehyde, then dehydrated through an acetone or ethanol series, and dried at the **critical point**. The dried samples are then mounted on a stub of metal with adhesive and coated with evaporated **gold palladium**.

When viewing the prepared specimen with the SEM, the electron beams do not pass through the specimen; instead, the specimen is scanned along its surface. The electrons that are reflected from the surface of the prepared specimen are then collected by detectors and processed as a black-and-white image of the surface of the specimen with a three-dimensional appearance.

This atlas contains a number of images obtained by using the transmission and scanning electron microscopes.

SECTION 2   Histologic Slide Interpretation

APPEARANCE OF HISTOLOGIC SECTIONS PREPARED BY DIFFERENT TYPES OF STAINS

Interpretation of histologic sections is greatly aided by the use of different stains, which selectively stain certain specific properties in different cells, tissues, and organs. The most prevalent stain that is used for preparation of histology slides is the hematoxylin and eosin (H&E) stain. Most of the images prepared for this atlas were taken from slides that were stained with H&E stain. To show other and more specific characteristic features of different cells, tissues, and organs, other stains are also used.

Figures 1.1 to 1.9 feature descriptions of the nine different stains that were used to prepare slides for this atlas, including their specific staining characteristics.

HEMATOXYLIN AND EOSIN STAIN

- Nuclei stain blue.
- Cytoplasm stains pink or red.
- Collagen fibers stain pink.
- Muscles stain pink.

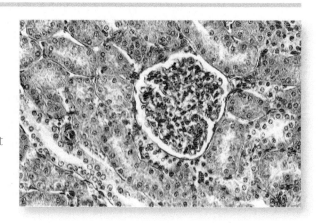

FIGURE 1.1 ■ Kidney cortex with a renal corpuscle and different convoluted tubules.

MASSON TRICHROME STAIN

- Nuclei stain black or blue-black.
- Muscles stain red.
- Collagen and mucus stain green or blue.
- Cytoplasm of most cells stains pink.

FIGURE 1.2 ■ Skeletal muscle sectioned in the longitudinal plane and cross section with surrounding blue-staining connective tissue.

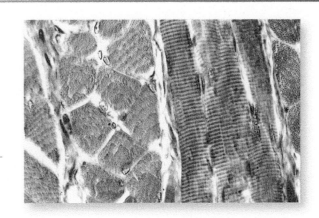

PERIODIC ACID–SCHIFF REACTION

- Glycogen stains deep red or magenta.
- Goblet cells in intestines and respiratory epithelia stain magenta-red.
- Basement membranes and brush borders in kidney tubules stain positive, or pink.

FIGURE 1.3 ■ Villus of a small intestine with brush border, columnar epithelium, and goblet cells.

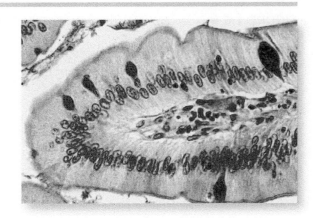

ELASTIC TISSUE STAIN

- Elastic fibers stain jet black.
- Nuclei stain gray.
- Remaining structures stain pink.

FIGURE 1.4 ■ Section of a wall from the aorta, showing the presence of dark-staining elastic fibers and pink smooth muscles.

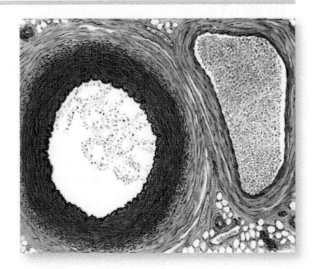

MALLORY-AZAN STAIN

- Fibrous connective tissue, mucus, and hyaline cartilage stain deep blue.
- Erythrocytes stain red-orange.
- Cytoplasm of liver and kidney stains pink.
- Nuclei stain red.

FIGURE 1.5 ■ Intramembranous ossification in skull bones showing blue connective tissue, red blood cells, and blood vessels with blood cells.

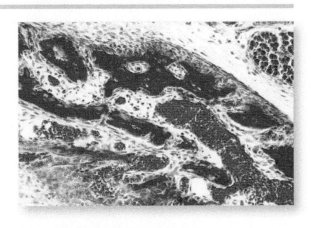

WRIGHT/GIEMSA STAIN

- Erythrocyte cytoplasm stains pink.
- Lymphocyte nuclei stain dark purple-blue with pale-blue cytoplasm.
- Monocyte cytoplasm stains pale blue, and the nucleus stains medium blue.
- Neutrophil nuclei stain dark blue.
- Eosinophil nuclei stain dark blue, and the granules stain bright pink.
- Basophil nuclei stain dark blue or purple, cytoplasm pale blue, and granules deep purple.
- Platelets stain light blue.

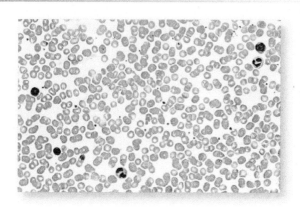

FIGURE 1.6 ■ Blood smear with different cells and platelets.

THE CAJAL AND DEL RIO HORTEGA METHODS (SILVER AND GOLD METHODS)

- Myelinated and unmyelinated fibers and neurofibrils stain blue-black.
- The general background is nearly colorless.
- Astrocytes stain black.
- Depending on the methods used, the end product can stain black, brown, or gold.

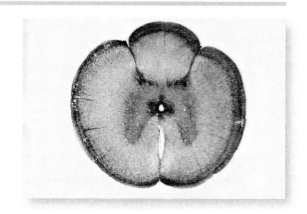

FIGURE 1.7 ■ Cross section of the spinal cord showing the gray and white matter.

OSMIC ACID (OSMIUM TETROXIDE) STAIN

- Lipids, in general, stain black.
- Lipids in a myelin sheath of nerves stain black.

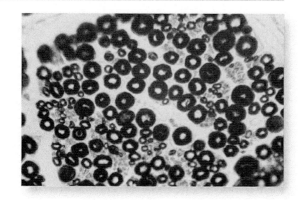

FIGURE 1.8 ■ Cross section of a peripheral nerve showing the myelin sheath of the axons.

IRON HEMATOXYLIN AND ALCIAN BLUE STAIN

- Connective tissue fibers stain dark blue.
- Smooth muscles stain light pink.
- Nuclei stain dark and cytoplasm light pink.

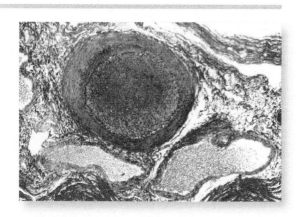

FIGURE 1.9 ■ Small artery and veins showing blood cells and the surrounding connective tissues.

INTERPRETATION OF HISTOLOGIC SECTIONS

One of the biggest challenges histology students encounter is interpreting what the two-dimensional histology sections represent in three dimensions. **Histologic sections** are thin, flat slices of fixed and stained tissues or organs mounted on flat glass slides. Such sections are normally composed of cellular, fibrous, and tubular structures that are cut in different planes. As a result, a variety of shapes, sizes, and layers may be visible, depending on the plane of section. **Fibrous** structures are solid and are found in connective, nervous, and muscle tissues. **Tubular** structures are hollow and represent various types of blood vessels, lymph vessels, glandular ducts, and glands of the body.

In tissues and organs, the cells, fibers, and tubes have a random orientation in space and are parts of a three-dimensional structure. During the preparation of histology slides, the thin sections cut from the specimen do not show much depth. In addition, the plane of section does not always bisect these structures in exact transverse or cross section. As a result, this produces a variation in the appearance of the cells, fibers, and tubes, depending on the angle of the plane of section. Consequently, it becomes difficult to correctly perceive the true three-dimensional structure of the specimen from which the sections were prepared on a flat slide. Therefore, correct visualization and interpretation of these sections in their proper three-dimensional perspective on the slide become an important criterion for understanding and mastering histology images. Figures 1.10 and 1.11 illustrate how the appearance of cells and tubes changes with different planes of section. Figure 1.12 is an actual histology slide of an organ that is filled with tubular structures that are highly convoluted. This section illustrates how the appearance of such tubular structures in the testis changes when they are sectioned in different planes.

FIGURE 1.10 | Planes of Section of a Round, Solid Object

To illustrate how the shape of a three-dimensional cell can be altered in a histologic section, a hard-boiled egg has been sectioned in longitudinal and transverse (cross) planes. The composition of a hard-boiled egg serves as a good example of a cell, with the yellow yolk representing the nucleus and the surrounding egg white (pale blue) representing the cytoplasm. Enclosing these structures are the soft eggshell membrane and a hard eggshell (red). At the rounded end of the egg is the air space (blue).

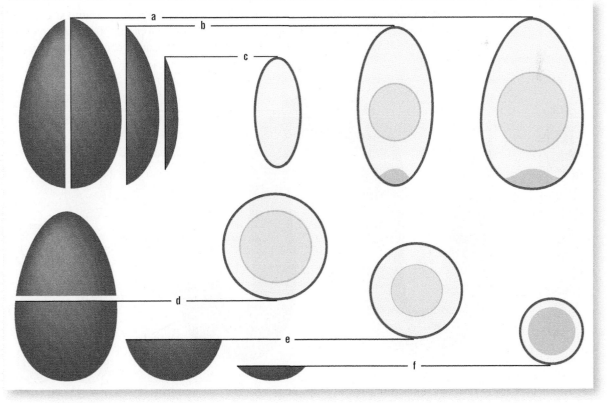

FIGURE 1.10 ■ Planes of sections through a round object, a hard-boiled, solid egg.

The **midline** sections of the egg in the **longitudinal** (**a**) and **transverse planes** (**d**) disclose its correct shape and size, as they appear in these planes of section. In addition, these two planes of section reveal the correct appearance, size, and distribution of the internal contents within the egg.

Similar but more **peripheral** sections of the egg in the **longitudinal** (**b**) and **transverse planes** (**e**) still show the external shape of the egg. However, because the section was cut peripherally and below the midline, the internal contents of the egg are not seen in their correct size or distribution within the egg white. In addition, the size of the egg appears smaller.

The **tangential plane** (**c** and **f**) of the section grazes or only passes through the outermost periphery of the egg. This section reveals that the egg is oval (c) or a small round (f) object. The egg yolk is not seen in either section because it was not located in the plane of section. As a result, such tangential section does not reveal sufficient detail for correct interpretation of the egg size or of its contents or their distribution within the internal membrane.

Thus, in a histological section, individual structure, shape, and size vary depending on the plane of section. Some cells may exhibit full cross sections of their nuclei, and they appear prominent in the cells. Other cells may exhibit only a fraction of the nucleus, and the cytoplasm appears large. Still other cells may appear only as clear cytoplasm, without any nuclei. All these variations are attributable to different planes of section through the nuclei. Understanding these variations in cell and tube morphology becomes important in interpreting different histological sections.

FIGURE 1.11 | Planes of Section through a Hollow Structure or a Tube

Tubular structures are often seen in histologic sections. Tubes are most easily recognized when they are cut in transverse (cross) sections. However, if the tubes are sectioned in planes other than transverse, their appearance is different. To be recognized as a hollow tube, they must first be visualized as three-dimensional structures. To illustrate how a blood vessel, duct, or a hollow glandular structure may vary in appearance in a histologic section, a curved tube with a simple (single) epithelial cell layer is sectioned in longitudinal, transverse, and oblique planes.

A **longitudinal** (**a**) plane of section that cuts the tube in the midline produces a U-shaped structure. The sides of the tube are lined by a single row of cuboidal (round) cells around an empty lumen except at the bottom, where the tube begins to curve; in this region, the cells appear multilayered.

Transverse (**d** and **e**) planes of section of the same tube produce round structures lined by a single layer of cells. The variations that are seen in the cytoplasm of different cells are related to the planes of section through the individual cells, as explained above. A transverse section of

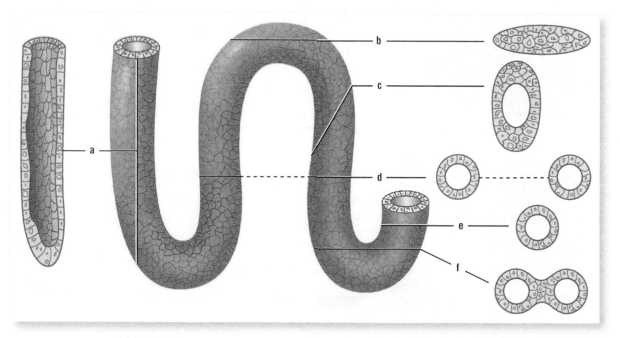

FIGURE 1.11 ■ Planes of section through a hollow object, a tube.

a straight tube can produce a single image (e). The double image (d) of the same structure can represent either two tubes running parallel to each other or a single tube that has curved in the space of the tissue or organ that is sectioned.

A **tangential** (**b**) plane of section through the tube with a single layer of cells produces a solid, multicellular, oval structure that does not resemble a tube. The reason for this is that the plane of section has grazed the outermost periphery of tube as it made a turn in space; the lumen was not present in the plane of section. An **oblique** (**c**) plane of section through the same tube and its single layer of cells produces an oval structure that includes an oval lumen in the center and multiple cell layers at the periphery.

A **transverse** (**f**) section in the region of a sharp curve in the tube grazes the innermost cell layer and produces two round structures connected by a multiple, solid layer of cells. These sections of the tube also contain round lumen, indicating that the plane of section passed perpendicular to the structure.

Figure 1.12 shows a section from the testis. This organ is filled with numerous and convoluted (twisted) tubular structures, the seminiferous tubules. Careful examination of this figure shows how individual tubular structures can change shape and appearance, depending on the plane of section through the tubules. Similar structural alteration is possible in solid structures, such as the muscle fibers, connective tissue fibers, or nerve fibers.

FIGURE 1.12 | Hollow Tubules of the Testis in Different Planes of Section

Organs such as the testes and kidneys consist primarily of highly twisted or convoluted tubules. When flat sections of such organs are seen on a histology slide, the cut tubules exhibit a variety of shapes because of the plane of section. To show how twisted tubules appear in a histologic slide, a portion of a testis was prepared for examination. Each testis consists of numerous, highly twisted seminiferous tubules that are lined by multilayered or stratified germinal epithelium.

A **longitudinal plane** (**1**) through a seminiferous tubule produces an elongated tubule with a long lumen. A **transverse plane** (**2**) through a single seminiferous tubule produces a round tubule. Similarly, a **transverse plane through a curve** (**3, 5**) of a seminiferous tubule produces two oval structures that are connected by solid layers of cells. An **oblique plane** (**4**) through a tubule produces an oval structure with an oval lumen in the center and multiple cell layers at the periphery. A **tangential plane** (**6**) of a seminiferous tubule passes through its periphery. As a result, this plane produces a solid, multicellular, oval structure that does not resemble a tube because the plane of section passed below the lumen.

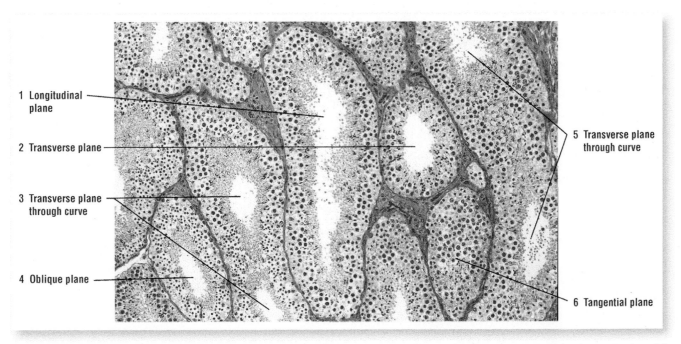

FIGURE 1.12 ■ Tubules of the testis in different planes of section. Stain: hematoxylin and eosin (plastic section). ×30.

PART II

Cell and Cytoplasm

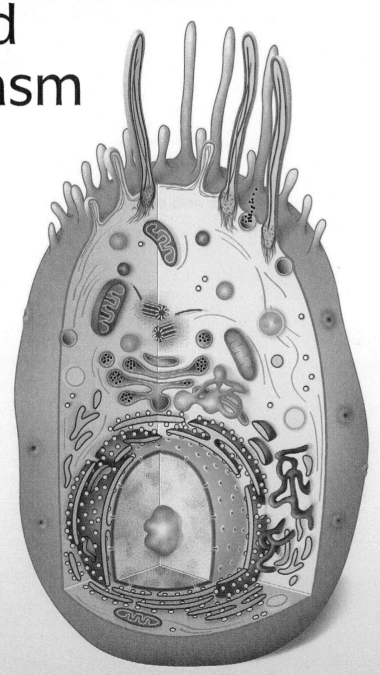

Light and Transmission Electron Microscopy

Histology, or microscopic anatomy, is a visual, colorful science. The light source for the early microscopes was sunlight. In modern microscopes, electric illumination is used as the main light source.

With the simplest light microscopes, examination of mammalian cells showed a nucleus and a cytoplasm, surrounded by some sort of a border or cell membrane. As microscopic techniques evolved, the use of various histochemical, immunocytochemical, and staining techniques revealed that the cytoplasm of different cells contained numerous subcellular elements called **organelles**. Although much initial information in histology was gained by examining tissue slides with a light microscope, its resolving power was too limited. To gain additional information called for increased resolution.

With the advent of transmission electron microscopy, superior resolution, and higher magnification of cells, the examination of the contents of the cytoplasm became possible. Histologists are now able to describe the ultrastructure of the cell, its membrane, and the numerous organelles that are present in the cytoplasm of different cells.

CELL AND CYTOPLASM

Some living organisms are single celled, whereas others contain a multitude of cells and cell types. The main function of these cells is to maintain a proper **homeostasis** in the organism, which is to maintain the internal environment in a relatively constant state. To perform this task, cells possess certain structural features in their cytoplasm that are common to all. As a result, it is possible to illustrate a cell in a more generalized, composite form with various cytoplasmic organelles. It is essential to remember, however, that the quantity, appearance, and distribution of the cytoplasmic organelles within a given cell depend on the cell type and its function.

CELL MEMBRANE

Except for mature red blood cells, erythrocytes, all mammalian cells contain a **nucleus**. In addition, all cells are surrounded by a **cell** or a **plasma membrane**, which forms an important barrier or boundary between the internal and the external environments. Internal to the cell membrane is the **cytoplasm**, a dense, fluidlike medium that contains numerous **organelles**, microtubules, microfilaments, and membrane-bound secretory granules or ingested material.

The membrane that surrounds the cell consists of a **phospholipid bilayer**, a double layer of **phospholipid molecules**. Interspersed within and embedded in the phospholipid bilayer of the cell membrane are the **integral membrane proteins** and **peripheral membrane proteins**, which make up almost half of the total mass of the membrane. The integral membrane proteins are incorporated within the lipid bilayer of the cell membrane. Some of the integral proteins span the entire thickness of the cell membrane. These are the **transmembrane proteins**, and they are exposed on the outer and the inner surface of the cell membrane. The membrane proteins participate in transporting molecules across the lipid bilayer, serve as membrane receptors for different hormones, attach to and support the internal cytoskeleton of the cell membrane, and

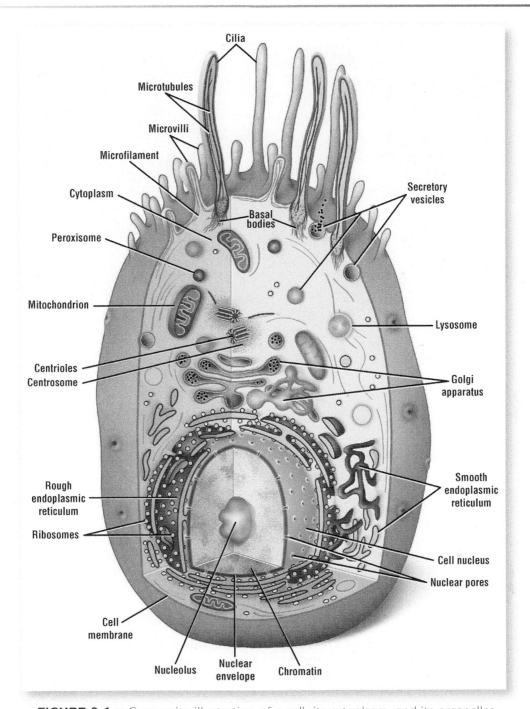

FIGURE 2.1 ■ Composite illustration of a cell, its cytoplasm, and its organelles.

possess specific enzyme activity. The peripheral proteins do not protrude into the phospholipid bilayer and are not embedded within the cell membrane. Instead, they are associated with the cell membrane on both its extracellular (outer) and intracellular (inner) surfaces. Some of the peripheral proteins are anchored to the network of tiny **microfilaments** of the cytoskeleton of the cell and are held firmly in place. Also present within the plasma membrane is the lipid molecule **cholesterol**. Cholesterol stabilizes the cell membrane, makes it more rigid, and regulates the fluidity of the phospholipid bilayer.

Located on the external surface of the cell membrane in certain specialized cells is a delicate, fuzzy cell coat called the **glycocalyx**, composed of carbohydrate molecules that are attached to the integral proteins of the cell membrane and that project from the external cell surface. The glycocalyx is seen on the microvilli of the absorptive cells in the small intestine

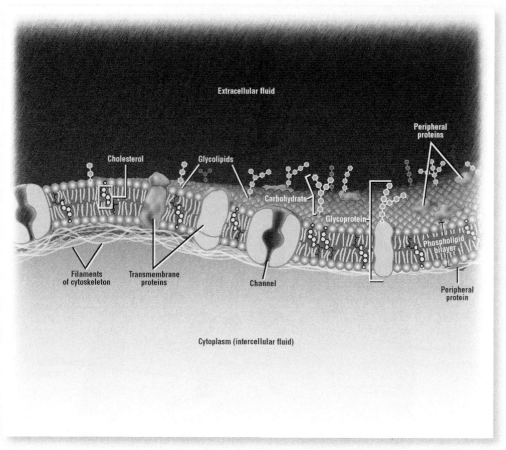

Extracellular fluid

Peripheral proteins

Cholesterol

Glycolipids

Carbohydrate

Glycoprotein

Phospholipid bilayer

Peripheral protein

Filaments of cytoskeleton

Transmembrane proteins

Channel

Cytoplasm (intercellular fluid)

FIGURE 2.2 ■ Composition of cell membrane.

and proximal convoluted tubules in the kidney. Glycocalyx is not seen with routine histological stain unless the sections are stained with periodic acid–Schiff or viewed with the electron microscope. The glycocalyx performs an important role in cell recognition, in cell-to-cell attachments or adhesions, and as a receptor or binding sites for different bloodborne hormones.

MOLECULAR ORGANIZATION OF THE CELL MEMBRANE

The lipid bilayer of the cell membrane has a fluid consistency, and as a result, the compositional structure of the cell membrane is characterized as a **fluid mosaic model**. The phospholipid molecules of the cell membrane are distributed as two layers. Their **polar heads** are arranged on both the inner and outer surfaces of the cell membrane. The **nonpolar tails** of the lipid layers face each other in the center of the membrane. Images of cell membrane viewed with the transmission electron microscope, however, appear as three distinct layers, consisting of outer and inner electron-dense layers and a less dense or lighter middle layer. This discrepancy is due to the osmic acid (osmium tetroxide) that is used to fix and stain tissues for electron microscopy. Osmic acid binds to the polar heads of the lipid molecules in the cell membrane and stains them very dense. The nonpolar tails in the middle of the cell membrane remain light and unstained.

CELL MEMBRANE PERMEABILITY AND MEMBRANE TRANSPORT

The phospholipid bilayer of the cell membrane is permeable to certain substances and impermeable to others. This property of the cell membrane is called **selective permeability**. Selective permeability forms an important barrier between the internal and external environments of the cell, which then maintains a constant intracellular environment.

The phospholipid bilayer is permeable to such molecules as oxygen, carbon dioxide, water, steroids, and other lipid-soluble chemicals. Other substances, such as glucose, ions, or proteins, cannot pass through the cell membrane and cross it only by specific **transport mechanisms**. Some of these substances are transported through the integral membrane proteins using pump molecules or through protein channels that allow the passage of specific molecules. A process called **endocytosis** performs the uptake and transfer of molecules and solids across the cell membrane into the cell interior. In contrast, the process of releasing material from the cell cytoplasm across the cell membrane to the exterior is called **exocytosis**.

Pinocytosis is the process by which cells ingest small molecules of extracellular fluids or liquids. **Phagocytosis** refers to the ingestion or intake by specialized cells of larger solid particles, such as bacteria, worn-out cells, or cellular debris. Examples of such cells are the neutrophils in the blood and macrophages or monocytes in the extracellular connective tissues. **Receptor-mediated endocytosis** is highly selective form of pinocytosis or phagocytosis. In this process, specific molecules in the extracellular fluid bind to receptors on the cell membrane and are then taken into the cell interior. These receptors cluster on the cell membrane, and the membrane indents at this point to form **coated pits** that are lined with peripheral membrane proteins called **clathrin**. The pit pinches off and forms a clathrin-coated vesicle that enters the cell cytoplasm. The clathrin molecules then separate from the coated vesicle and recycle back to the cell membrane to form new coated pits. Examples of receptor-mediated endocytosis include uptake of low-density lipoproteins and insulin from the blood.

CELLULAR ORGANELLES

Each cell cytoplasm contains numerous organelles, each of which performs a specialized metabolic function that is essential for maintaining cellular homeostasis and cell life. A membrane similar to the cell membrane surrounds such cytoplasmic organelles as nucleus, mitochondria, endoplasmic reticulum, Golgi apparatus or Golgi complex, lysosomes, and peroxisomes. Organelles that are not surrounded by membranes include ribosomes, basal bodies, centrioles, and centrosomes.

Mitochondria

Mitochondria are round, oval, or elongated structures whose variability and number depend on cell function. Each mitochondrion (singular) consists of an outer and inner membrane. The inner membrane exhibits numerous folds called **cristae**, which contain respiratory chain enzymes that produce the energy molecule **adenosine triphosphate** (**ATP**). In protein-secreting cells, these cristae project into the interior of the mitochondria as **shelves**. In steroid-secreting cells, such as the adrenal cortex or interstitial cells in the testes, the mitochondria cristae are **tubular** and contain enzymes for steroidogenesis (production of steroid hormones).

FUNCTIONAL CORRELATIONS 2.1 ■ Mitochondria

Mitochondria produce most of the high-energy molecule **adenosine triphosphate** (**ATP**) in cells and are, therefore, considered the powerhouses of the cells. The cristae in the mitochondria increase the surface area of the inner membrane. The cristae contain most of the respiratory chain enzymes as well as **ATP synthetase**, which is responsible for cell respiration (oxidative phosphorylation) and production of cell ATP. ATP is the chemical energy responsible for various metabolic cell activities.

The number of mitochondria in a given cell is directly related to the cell's energy needs. Thus, cardiac or skeletal muscle cells with continuous high-energy needs contain numerous mitochondria, whereas cells with low-energy needs have few mitochondria. Also, in these high-energy cells, the mitochondria exhibit large numbers of closely packed cristae, whereas in cells with low-energy metabolism, the cristae are less extensively developed. Surrounding the cristae is an amorphous **mitochondrial matrix**, which contains enzymes, ribosomes, and, unlike other cytoplasmic organelles, a small, circular DNA molecule called **mitochondrial DNA**. New mitochondria arise from preexisting mitochondria by growth and division.

Rough and Smooth Endoplasmic Reticulum

The **endoplasmic reticulum** in the cytoplasm is an extensive network of sacs, vesicles, and interconnected flat tubules called **cisternae**. Endoplasmic reticulum may be either rough or smooth. Their predominance and distribution in a given cell depends on cell function.

Rough endoplasmic reticulum (RER) is characterized by numerous flattened, interconnected cisternae, whose cytoplasmic surfaces are covered or studded with dark-staining granules called **ribosomes**. The presence of ribosomes distinguishes the rough endoplasmic reticulum, which extends from the outer membrane of the nuclear envelope to sites throughout the cytoplasm. In contrast, **smooth endoplasmic reticulum (SER)** is devoid of ribosomes, and it consists primarily of anastomosing or connecting tubules. In most cells, smooth endoplasmic reticulum, which is less abundant than the rough endoplasmic reticulum, is also continuous with rough endoplasmic reticulum.

FUNCTIONAL CORRELATIONS 2.2 ■ Rough and Smooth Endoplasmic Reticulum

Cells that synthesize large amounts of protein for export, such as pancreatic acinar cells or salivary gland cells, exhibit a highly developed and extensive **rough endoplasmic reticulum (RER)** with numerous stacks of flattened cisternae. Thus, the main function of RER is **protein synthesis**. Proteins that will be **transported** or **exported** either to the outside of the cell or packaged in organelles such as lysosomes are synthesized by the ribosomes attached to the surface of the RER. In addition, **integral membrane proteins** and **phospholipid molecules** are synthesized by the RER that become part of the cell membrane. In contrast, proteins for the cytoplasm, nucleus, and mitochondria utilization are synthesized by the **free ribosomes** that are scattered within the cell cytoplasm.

SMOOTH ENDOPLASMIC RETICULUM

Although the **smooth endoplasmic reticulum (SER)** is continuous with the RER, its membranes lack ribosomes, and therefore, its functions are completely different and unrelated to protein synthesis. SER is found in abundance in cells that synthesize **phospholipids** that constitute all cell membranes, **cholesterol**, and **steroid hormones**, such as estrogens, testosterone, and corticosteroids. When liver cells (hepatocytes) are exposed to potentially harmful drugs and chemicals, SER proliferates and inactivates or **detoxifies** the chemicals. Similarly, in hepatocytes, SER is involved in **carbohydrate metabolism** that converts glycogen to glucose. Skeletal and cardiac muscle fibers also exhibit an extensive network of SER, called **sarcoplasmic reticulum**, whose primary functions is **calcium storage** (sequestering) between contractions and calcium release for initiation of muscular contractions.

Golgi Apparatus

The **Golgi apparatus** (also known as **Golgi complex** or **Golgi body**) is also composed of a system of membrane-bound, smooth, flattened, stacked, and slightly curved **cisternae**. These cisternae, however, are separate from those of endoplasmic reticulum. In most cells, there is a polarity in the Golgi apparatus. Near the Golgi apparatus, numerous small vesicles with newly synthesized proteins bud off from the rough endoplasmic reticulum and move to the Golgi apparatus for further processing. The Golgi cisternae nearest the budding vesicles are the forming, convex, or the *cis* face of the Golgi apparatus. The opposite side of the Golgi apparatus is the maturing inner concave side or the *trans* face. Vesicles from the endoplasmic reticulum move through the cytoplasm to the *cis* side of the Golgi apparatus and bud off from the *trans* side for transport of proteins to different sites in the cell cytoplasm.

FUNCTIONAL CORRELATIONS 2.3 ■ Golgi Apparatus

The **Golgi apparatus** is present in all cells except mature red blood cells, the erythrocytes. Its size and development varies, depending on the cell function; however, it is most highly developed in **secretory cells**. Most of the new proteins synthesized by the cisternae of the rough endoplasmic reticulum (RER) are transported in the cell cytoplasm as **transfer vesicles** to the *cis* **face** of the Golgi apparatus, which faces the RER. Within the Golgi cisternae are different types of enzymes that modify, sort, and package proteins for different destinations in the cell. As the protein molecules move through the different Golgi cisternae, sugars are added to the proteins and lipids to form **glycoproteins** and **glycolipids**. Also, proteins are added to lipids to form lipoproteins. As the secretory molecules near the exit or trans face of the Golgi cisternae, they are further modified, sorted, and packaged as membrane-bound vesicles, which then separate from the Golgi cisternae. Some secretory vesicles become **lysosomes** and remain in the cytoplasm. Other proteins migrate to the cell membrane and are incorporated into the cell membrane itself, thus contributing proteins and phospholipids to the membrane. Still other secretory granules become vesicles that are filled with a secretory product destined for **exocytosis** (export) to the outside of the cell.

Ribosomes

The **ribosomes** are small, electron-dense granules found in the cytoplasm of the cell; ribosomes are not surrounded by a membrane. In a given cell, there are both **free ribosomes** and **attached ribosomes**, as seen on the endoplasmic reticulum cisternae. Ribosomes play an important role in **protein synthesis** and are most abundant in the cytoplasm of protein-secreting cells. Ribosomes perform an essential role in decoding or translating the **coded genetic messages** from the nucleus for amino acid sequence of proteins that are then synthesized by the cell. The **unattached** or free ribosomes synthesize proteins for use within the cell cytoplasm. In contrast, ribosomes that are **attached** to the membranes of the endoplasmic reticulum synthesize proteins that are packaged and stored in the cell as lysosomes or are released from the cell as secretory products. Ribosomal subunits and associated proteins are first synthesized in the nucleolus and then transported to the cytoplasm via the nuclear pores.

Lysosomes

Lysosomes are cytoplasmic organelles that contain many hydrolyzing or digestive enzymes called **acid hydrolases**. Lysosomal hydrolases are synthesized in the rough endoplasmic reticulum and transferred to the Golgi apparatus, where they are modified and packaged into membrane-bound lysosomes. They are highly variable in appearance and size. To prevent the lysosomes from digesting the cytoplasm and cell contents, a membrane separates the lytic enzymes in the lysosomes from the cell cytoplasm. The main function of lysosomes is the **intracellular digestion** or **phagocytosis** of substances taken into the cells. Lysosomes digest phagocytosed microorganisms, cell debris, cells, and damaged, worn-out, or excessive cell organelles, such as rough endoplasmic reticulum or mitochondria. During intracellular digestion, a membrane surrounds the material to be digested. The membrane of the lysosome then fuses with the ingested material, and their hydrolytic enzymes are emptied into the formed vacuole. After digestion of the lysosomal contents, the indigestible debris in the cytoplasm is retained in large membrane-bound vesicles called **residual bodies**. Lysosomes are very abundant in such phagocytic cells as tissue macrophages and specific white blood cells (leukocytes) such as neutrophils.

Peroxisomes

Peroxisomes are cell organelles that appear similar to lysosomes, but are smaller. They are found in nearly all cell types. Peroxisomes contain several types of **oxidases**, which are enzymes that oxidize various organic substances to form **hydrogen peroxide**, a highly cytotoxic product.

Peroxisomes also contain the enzyme **catalase**, which eliminates excess hydrogen peroxide by breaking it down into water and oxygen molecules. Because the degradation of hydrogen peroxide takes place within the same organelle, peroxisomes protect other parts of the cells from this cytotoxic product. Peroxisomes are abundant in the cells of the liver and kidney, where much of the toxic substances are removed from the body. They detoxify, degrade alcohol, oxidize fatty acids, and metabolize various compounds.

CELL CYTOSKELETON

The **cytoskeleton** of a cell consists of a network of tiny protein filaments and tubules that extend throughout the cytoplasm. The cytoskeleton serves the cell's structural framework. Three types of filamentous proteins, microfilaments, intermediate filaments, and microtubules, form the cytoskeleton of a cell.

Microfilaments, Intermediate Filaments, and Microtubules

Microfilaments are the thinnest structures of the cytoskeleton. They are composed of the protein **actin** and are most prevalent on the peripheral regions of the cell membrane. These structural proteins shape the cells and contribute to cell movement and movement of the cytoplasmic organelles. The microfilaments are distributed throughout the cells and are used as anchors at cell junctions. The actin microfilaments also form the structural **core** of microvilli and the **terminal web** just inferior to the plasma membrane. In muscle tissues, the actin filaments fill the cells and are associated with **myosin** proteins to induce muscle contractions.

As their name implies, the **intermediate filaments** are thicker than microfilaments and are more stable. Several cytoskeletal proteins that form the intermediate filaments have been identified and localized. The intermediate filaments vary among cell types and have specific distribution in different cell types. Epithelial cells contain the intermediate filaments **keratin**. In skin cells, these filaments terminate at cell junctions, the **desmosomes** and **hemidesmosomes**, where they stabilize the shape of the cell and form attachments to adjacent cells. **Vimentin** filaments are found in many mesenchymal cells. **Desmin** filaments are found in both smooth and striated muscles. **Neurofilament** proteins are found in the nerve cells and their processes. **Glial filaments** are found in astrocytic glial cells of the nervous system. **Nuclear lamin** intermediate filaments are found on the inner layer of the nuclear membrane.

Microtubules are found in almost all cell types except mature red blood cells. They are the largest elements of the cytoskeleton. Microtubules are hollow, unbranched cylindrical structures composed of the two-protein subunits, α and β **tubulin**. All microtubules originate from the microtubule-organizing center, the **centrosome** in the cytoplasm, which contains a pair of **centrioles**. In the centrosome, the tubulin subunits polymerize and radiate from the centrioles in a starlike pattern from the center. Microtubules determine cell shape and function in intracellular movement of organelles and secretory granules, such as axoplasmic transport in neurons. Microtubules are also essential in cell mitosis where they form the spindles that separate the duplicated chromosomes and remodel the cell during mitosis. These tubules are most visible and are predominant in **cilia** and **flagella**, where they are responsible for their beating movements. Microtubules also form the basis of centrioles and basal bodies of the cilia.

CENTROSOME AND CENTRIOLES

The **centrosome** is an area of the cytoplasm located near the nucleus. It is the major **microtubule-forming center** and the site for generating new microtubules and mitotic spindles. The centrosome consists of two small cylindrical structures called **centrioles** and the surrounding matrix; the centrioles are oriented at right angles to each other. Each centriole consists of nine evenly spaced clusters of three sets of fused microtubules arranged in a circle or a ring. The microtubules exhibit longitudinal orientation and are parallel to each other.

Before mitosis, the centrioles in the centrosome replicate and form two pairs. During mitosis, each pair moves to the opposite poles of the cell, where they become microtubule-organizing centers for **mitotic spindles** that control the distribution of chromosomes to the daughter cells. Beneath the cell membrane, the centrioles induce the formation of **basal bodies** and organize the development of the microtubules in cilia and flagella.

CYTOPLASMIC INCLUSIONS

The **cytoplasmic inclusions** are temporary structures that accumulate in the cytoplasm of certain cells. **Lipids**, **glycogen**, **crystals**, **pigment**, or byproducts of metabolism are inclusions and represent the nonliving parts of the cell.

NUCLEUS, NUCLEAR ENVELOPE, AND NUCLEAR PORES

The **nucleus** is the largest organelle of a cell. Most cells contain a single nucleus, but other cells may exhibit multiple nuclei. Skeletal muscle cells have multiple nuclei, whereas mature red blood cells of mammals do not have a nucleus or are nonnucleated.

The nucleus consists of **chromatin**, one or more **nucleoli** (singular, nucleolus), and **nuclear matrix**. The nucleus contains the cellular genetic material **deoxyribonucleic acid (DNA)**, which encodes all cell structures and functions. A double membrane called the **nuclear envelope** surrounds the nucleus, whereas the nucleolus is not surrounded by a membrane. Both the inner and outer layers of the nuclear envelope have a structure similar to the lipid bilayer of the cell membrane. The outer nuclear membrane is studded with ribosomes and is continuous with the rough endoplasmic reticulum of the cytoplasm. The inner nuclear membrane lacks ribosomes and is in contact with the nuclear chromatin.

At intervals around the periphery of the nucleus, the outer and inner membranes of the nuclear envelope fuse to form numerous **nuclear pores**. These pores function in controlling the movement of metabolites, macromolecules, and ribosomal subunits between the nucleus and cytoplasm.

thePoint®   Supplemental micrographic images are available at **www.thePoint.com/Eroschenko13e** under Cell and Cytoplasm.

FUNCTIONAL CORRELATIONS 2.4 ■ Cilia and Microvilli

Cilia are highly motile surface modifications in cells that line the respiratory organs, oviducts or uterine tubes, and efferent ducts in the testes. Cilia are inserted into the **basal bodies** beneath the cell membrane. The main function of cilia is to sweep or move fluids, cells, or particulate matter across cell surfaces. In the lungs, the cilia rid the air passages of particulate matter or mucus. In the oviduct, cilia move eggs and sperm along the passageway, and in the testes, cilia move mature sperm into the epididymis.

The motility exhibited by cilia is caused by the sliding of adjacent microtubule doublets in the core of the cilia. Each of the nine doublets in the cilia consists of two subfibers called A and B. Extending from the A subfiber are two armlike filaments containing the **motor protein dynein**, which exhibits ATPase activity. This protein uses the energy of ATP hydrolysis to move cilia. Dynein armlike extensions from one doublet temporarily attach and detach from the subfiber B of the adjacent doublet, producing a sliding force between the doublets. These rapid back-and-forth changes between adjacent doublets produce cilia motility.

MICROVILLI

In contrast to cilia, **microvilli** are nonmotile. Microvilli are highly developed on the apical surfaces of epithelial cells of the small intestine and kidney. Here, the main functions of the microvilli are to absorb nutrients from the digestive tract of the small intestine or the glomerular filtrate in the kidney.

FIGURE 2.3 | Internal and External Morphology of Ciliated and Nonciliated Epithelium

A low-magnification electron micrograph shows the internal morphology and surfaces of ciliated and nonciliated cells in the epithelium of the efferent ductules of the testis. The numerous **cilia (2)** in the ciliated cells are attached to the dense **basal bodies (8)** at the cell apices, from which they extend into the **lumen (1)** of the duct. In contrast to cilia, the **microvilli (7)** in the nonciliated cells are much shorter and have a different internal structure than the cilia (see Fig. 2.7 for details and comparison).

Note also the dense structures in the apices between the adjacent epithelial cells. These are the **junctional complexes (3, 9)** that hold the cells tightly together. Distinct **cell membranes (10)** separate the individual cells. Located in the cytoplasm of these cells are numerous, elongated or rod-shaped **mitochondria (4, 11)** and numerous light-staining **vesicles (6)**. Each cell also contains various shaped **nuclei (12)** with dispersed, dense-staining nuclear **chromatin (5)** that is arranged around the nuclear periphery.

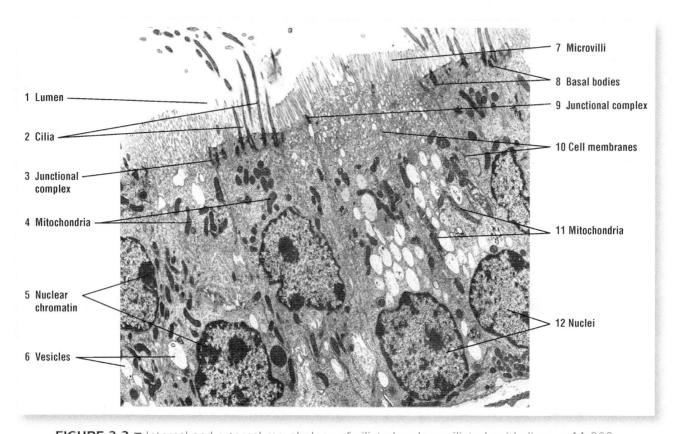

1 Lumen
2 Cilia
3 Junctional complex
4 Mitochondria
5 Nuclear chromatin
6 Vesicles
7 Microvilli
8 Basal bodies
9 Junctional complex
10 Cell membranes
11 Mitochondria
12 Nuclei

FIGURE 2.3 ◼ Internal and external morphology of ciliated and nonciliated epithelium. ×11,000.

FIGURE 2.4 | Junctional Complex Between Epithelial Cells

A high-magnification electron micrograph illustrates a junctional complex between two adjacent epithelial cells. In the upper or apical region of the cells, the opposing cell membranes fuse to form a **tight junction** or **zonula occludens** (**2a**), which extends around the cell peripheries like a belt. Inferior to the zonula occludens (2a) is another junction called the **zonula adherens** (**2b**). It is characterized by a dense layer of proteins on the inside of the plasma membranes of both cells, which attach to the cytoskeleton filaments of each cell. A small intercellular space with transmembrane adhesion proteins separates the two membranes. This type of junction also extends around the cells like a belt. Below the zonula adherens is a **desmosome** (**2c**). Desmosomes (2c) do not encircle the cells, but are spotlike structures that have random distribution in the cells. The cytoplasmic side of each desmosome exhibits dense areas composed of attachment proteins. Transmembrane glycoproteins extend into the intercellular space between opposing cells membranes of the desmosome and attach the cells to each other.

Note also in the micrograph the distinct **cell membranes** (**3**) of each cell, the numerous **mitochondria** (**1**) in cross section, and a variety of **vesicular structures** (**6**) in their cytoplasm. Visible on the cell apices are sections of **cilia** (**5**) with a core of **microtubules** and a few **microvilli** (**4**).

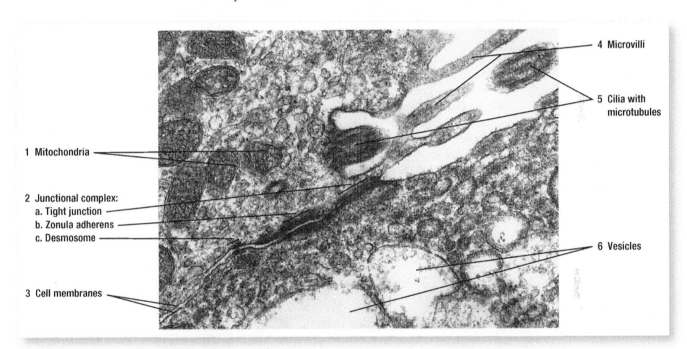

1 Mitochondria

2 Junctional complex:
  a. Tight junction
  b. Zonula adherens
  c. Desmosome

3 Cell membranes

4 Microvilli

5 Cilia with microtubules

6 Vesicles

FIGURE 2.4 ■ A junctional complex between epithelial cells. ×31,200.

FUNCTIONAL CORRELATIONS 2.5 ■ Junctional Complex

Junctional complexes have a variety of functions, depending on their morphology, shape, and location. In the epithelium that lines the stomach, intestines, and urinary bladder, the **zonulae occludentes** or tight junctions are the most apical junctions that prevent the passage of corrosive chemicals or waste products between cells and into the bloodstream. The tight junctions consist of **transmembrane proteins** called **claudin** that fuse the outer membranes of adjacent cells. In this manner, the cells form a tight, beltlike epithelial barrier. Similarly, the **zonula adherens** or adhering junctions assist these cells in resisting separation; the transmembrane proteins attach to the cytoskeleton proteins and bind adjacent cells. **Actin filaments** attach to zonula adherens. **Desmosomes** are spotlike structures that are most commonly seen in the epithelium of the skin and in cardiac muscle fibers. Here, the cells are subjected to great mechanical stresses. In these organs, desmosomes

FUNCTIONAL CORRELATIONS 2.5 ■ Junctional Complex (*Continued*)

prevent skin cells from separating and cardiac muscle cells from pulling apart during the powerful heart contractions. The desmosomes are bound to **intermediate filaments** and form strong attachment sites between adjacent the cells.

Other junctional complexes are **hemidesmosomes** and **gap junctions**. Hemidesmosomes are one half of the desmosome and are present at the base of epithelial cells where strong adhesion to the connective tissue is required to prevent tearing of the epithelium from the underlying connective tissue layers as in the basal layers of the skin. Here, hemidesmosomes anchor the epithelial cells to the basement

membrane and the adjacent extracellular connective tissue. Basement membrane consists of a basal lamina and reticular fibers of the connective tissue.

Gap junctions are also spotlike in structure. The plasma membranes at gap junctions are closely apposed, and tiny fluid channels called **connexons** connect the adjacent cells. Molecules, ions, and low-resistance electrical communication occurs through these connexons between adjacent cells. These fluid channels are vital in cardiac muscle cells and nerve cells, where fast impulse transmission through the adjacent cells or axons is essential for synchronization and coordination of normal functions.

FIGURE 2.5 | **Basal Regions of Epithelial Cells**

A medium-magnification electron micrograph illustrates the appearance of the basal region or the base of epithelial cells. Note that the basal regions of the cells are attached to a thin, moderately electron-dense layer called the **basal lamina** (**3**). Deep to the basal lamina (**3**) is a **connective tissue** (**2**) layer of fine reticular fibers. The basal lamina (**3**) is seen only with the electron microscope. Basal lamina (**3**) and the reticular fibers of connective tissue (**2**) are recognized under the light microscope as a basement membrane.

Inferior to the epithelial cells is an elongated, spindle-shaped **fibroblast** (**4**) with its **nucleus** (**4**) and dispersed **chromatin** (**5**), surrounded by numerous connective tissue fibers (**2**) produced by the fibroblasts. In the cytoplasm of one of the epithelial cells is also seen a **nucleus** (**8**), dispersed **chromatin** (**9**), and a dense, round **nucleolus** (**7**). **Cisternae** of **rough endoplasmic reticulum** (**11**), elongated **mitochondria** (**14**), and various types of **dense bodies** (**6**) are visible in different cells. Between the individual epithelial cells is a distinct **cell membrane** (**1, 10**). Hemidesmosomes are not illustrated but attach the basal membrane of the cells to the basal lamina (**3**).

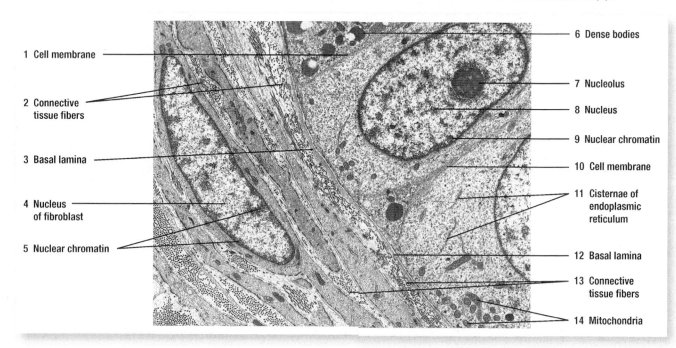

1 Cell membrane

2 Connective tissue fibers

3 Basal lamina

4 Nucleus of fibroblast

5 Nuclear chromatin

6 Dense bodies

7 Nucleolus

8 Nucleus

9 Nuclear chromatin

10 Cell membrane

11 Cisternae of endoplasmic reticulum

12 Basal lamina

13 Connective tissue fibers

14 Mitochondria

FIGURE 2.5 ■ Basal regions of epithelial cells. ×9,500.

FIGURE 2.6 | Basal Region of Ion-Transporting Cell

A medium-magnification electron micrograph illustrates the basal region of a cell from the distal convoluted tubule of the kidney. In contrast to the basal regions of epithelial cells, the basal regions of cells in convoluted kidney tubules are characterized by numerous and complex **infoldings** of the **basal cell membrane** (5). These infoldings then form numerous **basal membrane interdigitations** (10) with the similar infoldings of the neighboring cell. Numerous and long **mitochondria** (4, 9) with vertical or apical–basal orientations are located between the cell membrane infoldings.

A portion of a large **nucleus** (1) is visible with its dispersed **chromatin** (8). Surrounding the nucleus is a distinct **nuclear envelope** (2), which consists of a double membrane. Both the outer and inner membranes of the nuclear envelope (2) fuse at intervals around the periphery of the nucleus to form numerous **nuclear pores** (3).

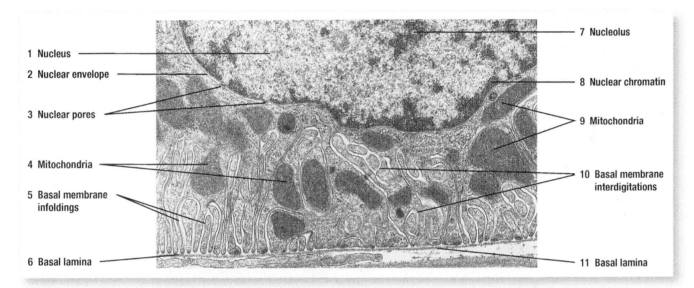

1 Nucleus

2 Nuclear envelope

3 Nuclear pores

4 Mitochondria

5 Basal membrane infoldings

6 Basal lamina

7 Nucleolus

8 Nuclear chromatin

9 Mitochondria

10 Basal membrane interdigitations

11 Basal lamina

FIGURE 2.6 ■ Basal region of an ion-transporting cell. ×16,600.

FUNCTIONAL CORRELATIONS 2.6 ■ Infolded Basal Regions of the Cell

The deep **infoldings** of the basal and lateral cell membranes are seen only with electron microscopy. These infoldings are found in certain cells of the body, whose main function is to transport **ions** across the cell membrane. The cells in the tubular portions of the kidney (proximal convoluted tubules and distal convoluted tubules) selectively absorb useful or nutritious components from the glomerular filtrate and retain them in the body. At the same time, these cells eliminate toxic or nonuseful metabolic waste products such as urea and drug metabolites.

Because these cells transport numerous ions across their membranes, increased amounts of energy are needed, which is generated by **Na⁺/K⁺ ATPases (sodium pumps)** embedded in the infolded basal and lateral cell membranes. To perform these vital functions, numerous long mitochondria that are located in these basal infoldings continually supply the cells with the energy source (ATP) that operates these pumps for membrane transport. Similar basal cell membrane infoldings are seen in the striated ducts of the salivary glands. These glands produce saliva, which is then modified by selective transport of various ions across the cell membrane as it moves through these ducts to the larger excretory ducts.

FIGURE 2.7 | Cilia and Microvilli

This high-magnification electron micrograph illustrates the ultrastructural differences between cilia (singular, cilium) and microvilli (singular, microvillus). Both **cilia (1)** and **microvilli (2)** project from the apical surfaces of certain cells in the body. The cilia (1) are long, motile structures, with a core of uniformly arranged **microtubules (3)** in longitudinal orientation. The core of each cilium contains a constant number of nine microtubule doublets located peripherally and two single microtubules in the center. Each cilium is attached to and extends from the **basal body (4)** in the apical region of the cell. Instead of nine microtubule doublets, the basal bodies exhibit nine microtubule triplets and no central microtubules.

In contrast to cilia, microvilli (2) are smaller, shorter, closely packed finger-like extensions that greatly increase the surface area of certain cells. Microvilli (2) are nonmotile and exhibit a core of thin microfilaments called actin. The actin filaments extend from the microvilli (2) into the apical cytoplasm of the cell to form a terminal web, a complex network of actin filaments.

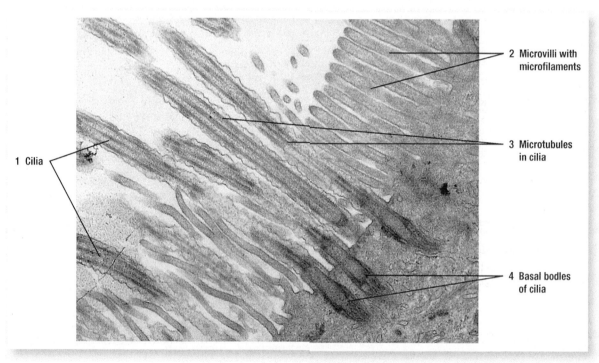

1 Cilia

2 Microvilli with microfilaments

3 Microtubules in cilia

4 Basal bodies of cilia

FIGURE 2.7 ■ Cilia and microvilli. ×20,000.

FIGURE 2.8 | **Nuclear Envelope and Nuclear Pores**

A high-magnification electron micrograph illustrates in detail part of a **nucleus (8)** and the surrounding membrane, the **nuclear envelope (3)**, which consists of an **outer nuclear membrane (3a)** and an **inner nuclear membrane (3b)**. Between the two nuclear membranes (3a, 3b) is a space. The outer nuclear membrane (3a) is in contact with the **cell cytoplasm (4)**, whereas the inner nuclear membrane (3b) is associated with the **nuclear chromatin (7)**. The nuclear envelope is continuous with the **rough endoplasmic reticulum (1)**, and the outer nuclear membrane (3a) usually contains ribosomes. At certain intervals around the nucleus, the two membranes of the nuclear envelope (3) fuse and form numerous **nuclear pores (2, 6)**.

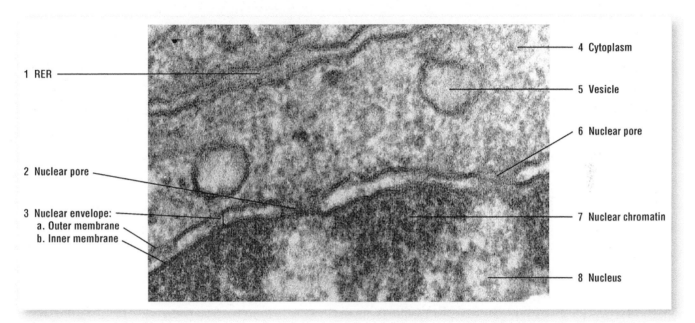

FIGURE 2.8 ■ Nuclear envelope and nuclear pores. ×110,000.*

FUNCTIONAL CORRELATIONS 2.7 ■ Nucleus, Nucleolus, and Nuclear Pores

The **nucleus** is the control center of the cell; it stores and processes most of the cell's genetic information. The nucleus directs all of the activities of the cell through the process of protein synthesis and ultimately controls the structural and functional characteristics of each cell. The cell's genetic material, **deoxyribonucleic acid (DNA)**, is visible in the cell in the form of **chromatin**. When the cells are not actively producing protein, the DNA is not condensed and does not stain.

The **nucleolus** is a dense-staining, nonmembrane-bound structure within the nucleus. One or more nucleoli may be visible in a given cell. The nucleolus functions in synthesis, processing, and assembly

of **ribosomes**. In nucleoli, the ribosomal **ribonucleic acid (RNA)** is produced and combined with proteins to form ribosomal subunits. These ribosomal subunits are then transported to the cell cytoplasm through the nuclear pores to form complete ribosomes. Consequently, nucleoli are prominent in cells that synthesize large amounts of proteins.

Nuclear pores control the transport of macromolecules between the nucleus and the cytoplasm. The nuclear pore membrane, like other cell membranes, shows selective permeability. As a result, some of the larger molecules travel through the pores via an active transport mechanism.

FIGURE 2.9 | Mitochondria

A high-magnification electron micrograph illustrates the ultrastructure of **mitochondria** (**1, 4**) in a **longitudinal section** (**1**) and in **cross section** (**4**). Note that the mitochondria (1, 4) also exhibit two membranes. The **outer mitochondrial membrane** (**5, 9**) is smooth and surrounds the entire organelle. The inner mitochondrial membrane is highly folded, surrounds the matrix of the mitochondria, and projects inward into the organelle to form the numerous, shelflike **cristae** (**6**). Some mitochondrial matrix may contain dense-staining granules. Also visible in the **cytoplasm** (**8**) of the cell are variously sized, light-staining **vacuoles** (**7**), a section of **rough endoplasmic reticulum** (**2**), and free **ribosomes** (**3**). This type of mitochondria with shelflike cristae (6) is normally found in protein-secreting cells and muscle cells.

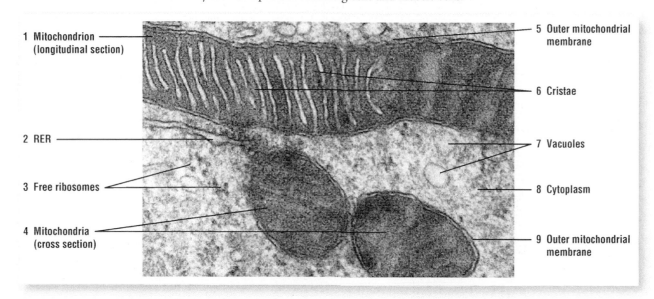

1 Mitochondrion (longitudinal section)

2 RER

3 Free ribosomes

4 Mitochondria (cross section)

5 Outer mitochondrial membrane

6 Cristae

7 Vacuoles

8 Cytoplasm

9 Outer mitochondrial membrane

FIGURE 2.9 ◼ Mitochondria (longitudinal and cross section). ×49,500.

FIGURE 2.10 | Rough Endoplasmic Reticulum

A high-magnification electron micrograph illustrates the components of the **rough endoplasmic reticulum** (**3**) in the cytoplasm of a cell. It consists of stacked layers of membranous cavities called **cisternae** (**3**). In the rough endoplasmic reticulum, ribosomes are attached to the outer surface of

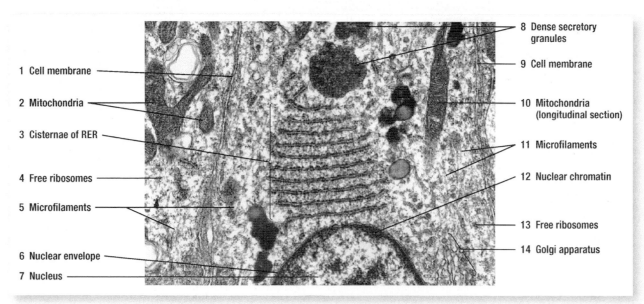

1 Cell membrane

2 Mitochondria

3 Cisternae of RER

4 Free ribosomes

5 Microfilaments

6 Nuclear envelope

7 Nucleus

8 Dense secretory granules

9 Cell membrane

10 Mitochondria (longitudinal section)

11 Microfilaments

12 Nuclear chromatin

13 Free ribosomes

14 Golgi apparatus

FIGURE 2.10 ◼ Rough endoplasmic reticulum. ×32,000.

the membranes. Also present in the cytoplasm are **free ribosomes** (**4, 13**), some of which attach to other ribosome and form ribosome groups called **polyribosomes** (**4, 13**). Visible in the cytoplasm are also numerous **mitochondria** (**2, 10**), in longitudinal (**10**) and **cross section** (**2**), **dense secretory granules** (**8**), and very thin strands of **microfilaments** (**5, 11**). In the lower right corner of the micrograph, the smooth cisternae and associated vesicles of the **Golgi apparatus** (**14**) are visible. Note the **cell membranes** (**1, 9**) of adjacent cells, **nuclear envelope** (**6**), and portions of the **nucleus** (**7**) and nuclear **chromatin** (**12**).

FIGURE 2.11 | Smooth Endoplasmic Reticulum

This high-magnification electron micrograph illustrates the structure of the **smooth endoplasmic reticulum** (**2**) in two adjacent cells. Smooth endoplasmic reticulum (**2**) is devoid of ribosomes and consists primarily of smooth, anastomosing tubules. In this micrograph, the tubules of the smooth endoplasmic reticulum (**2**) are primarily seen in cross section. In other sections, the smooth endoplasmic reticulum (**2**) can be seen as flattened vesicles. In some cells, smooth endoplasmic reticulum is continuous with **cisternae** of the **rough endoplasmic reticulum** (**7**), as seen in this micrograph.

Also seen in the micrograph are the **cell membranes** (**6, 11**) of the two cells, the **cell membrane interdigitations** (**10**), and the **extracellular matrix** (**9**) between the two cell membranes. A section of the **nucleus** (**4, 5**), **nuclear envelope** (**8**), **nuclear chromatin** (**3**), and **mitochondrion** (**1**) in cross section are also visible in the two cells. The mitochondria (**1**) in these cells contain tubular cristae, indicating that the cells synthesize products other than proteins.

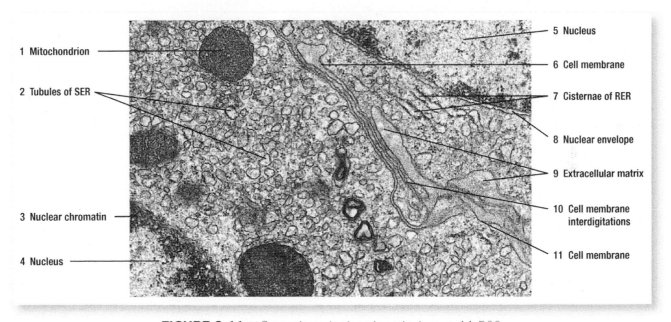

1 Mitochondrion

2 Tubules of SER

3 Nuclear chromatin

4 Nucleus

5 Nucleus

6 Cell membrane

7 Cisternae of RER

8 Nuclear envelope

9 Extracellular matrix

10 Cell membrane interdigitations

11 Cell membrane

FIGURE 2.11 ■ Smooth endoplasmic reticulum. ×11,500.

FIGURE 2.12 | Golgi Apparatus

A high-magnification electron micrograph illustrates the components of the **Golgi apparatus** (**2**). This apparatus consists of membrane-bound **Golgi cisternae** (**2**) with numerous membranous **Golgi vesicles** (**1**) located near the end of the cisternae. The Golgi apparatus (**2**) usually exhibits a crescent shape. Its convex side is called the *cis* **face** (**3**), and the opposite, concave side is the *trans* **face** (**9**) of the Golgi apparatus (**2**). This micrograph illustrates the Golgi apparatus (**2**) in the seminiferous tubule of the testis, where a spermatid is undergoing transformation into a sperm. At this stage of the transformation, the Golgi apparatus (**2**) is packaging and condensing the secretory product into an electron-dense **acrosome granule** (**7**). The acrosome granule (**7**) is located in the **acrosomal vesicle** (**8**) that adheres to the **nuclear envelope** (**6**) at the anterior pole of the spermatid. In the left corner of the micrograph, note a short cisterna of the **granular** (**rough**) **endoplasmic reticulum** (**4**) and some **free ribosomes** (**5**) in the **cytoplasm** (**11**) of the spermatid. A **cell membrane** (**10**) surrounds the cell.

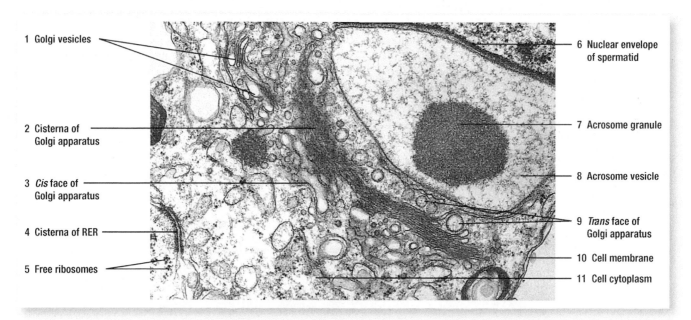

1 Golgi vesicles

2 Cisterna of Golgi apparatus

3 *Cis* face of Golgi apparatus

4 Cisterna of RER

5 Free ribosomes

6 Nuclear envelope of spermatid

7 Acrosome granule

8 Acrosome vesicle

9 *Trans* face of Golgi apparatus

10 Cell membrane

11 Cell cytoplasm

FIGURE 2.12 ■ Golgi apparatus. ×23,000.

FIGURE 2.13 | Ultrastructure of Lysosomes and Residual Bodies in Cytoplasm of Tissue Macrophage

A medium-magnification electron micrograph illustrates numerous dense-staining **lysosomes** (**3**) in the cytoplasm of a tissue macrophage. The lysosomes (**3**) show great variation in size, appearance, density, and the contents. Also visible in the cell cytoplasm are what appear to be the **residual bodies** (**1, 4**), consisting of lipid-like material and dense undigested matter enclosed in a membrane. Distinguishing between material being digested in the lysosomes and the residual bodies is often quite difficult. Located also in the cytoplasm are numerous **mitochondria** (**2**), sectioned in different planes. Note also the difference in size between the mitochondria and the variably sized lysosomes. In the left hand corner is a section of a cytoplasm from an adjacent cell.

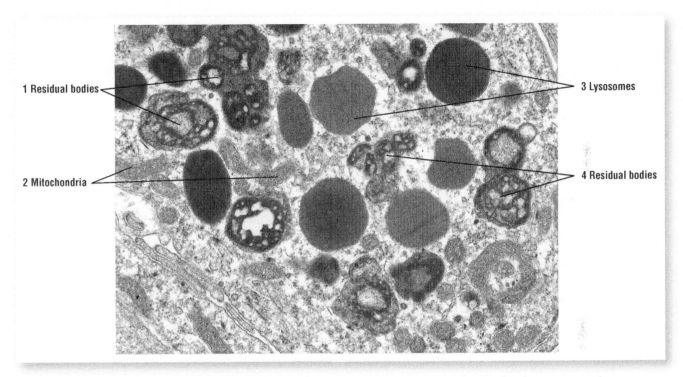

FIGURE 2.13 ■ Ultrastructure of lysosomes and residual bodies in the cytoplasm of a tissue macrophage. Courtesy of Dr. Rex A. Hess, Professor Emeritus, Comparative Biosciences, College of Veterinary Medicine, University of Illinois, Urbana, IL. ×16,000.

Chapter 2 Summary

Light and Transmission Electron Microscopy

CELL AND CYTOPLASM

- Cells maintain proper homeostasis of the body
- Structural features are common to all cells

CELL MEMBRANE

- Consists of phospholipid bilayer and integral (transmembrane) membrane proteins
- Peripheral membrane proteins located on external and internal cell surfaces
- Peripheral proteins anchored to microfilaments of cytoskeleton
- Transmembrane proteins are located within lipid bilayer of the cell membrane
- Transmembrane proteins transport molecules across lipid bilayer
- Cholesterol molecules within the cell membrane stabilize the cell membrane
- Carbohydrate glycocalyx covers cell surfaces (microvilli) in specialized absorptive cells
- Glycocalyx important for cell recognition, cell adhesion, and receptor binding sites

MOLECULAR ORGANIZATION OF CELL MEMBRANE

- Lipid bilayer is in fluid state, hence the fluid mosaic model
- Phospholipids form two layers with polar heads facing inner and outer surfaces
- Nonpolar tails are in center of membrane

CELL MEMBRANE PERMEABILITY AND TRANSPORT

- Cell membrane shows selective permeability and forms a barrier between internal and external cell environments
- Permeable to oxygen, carbon dioxide, water, steroids, and lipid-soluble chemicals
- Larger molecules enter cell by specialized transport mechanisms
- Endocytosis is ingestion of extracellular material into the cell
- Exocytosis is release of material from the cell
- Pinocytosis is ingestion of extracellular fluid into the cell
- Phagocytosis is uptake of large, solid particular matter into the cell

- Receptor-mediated endocytosis involves pinocytosis or phagocytosis via receptors on cell membrane and formation of clathrin-coated pits
- Uptake of low-density lipoproteins and insulin as example of receptor-mediated endocytosis

CELLULAR ORGANELLES

- Membrane bound: nucleus, mitochondria, endoplasmic reticulum, Golgi complex, lysosomes, and peroxisomes
- Nonmembrane bound: ribosomes, basal bodies, and centrosomes

Mitochondria

- Surrounded by cell membrane
- Shelflike cristae in protein-secreting cells and tubular cristae in steroid-secreting cells
- Present in all cells, except mature red blood cells, and is especially numerous in highly metabolic cells
- Produce high-energy ATP molecules
- Cristae contain respiratory chain enzymes for ATP production
- Matrix contains enzymes, ribosomes, and circular mitochondrial DNA
- Arise from preexisting mitochondria by growth and division

Rough Endoplasmic Reticulum

- Exhibits interconnected cisternae that are covered with ribosomes
- Highly developed in protein-synthesizing cells
- Synthesizes proteins for export or lysosomes
- Synthesizes integral membrane proteins and phospholipids for cell membrane
- Free ribosomes synthesize proteins for cell cytoplasm

Smooth Endoplasmic Reticulum

- Devoid of ribosomes and consists of anastomosing tubules
- Found in cells that synthesize phospholipids, cholesterol, and steroid hormones
- In liver cells, proliferates to deactivate or detoxify harmful chemicals
- In liver cells is involved with carbohydrate metabolism and converts glycogen to glucose
- In skeletal and cardiac muscle fibers, stores and releases calcium between contractions

Golgi Apparatus

- Present in all cells, except mature red blood cells
- Consists of stacked, curved cisternae with convex side as the *cis* face
- Mature concave side is the *trans* face
- New synthesized protein transported in transfer vesicles to Golgi apparatus
- Cisternae modify enzymes and sort and package proteins
- Adds sugars to proteins and lipids to form glycoproteins, glycolipids, and lipoproteins
- Secretory granules are modified, sorted, and packaged in membranes for export outside of cell or for lysosomes
- Other proteins and phospholipids are incorporated into cell membrane

Ribosomes

- Appear as free or attached (as to endoplasmic reticulum)
- Most abundant in protein-synthesizing cells
- Decode genetic messages from nucleus for amino acid sequence of protein synthesis
- Free ribosomes synthesize proteins for cell use
- Attached ribosomes synthesize proteins that are packaged for export or lysosomes use
- Ribosomal subunits synthesized in nucleolus and transported to cytoplasm via nuclear pores

Lysosomes

- Membrane-bound vesicles filled with hydrolyzing or digesting enzymes called acid hydrolases
- Synthesized in rough endoplasmic reticulum and packaged in Golgi apparatus
- Separated from cytoplasm by membrane to prevent damage to cell
- Functions in intracellular digestion or phagocytosis
- Digest microorganisms, cellular debris, worn-out cells, or cell organelles
- Residual bodies seen after phagocytosis
- Very abundant in tissue macrophages and white blood cells neutrophils

Peroxisomes

- Contain oxidases that form cytotoxic hydrogen peroxide
- Contain enzyme catalase to eliminate excess hydrogen peroxide
- Abundant in liver and kidney cells, which remove much of the toxic material
- Detoxify, degrade alcohol, oxidize fatty acids, and metabolize compounds

CELL CYTOSKELETON

Microfilaments

- Thinnest microfilaments in the cytoskeleton
- Composed of protein actin and contribute to cell and organelle movements
- Distributed throughout cell and used as anchors at cell junctions
- Form core of microvilli and terminal web at cell apices
- Actin–myosin interactions produce muscle contractions

Intermediate Filaments

- Thicker than microfilaments
- Epithelial cells contain keratin filaments
- In skin cells, they terminate at desmosomes and hemidesmosomes
- Vimentin filaments found in mesenchymal cells
- Desmin filaments found in smooth and skeletal muscles
- Glial filaments found in astrocytic cells of the nervous system
- Lamin filaments found in nuclear membrane

Microtubules

- Largest filaments in cytoskeleton and found in most cells except red blood cells
- Composed of α and β tubulin
- Originate from centrosome
- Determine cell shape and function in intracellular transport
- Form spindles and separate duplicated chromosomes during cell mitosis
- Present in cilia, flagella, centrioles, and basal bodies

Centrosome and Centrioles

- Centrosome located near nucleus and contain two centrioles
- Major microtubule-forming center and mitotic spindles
- Centrioles perpendicular to one another; contain nine clusters of three microtubules each arranged in a circle
- Before mitosis, centrioles replicate
- During mitosis, centrioles form mitotic spindles to control distribution of chromosomes
- Centrioles induce formation of basal bodies and microtubules in cilia and flagella

CYTOPLASMIC INCLUSIONS

- Temporary structures such as lipids, glycogen, crystals, and pigment

NUCLEUS AND NUCLEAR ENVELOPE

- Nucleus contains chromatin, nucleoli, nuclear matrix, and cellular DNA
- Double membrane called the nuclear envelope surrounds the nucleus
- Nucleolus is not membrane bound
- Outer membrane of nuclear envelope contains ribosomes and is continuous with rough endoplasmic reticulum
- Nuclear pores at intervals in the nuclear envelope
- Nuclear pores control movements of material between nucleus and cytoplasm

SURFACES OF CELLS

Junctional Complex

- Zonula occludens or tight junctions form an effective epithelial barrier
- Transmembrane proteins claudin fuse the outer membranes of adjacent cells to form tight junctions
- In zonula adherens or adhering junctions, transmembrane proteins attach to cytoskeleton and bind adjacent cells
- Actin filaments attach zonula adherens
- Desmosomes are spotlike structures, very prominent in skin and cardiac cells
- Desmosomes anchor cells through extension of transmembrane proteins into intercellular space between adjacent cells
- Desmosomes bound to intermediate filaments
- Hemidesmosomes are present at base of epithelial cells to prevent separation from connective tissue layer, as in basal layer of skin
- Gap junctions are spotlike structures with fluid channels called connexons
- Ions and chemicals diffuse through connexons from cell to cell
- Gap junctions allow rapid communications between cells for synchronized action

Basal Regions of Cells

Infolded Basal Regions

- Infolded basal and lateral cell membranes function in ionic transport
- Found in kidney and salivary gland cells
- Na^+/K^+ ATPase (sodium pumps) embedded in infolded membranes
- Numerous and long mitochondria in infoldings supply ATP for ion transport

Cilia

- Motile apical surface modifications that are inserted into basal bodies
- Line cells in the respiratory organs, uterine tubes, and efferent ducts in testes
- Motility caused by sliding microtubule doublets
- Motor protein dynein uses ATP to move cilia

Microvilli

- Nonmotile apical surface modifications
- Well developed in small intestines and kidney
- Main function is absorption of nutrients from intestines and glomerular filtrate

Chapter 2 Review Questions

QUESTIONS

In the following multiple-choice questions, choose the letter corresponding to the one best answer.

1. **What type of junctional cell complex prevents passage of chemicals between cells?**

   A. Desmosome
   B. Hemidesmosome
   C. Gap junction
   D. Zonula adherens (adhering junction)
   E. Zonula occludentes (tight junction)

2. **Rapid communications between cells is provided by what junctional cell complex?**

   A. Desmosome
   B. Hemidesmosome
   C. Zonula occludentes
   D. Gap junction
   E. Zonula adherens

3. **Which cell organelles contain the motor protein dynein?**

   A. Centrosomes
   B. Mitochondria
   C. Cilia
   D. Microvilli
   E. Centrioles

4. **What controls the transport of macromolecules in and out of the nucleus?**

   A. Nuclear pores
   B. Nucleolus
   C. Nuclear membrane
   D. Nuclear chromatin
   E. Surrounding cytoplasm

5. **The major microtubule-forming center in the cell is the:**

   A. centriole.
   B. mitotic spindle.
   C. cilia.
   D. centrosome.
   E. basal body.

ANSWERS

1. **Correct Answer: E.** Zonula occludentes (tight junction). These structures are located at the apical regions of the cells and play an important role in the epithelium of the digestive organs, where they prevent the passage of corrosive chemicals between cells.

2. **Correct Answer: D.** Gap junction. Of the junctional complexes, the spotlike gap junctions exhibit tiny channels (connexons) that connect adjacent cells and allow for communication between them. Such junctions are vital for rapid communication in cardiac muscle cells and nerve cells.

3. **Correct Answer: C.** Cilia. The motor protein dynein exhibits ATPase activity and uses the energy of ATP hydrolysis to induce cilia motility.

4. **Correct Answer: A.** Nuclear pores. A selective permeability membrane with nuclear pores surrounds the nuclei of different cells. The nuclear pores control the transport of molecules between the nucleus and cytoplasm.

5. **Correct Answer: D.** Centrosome. All microtubules originate from the microtubule-organizing center in the cytoplasm called the centrosome.

ADDITIONAL HISTOLOGIC IMAGES

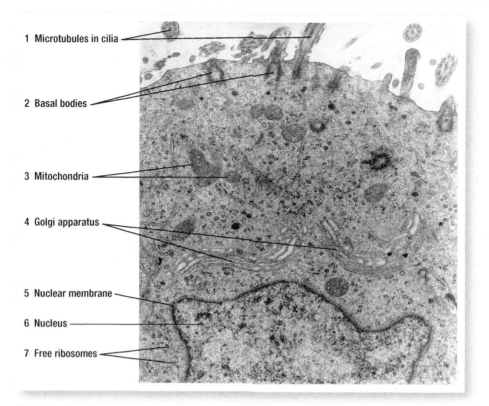

1 Microtubules in cilia

2 Basal bodies

3 Mitochondria

4 Golgi apparatus

5 Nuclear membrane

6 Nucleus

7 Free ribosomes

FIGURE 2.14 ■ Cytoplasmic contents and organelles of a ciliated cell from an avian oviduct. ×15,000.

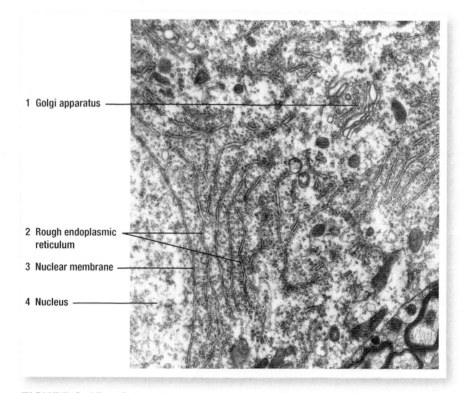

1 Golgi apparatus

2 Rough endoplasmic reticulum

3 Nuclear membrane

4 Nucleus

FIGURE 2.15 ■ Cell and cytoplasmic organelles in a cell from a rodent spinal cord. ×10,000. Courtesy of Dr. Mark DeSantis, Professor Emeritus, WWAMI Medical Program, University of Idaho, Moscow, ID.

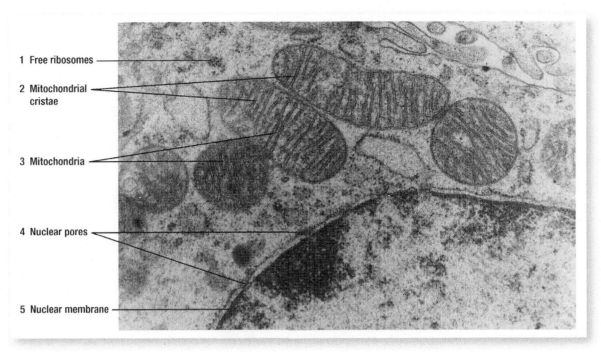

1 Free ribosomes

2 Mitochondrial cristae

3 Mitochondria

4 Nuclear pores

5 Nuclear membrane

FIGURE 2.16 ■ A section of a cell nucleus and the adjacent cytoplasmic organelles. ×45,000.

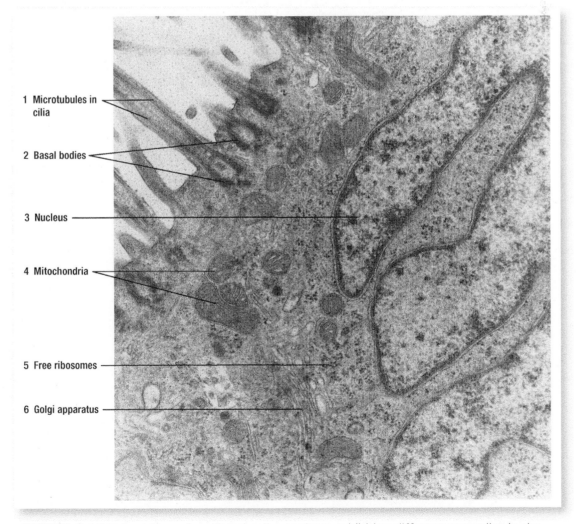

1 Microtubules in cilia

2 Basal bodies

3 Nucleus

4 Mitochondria

5 Free ribosomes

6 Golgi apparatus

FIGURE 2.17 ■ A section of a ciliated cell cytoplasm exhibiting different organelles in the epithelium of an avian oviduct. ×15,000.

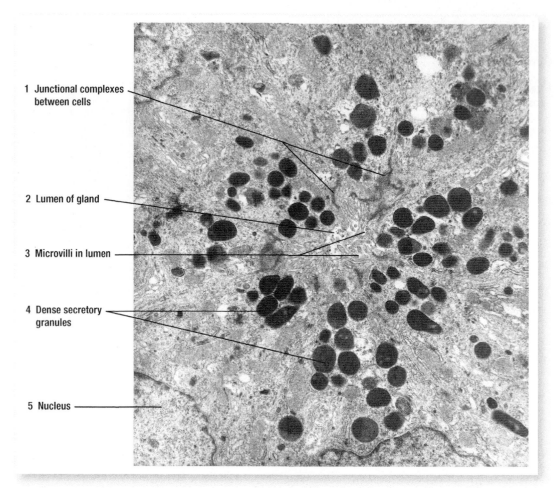

1 Junctional complexes
  between cells

2 Lumen of gland

3 Microvilli in lumen

4 Dense secretory
  granules

5 Nucleus

FIGURE 2.18 ■ Secretory cells with dense secretory granules in the apical regions of a gland from a section of an avian oviduct. ×5,500.

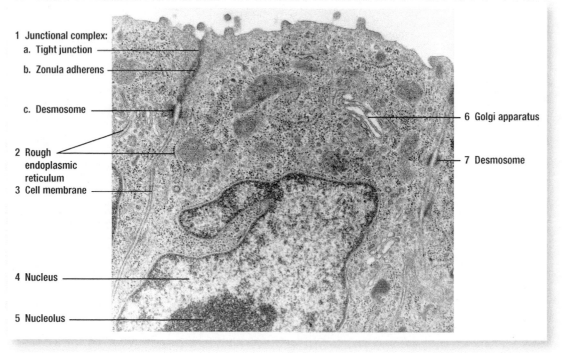

1 Junctional complex:
  a. Tight junction
  b. Zonula adherens

  c. Desmosome

2 Rough
  endoplasmic
  reticulum

3 Cell membrane

4 Nucleus

5 Nucleolus

6 Golgi apparatus

7 Desmosome

FIGURE 2.19 ■ Apical section of cells from the lining epithelium of an avian oviduct showing different cytoplasmic organelles. ×15,000.

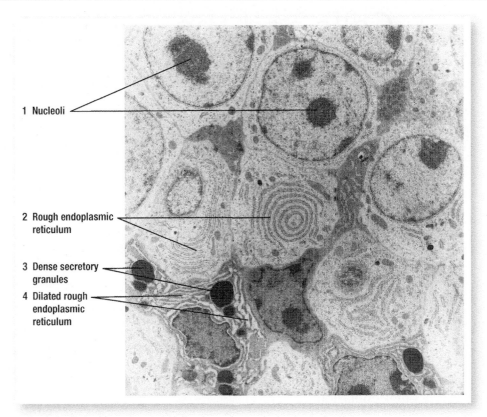

1 Nucleoli

2 Rough endoplasmic
reticulum

3 Dense secretory
granules

4 Dilated rough
endoplasmic
reticulum

FIGURE 2.20 ■ Transverse section of a secretory epithelium from an avian oviduct showing the developed rough endoplasmic reticulum. ×5,000.

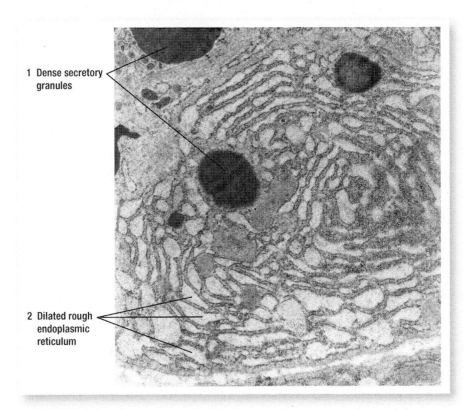

1 Dense secretory
granules

2 Dilated rough
endoplasmic
reticulum

FIGURE 2.21 ■ Secretory cell with dense secretory granules and the dilated rough endoplasmic reticulum in the glandular epithelium of an avian oviduct. ×45,000.

Cells and the Cell Cycle

During embryonic development, the cells divide and multiply to form new cells, tissues, and organs. In an adult organism, however, not all cells retain the ability to further divide and reproduce. As a result, different populations of cells are recognized based on their ability or inability to divide and reproduce.

PERMANENT CELL POPULATION IN ADULT ORGANISMS

Nerve cells in the nervous system and muscle cells (skeletal and cardiac) continue to divide during embryonic development. Once these cells establish the organs in postnatal life, however, their ability to further divide ceases, and they cannot be replaced if they are damaged or destroyed.

Stable Cell Population

In such organs as the **liver**, cells remain relatively stable in postnatal life and exhibit a slow rate of replacement under normal conditions. However, when part of the liver is surgically removed or is damaged by toxic substances, the liver cells exhibit regenerative capabilities. They regenerate, proliferate, and replace lost cells in order to maintain the normal functions of the organ. The life span of normal and healthy liver cells is about 5 months, in contrast to the life spans of cells in organs where cell renewal is continuous.

Renewing Cell Population

These cells are continuously dividing to replace lost or worn-out cells in different tissues and organs of the body. **Skin cells** and **gastrointestinal epithelium** (**oral cavity**, **esophagus**, **stomach**, **small** and **large intestine**) **cells** continually divide. Similarly, numerous **blood cells** have short life spans and are continually reproduced in red bone marrow of different bones to replace the worn-out cells. Also, **germ cells** (**spermatogonia**) in the **testes** are continuously dividing to produce new sperm.

CELL CYCLE: INTERPHASE AND MITOSIS

The time interval between two successive cell divisions represents the **cell cycle**. It involves cell replication by duplicating the cell's genetic contents and producing two identical daughter cells. The cell cycle is divided into two main phases: **interphase** and **mitosis**. Interphase consists of a prolonged interval comprising different phases during which time the cell size and its contents increase. In addition, DNA, centrioles, and chromosomes replicate, and the cell prepares for division, or mitosis, which exhibits four distinct and histologically recognizable stages or phases.

Prophase

During this first prolonged phase of mitosis, the **chromosomes** condense and become histologically visible. Each chromosome consists of two genetically identical sister **chromatids** that are joined together at a pinched area called the **centromere**. With the condensation of the chromosomes, the nuclear envelope and nucleolus disappear (fragment) with only fragments visible in the cell. The **centrosome** divides, and the **centrioles** migrate to the opposite poles of the cell to form **microtubules** of the **mitotic spindle** (Fig. 3.1A). The microtubule spindles continue to grow toward the chromosomes, where some of them attach to a platelike protein complex called the **kinetochore**, which appears on each side of the centromere. These **kinetochore microtubules** eventually align the chromosomes in the middle of the cell. The microtubules that do not attach to the chromosomes at the kinetochore become the **polar microtubules**.

Metaphase

In this short phase, the chromosomes become highly condensed. The chromosomes are aligned along the equator of the cell as a result of their attachment to the **kinetochore microtubules** of the mitotic spindles that radiate from both spindle poles. The kinetochore microtubules direct the movement of chromosomes toward the middle of the cells, forming the **metaphase** or **equatorial plate** (Fig. 3.1A, B).

Anaphase

During this phase, the chromatid pairs separate at the centromere because of an enzymatic action, and each chromatid now becomes a separate chromosome. These chromosomes now begin their migration to the opposite poles of the cell, pulled by the shortening of the kinetochore microtubules, which are attached to the centromeres. The migrating or pulled chromosomes exhibit a V shape in the cell. In late anaphase, a **cleavage furrow** in the cell membrane appears at the cell equator, indicating the area where the cell will divide (Fig. 3.1C).

Telophase

This is the terminal phase of mitosis. It begins when the chromosomes complete their migration to the opposite side of the mitotic spindle and the chromosomes decondense into the chromatin of the interphase cell. Also, the **nucleolus** reappears, and the rough endoplasmic reticulum begins to form a new **nuclear envelope**. A constriction of the cytoplasm is formed by the **contractile ring** composed of **actin** filaments, which becomes the site of cleavage for the separation of daughter cells. **Cleavage** of the joined daughter cells follows. **Cytokinesis** is the process by which the cytoplasm is divided into two genetically identical cells (Fig. 3.1D, E).

Interphase

Mitosis is now complete, and the cell is ready for the new interphase to begin. The chromosomes have unraveled to become visible as **chromatin** material in the nucleus. The resulting cell division has produced two new cells that are identical in their genetic content to the parent cell (Fig. 3.1E).

MEIOSIS

Meiosis is a special type of cell division that is restricted to **male** and **female germ cells**. This type of division produces an ovum and a spermatozoon whose chromosome numbers have been reduced from **diploid** (46 chromosomes) to **haploid** (23 chromosomes).

The process of meiosis involves two successive cell divisions after one DNA replication. This ensures that haploid cells are produced from every cell that enters meiosis. The recombination of genes and the establishment of a full chromosome count occur at fertilization of the ovum by the sperm, thus ensuring viability of the progeny. Additional information concerning the meiotic process is described in Chapters 20 and 21.

the**Point**   Supplemental micrographic images are available at **www.thePoint.com/Eroschenko13e** under Cell and Cytoplasm.

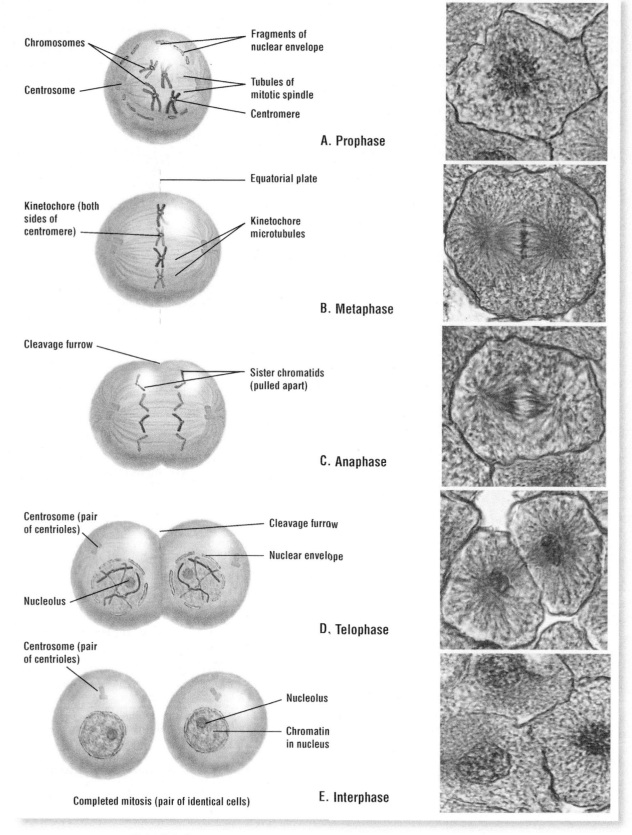

Chromosomes

Centrosome

Fragments of
nuclear envelope

Tubules of
mitotic spindle

Centromere

A. Prophase

Equatorial plate

Kinetochore (both
sides of
centromere)

Kinetochore
microtubules

B. Metaphase

Cleavage furrow

Sister chromatids
(pulled apart)

C. Anaphase

Centrosome (pair
of centrioles)

Cleavage furrow

Nuclear envelope

Nucleolus

D. Telophase

Centrosome (pair
of centrioles)

Nucleolus

Chromatin
in nucleus

Completed mitosis (pair of identical cells)

E. Interphase

FIGURE 3.1 ■ **A–E.** Different phases of mitosis and cytokinesis.

Chapter 3 Summary

Cells and the Cell Cycle

CELL POPULATIONS IN ADULTS

- Permanent—nerve and muscle cells are not replaced when damaged
- Stable cell population—liver cells can proliferate to replace removed or damaged cells
- Renewing cell population—skin, gastrointestinal organs, blood cells in red bone marrow, and germ cells in testes are constantly replaced

CELL CYCLE: INTERPHASE AND MITOSIS

- Divided into interphase and mitosis
- Interphase is prolonged and consists of different phases that replicate cell contents
- Mitosis consists of four phases—prophase, metaphase, anaphase, and telophase

Prophase

- Condensation of chromosomes to form two identical chromatids
- Chromatids are joined together at the centromere
- Nuclear envelope and nucleolus disappear
- Centrosome divides, and centrioles move to the opposite poles of the cell
- Centrioles form microtubules of the mitotic spindle
- Microtubules attach to kinetochores of chromatids and align chromosomes in the middle of the cell

Metaphase

- Chromosomes highly condensed
- Kinetochore aligns chromosomes along the equator of the cell
- Formation of equatorial plate

Anaphase

- Chromatid pairs separate at the centromere because of enzymatic action and become chromosomes
- Chromosomes migrate to opposite poles of the cell because of shortening of kinetochore microtubules
- Migrating chromosomes form a V shape in the cell
- Cleavage furrow appears at the cell equator

Telophase

- Terminal phase of mitosis
- Chromosomes complete their migration to the opposite side of the mitotic spindle
- Chromosomes condense to form chromatin of the interphase cell
- Nucleolus reappears, and a nuclear envelope is formed
- Contractile ring becomes the site of cleavage for separation of daughter cells
- Cytokinesis is the division of genetically identical cells during mitosis

MEIOSIS

- Specialized cell division restricted to male and female germ cells
- Produces ova and sperm with a haploid number (23) of chromosomes
- Recombination of genes occurs at fertilization of ovum by sperm

Chapter 3 Review Questions

QUESTIONS

In the following multiple-choice questions, choose the letter corresponding to the one best answer.

1. **The terminal phase of the cell cycle is:**

   A. telophase.
   B. interphase.
   C. anaphase.
   D. prophase.
   E. metaphase.

2. **A contractile ring and cytokinesis are seen during:**

   A. interphase (initial phase).
   B. telophase.
   C. equatorial plate formation.
   D. mitotic spindle formation.
   E. centrosome division.

3. **The cleavage furrow is formed during:**

   A. interphase.
   B. telophase.
   C. anaphase.
   D. metaphase.
   E. prophase.

4. **Kinetochores are located:**

   A. in the mitotic spindle.
   B. on the chromosomes.
   C. on each side of the centromere.
   D. on the centrosome.
   E. on the nuclear membrane.

5. **What pulls the chromosomes apart during mitosis?**

   A. Centrioles
   B. Kinetochore microtubules
   C. Cleavage furrow
   D. Centromeres
   E. Mitotic spindle

ANSWERS

1. **Correct Answer: A.** Telophase. At this stage, the chromosomes condense into chromatin. The nucleolus reappears, and a new nuclear envelope is formed.

2. **Correct Answer: B.** Telophase. During this phase, cleavage of the joined cells follows. Cytokinesis is the process resulting in two genetically identical cells.

3. **Correct Answer: C.** Anaphase. During late anaphase of cell division, the migrating chromosomes exhibit a cleavage furrow that indicates where the cells will divide.

4. **Correct Answer: A.** Mitotic spindle. Microtubules of the mitotic spindle attach to the platelike protein complex, the kinetochore.

5. **Correct Answer: B.** Kinetochore microtubules. Shortening of the kinetochore microtubules pulls the chromosomes apart toward the opposite poles of the cell during the continuing mitotic process.

PART III

Tissues

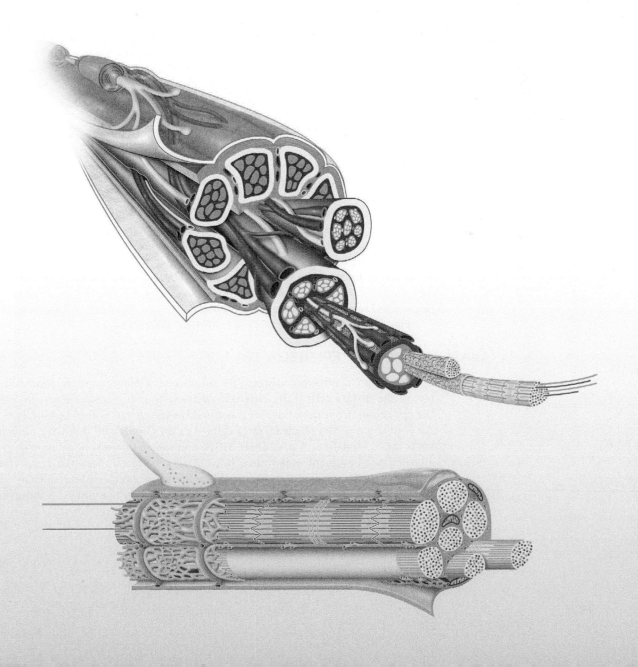

Epithelial Tissue

SECTION 1 Classification of Epithelial Tissue

LOCATION OF EPITHELIUM

The four basic tissue types in the body are the epithelial, connective, muscular, and nervous tissue. These tissues exist and function in close association with one another.

The **epithelial tissue**, or **epithelium**, consists of sheets of cells that cover the **external surfaces** of the body, line the **internal cavities** and the **organs**, form various **organs** and **glands**, and line their **ducts**. Epithelial cells are in contact with each other, either in a single cells layer or in multiple cell layers. The morphology of any epithelium, however, differs from organ to organ, depending on its location and its function. For example, epithelium that covers the outer surfaces of the body and serves as a protective layer differs from the epithelium that lines the internal organs or their ducts. In certain organs, epithelial lining has a specific name. As an example, the epithelium that lines the interior of all the blood and lymph vessels is called **endothelium**. Epithelium that lines the abdominal, pericardial, and pleural (lung) cavities is called **mesothelium**. Both endothelium and mesothelium in most cases exhibit thin or simple squamous epithelium.

Epithelium is **avascular** in most areas of the body; it does not have a direct blood supply except in the inner ear. Here, an area called **stria vascularis** exhibits a rich **capillary network** and is, therefore, vascular epithelium in contrast to other nonvascular epithelial lining. In areas where epithelium does not receive direct blood supply, oxygen, nutrients, and metabolites **diffuse** into the epithelial linings from the blood capillaries located in the underlying connective tissue. In contrast to the other basic tissues, epithelial cells exhibit a high **mitotic rate** with continuous cell renewal and replacement of the worn-out cells.

Figure 4.1 shows different types of epithelia in selected organs.

CLASSIFICATION OF EPITHELIA

Epithelium is classified according to the number **of cell layers** and the **morphology** or structure of the **surface cells**. A **basement membrane** is a thin, noncellular region that separates the epithelium from the underlying **connective tissue** and is seen with a light microscope. An epithelium with a single layer of cells is called **simple** and that with numerous cell layers is called **stratified**. A **pseudostratified** epithelium consists of a single layer of cells that attaches to a **basement membrane**, but not all cells reach the surface. An epithelium that exhibits flat cells is called **squamous**. When the surface cells are round, or as tall as they are wide, the epithelium is **cuboidal**. When the cells are taller than they are wide, the epithelium is called **columnar**.

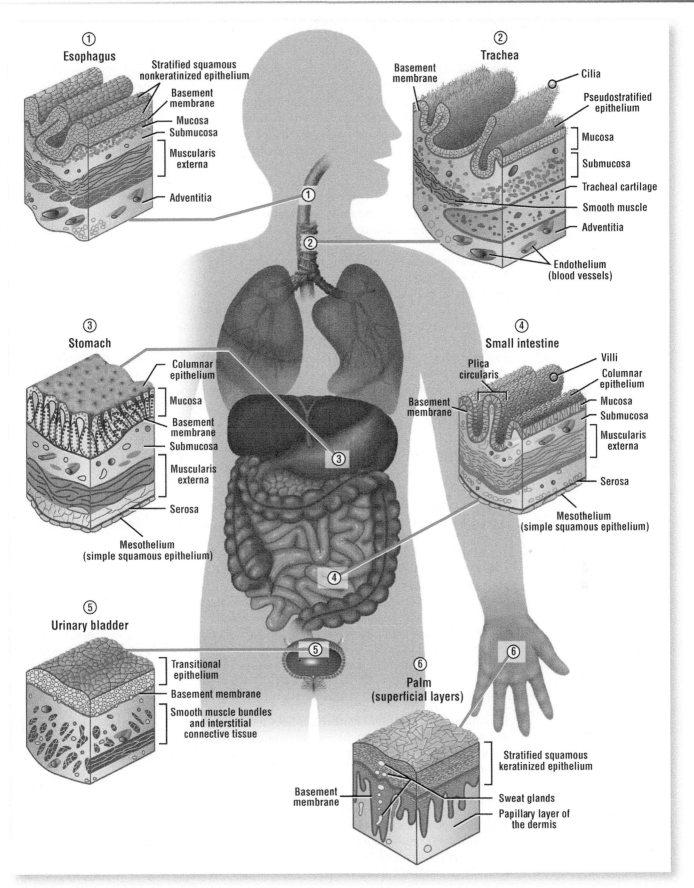

FIGURE 4.1 ■ Different types of epithelia in selected organs.

SPECIAL SURFACE MODIFICATIONS AND JUNCTIONAL COMPLEXES IN EPITHELIAL CELLS

Epithelial cells in different organs exhibit special cell membrane modifications on their **apical (upper) surfaces**. These modifications are cilia, stereocilia, or microvilli. **Cilia** are motile structures found on certain cells in the **uterine tubes, uterus, efferent ducts** in the **testes**, and **conducting tubes** of the **respiratory system**. **Microvilli** are small, nonmotile projections that cover the surfaces of all absorptive cells in the small intestine and the proximal convoluted tubules in the kidney. Their function in these organs is the absorption of fluid and nutrients during the digestive processes.

In addition to microvilli, certain cells exhibit long apical processes that extend from their surfaces into the lumina. These structures are the nonmotile **stereocilia**. They are longer than the microvilli and are found in the **epididymis, vas deferens**, and in the **sensory organ** of the **inner ear**. In the epididymis, the stereocilia increase the cell surfaces and facilitate **absorption** of testicular fluid produced in the seminiferous tubules of the testes. In the inner ear, stereocilia are located in the auditory and vestibular systems where they perform sensory functions that respond to **sound** and **balance**.

Various specialized structures in the epithelium link individual cells into a functional unit that provides strong adhesion to and rapid communication between neighboring cells. The apical **zonulae occludentes** (singular, zonula occludens), or **tight junctions**, form a seal that prevents the entrance of material between the epithelial cells. The **zonulae adherens (adhering junctions)** provide firm adhesion between cells, whereas the strong attachment sites of **desmosomes** provide stability to cells subject to shearing stresses. At the base of some epithelial cells, **hemidesmosomes** attach the cells to the basement membrane, whereas the **gap junctions** allow for selective diffusion of molecules between cells as well as rapid cell-to-cell communication.

TYPES OF EPITHELIA

Simple Epithelium

Simple squamous epithelium, called **mesothelium**, covers the external surfaces of the digestive organs, lungs, and heart. Simple squamous epithelium, called **endothelium**, lines the lumina of the heart chambers and all blood and lymphatic vessels.

Simple cuboidal epithelium lines small excretory ducts in various organs. In the proximal convoluted tubules of the kidney, the apical surfaces of the simple cuboidal epithelium are lined with a **brush border** consisting of **microvilli**.

Simple columnar epithelium lines the lumina of the **digestive organs** (stomach, small and large intestines, and gallbladder). In the small intestine, simple columnar absorptive cells that line the villi also exhibit **microvilli**, or a brush border. Villi are finger-like structures that project into the lumen of the small intestine. In uterine tubes and the uterine cavity of the reproductive tract, the simple columnar epithelium also contains cells with motile **cilia**.

Pseudostratified Columnar Epithelium

Pseudostratified columnar epithelium lines the **respiratory passages** and lumina of the **epididymis** and **vas deferens**. In the trachea, bronchi, and larger bronchioles, some surface cells are lined with motile **cilia**; in the epididymis and vas deferens, the surface cells exhibit long, nonmotile **stereocilia**.

Stratified Epithelium

Stratified squamous epithelium contains multiple cell layers. The basal cells are cuboidal to columnar; these cells produce cells that migrate toward the surface and become squamous. There are two types of stratified squamous epithelia: nonkeratinized and keratinized.

Nonkeratinized epithelium exhibits live surface or luminal cells and covers moist cavities, such as the mouth, pharynx, esophagus, vagina, and anal canal. **Keratinized epithelium** lines the external surfaces of the body. The surface layers contain nonliving, keratinized cells that are filled with the protein **keratin**. The exposed epithelium that covers the palms and soles exhibits especially thick layers of keratinized cells for added protection against abrasion.

Stratified cuboidal epithelium and **stratified columnar epithelium** have a limited distribution in the body. Both types of epithelia line the larger **excretory ducts** of the pancreas, salivary glands, and sweat glands. In these ducts, the epithelium exhibits two or more layers of cells.

Transitional epithelium lines the minor and major calyces, pelvis, ureters, and the bladder of the **urinary system**. Transitional epithelium changes shape that can resemble either stratified squamous or stratified cuboidal epithelium, depending on whether it is stretched or contracted. When transitional epithelium is **contracted**, the surface cells appear **dome shaped**; when **stretched**, the epithelium appears **squamous** and resembles the stratified epithelium of other organs.

BASEMENT MEMBRANE/BASAL LAMINA

Located between the epithelial cells and the underlying connective tissue is a supportive noncellular layer called **basement membrane** or **basal lamina**. The use of the terms basement membrane and basal lamina is inconsistent and interchangeable in the literature. Using different tissue stains, basement membrane was initially recognized and described with the light microscope. With the advent of transmission electron microscopy (TEM), the basement membrane was observed to consist of two major components, **basal lamina** and **reticular lamina**. Basal lamina consists of fine fibrils and has direct contact with basal poles of the epithelial cells. Reticular lamina is located beneath basal lamina, is formed by collagen fibers, and is more diffuse. This layer supports the basal lamina and is continuous with the connective tissue.

thePoint' Supplemental micrographic images are available at **www.thePoint.com/Eroschenko13e** under Epithelial Tissue.

FIGURE 4.2 | **Simple Squamous Epithelium: Surface View of Peritoneal Mesothelium**

To examine the surface of the simple squamous epithelium, a piece of mesentery was fixed and treated with silver nitrate and then counterstained with hematoxylin. The cells of the simple squamous epithelium (**mesothelium**) appear flat, adhere tightly to each other, and form a sheet with the thickness of a single cell layer. The irregular **cell boundaries** (1) of the epithelium stain dark and are highly visible owing to silver deposition between the cell boundaries; they form a characteristic mosaic pattern. The blue-gray **cell nuclei** (2) are centrally located in the yellow-to-brown-stained **cytoplasm** (3).

Simple squamous epithelium covers the surfaces that allow passive transport of gases or fluids and lines the pleural (thoracic), pericardial (heart), and peritoneal (abdominal) cavities.

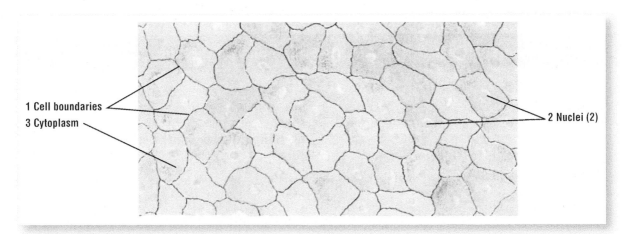

1 Cell boundaries
3 Cytoplasm
2 Nuclei (2)

FIGURE 4.2 ■ Simple squamous epithelium: surface view of peritoneal mesothelium. Stain: silver nitrate with hematoxylin. High magnification.

FIGURE 4.3 | **Simple Squamous Epithelium: Peritoneal Mesothelium Surrounding Small Intestine (Transverse Section)**

The simple squamous epithelium lining the pleural and peritoneal cavities is called mesothelium. A transverse section of a wall of the small intestine illustrates **mesothelium (1)**, a thin layer of spindle-shaped cells with prominent and oval nuclei. A thin **basement membrane (2)** is located directly under the mesothelium (1). In a surface view, the disposition of these cells would appear similar to those shown in Figure 4.2.

Mesothelium (1) and the underlying irregular **connective tissue (5)** form the serosa of the peritoneal cavity. Serosa is attached to a layer of **smooth muscle fibers (6)** called the muscularis externa **serosa** (see Fig. 4.1 parts 3 and 4). In this illustration, the bundles of smooth muscle fibers (6) are cut in the transverse plane. Also present in the connective tissue are small **blood vessels (4)**, lined also by a simple squamous epithelium called the endothelium (4), and numerous **fat (adipose) cells (3)**.

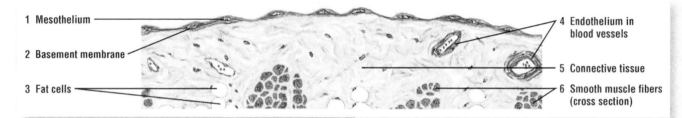

1 Mesothelium
2 Basement membrane
3 Fat cells
4 Endothelium in blood vessels
5 Connective tissue
6 Smooth muscle fibers (cross section)

FIGURE 4.3 ■ Simple squamous epithelium: peritoneal mesothelium surrounding the small intestine (transverse section). Stain: hematoxylin and eosin. High magnification.

FIGURE 4.4 | Different Epithelial Types in Kidney Cortex

This high-power photomicrograph of the kidney illustrates the different types of epithelia that are present in the kidney cortex (peripheral region). **Simple squamous epithelium** (**1**) lines the outer portion of the double-layered epithelial capsule called the **Bowman capsule** (**5**). The inner layer of the capsule surrounds the **capillaries** (**3**) of the **glomerulus** (**2**). The glomerulus (**2**) is a tuft of capillaries (**3**) where blood filtration takes place. Simple squamous epithelium called **endothelium** (**4, 9**) also lines the capillaries (**3**) and all **blood vessels** (**8**). **Simple cuboidal epithelium** (**6**) lines the lumina of the surrounding **convoluted tubules** (**7**). The blue-staining fibers surrounding the Bowman capsule (**5**), convoluted tubules (**7**), and blood vessels (**8**) in the kidney cortex are the collagen fibers of the **connective tissue** (**10**).

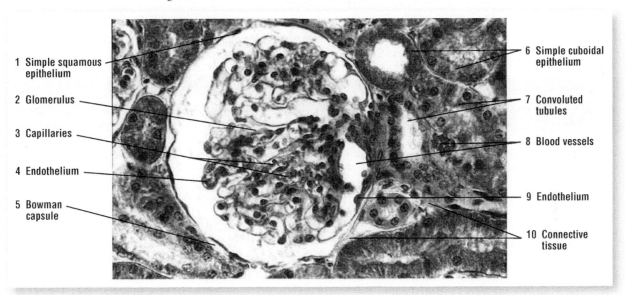

1 Simple squamous epithelium

2 Glomerulus

3 Capillaries

4 Endothelium

5 Bowman capsule

6 Simple cuboidal epithelium

7 Convoluted tubules

8 Blood vessels

9 Endothelium

10 Connective tissue

FIGURE 4.4 ■ Different epithelial types in the kidney cortex. Stain: Masson trichrome. ×120.

FIGURE 4.5 | Simple Columnar Epithelium: Stomach Surface

The surface of the stomach is covered by a tall, **simple columnar epithelium** (**1**). The illustration shows the light-staining **apical cytoplasm** (**1a**) and the dark-staining **basal nuclei** (**1b**) of the simple columnar epithelium (**1**). The epithelial cells are in close contact with each other and are arranged in

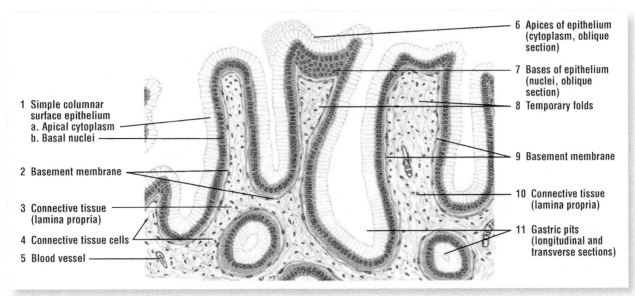

1 Simple columnar surface epithelium
   a. Apical cytoplasm
   b. Basal nuclei

2 Basement membrane

3 Connective tissue (lamina propria)

4 Connective tissue cells

5 Blood vessel

6 Apices of epithelium (cytoplasm, oblique section)

7 Bases of epithelium (nuclei, oblique section)

8 Temporary folds

9 Basement membrane

10 Connective tissue (lamina propria)

11 Gastric pits (longitudinal and transverse sections)

FIGURE 4.5 ■ Simple columnar epithelium: surface of the stomach. Stain: hematoxylin and eosin. Medium magnification.

a single row. A thin, connective tissue **basement membrane** (**2, 9**) separates the surface epithelium (**1**) from the underlying collagen fibers and cells of the **connective tissue** (**3, 10**), called the **lamina propria**. Small **blood vessels** (**5**), lined with endothelium, are present in the connective tissue (**3, 10**).

In some areas, the surface epithelium has been sectioned in a transverse or oblique plane. When a plane of section passes close to the free surface of the epithelium, the sectioned apices (**6**) of the epithelium resemble a layer of stratified, enucleated polygonal cells. When a plane of section passes through **bases** (**7**) of the epithelial cells, the nuclei resemble a stratified epithelium.

The surface cells of the stomach secrete a protective coat of mucus. The pale appearance of cytoplasm is caused by the routine histologic preparation of the tissues. The mucigen droplets that filled the apical cytoplasm (**1a**) were lost during section preparation. The more granular cytoplasm is located basally (**1b**) and stains more acidophilic.

In an empty stomach, the stomach wall exhibits numerous **temporary folds** (**8**) that disappear when the stomach is filled with solid or fluid material. Also, the surface epithelium extends downward to form numerous indentations or pits in the surface of the stomach called **gastric pits** (**11**), seen in both longitudinal section and transverse section.

FUNCTIONAL CORRELATIONS 4.3 ■ Simple Cuboidal Epithelium and Simple Columnar Epithelium

Simple cuboidal epithelium lines ducts of glands in organs for sturdiness and **protection**. In kidneys, this epithelium functions in transport, absorption of filtered substances, and active secretion of substances into the filtrate.

Simple columnar epithelium covers the surface of the stomach where the cells secrete **mucus**. The mucus lines the stomach surface and protects its lining from the corrosive gastric secretions found in the stomach during food processing and digestion.

FIGURE 4.6 | **Simple Columnar Epithelium on Villi in Small Intestine: Cells with Microvilli (Brush Borders) and Goblet Cells**

The intestinal **villi** (**1**), illustrated in transverse section and longitudinal section, are covered by simple columnar epithelium. In the small intestine, the epithelium consists of two cell types: columnar cells with microvilli or brush borders (**5, 7**) and oval-shaped **goblet cells** (**6, 13**).

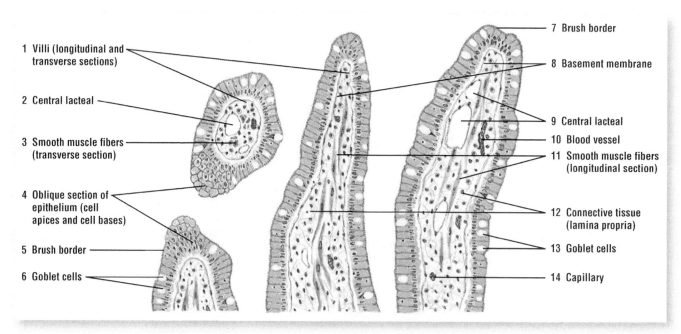

1 Villi (longitudinal and transverse sections)

2 Central lacteal

3 Smooth muscle fibers (transverse section)

4 Oblique section of epithelium (cell apices and cell bases)

5 Brush border

6 Goblet cells

7 Brush border

8 Basement membrane

9 Central lacteal

10 Blood vessel

11 Smooth muscle fibers (longitudinal section)

12 Connective tissue (lamina propria)

13 Goblet cells

14 Capillary

FIGURE 4.6 ■ Simple columnar epithelium on villi in the small intestine: cells with brush borders (microvilli) and goblet cells. Stain: hematoxylin and eosin. Medium magnification.

The **brush border** (5, 7) is seen as a reddish outer cell layer with faint vertical striations; these striations represent microvilli on the apices of columnar cells.

Pale-staining goblet cells (6, 13) are interspersed among the columnar cells. During routine histologic preparation, the mucus is lost; hence, the goblet cell cytoplasm appears clear or only lightly stained (6, 13). Normally, the mucigen droplets occupy **cell apices** (4) and the nucleus cell bases (4).

When the epithelium at the tip of a villus is sectioned in an oblique plane, the cell apices (4) of the columnar cells appear as a mosaic of enucleated cells, whereas the cell bases (4) appear as stratified epithelium.

A thin connective tissue **basement membrane** (8) is visible directly under the epithelium. The connective tissue **lamina propria** (**12**) contains an empty lymphatic vessel with a very thin endothelium called the **central lacteal** (**2, 9**). Also present in the lamina propria (12) are numerous **blood vessels** (**10**) and a **capillary** (**14**) lined with endothelium. **Smooth muscle fibers** (**3, 11**) extend into the villi. In this illustration, smooth muscle fibers (3, 11) are cut in transverse section (3) and longitudinal section (11).

The connective tissue lamina propria also contains numerous other connective tissue cells, such as plasma cells, lymphocytes, macrophages, and fibroblasts. These cells are normally seen with higher magnification.

FUNCTIONAL CORRELATIONS 4.4 ■ Epithelium with Brush Borders (Microvilli) in Small Intestine and Kidney

The main function of the epithelium in the small intestine is **absorption** of nutrients. This function is enhanced by the presence of finger-like **villi**, which increase the absorptive surface area. The villi, in turn, are covered by simple columnar epithelium with **brush borders**, or **microvilli**. These microvilli absorb nutrients and fluids from the intestinal contents. The intestinal epithelium also contains numerous **goblet cells** that secrete **mucus**, which **protects** the intestinal epithelium from corrosive secretions that enter the small intestine from the stomach during digestion.

Production of urine by the kidney involves filtration, absorption, and excretion. The apical surfaces of the simple cuboidal epithelium in the proximal convoluted tubules of the kidney are also covered with extensive **brush borders** or **microvilli**. The main function of these microvilli is to **absorb** the nutrient material and fluid from the filtrate that passes through the tubules.

FIGURE 4.7 | Pseudostratified Columnar Ciliated Epithelium: Respiratory Passages—Trachea

Pseudostratified columnar ciliated epithelium lines the upper respiratory passages, such as the trachea and bronchi. In this type of epithelium, the cells appear to form several layers. Serial sections show that all cells reach the **basement membrane (4, 13)**; however, because the epithelial cells are of different shapes and heights, not all reach the surface. For this reason, this type of epithelium is called pseudostratified rather than stratified.

Numerous motile and closely spaced **cilia (1, 8)** (cilium, singular) cover all cell apices of the ciliated cells, except those of the light-staining, oval **goblet cells (3, 11)** that are interspersed among the ciliated cells. Each cilium arises from a **basal body (9)**, whose internal morphology is identical to the centriole. The basal bodies **(9)** are located directly beneath the apical cell membrane and are adjacent to each other; they often give the appearance of a continuous dark, apical membrane **(9)**.

In pseudostratified epithelium, the deeper nuclei belong to the intermediate and short **basal cells (12)**. The more superficial, oval nuclei belong to the columnar ciliated cells **(1, 8)**. The small, round, heavily stained nuclei, without any visible surrounding cytoplasm, are those of **lymphocytes (2, 10)**. These cells migrate from the underlying **connective tissue (5)** through the epithelium.

A clearly visible basement membrane **(4, 13)** separates the pseudostratified epithelium from the underlying connective tissue **(5)**. Visible in the connective tissue **(5)** are **fibrocytes (5a)**, dense **collagen fibers (5b)**, scattered lymphocytes, and small **blood vessels (14)**. Deeper in the connective tissue are glands with **mucous acini (6)** and **serous acini (7, 15)**. These provide secretions that moisten the respiratory passages.

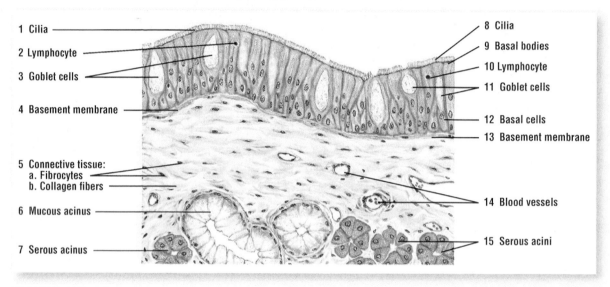

1 Cilia
2 Lymphocyte
3 Goblet cells
4 Basement membrane
5 Connective tissue:
  a. Fibrocytes
  b. Collagen fibers
6 Mucous acinus
7 Serous acinus

8 Cilia
9 Basal bodies
10 Lymphocyte
11 Goblet cells
12 Basal cells
13 Basement membrane
14 Blood vessels
15 Serous acini

FIGURE 4.7 ■ Pseudostratified columnar ciliated epithelium: respiratory passages—trachea. Stain: hematoxylin and eosin. High magnification.

FUNCTIONAL CORRELATIONS 4.5 ■ **Epithelium with Cilia or Stereocilia**

In **trachea and bronchi, pseudostratified epithelium** contains both **goblet cells** and **ciliated cells**. The motile cilia on the ciliated cells cleanse the inspired air and transport mucus and entrapped **particulate material** across the cell surfaces to the oral cavity for either swallowing or spitting out.

Simple columnar cells with motile cilia in the **uterine tubes** facilitate the conduction of oocyte and sperm across their surfaces. In the **efferent ductules** of the **testes**, ciliated cells assist in **transporting** sperm out of the testis and into the ducts of the epididymis.

The lumina of the **epididymis** and **vas deferens** are lined by pseudostratified epithelium with prominent **stereocilia**. These are long nonmotile structures, and their structure is highly different from that of the motile cilia. However, the major function of stereocilia in these organs, like that of microvilli, is to absorb the testicular fluid in the epididymis and vas deferens that was produced by cells in the testes. Stereocilia are also present in the inner ear, where their function is quite different; here, they perform sensory functions for hearing and balance or equilibrium.

FIGURE 4.8 | **Transitional Epithelium: Bladder (Unstretched or Relaxed)**

Transitional epithelium (1) is found exclusively in the excretory passages of the urinary system. It covers the lumina of renal calyces, pelvis, ureters, and bladder. This stratified epithelium is composed of several layers of similar cells. In an empty bladder, the epithelial cells appear cuboidal and extend into the lumen. These cells are frequently called umbrella or dome cells. The epithelium continuously changes its shape in response to either stretching, as a result of fluid accumulation, or contraction during voiding of urine.

In a relaxed, unstretched condition, the **surface cells** (7) are usually cuboidal and bulge out into the lumen. Frequently, **binucleate** (**two nuclei**) **cells** (6) are visible in the superficial layers or surface cells (7) of the bladder.

Transitional epithelium (1) rests on a **connective tissue** (3, 8) layer, composed primarily of **fibroblasts** (**8a**) and **collagen fibers** (**8b**). Between the connective tissue (3, 8) and the transitional epithelium (1) is a thin **basement membrane** (2). The base of the epithelium is not indented by connective tissue papillae, and it exhibits an even contour.

Small **blood vessels**, **venules** (4, 11), and **arterioles** (9) of various sizes are present in the connective tissue (3, 8). Deeper in the connective tissue are strands of **smooth muscle fibers** (5, 10), sectioned in both cross (5) and longitudinal (10) planes. The muscle layers in the bladder are located deep to the connective tissue (3, 8).

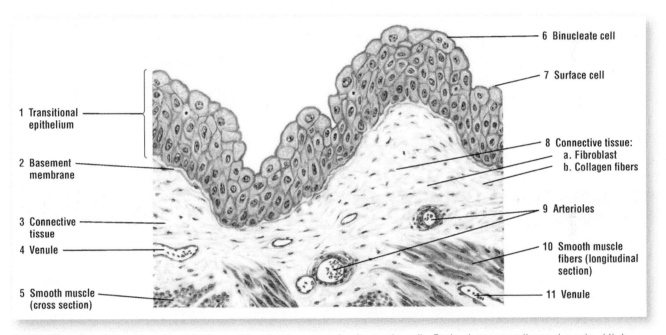

FIGURE 4.8 ■ Transitional epithelium: bladder (unstretched or relaxed). Stain: hematoxylin and eosin. High magnification.

FIGURE 4.9 | Transitional Epithelium: Bladder (Stretched)

When fluid begins to fill the bladder, the **transitional epithelium (1)** changes its shape. Increased volume in the bladder appears to reduce the number of cell layers because the **surface cells (5)** flatten to accommodate increasing surface area. In the stretched condition, the transitional epithelium (1) may resemble stratified squamous epithelium found in other regions of the body. Note also that the folds in the bladder wall disappear, and the **basement membrane (2)** is smoother. As in the empty bladder (see Fig. 4.8), the underlying connective tissue (6) contains **venules (3)** and **arterioles (7)**. Below the **connective tissue (6)** are **smooth muscle fibers (4, 8)**, sectioned in cross (4) and longitudinal (8) planes. (Compare transitional epithelium with the stratified squamous epithelium of the esophagus, shown in Fig. 4.10.)

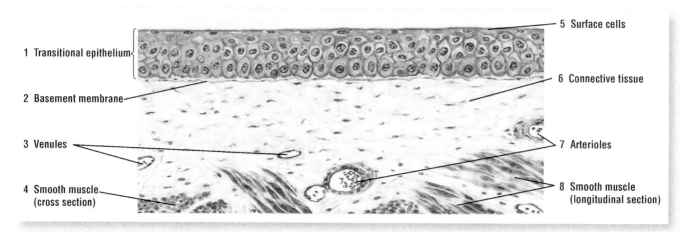

1 Transitional epithelium
2 Basement membrane
3 Venules
4 Smooth muscle (cross section)
5 Surface cells
6 Connective tissue
7 Arterioles
8 Smooth muscle (longitudinal section)

FIGURE 4.9 ■ Transitional epithelium: bladder (stretched). Stain: hematoxylin and eosin. High magnification.

FUNCTIONAL CORRELATIONS 4.6 ■ Transitional Epithelium

Transitional epithelium allows **distension** of the urinary organs (calyces, pelvis, ureters, bladder) during urine accumulation and **contraction** of these organs during the emptying process without breaking the cell contacts in the epithelium. This change in cell shape is due to the unique feature of the cell membrane in the transitional epithelium. Here are found specialized regions called **plaques** that act like hinges during different bladder functions. When the bladder is empty, the plaques are folded into irregular contours. During bladder filling, these structures unfold allowing the cells to stretch and flatten. The membrane plaques are impermeable to fluids, salts, and hypertonic urine. Transitional epithelium forms a **protective osmotic barrier** against the hypertonic and cytotoxic effect of urine in the bladder and underlying connective tissue.

FIGURE 4.10 | **Stratified Squamous Nonkeratinized Epithelium: Esophagus**

Stratified squamous epithelium is characterized by numerous cell layers, with the outermost layer consisting of flat or squamous cells, which contain nuclei and are alive. The thickness of the epithelium varies among different regions of the body, and, as a result, the composition of the epithelium also varies. Illustrated in this figure is an example of the moist, **nonkeratinized stratified squamous epithelium** (1) that lines the esophagus as well as the oral cavity, vagina, and anal canal.

Cuboidal or low columnar **basal cells** (5) are located at the base of the stratified epithelium. The cytoplasm is finely granular, and the oval, chromatin-rich nucleus occupies most of the cell. Cells in the intermediate layers of the epithelium are **polyhedral** (4) with round or oval nuclei and more visible cell cytoplasm and membranes. **Mitoses** (6) are frequently observed in the deeper cell layers and in the basal cells (5). Cells and their nuclei become progressively flatter as the cells migrate toward the free surface of the epithelium. Above the polyhedral cells (4) are several rows of flattened or **squamous cells** (3).

A fine **basement membrane** (7) separates the epithelium (1) from the underlying **connective tissue**, the **lamina propria** (2). **Papillae** (10) or extensions of connective tissue indent the lower surface of the epithelium (1), giving it a characteristic wavy appearance. The connective tissue (2) contains **collagen fibers** (11), **fibrocytes** (9), **capillaries** (12), and **arterioles** (8).

In areas where stratified squamous epithelium is exposed to increased wear and tear, the outermost layer, called the stratum corneum, becomes thick and keratinized, as illustrated in the epidermis of the palm in Figure 4.11.

An example of thin, stratified squamous epithelium without connective tissue papillae indentation is found in the cornea of the eye; the surface underlying the epithelium is smooth. This type of epithelium is only a few cell layers thick, but it has the characteristic arrangement of basal columnar, polyhedral, and superficial squamous cells.

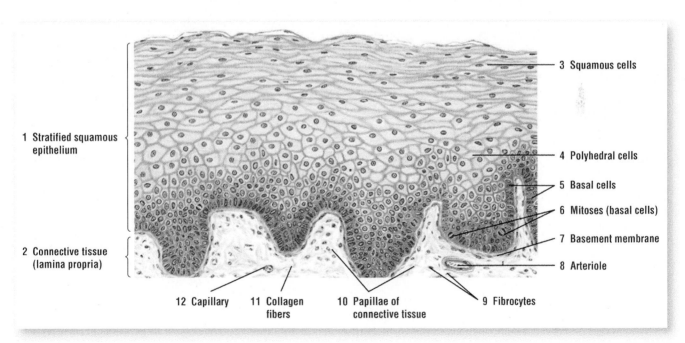

FIGURE 4.10 ■ Stratified squamous nonkeratinized epithelium: esophagus. Stain: hematoxylin and eosin. Medium magnification.

FIGURE 4.11 | Stratified Squamous Keratinized Epithelium: Palm of the Hand

The skin is covered with **stratified squamous keratinized epithelium** (1). The outermost layer of the skin contains dead cells and is called the **stratum corneum** (5). In the palms and soles, the stratum corneum (5) is thick, whereas in the rest of the body, it is thinner. Inferior to the stratum corneum (5) are the different cell layers that give rise to the stratum corneum (5).

This medium-power photomicrograph illustrates the stratified squamous keratinized epithelium (1) of the palm and the cell layers **stratum granulosum** (6) and **stratum spinosum** (7) as well as the basal cell layer, **stratum basale** (8). The epithelium is attached to the underlying **connective tissue** (3) layer composed of dense collagen fibers and fibroblasts. The underlying surface of the epithelium (1) is indented by connective tissue (3) extensions called **papillae** (2) that form the characteristic wavy boundary between the epithelium (1) and the connective tissue (3). Passing through the connective tissue (3) and the epithelium (1) are **excretory ducts of the sweat glands** (4) that are located deep to the epithelium.

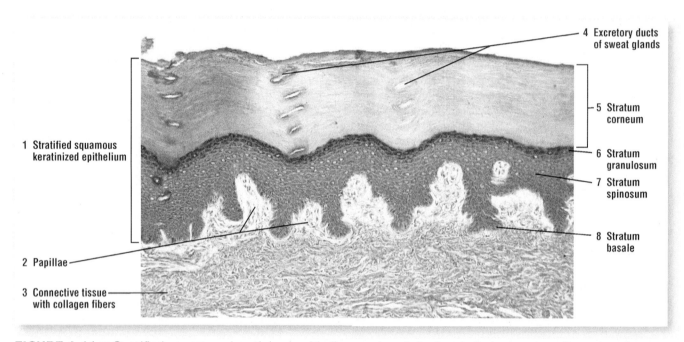

FIGURE 4.11 ■ Stratified squamous keratinized epithelium: palm of the hand. Stain: hematoxylin and eosin. ×40.

FIGURE 4.12 | Stratified Cuboidal Epithelium: Excretory Duct in Salivary Gland

The stratified cuboidal epithelium has a limited distribution and is seen in only a few organs. The larger excretory ducts in the salivary glands and in the pancreas are lined with stratified cuboidal epithelium. This figure illustrates a high-power photomicrograph of a large excretory duct of a salivary gland. The luminal lining consists of two layers of cuboidal cells, forming the **stratified cuboidal epithelium** (1). Surrounding the excretory duct are collagen fibers of the **connective tissue** (2, 7) and **blood vessels** (3, 5) that are lined by simple squamous epithelium called **endothelium** (4, 6).

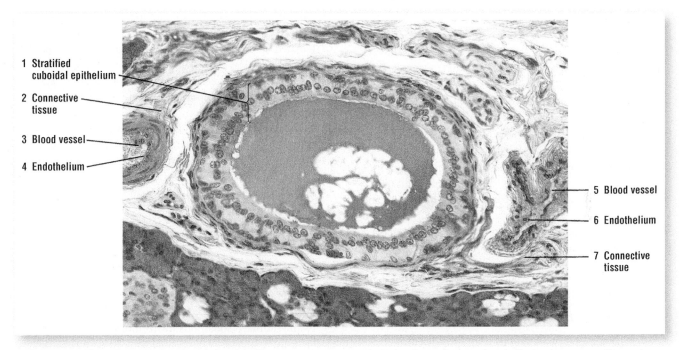

1 Stratified cuboidal epithelium
2 Connective tissue
3 Blood vessel
4 Endothelium
5 Blood vessel
6 Endothelium
7 Connective tissue

FIGURE 4.12 ■ Stratified cuboidal epithelium: an excretory duct in the salivary gland. Stain: hematoxylin and eosin. ×100.

Chapter 4 Summary

SECTION 1 • Classification of Epithelial Tissue

EPITHELIAL TISSUE

Major Features

- Classification is based on number of cell layers and cell morphology
- Basement membrane separates epithelium from connective tissue
- Almost all epithelia are nonvascular, except the epithelium in the inner ear, which is vascular
- Delivery of nutrients to epithelial cells and removal of metabolic waste occur via diffusion from adjacent capillaries
- Surface modifications include motile cilia, microvilli, and nonmotile stereocilia
- Lateral cell surface modification includes zonulae occludentes, zonulae adherens, desmosomes, gap junctions, and hemidesmosomes basally

Types of Epithelia

Simple Squamous Epithelium

- Single layer of flat or squamous cells; includes mesothelium and endothelium
- Mesothelium lines external surfaces of digestive organs, lung, and heart
- Endothelium lines inside of heart chambers, blood vessels, and lymphatic vessels
- Functions in filtration, diffusion, transport, secretion, and reduction of friction

Simple Cuboidal Epithelium

- Single layer of round cells
- Lines small ducts and kidney tubules
- Protects ducts; transports and absorbs filtered material in kidney tubules

Simple Columnar Epithelium

- All cells are tall, some lined by microvilli
- Lines the lumina of digestive organs
- Secretes protective mucus for stomach lining
- Absorption of nutrients in small intestine

Pseudostratified Columnar Epithelium, Epithelium with Cilia or Stereocilia

- All cells reach basement membrane, but not all reach the surface
- Ciliated cells interspersed among mucus-secreting goblet cells
- In respiratory passages, ciliated and mucus cells clean inspired air and transport particulate matter across cell surfaces
- In uterine tubes and the efferent ducts of testes, ciliated cells transport oocytes and sperm across cell surfaces, respectively In the epididymis and vas deferens, the lining stereocilia absorb testicular fluid
- In the inner ear, stereocilia perform sensory functions for hearing and balance

Stratified Epithelium

- Formed by multiple layers of cells, the superficial cell layer determining epithelial type
- Nonkeratinized squamous epithelium contains live superficial cell layer
- Nonkeratinized squamous forms moist and protective layer in esophagus, vagina, anal canal, and oral cavity
- Keratinized epithelium contains dead superficial cell layer
- Keratinized epithelium provides protection against abrasion, bacterial invasion, and desiccation
- Cuboidal epithelium lines large excretory ducts in different organs
- Cuboidal epithelium provides protection for the ducts

Transitional Epithelium

- Found exclusively in renal calyces, renal pelvis, ureters, and bladder
- Changes shape in response to distensions caused by fluid accumulation
- Plaques in the cells allow extensions of the epithelium during fluid accumulation
- During extension or contraction, cell-to-cell contact remains unbroken
- Forms protective osmotic barrier between hypertonic urine and underlying tissue

Chapter 4 Review Questions: Section 1

QUESTIONS

In the following multiple choice questions, choose the letter corresponding to the one best answer.

1. What lies directly under the epithelium?

A. Blood vessels
B. Muscle tissue
C. Basement membrane
D. Nervous tissue
E. Connective tissue

2. The epithelium that protects the skin from abrasion and bacterial invasion is:

A. pseudostratified.
B. stratified squamous keratinized.
C. striated.
D. stratified squamous nonkeratinized.
E. stratified columnar.

3. What modification would be best suited for cells transporting materials across their surfaces?

A. Microvilli
B. Stereocilia
C. Cilia
D. Brush border
E. Microfilaments

4. The epithelium that allows distension in an organ is:

A. transitional.
B. squamous.
C. cuboidal.
D. columnar.
E. pseudostratified.

5. A function attributed to the basement membrane/basal lamina is:

A. forming tight junctions in the apical regions of the cells.
B. facilitating increased absorption of fluids and nutrients by epithelial cells.
C. forming hemidesmosomes for the attachment of cells to the connective tissue.
D. attaching to and supporting epithelial cells.
E. forming desmosomes in epithelial cells.

ANSWERS

1. **Correct Answer: C.** Basement membrane. This membrane, when stained with the right chemicals, is seen with the light microscope. With the transmission electron microscope, the basement membrane consists of basal lamina and lamina reticularis.

2. **Correct answer: B.** Stratified squamous keratinized. The keratin on the epithelial surface forms a protective shield that prevents abrasion and bacterial invasion.

3. **Correct Answer: C.** Cilia. Cilia are motile structures that line cells in respiratory tracts, uterine tubes, and efferent ducts of the testes, and they can move objects across their surfaces.

4. **Correct Answer: A.** Transitional. This type of epithelium lines the bladder and urinary passages. When the bladder is beginning to fill with urine, transitional epithelium allows for distension of the organ to accommodate more fluid before voiding.

5. **Correct Answer: D.** Attaching to and supporting epithelial cells.

SECTION 2 Classification of Glandular Tissue

The body contains a variety of glands. They are classified as either **exocrine glands** or **endocrine glands**. These glands develop from epithelial cells that extend from the surface into the underlying connective tissue. Exocrine glands are connected to the surface epithelium by excretory **ducts**, into which their secretory products pass to the external surface. In contrast, the endocrine glands have lost their connection to the surface epithelium, and their secretory products are delivered directly into the capillaries of the connective tissue that surrounds the **circulatory system**.

EXOCRINE GLANDS

Exocrine glands are either **unicellular** or **multicellular**. Unicellular glands consist of single cells. The mucus-secreting **goblet cells** found in the epithelia of the small and large intestines and in the respiratory passages are the best examples of unicellular glands.

Multicellular glands are characterized by a **secretory portion**, an end piece where the epithelial cells secrete a product, and an epithelium-lined excretory **ductal portion**, through which the secretion is delivered to the exterior of the gland. Larger excretory ducts are usually lined by stratified epithelium, either cuboidal or columnar.

Simple and Compound Exocrine Glands

Multicellular exocrine glands are divided into two major categories depending on the structure of their ductal portion. A **simple exocrine gland** exhibits an unbranched duct, which may be straight or coiled. Also, if the terminal secretory portion of the gland is shaped in the form of a tube, the gland is called a **tubular gland**.

An exocrine gland that shows a repeated branching pattern of the ducts that drain the secretory portions is called a **compound exocrine gland**. Furthermore, if the secretory portions of the gland are shaped like a flask or a tube, the glands are called **acinar (alveolar) glands** or **tubular glands**, respectively. Certain exocrine glands exhibit a mixture of both tubular and acinar secretory portions. Such glands are called **tubuloacinar glands**.

Exocrine glands may also be classified on the basis of the secretory products of their cells. Glands with cells that produce a viscous secretion that lubricates or protects the inner lining of the organs are **mucous glands**. These glands produce the lubricating product **mucus**. Glands with cells that produce watery secretions that are often rich in enzymes are **serous glands**. Certain glands in the body contain a mixture of both mucous and serous secretory cells; these are **mixed (seromucous) glands**.

Merocrine and Holocrine Glands

Exocrine glands may also be classified on the basis of how their secretory product is discharged. **Merocrine glands**, such as exocrine acinar cells of the pancreas and the salivary glands, release their secretion by exocytosis without any loss of cellular components. Most exocrine glands in the body secrete their product in this manner. In **holocrine glands**, such as the sebaceous glands of the skin, the cells themselves become the secretory product that accumulates in the glands. Here, gland cells accumulate lipids, die, and degenerate to become **sebum**, the secretory product. In another type of gland, called **apocrine glands (mammary glands)**, a portion of the apical part of the secretory cell is discharged as the secretory product. However, almost all glands that were once classified as apocrine are now regarded as merocrine glands.

ENDOCRINE CELLS, TISSUES, AND GLANDS

Endocrine glands differ from exocrine glands in that they do not have excretory ducts for releasing their secretory products. Instead, endocrine glands exhibit increased vascularity, and their secretory cells are surrounded by rich capillary networks. This close proximity to the capillary networks allows for efficient release of the secretory products from these cells directly into the bloodstream and their distribution to different organs via the systemic circulation.

The endocrine system can be separated into the following three parts.

Endocrine Cells

Endocrine glands can be also considered as **individual cells** (**unicellular glands**) that are scattered throughout different organs including the digestive organs (**enteroendocrine cells**), respiratory tract, pancreatic ducts, and others. Collectively, these scattered individual endocrine cells constitute the **diffuse neuroendocrine system** (**DNES**). These cells are considered neuroendocrine because they produce and release hormones similar to those of neurosecretory cells in the central nervous system (CNS).

Endocrine Tissues

In certain organs, such as the pancreas and the reproductive organs of both sexes, endocrine cells are seen as clusters mixed together with exocrine glands. The **endocrine tissues** are surrounded by capillary networks, whereas the cells of exocrine glands are attached to excretory ducts.

Major Endocrine Organs

The **major endocrine organs** in the organism are the separate **pituitary gland**, **thyroid glands**, **parathyroid glands**, and **adrenal glands**. The primary functions of these organs are to synthesize, store, and release the specific hormones into the systemic circulation as needed.

thePoint'   Supplemental micrographic images are available at **www.thePoint.com/Eroschenko13e** under Cell and Cytoplasm.

FIGURE 4.13 | **Unbranched Simple Tubular Exocrine Glands: Intestinal Glands**

Unbranched simple tubular glands without excretory ducts are best represented by the **intestinal glands** (**crypts of Lieberkühn**) in the **large intestine** (**A** and **B**) and **rectum**. The **surface epithelium** and the **secretory cells** of these glands are lined with numerous goblet cells; these are unicellular exocrine glands. Similar but shorter intestinal glands with goblet cells are also found in the small intestine.

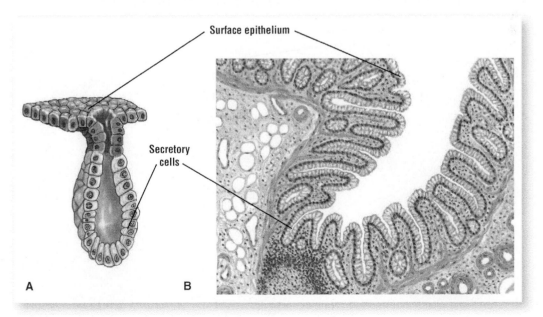

FIGURE 4.13 ■ Unbranched simple tubular exocrine glands: intestinal glands.
A. Diagram of the gland. **B.** Transverse section of the large intestine. Stain: hematoxylin and eosin. Medium magnification.

FIGURE 4.14 | Simple Branched Tubular Exocrine Glands: Gastric Glands

Simple or slightly branched tubular glands without excretory ducts are found in the stomach. These are the **gastric glands** (**A** and **B**). In the fundus and body of the stomach, they are lined with modified columnar cells that are specialized for secreting hydrochloric acid and the precursor for the proteolytic enzyme pepsin.

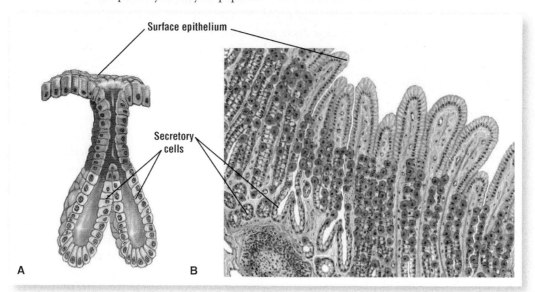

FIGURE 4.14 ■ Simple branched tubular exocrine gland: gastric glands. **A.** Diagram of the gland. **B.** Transverse section of the stomach. Stain: hematoxylin and eosin. Low magnification.

FIGURE 4.15 | Coiled Tubular Exocrine Glands: Sweat Glands

Sebaceous glands in the skin are coiled tubular glands with long, unbranched ducts (**A** and **B**). Note the **secretory cells** of the gland and the **excretory duct**, which delivers the secretory product to the surface. Note also the transition from single layer of cells in the secretory portion of the gland and the stratified cuboidal epithelium in the excretory duct.

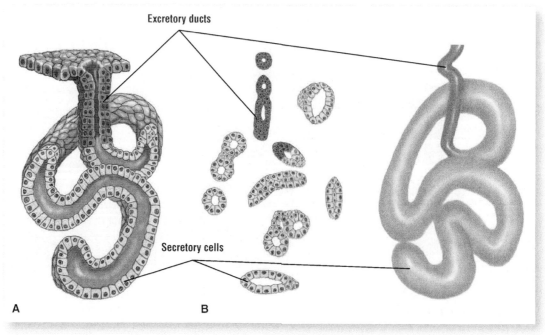

FIGURE 4.15 ■ Coiled tubular exocrine glands: sweat glands. **A.** Diagram of the gland. **B.** Transverse and three-dimensional view of a coiled sweat gland. Stain: hematoxylin and eosin. Medium magnification.

FIGURE 4.16 | Compound Acinar (Exocrine) Gland: Mammary Glands

The mammary gland is an example of a **compound acinar (alveolar) gland** (**A** and **B**). The lactating mammary gland contains enlarged **secretory acini** (**alveoli**) with large lumina that are filled with milk. Draining these acini (alveoli) are **excretory ducts**, some of which contain secretory material and are lined by stratified epithelium.

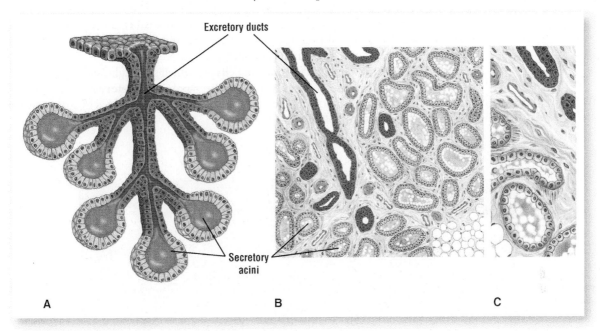

FIGURE 4.16 ■ Compound acinar exocrine gland: mammary gland. **A.** Diagram of the gland. **B and C.** A mammary gland during lactation. Stain: hematoxylin and eosin. **B.** Low magnification. **C.** Medium magnification.

FIGURE 4.17 | Compound Tubuloacinar (Exocrine) Gland: Salivary Glands

The salivary glands (parotid, submandibular, and sublingual) best illustrate **compound tubuloacinar glands** (**A** and **B**). The glands contain **secretory acinar elements** and **secretory tubular elements**. In addition, the submandibular and sublingual salivary glands contain both serous and

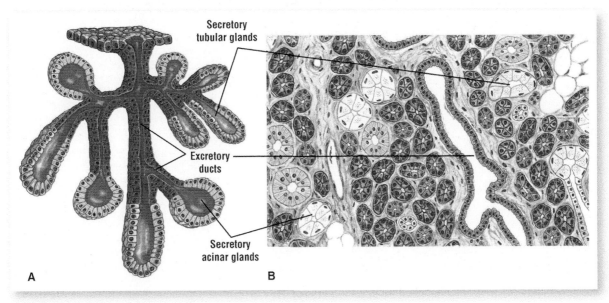

FIGURE 4.17 ■ Compound tubuloacinar (exocrine) gland: salivary gland. **A.** Diagram of the gland. **B.** A submandibular salivary gland. Stain: hematoxylin and eosin. Low magnification.

mucous acini. Details and comparisons of these acini are described in Chapter 13. The **excretory ducts** are lined with cuboidal, columnar, or stratified epithelium and are named according to their location in the gland.

FIGURE 4.18 | Compound Tubuloacinar (Exocrine) Gland: Submaxillary Salivary Gland

A photomicrograph of a submaxillary salivary gland shows the secretory units of a compound tubuloacinar gland. The grapelike **secretory acinar elements** (1) are circular in transverse section and are distinguished from the longer **secretory tubular elements** (7) of the gland. Empty lumina can be seen in some sections of both types of secretory elements. This salivary gland is a mixed gland and contains both the **mucous cells** (4), which stain light, and **serous cells** (5), which stain dark. Draining the secretory elements of the gland are **excretory ducts** (3, 6, 8). The small excretory ducts are lined by simple cuboidal epithelium and surrounded by **connective tissue** (2), which also surrounds all of the secretory elements.

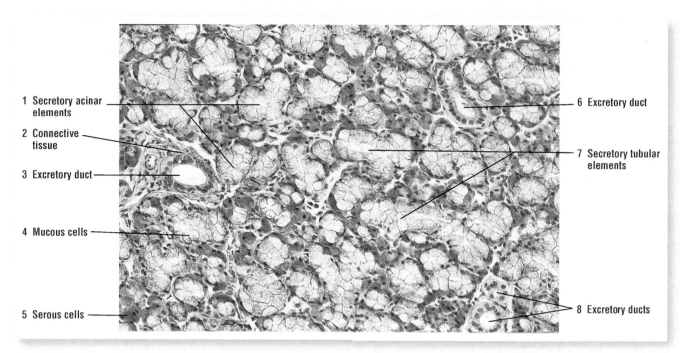

1 Secretory acinar elements

2 Connective tissue

3 Excretory duct

4 Mucous cells

5 Serous cells

6 Excretory duct

7 Secretory tubular elements

8 Excretory ducts

FIGURE 4.18 ■ Compound tubuloacinar (exocrine) gland: submaxillary salivary gland. Stain: hematoxylin and eosin. ×64.

FIGURE 4.19 | Endocrine Gland: Pancreatic Islet

An example of an endocrine gland is illustrated as a pancreatic islet from the pancreas. The pancreas is a mixed gland, containing both an **exocrine portion** and **endocrine portion**. Here, the exocrine acini surround the endocrine pancreatic islets (**A** and **B**).

The structure and function of other endocrine organs (glands) are presented in greater detail in Chapter 19.

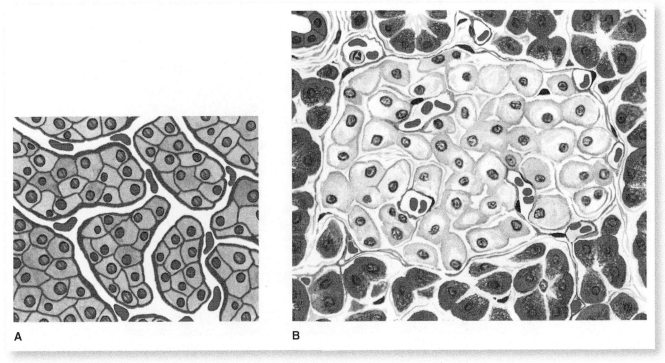

A   B

FIGURE 4.19 ■ Endocrine gland: pancreatic islet. **A.** Diagram of a pancreatic islet. **B.** High magnification of the endocrine and exocrine pancreas. Stain: hematoxylin and eosin. High magnification.

FIGURE 4.20 | Endocrine and Exocrine Pancreas

A photomicrograph of the pancreas shows a mixed gland with both endocrine and exocrine portions. The **exocrine pancreas (3)** consists of numerous secretory acini that deliver their secretory material into the **excretory duct (1)**, which is lined by simple cuboidal epithelium and surrounded by a layer of connective tissue. The **endocrine pancreas (5)** is called the pancreatic islet (5) because it is separated from the cells of the exocrine pancreas (3) by a thin **connective tissue capsule (4)**. The endocrine pancreatic islet (5) does not contain excretory ducts. Instead, it is highly vascularized, and all of the secretory products leave the pancreatic islet via numerous **blood vessels (capillaries) (2)**.

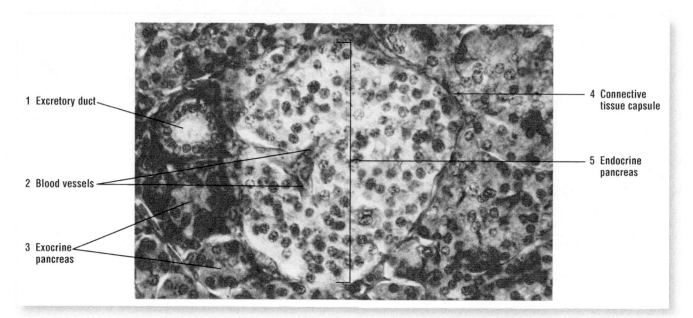

1 Excretory duct

2 Blood vessels

3 Exocrine pancreas

4 Connective tissue capsule

5 Endocrine pancreas

FIGURE 4.20 ■ Endocrine and exocrine pancreas. Stain: Mallory-Azan. ×100.

Chapter 4 Summary

SECTION 2 • Classification of Glandular Tissue

GLANDULAR TISSUE

Exocrine Glands

- Can be unicellular or multicellular
- Multicellular glands contain secretory portion and ductal portion
- Secretions enter the ductal system
- Simple tubular glands exhibit unbranched duct; found in intestinal glands
- Coiled tubular glands seen in sweat glands
- Compound glands exhibit repeated ductal branching with either acinar (alveolar) or tubular secretory portions
- Compound acinar glands seen in mammary glands
- Compound tubuloacinar glands seen in salivary glands
- Mucous glands lubricate and protect inner linings of organs
- Serous glands produce watery secretions that contain enzymes
- Mixed glands contain both serous and mucous cells
- Merocrine glands, like pancreas, release secretion without cell loss
- Holocrine glands, like sebaceous skin glands, release secretion with cell components

Endocrine Cells, Tissues, and Glands

- Diffuse neuroendocrine system (DNS): individual cells as endocrine glands in digestive organs and respiratory system
- Endocrine tissues: isolated endocrine tissues mixed with exocrine glands as in pancreas and reproductive organs
- Major endocrine organs: pituitary, thyroid, and adrenal glands
- Do not have excretory ducts and are highly vascularized
- Secretory products enter bloodstream (capillaries) for systemic distribution

Chapter 4 Review Questions: Section 2

QUESTIONS

In the following multiple choice questions, choose the letter corresponding to the one best answer.

1. Exocrine glands are connected to the surface epithelium by:

A. blood vessels.
B. connective tissue.
C. excretory ducts.
D. tubular glands.
E. adjacent glands.

2. The unicellular endocrine glands are primarily found in the:

A. pituitary gland.
B. thyroid gland.
C. mammary glands.
D. digestive organs.
E. bladder.

3. An example of a mixed gland containing both endocrine and exocrine cells is seen in the:

A. pituitary gland.
B. salivary gland.
C. pancreas.
D. sweat gland.
E. sebaceous gland.

4. An example of a gland that produces holocrine secretions is the:

A. sebaceous gland.
B. sweat gland.
C. salivary gland.
D. pancreas.
E. mammary gland.

5. Tubuloacinar glands are seen in the:

A. sweat glands.
B. stomach.
C. mammary glands.
D. pancreas.
E. salivary glands.

ANSWERS

1. Correct Answer: C. Excretory ducts. Excretory ducts lead from the exocrine glands toward the epithelial surface to discharge secretory products.

2. Correct Answer: D. Digestive organs. The lining of the digestive tract contains numerous individual and unicellular endocrine glands that play an important role in digestive processes.

3. Correct Answer: C. Pancreas. The pancreas has both types of cells—the endocrine cell as separate islands surrounded by exocrine cells.

4. Correct Answer: A. Sebaceous gland. In these glands, the cells degenerate and become part of the holocrine secretion process.

5. Correct Answer: E. Salivary glands. These glands exhibit both tubular and acinar glandular structures.

ADDITIONAL HISTOLOGIC IMAGES

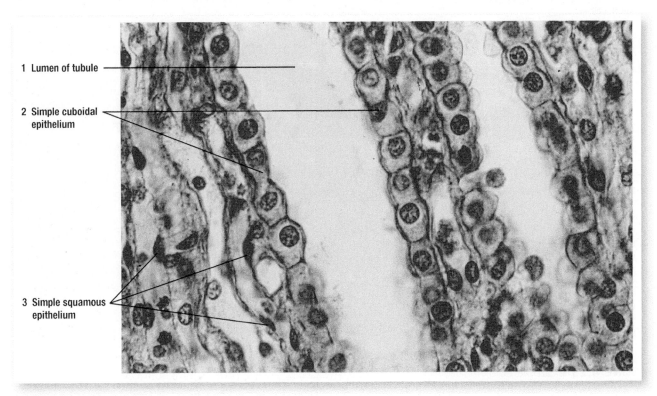

1 Lumen of tubule

2 Simple cuboidal epithelium

3 Simple squamous epithelium

FIGURE 4.21 ■ Simple cuboidal and simple squamous epithelium in different tubules of a rodent kidney. Stain: hematoxylin and eosin. ×165.

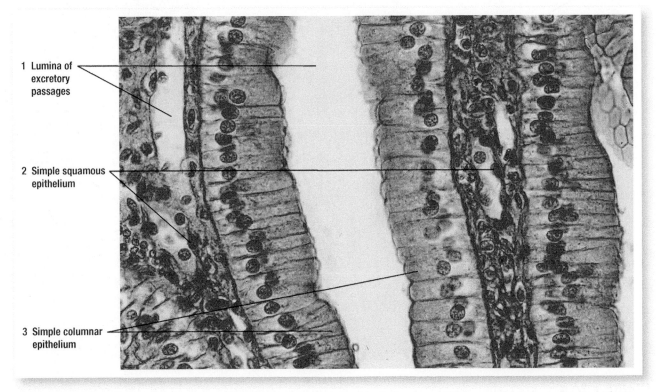

1 Lumina of excretory passages

2 Simple squamous epithelium

3 Simple columnar epithelium

FIGURE 4.22 ■ Simple columnar and simple squamous epithelia in the papillary region of a primate kidney. Stain: hematoxylin and eosin. ×165.

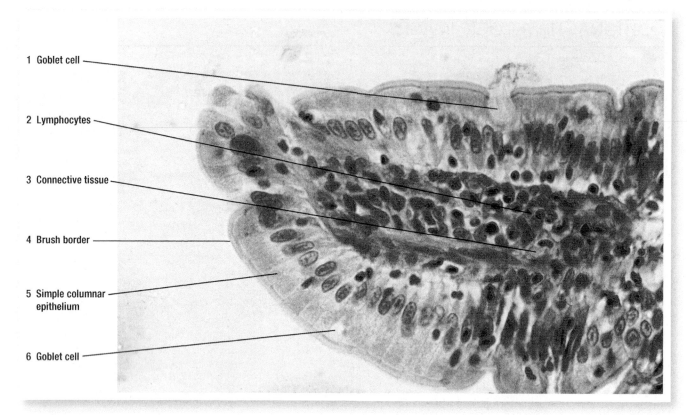

1 Goblet cell
2 Lymphocytes
3 Connective tissue
4 Brush border
5 Simple columnar epithelium
6 Goblet cell

FIGURE 4.23 ■ Simple columnar epithelium with brush border, goblet cells, and lymphocytes in the connective tissue of a rodent intestinal villus. Stain: hematoxylin and eosin. ×205.

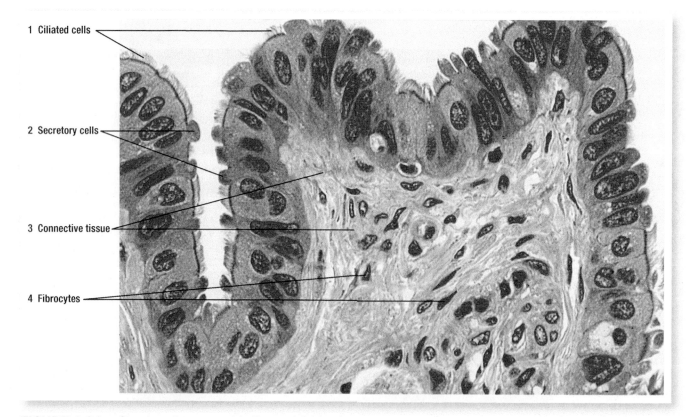

1 Ciliated cells
2 Secretory cells
3 Connective tissue
4 Fibrocytes

FIGURE 4.24 ■ Simple columnar epithelium exhibiting both ciliated and secretory cells overlying connective tissue with fibrocytes in a primate oviduct. Stain: hematoxylin and eosin. ×205.

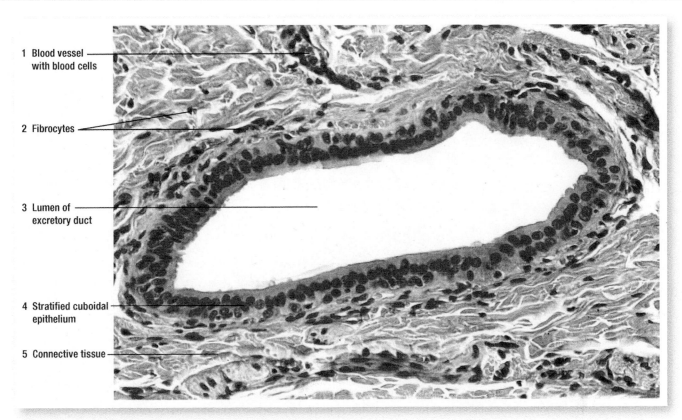

1 Blood vessel with blood cells

2 Fibrocytes

3 Lumen of excretory duct

4 Stratified cuboidal epithelium

5 Connective tissue

FIGURE 4.25 ■ Stratified cuboidal epithelium lining the excretory duct of a primate salivary gland and surrounded by connective tissue fibers and cells. Stain: hematoxylin and eosin. ×165.

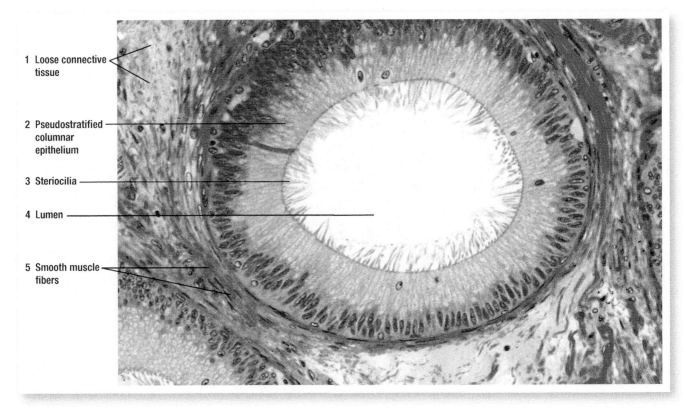

1 Loose connective tissue

2 Pseudostratified columnar epithelium

3 Steriocilia

4 Lumen

5 Smooth muscle fibers

FIGURE 4.26 ■ Pseudostratified columnar epithelium with stereocilia surrounded by smooth muscle fibers in a primate epididymis. Stain: hematoxylin and eosin. ×200.

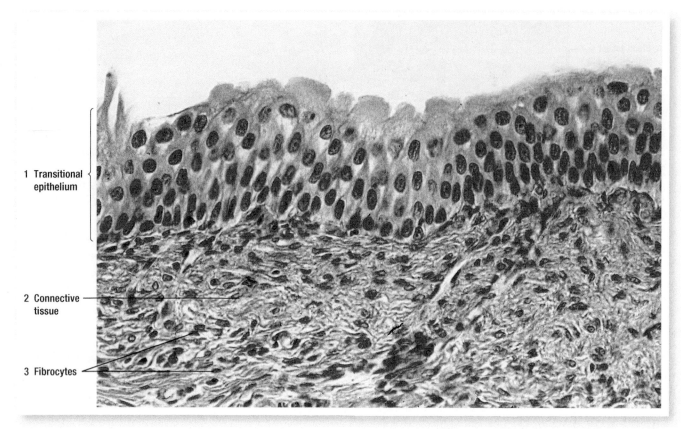

1 Transitional
  epithelium

2 Connective
  tissue

3 Fibrocytes

FIGURE 4.27 ■ Transitional epithelium in a relaxed primate bladder overlying connective tissue with fibrocytes. Stain: hematoxylin and eosin. ×205.

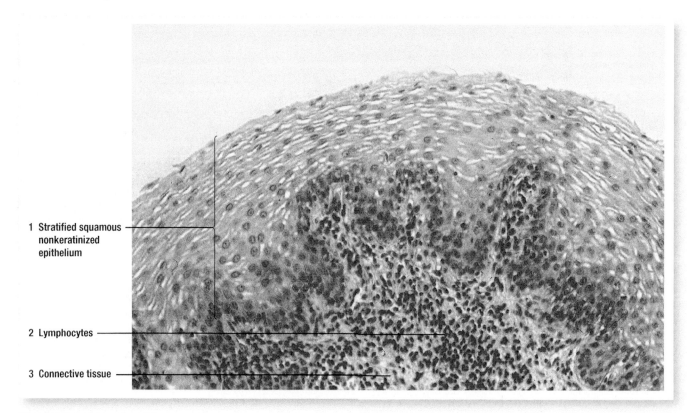

1 Stratified squamous
  nonkeratinized
  epithelium

2 Lymphocytes

3 Connective tissue

FIGURE 4.28 ■ Stratified squamous nonkeratinized (moist) vaginal primate epithelium with underlying connective tissue filled with numerous dark-staining lymphocytes. Stain: hematoxylin and eosin. ×165.

Connective Tissue

Connective tissue originates from embryonic **mesenchyme cells** that differentiate during development into cell types that include **cartilage**, **bone**, and **blood**. Because mesenchyme cells can differentiate into different cells, they can also serve as **stem cells**. With the exceptions of blood and lymph, the connective tissue consists of different cell types and **extracellular material** called **matrix**. The extracellular matrix consists of protein **collagen**, **reticular**, and **elastic fibers** and the **ground substance** within which are embedded the different protein fibers. The ground substance has a gellike characteristic that contains a mixture of **glycoproteins** and **carbohydrates** with a high **water-binding** affinity (hydration). As a result, the highly hydrated state of the ground substance allows for efficient **exchange** of nutrients, oxygen, and metabolic waste between the cells and the blood vessels. The connective tissue also binds, anchors, and supports various cells, tissues, and organs of the body. In addition, the connective tissue matrix contains numerous cell types that provide essential **protection** and **defense** against bacterial invasion and foreign bodies. The connective tissue is classified as either loose connective tissue or dense connective tissue, depending on the amount, type, arrangement, and abundance of cells, fibers, and ground substance.

CLASSIFICATION OF CONNECTIVE TISSUE

Loose Connective Tissue

Loose connective tissue is more prevalent in the body than dense connective tissue. It is characterized by a loose, irregular arrangement of connective tissue fibers and abundant ground substance. Various connective tissue cells and fibers are found in the matrix. **Collagen fibers**, **fibroblasts**, **fibrocytes**, **adipose cells**, **mast cells**, **plasma cells**, and **macrophages** predominate in the loose connective tissue, with fibroblasts being the most common cell types. Figure 5.1 shows the various types of cells and fibers that are usually found in loose connective tissue.

Dense Connective Tissue

In contrast to loose connective tissue, **dense irregular connective tissue** contains thicker and more densely packed collagen fibers, with fewer cell types in the matrix and less ground substance. The collagen fibers in this tissue type exhibit a random and irregular orientation. **Dense irregular connective tissue** is present in the dermis of skin, in capsules of different organs, and in areas of the body where strong binding and support are needed.

In contrast, the dense regular connective tissue contains densely packed collagen fibers that exhibit a uniform, regular, and parallel arrangement. This type of tissue is primarily found in the **tendons** and **ligaments**. In both dense connective tissue types, **fibroblasts** are the most abundant cells; these are scattered between the dense collagen bundles.

CELLS OF THE CONNECTIVE TISSUE

The two most common cell types in the connective tissue are the active **fibroblasts** and the inactive or resting fibroblasts, the **fibrocytes**. Fusiform fibroblasts synthesize all the connective tissue fibers (collagen, elastic, and reticular) and the extracellular ground substance, including proteoglycans, glycosaminoglycans, and adhesive glycoproteins.

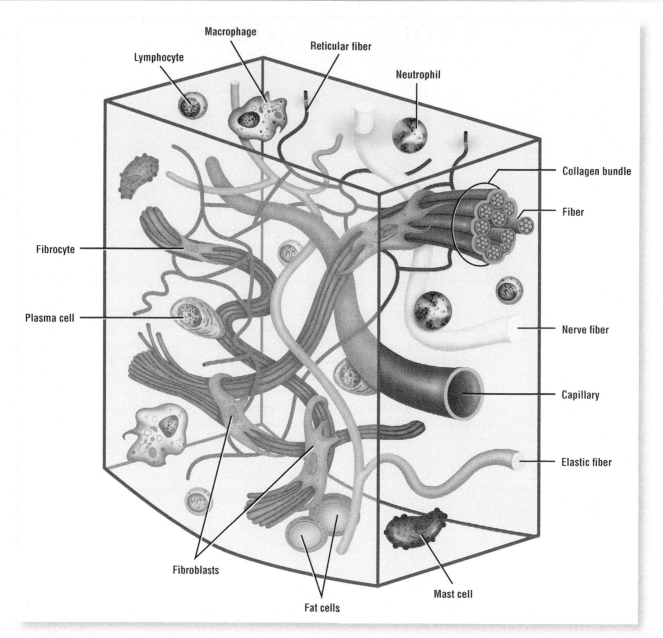

FIGURE 5.1 ■ Composite illustration of loose connective tissue with its predominant cells and fibers.

Adipose (fat) cells store fat and may occur singly or in groups in the connective tissue. There are two types of adipose cells. Cells with a large, single, or unilocular lipid droplet in the cytoplasm are **white adipose tissue**, whereas cells with numerous or multilocular lipid droplets are **brown adipose tissue**. White adipose tissue is more abundant than brown adipose tissue, and when adipose cells predominate, the connective tissue is called **adipose tissue**.

Macrophages or **histiocytes** are phagocytic cells that ingest foreign material or dead cells and are most numerous in loose connective tissue, after fibroblasts. They are difficult to distinguish from fibroblasts, unless they are performing phagocytic activity and contain ingested material in their cytoplasm. The macrophages, however, are called by different names in different tissues/organs.

Mast cells are normal elements of the connective tissue, usually closely associated with blood vessels. They are widely distributed in the connective tissue of the skin, the digestive, and respiratory organs. Mast cells are ovoid cells filled with fine, regular, dark-staining, basophilic granules. However, mast cells can exhibit variable sizes and granular content.

Plasma cells arise from the lymphocytes that migrate into the connective tissue and have a wide distribution in the body. They are especially abundant in the loose connective tissue and lymphatic tissue of the respiratory and digestive tracts, respectively.

Leukocytes (white blood cells), neutrophils, and eosinophils migrate from the blood vessels and capillaries to reside in the connective tissue. Their main function is to defend the organism against bacterial invasion or foreign matter.

Fibroblasts and adipose cells are permanent or resident connective tissue cells. Neutrophils, eosinophils, plasma cells, mast cells, and macrophages migrate from the blood vessels and take up residence in the connective tissue of different regions of the body.

FUNCTIONAL CORRELATIONS 5.1 ■ Cells in Connective Tissue

Fibroblasts are the dominant cells in the connective tissue. These highly active cells with irregularly branched cytoplasm synthesize collagen, reticular, and elastic fibers as well as carbohydrates, such as glycosaminoglycans, proteoglycans, and adhesive glycoproteins of the extracellular matrix. The spindle-shaped **fibrocytes** are smaller than the fibroblasts and are the mature and less active cells of the fibroblast line.

Macrophages or histiocytes are **phagocytes** that are attracted to the sites of **inflammation**. They ingest bacteria, dead cells, cell debris, and other foreign matter that enters the connective tissue. Macrophages are part of the **mononuclear phagocyte system**, derived from circulating blood monocytes that are formed in the bone marrow, take up residence in the connective tissue, and differentiate into macrophages. These cells also enhance **immunologic** activities of the **lymphocytes**. Macrophages are **antigen-processing** cells to lymphocytes that are then stimulated to perform specific immune responses. Although present throughout connective tissue of the body, the macrophages have specific names in different organs. **Dusts cells** are found in the alveoli of the lungs, **Kupffer cells** line the sinusoids in the liver, **Langerhans cells** are in the epidermis of the skin, **microglia** in the tissues of the brain, **monocytes** in the circulating blood, and the **osteoclasts** in the bone.

Lymphocytes are the most numerous cells in the loose connective tissue of the respiratory and gastrointestinal tracts. They do not have any function in the bloodstream, but leave the circulatory system and enter the connective tissue through the capillaries. They mediate immune responses to antigens that enter these organs and, once activated, produce antibodies that kill cells by inducing cell death (apoptosis). There are three functional types of lymphocytes: T lymphocytes, B lymphocytes, and NK (natural killer) cells. These lymphocytes are primarily identified by the specific marker proteins on the cell membrane.

Plasma cells are derived from B lymphocytes that enter the connective tissue from blood vessels and then differentiate into plasma cells when they are exposed to **antigens**. Thus, plasma cells become mature cells highly specialized for **antibody (immunoglobulin) synthesis** that is released into the blood stream to destroy specific antigens and defend the organism against infections.

Adipose cells store fat (lipid) and are mostly found in loose connective tissue. There are **white adipose cells** and **brown adipose cells**. Their main function is to provide protective packing material and insulation in and around numerous vital organs. Additional information concerning both types of adipose cells and a histological image of adipose tissue are provided in Functional Correlations Box 5.4 and in Figure 5.13.

Neutrophils are active and powerful phagocytes; they leave the bloodstream and enter connective tissue to engulf and destroy bacteria at sites of infections.

Eosinophils become activated and increase in number after parasitic infections or allergic reactions. They **phagocytize antigen–antibody complexes** formed during allergic reactions.

Mast cells reside in the connective tissue. Their location near small blood vessels and capillaries allows them to perform numerous defensive functions. The cytoplasm of mast cells contains numerous dense-staining granules, which upon release function in local inflammatory and immune responses. Exposure of mast cells to allergens causes rapid release of **histamine** and other **vasoactive** mediators. Histamine causes dilation of blood vessels and increases the permeability of capillaries and venules, thereby causing local **edema**. Release of histamine also induces symptoms of allergic reactions known as **immediate hypersensitive reactions**. Mast cells also contain the chemical **heparin**, which acts locally as a weak anticoagulant.

FIBROUS COMPONENTS OF THE CONNECTIVE TISSUE

There are three distinctive types of connective tissue fibers: **collagen**, **elastic**, and **reticular**. The amount and arrangement of these fibers depend on the function of the tissues or organs in which they are found. **Fibroblasts** synthesize all the collagen, elastic, and reticular fibers. The primary function of the fibrous components within the connective tissue is to provide strength and resistance to stretching and deformation. Thus, the mechanical and physical properties of the fibrous components of the connective tissue primarily depend on the mixture of the fibers in the extracellular matrix and the predominance of fiber type.

Types of Collagen Fibers

Collagen fibers are tough, thick, fibrous proteins that do not branch. They are the most abundant fibers and are found in almost all the connective tissues of all organs. There are at least 28 different types of genetically distinct collagens found in vertebrates. The collagen types are based on their molecular or amino acid composition, morphology, distribution, and function. Listed below are the most frequently recognized fibers in histologic slides that are illustrated in the atlas:

- **Type I collagen fibers:** These are the most common connective tissue fibers and are found in the dermis of the skin, tendons, ligaments, fasciae, fibrocartilage, the capsules of organs, and bones. They are very strong and offer great resistance to tensile stresses.
- **Type II collagen fibers:** These are present in hyaline cartilage, in elastic cartilage, and in the vitreous body of the eye. The fibers provide support to resist pressure.
- **Type III collagen fibers:** These are the thin, branching reticular fibers that form the delicate supporting meshwork in such organs as the lymph nodes, spleen, and bone marrow, where they form the main extracellular matrix to support the cells of these organs.
- **Type IV collagen fibers:** These are present in and form the supportive meshwork in the basal lamina of the basement membrane, to which the basal regions of the cells attach.

Reticular Fibers

Reticular fibers consisting mainly of type III collagen are thin and form a delicate netlike support framework in the liver, lymph nodes, spleen, hemopoietic organs, and other locations where blood and lymph are filtered. Reticular fibers also support capillaries, nerves, and muscle cells. These fibers become visible only when the tissue or organ is stained with silver stain.

Elastic Fibers

Elastic fibers are thin, small, branching fibers that are capable of stretching and returning to their original length. They have less tensile strength than collagen fibers and are composed of microfibrils and the protein **elastin**. When stretched, elastic fibers return to their original size (recoil) without deformation. Elastic fibers are found in abundance in the lungs, bladder wall, and skin. In the walls of the aorta and pulmonary trunk, the presence of elastic fibers allows for stretching and recoiling of these vessels during powerful blood ejections from the heart ventricles. In the walls of the large vessels, the smooth muscle cells synthesize the elastic fibers; in other organs, fibroblasts synthesize elastic fibers.

the**Point**   Supplemental micrographic images are available at **www.thePoint.com/Eroschenko13e** under Connective Tissue.

FIGURE 5.2 | Loose Connective Tissue (Spread)

This composite image of mesentery was stained to show different fibers and cells. Mesentery is a thin sheet of loose connective tissue that supports the intestines of the digestive tract.

The pink **collagen fibers** (**3**) are the thickest, largest, and most numerous fibers, and, in this preparation, the collagen fibers (3) course in all directions.

The **elastic fibers** (**5, 10**) are thin, fine, single fibers that are usually straight; however, after tissue preparation, the fibers may become wavy as a result of the release of tension. Elastic fibers (5, 10) form branching and anastomosing networks. Fine reticular fibers are also present in loose connective tissue, but these are not included in this illustration.

The permanent cells of connective tissues are the **fibroblasts** (**2**) that appear flattened with an oval nucleus, sparse chromatin, and one or two nucleoli. Fixed **macrophages**, or **histiocytes** (**12**), are always present in the connective tissue. When inactive, they appear similar to fibroblasts, although their processes may be more irregular and their nuclei smaller. Phagocytic inclusions, however, alter the cytoplasm of the macrophages. In this illustration, the cytoplasm of different macrophages (12) is filled with ingested, dense-staining particles.

Mast cells (**1, 9**) are also present in the loose connective tissue and are seen as single or grouped cells along small blood vessels (**capillary, 7**). The mast cells (1, 9) are usually ovoid, with a small, centrally placed nucleus and cytoplasm filled with fine, closely packed granules that stain dense or deep red with neutral red stain.

Different blood cells are also seen in the loose connective tissue. **Small lymphocytes** (**6**) exhibit a dense-staining nucleus that occupies most of the cell cytoplasm. **Large lymphocytes** (**8**) also exhibit a dense nucleus with more cytoplasm. Loose connective tissue also contains blood cells eosinophils and neutrophils and adipose cells. These are illustrated in greater detail in Figure 5.3, in the loose connective tissue in Figure 5.5, and in the mesentery of an intestine in Figure 5.13.

The faint background around the fibers and cells is the ground substance.

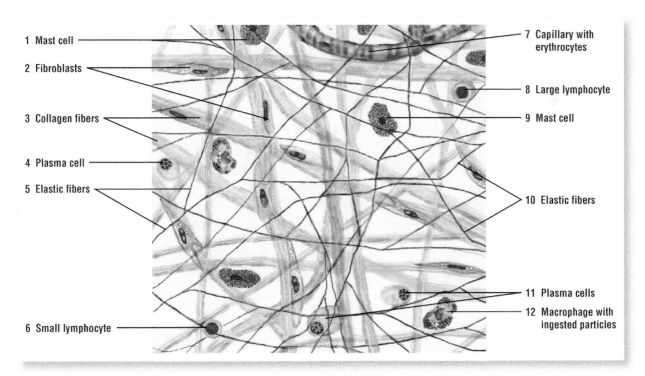

FIGURE 5.2 ■ Loose connective tissue (spread). Stained for cells and fibers. High magnification.

FIGURE 5.3 | Individual Cells of Connective Tissue

The main cells of the connective tissue are the fibroblasts and fibrocytes. The **fibroblast** (1) is an elongated cell with cytoplasmic projections, an ovoid nucleus with sparse chromatin, and one or two nucleoli. The **fibrocyte** (6) is a more mature, smaller spindle-shaped cell without cytoplasmic projections; the nucleus is similar but smaller than that in the fibroblast.

The **plasma cell** (2) exhibits a smaller, eccentrically placed nucleus with condensed, coarse chromatin clumps distributed peripherally in a characteristic radial (cartwheel) pattern and one central mass. A prominent, clear area in the cytoplasm is adjacent to the nucleus.

The large white **adipose cell** (3) exhibits a narrow rim of cytoplasm and a flattened, eccentric nucleus. In histologic sections, the large fat globules of adipose cells have been dissolved by different chemicals, leaving a large, highly characteristic empty space.

The **large lymphocyte** (4) and **small lymphocyte** (10) are spherical cells that differ primarily in the amount of cytoplasm that is present in the large lymphocyte (4). The dense-staining nuclei of all lymphocytes have condensed chromatin but no nucleoli.

The free **macrophage** (5) usually appears round with irregular cell outlines and a variable appearance. In the illustration, the macrophage exhibits a small nucleus rich in chromatin and cytoplasm filled with dense, ingested particles.

An **eosinophil** (7) is a large blood cell with a bilobed nucleus and large, eosinophilic cytoplasmic granules that fill the cytoplasm.

A **neutrophil** (8) is also a large blood cell, characterized by a multilobed nucleus and a lack of distinct stained granules in the cytoplasm when viewed with a light microscope.

Cells with **pigment granules** (9) may be seen in the connective tissue. Also, the basal epithelial cells of the skin contain brown-staining pigment or melanin granules.

A **mast cell** (11) is usually ovoid, with a small, centrally placed nucleus. The cytoplasm is normally filled with fine, closely packed, dense-staining granules.

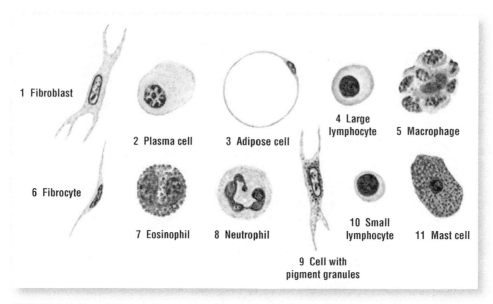

FIGURE 5.3 ■ Cells of the connective tissue. Stain: hematoxylin and eosin. High magnification or oil immersion.

FIGURE 5.4 | Connective Tissue, Capillary, and Mast Cell in Mesentery of Small Intestine

This micrograph illustrates the connective tissue from the mesentery of a small intestine. Closely associated with the **capillary** (3) and sectioned in a longitudinal plane is a **mast cell** with **dense granules** (5) in its cytoplasm and a red-staining nucleus. The capillary (3) is packed with **red blood cells** (6). Because the lumen of the capillary is about the size of a red blood cell (RBC), the RBCs in its lumen are lined up in a row. Located above the capillary (3) is a larger vessel, a **venule** (2), sectioned in a transverse plane and also packed with RBCs. Surrounding the blood vessels (2, 3) are numerous **adipose cells** (1) with their lipid contents washed out during slide preparation. Also present are the dense layers of blue-staining **collagen fibers** (4) and **fibrocytes** (7) that are closely associated with the blood vessels and the capillaries.

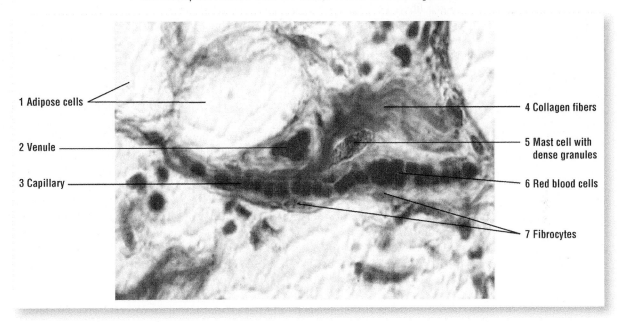

FIGURE 5.4 ■ A connective tissue, a capillary, and a mast cell in the mesentery of a small intestine. Stain: Mallory-Azan. ×205.

FIGURE 5.5 | Embryonic Connective Tissue

The embryonic connective tissue resembles the mesenchyme or mucous connective tissue; this is loose and irregular connective tissue. The difference in ground substance (semifluid vs. jelly-like) is not apparent in these sections.

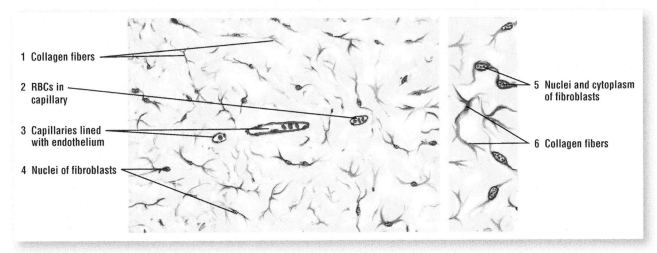

FIGURE 5.5 ■ Embryonic connective tissue. Stain: hematoxylin and eosin. *Left*, low magnification; *right*, high magnification.

The **fibroblasts** (4) are numerous, and fine **collagen fibers** (1) are found between them, some coming in close contact with fibroblasts. The embryonic connective tissue is vascular. **Capillaries** (3) lined with endothelium and filled with **RBCs** (2) are visible in the ground substance.

At higher magnification, primitive **fibroblasts** (5) are seen as large, branching cells with cytoplasm, prominent cytoplasmic processes, an ovoid nucleus with fine chromatin, and one or more nucleoli. The widely separated **collagen fibers** (6) are more apparent at this magnification.

FIGURE 5.6 | Loose Connective Tissue

Collagen fibers (9) predominate in loose connective tissue, course in different directions, and form a loose fiber meshwork. Surrounding the connective tissue fibers and cells are clear spaces of the ground substance. In the illustration, collagen fibers (9) are sectioned in various planes, and transverse ends may be seen. The fibers are acidophilic and stain pink with eosin. Thin elastic fibers are also present in loose connective tissue but are difficult to distinguish with this stain and at this magnification.

The **fibroblasts** (2) are the most numerous cells in the loose connective tissue and may be sectioned in various planes, so that only parts of the cells may be seen. Also, during section preparation, the cytoplasm of these cells may shrink. A typical fibroblast (2) shows an oval nucleus with sparse chromatin and lightly acidophilic cytoplasm, with a few short processes.

Also present in loose connective tissue are blood cells such as the **neutrophils** (6) with lobulated nuclei, **eosinophils** (3) with red-staining granules, and small lymphocytes (7) with dense-staining nuclei and sparse cytoplasm. The **fat** (**adipose**) **cells** (5) appear characteristically empty with a thin rim of cytoplasm and peripherally displaced flat **nuclei** (4).

The loose connective tissue is also highly vascular; **capillaries** (8) sectioned in different planes (t.s., transverse section; l.s., longitudinal section) are visible. A larger **arteriole** (1) with RBCs is also seen.

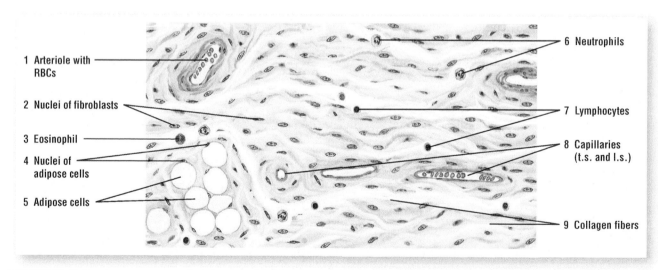

1 Arteriole with RBCs

2 Nuclei of fibroblasts

3 Eosinophil

4 Nuclei of adipose cells

5 Adipose cells

6 Neutrophils

7 Lymphocytes

8 Capillaries (t.s. and l.s.)

9 Collagen fibers

FIGURE 5.6 ■ Loose connective tissue with blood vessels and adipose cells. Stain: hematoxylin and eosin. High magnification.

FIGURE 5.7 | Dense Irregular and Loose Irregular Connective Tissue (Elastin Stain)

This figure illustrates a transition zone between loose irregular connective tissue in the upper region and denser irregular connective tissue in the lower region of the illustration. In addition, the tissue section has been specially prepared to show the presence and distribution of elastic fibers mixed with the collagen fibers in the connective tissue.

The **elastic fibers** (**1, 7**) have been selectively stained a deep blue using the Verhoeff method. Using Van Gieson stain as a counterstain, acid fuchsin stains **collagen fibers** (**2, 6**) red. Cellular details of fibroblasts are not obvious, but the **fibroblast nuclei** (**3, 5**) stain deep blue. **Blood vessels** (**4**) are also present.

The characteristic features of dense irregular and loose connective tissues become apparent with this staining technique. In dense irregular connective tissue, the collagen fibers (6) are larger, more numerous, and more concentrated. Elastic fibers are also larger and more numerous (7). In contrast, in the loose connective tissue, both fiber types are smaller (1, 2) and more loosely arranged. Fine elastic networks are seen in both types of connective tissue.

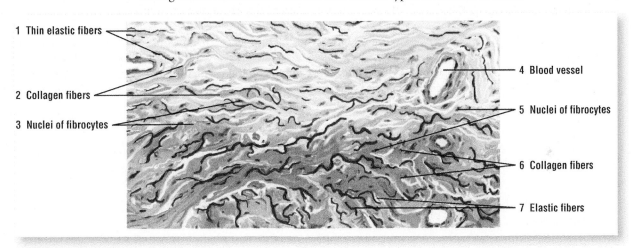

1 Thin elastic fibers
2 Collagen fibers
3 Nuclei of fibrocytes
4 Blood vessel
5 Nuclei of fibrocytes
6 Collagen fibers
7 Elastic fibers

FIGURE 5.7 ■ Dense irregular and loose irregular connective tissue. Stains: Verhoeff and Van Gieson. Medium magnification.

FIGURE 5.8 | Loose Irregular and Dense Irregular Connective Tissue

This figure illustrates a gradual transition from **loose irregular connective tissue** (**5**) to **dense irregular connective tissue** (**1**). Where firmer support and more strength are required, dense irregular connective tissue with increased presence of collagen fibers replaces the loose type.

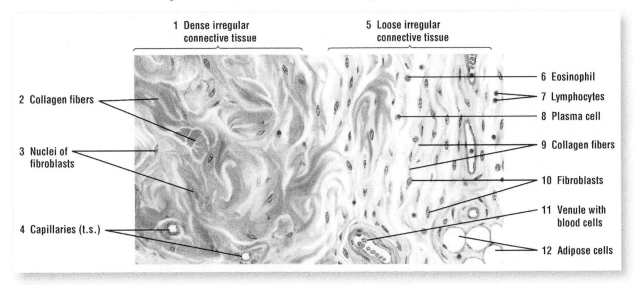

1 Dense irregular connective tissue
5 Loose irregular connective tissue
2 Collagen fibers
3 Nuclei of fibroblasts
4 Capillaries (t.s.)
6 Eosinophil
7 Lymphocytes
8 Plasma cell
9 Collagen fibers
10 Fibroblasts
11 Venule with blood cells
12 Adipose cells

FIGURE 5.8 ■ Dense irregular and loose irregular connective tissue. Stain: hematoxylin and eosin. High magnification.

The **collagen fibers (2, 9)** in both types of tissues are large, typically in bundles, and sectioned in several planes because they course in various directions. Also visible are thin, wavy elastic fibers that form fine networks. However, these fibers are not obvious in routine histologic preparations.

In the dense connective tissue (1), the **fibroblasts (nuclei) (3)** are often found compressed among the collagen fibers (2). In the loose connective tissue (5), the collagen fibers (9) are less compressed and the **fibroblasts (10)** are more visible. Also illustrated are **capillaries (4)**, a small **venule (11)**, an **eosinophil (6)** with lobulated nucleus, **lymphocytes (7)** with large round nuclei without visible cytoplasm, a **plasma cell (8)**, and numerous **adipose cells (12)**.

FIGURE 5.9 | Dense Irregular Connective Tissue and Adipose Tissue

This photomicrograph illustrates a deeper section of the skin called the dermis. This region contains **dense irregular connective tissue (1)** and the collagen-producing **fibroblasts (3)**. Here, the **collagen fibers (2)** show a very random and irregular orientation. Adjacent to the dense irregular connective tissue (1) is **adipose tissue (4)** with its numerous **adipose cells (5)**. Tissue preparation dissolves the lipids in individual adipose cells, and cell cytoplasm appears empty with only flattened, dense-staining nuclei in the peripheries. Dermis of the skin also contains numerous sweat glands. The light-staining regions are the **secretory cells** of the **sweat gland (7)**, whereas the dark-staining cells form the **stratified cuboidal epithelium** of the **excretory ducts (6, 8)**, which continue through the connective tissue and the stratified squamous epithelium of the skin to the surface of the skin (see Fig. 4.11).

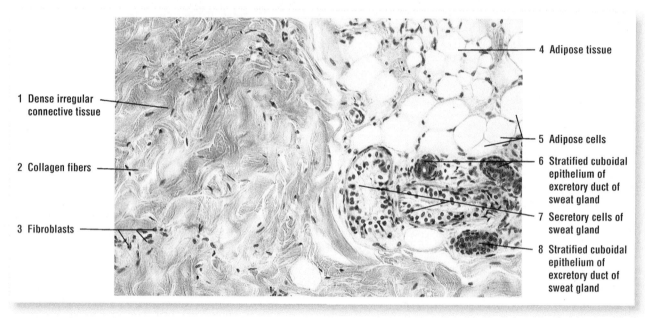

1 Dense irregular connective tissue

2 Collagen fibers

3 Fibroblasts

4 Adipose tissue

5 Adipose cells

6 Stratified cuboidal epithelium of excretory duct of sweat gland

7 Secretory cells of sweat gland

8 Stratified cuboidal epithelium of excretory duct of sweat gland

FIGURE 5.9 ■ Dense irregular connective tissue and adipose tissue. Stain: hematoxylin and eosin. ×64.

FUNCTIONAL CORRELATIONS 5.2 ■ Ground Substance and Connective Tissue

The **ground substance** in connective tissue consists primarily of amorphous, transparent, and colorless **extracellular matrix**, which has the properties of a semifluid gel and high water content. The matrix supports, surrounds, and binds all the connective tissue cells and their fibers. The ground substance of the connective tissue contains different types of mixed, unbranched polysaccharide chains of **glycosaminoglycans**, **proteoglycans**, and **adhesive glycoproteins**. **Hyaluronic acid** constitutes the principal glycosaminoglycan of connective tissue. Except for hyaluronic acid, the various glycosaminoglycans are bound to a core protein to form much larger molecules called **proteoglycan aggregates**. These proteoglycans attract increased amounts of water, which produces the hydrated gel of the ground substance.

FUNCTIONAL CORRELATIONS 5.2 ■ Ground Substance and Connective Tissue (*Continued*)

The semifluid consistency of the ground substance in the connective tissue facilitates **diffusion** of oxygen, electrolytes, nutrients, fluids, metabolites, and other water-soluble molecules between the cells and the blood vessels. Similarly, waste products from the cells diffuse through the ground substance back into the blood vessels. Also, because of its viscosity, the ground substance serves as an efficient **barrier**. It prevents movement of large molecules and the spread of pathogens from the connective tissue into the bloodstream. However, certain bacteria can produce hyaluronidase, an enzyme that hydrolyzes hyaluronic acid and reduces the viscosity of the gellike ground substance, allowing pathogens to invade the surrounding tissues.

The density of ground substance depends on the amount of extracellular tissue fluid or water that it contains. Mineralization of ground substance, as a result of increased calcium deposition, changes its density, rigidity, and permeability to diffusion, as seen in developing cartilage models and bones.

In addition to proteoglycans, connective tissue also contains several large cell **adhesive glycoproteins**, which have binding sites for cell receptors and matrix molecules. The adhesive glycoproteins bind cells to the fibers. The glycoprotein **fibronectin** binds connective tissue cells, collagen fibers, and proteoglycans, thereby interconnecting all three components of the connective tissue. Integral proteins of the plasma membrane, the **integrins**, bind to extracellular collagen fibers and to actin filaments in the cytoskeleton, thus establishing a structural continuity between the cytoskeleton and the extracellular matrix. **Laminin** is a large glycoprotein and a major component of the cell basement membrane. This protein binds epithelial cells to the basal lamina and has binding sites for integrin, type IV collagen, and other proteoglycans.

FIGURE 5.10 | Dense Regular Connective Tissue: Tendon (Longitudinal Section)

Dense regular connective tissue is present in ligaments and tendons. Shown here is a section of a tendon in the longitudinal plane showing the regular arrangement of the collagen fibers.

The **collagen fibers** (**2**, **5**, **8**) are arranged in compact, dense parallel bundles between which are thin partitions of looser connective tissue that contain parallel rows of **fibroblasts** (**1**, **3**). The fibroblasts (**1**, **3**) have short processes (not visible here) and nuclei that appear ovoid when seen in **surface view** (**3**) or flat and **rodlike in lateral view** (**1**).

Dense irregular connective tissue with less regular fiber arrangement than in the tendon surrounds and partitions the collagen bundles as the **interfascicular connective tissue** (**4**). Here are also found **fibroblasts** (**6**) and numerous blood vessels, such as this **arteriole** (**7**), that supply the connective tissue cells.

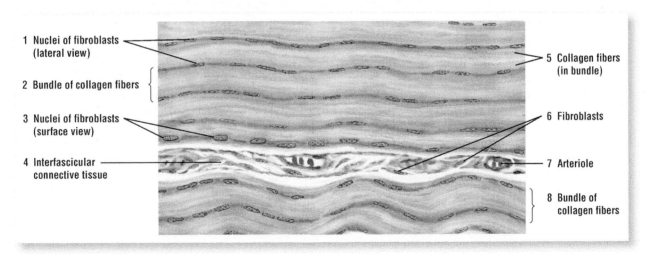

1 Nuclei of fibroblasts (lateral view)
2 Bundle of collagen fibers
3 Nuclei of fibroblasts (surface view)
4 Interfascicular connective tissue
5 Collagen fibers (in bundle)
6 Fibroblasts
7 Arteriole
8 Bundle of collagen fibers

FIGURE 5.10 ■ Dense regular connective tissue: tendon (longitudinal section). Stain: hematoxylin and eosin. Medium magnification.

FIGURE 5.11 | Dense Regular Connective Tissue: Tendon (Longitudinal Section)

A photomicrograph of dense regular connective tissue of a tendon shows the compact, regular, and parallel arrangement of **collagen fibers** (1). Between the densely packed collagen fibers are seen flattened nuclei of the **fibroblasts** (2). A small **blood vessel** (3) with blood cells courses between the dense bundles of collagen fibers to supply the connective tissue cells of the tendon.

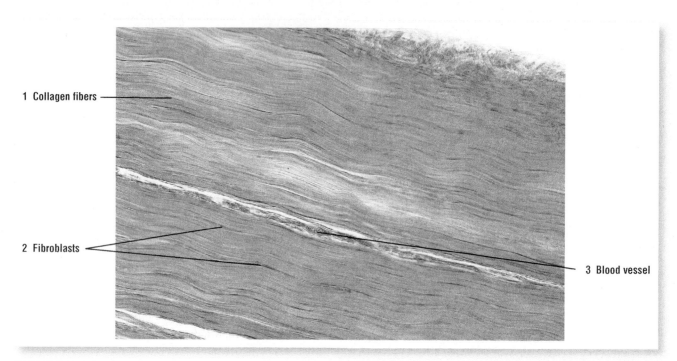

1 Collagen fibers

2 Fibroblasts

3 Blood vessel

FIGURE 5.11 ■ Dense regular connective tissue: tendon (longitudinal section). Stain: hematoxylin and eosin. ×64.

FUNCTIONAL CORRELATIONS 5.3 ■ Dense Connective Tissue

DENSE IRREGULAR CONNECTIVE TISSUE

Dense irregular connective tissue consists primarily of **collagen fibers** (**type I collagen**) with minimal amounts of surrounding ground substance. Except for the **fibroblasts** and/or **fibrocytes**, other cell types in dense connective tissue are sparse. Collagen fibers exhibit great **tensile strength**, and their main function is **support**. In dense irregular connective tissue, collagen fibers exhibit **random orientation** and are most highly concentrated in those areas of the body where strong support is needed to resist pulling forces or stress from different directions.

DENSE REGULAR CONNECTIVE TISSUE

Dense regular connective tissue exhibits a predominance of **collagen fibers** (**type I collagen**) and is present where great **tensile strength** is required, such as in **ligaments** and **tendons**. The parallel and dense arrangements of collagen fibers offer strong resistance to forces pulling along a **single axis** or direction.

Tendons and ligaments are attached to bones and are constantly subjected to strong pulling forces. Because of the dense arrangement of collagen fibers, little ground substance is present, and the predominant cell types that synthesize the collagen fibers are the **fibroblasts** that are located between rows of parallel collagen fibers.

FIGURE 5.12 | Dense Regular Connective Tissue: Tendon (Transverse Section)

A transverse section of a tendon is illustrated at a lower magnification (*left side*) and a higher magnification (*right side*). Within each large bundle of **collagen fibers** (**3, 7**) are **fibroblasts** (**nuclei**) (**1, 8**) sectioned transversely. The fibroblasts are located between the bundles of collagen fibers (**3, 7**). These fibroblasts (**8**) are better distinguished at the higher magnification on the right side, which shows bundles of collagen fibers (**7**) and the branched shape of fibroblasts (**8**) in transverse section.

Between the large collagen bundles are the **interfascicular connective tissue** (**2**) partitions. These partitions contain blood vessels, an **arteriole** and **venules** (**6**), nerves, and, occasionally, the sensitive pressure receptors **Pacinian corpuscles** (**9**).

Also illustrated on the left side of the figure is a transverse section of several **skeletal muscle fibers** (**4**). These are adjacent to the tendon but are separated from it by a connective tissue partition. Note that the **nuclei** (**5**) of skeletal muscle fibers (**4**) are located on the periphery of the fibers, whereas the fibroblasts (**1, 8**) are located between bundles of collagen fibers (**3, 7**).

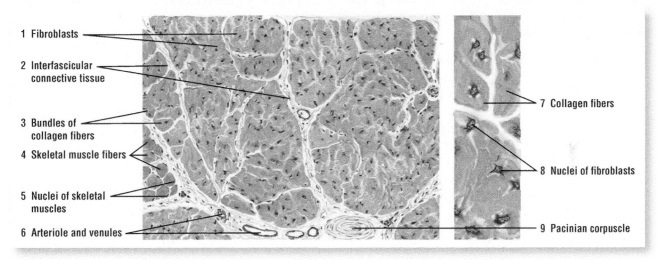

1 Fibroblasts
2 Interfascicular connective tissue
3 Bundles of collagen fibers
4 Skeletal muscle fibers
5 Nuclei of skeletal muscles
6 Arteriole and venules
7 Collagen fibers
8 Nuclei of fibroblasts
9 Pacinian corpuscle

FIGURE 5.12 ■ Dense regular connective tissue: tendon (transverse section). Stain: hematoxylin and eosin. *Left*, low magnification; *right*, high magnification.

FIGURE 5.13 | Adipose Tissue: Intestine

A section of intestinal mesentery is illustrated, in which accumulations of **adipose** (**fat**) **cells** (**4, 8**) are organized into adipose tissue. The **connective tissue** (**9**) that surrounds the adipose tissue is covered by a simple squamous epithelium called **mesothelium** (**10**).

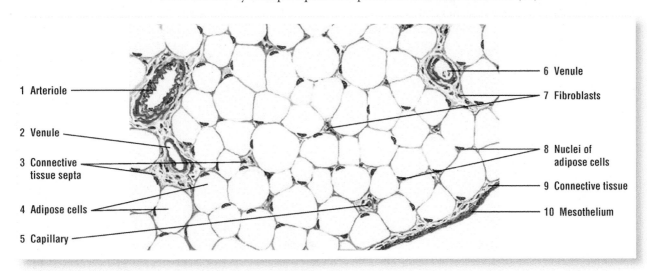

1 Arteriole
2 Venule
3 Connective tissue septa
4 Adipose cells
5 Capillary
6 Venule
7 Fibroblasts
8 Nuclei of adipose cells
9 Connective tissue
10 Mesothelium

FIGURE 5.13 ■ Adipose tissue in the intestine. Stain: hematoxylin and eosin. Medium magnification.

Adipose cells (4, 8) are closely packed and separated by thin strips of **connective tissue septa** (3), in which are compressed **fibroblasts** (7), **arterioles** (1), **venules** (2, 6), **nerves**, and **capillaries** (5).

Individual adipose cells (4) appear as empty cells because the fat was dissolved by chemicals during preparation of the tissue. The **adipose cell nuclei** (8) are compressed to the peripheral rim of the cytoplasm, and, in certain sections, it is difficult to distinguish between fibroblast nuclei (7) and adipose cell nuclei (8).

FUNCTIONAL CORRELATIONS 5.4 ■ Adipose Tissue

The two distinct types of adipose tissues in the body are **white adipose tissue** and **brown adipose tissue**. These adipose tissues represent the main sites of **lipid storage** and **metabolism** in the body.

WHITE ADIPOSE TISSUE (UNILOCULAR)

White adipose tissue is the more common type. Cells of white adipose tissue, the **adipocytes**, are large and store lipids as a single, large droplet (unilocular). The stored lipids are primarily **triglycerides** (fatty acids and glycerol) derived from the intestinal lipoproteins and the very-low-density lipoproteins from the liver. This adipose tissue also exhibits a wider distribution than brown adipose tissue. White adipose tissue is distributed throughout the body, with the distribution pattern showing variations that are dependent on the gender and age of the individual. In addition to serving as an energy source, white adipose tissue provides **insulation** under the skin and forms cushioning **fat pads** around different organs. This tissue is also highly vascularized because of its high metabolic activity. The white adipose cells also have receptors for insulin, glucocorticoids, growth hormone, and other factors that influence adipose tissue to accumulate and release lipids. Furthermore, white adipose tissue is also considered as an important endocrine organ. These cells are the sole source of a hormone called **leptin**, which increases carbohydrate and lipid metabolism in cells. This hormone also influences cells in the **hypothalamus** and regulates appetite, energy balance, food intake, and the formation of new adipose tissue.

BROWN ADIPOSE TISSUE (MULTILOCULAR)

In contrast to the white adipose tissue, which is present throughout the body, brown adipose tissue has a more limited distribution. These cells are smaller than white adipose tissue cells and store lipids as multiple small droplets (multilocular). Brown adipose tissue is found in all mammals, but is best developed in **hibernating animals**. The main function of brown adipose tissue is to supply the body with heat through **nonshivering thermogenesis**. In newborn humans exposed to cold and in fur-bearing animals emerging from hibernation, brown adipose tissue generates and increases body heat during these critical periods as a protective measure. The sympathetic nervous system regulates the production of heat by brown adipose, which releases **norepinephrine** to hydrolyze lipids into fatty acids and glycerol. The amount of brown adipose tissue gradually decreases in older individuals and is mainly found around the adrenal glands, great vessels, and in the neck region. However, as an adaptation, the cold environment activates the development of brown adipose cells and tissue.

Chapter 5 Summary

Connective Tissue

- Develops from mesenchyme and consists of cells and extracellular matrix
- Matrix consists of tissue fluid, the ground substance
- Embryonic connective tissue is present in the umbilical cord and developing teeth
- Ground substance is a medium for exchange of nutrients, oxygen, and waste
- Because of its consistency, ground substance serves as a barrier to pathogenic molecules
- Contains numerous cells that protect and defend body against bacteria and foreign bodies
- Classified as loose or dense connective tissue

CLASSIFICATION

Loose Connective Tissue

- More prevalent in body and exhibits a loose, irregular arrangement of cells and fibers
- Contains abundant ground substance that surrounds cells and fibers
- Collagen fibers, fibroblasts, fibrocytes, adipose cells, mast cells, plasma cells, and macrophages predominate

Dense Irregular Connective Tissue

- Consists primarily of fibroblasts and thick, densely packed collagen fibers (type I)
- Fewer other cell types and minimal ground substance
- Collagen fibers exhibit random orientation and provide strong tissue support
- Concentrated in areas where resistance to forces from different directions is needed

Dense Regular Connective Tissue

- Fibers densely packed with regular, parallel orientation
- Present in tendons and ligaments that are attached to bones
- Great resistance to forces pulling along single axis or direction
- Minimal ground substance; predominant cell type is fibroblast

CELLS OF CONNECTIVE TISSUE

Fibroblasts

- Are active permanent cells that synthesize collagen, reticular, and elastic connective tissue fibers
- Synthesize glycosaminoglycans, proteoglycans, and adhesive glycoproteins of ground substance

Fibrocytes

- Smaller than fibroblasts
- Inactive or resting connective tissue cells

White Adipose (Fat) Cells

- Most common type of adipose tissue with wide distribution
- Occur singly or in groups and exhibit single or unilocular lipid droplet
- When adipose cells predominate, the connective tissue is adipose tissue
- Store fat (lipid) as a single large droplet, primarily as triglycerides
- Lipids derived from intestinal lipoproteins and low lipid lipoproteins from liver
- Appear as empty cells because lipid is dissolved during tissue preparation
- Distributed throughout the body, serves as insulation, and forms fat pads for organ protection
- Highly vascularized owing to high metabolic activity
- Exhibit receptors for hormones that influence accumulation and release of lipid
- Sole source of hormone leptin that increases lipid metabolism and regulates appetite and food intake

Brown Adipose Cells

- Exhibits more limited distribution
- Cells smaller than white adipose cells; store fat as multiple lipid droplets (multilocular)
- Best developed in hibernating animals and newborn individuals
- In newborns or animals emerging from hibernation, generates body heat

- Norepinephrine from sympathetic nervous system promotes hydrolysis of lipids
- As an adaptation to cold environment, cell numbers and tissue increase

Macrophages

- Most numerous in loose connective tissue
- Ingest bacteria, dead cells, cell debris, and foreign matter
- Are antigen-presenting cells to lymphocytes for immunologic response
- Derived from circulating blood monocytes
- Called Kupffer cells in liver, osteoclasts in bone, microglia in central nervous system, Langerhans cells in skin, monocytes in blood, and osteoclasts in bone

Lymphocytes

- Most numerous in loose connective tissue of respiratory and gastrointestinal tracts
- Produce antibodies to kill infecting cells

Plasma Cells

- Characterized by chromatin distributed in radial pattern
- Derived from B lymphocytes exposed to antigens
- Produce antibodies to destroy specific antigens

Mast Cells

- Closely associated with blood vessels
- Found in skin, respiratory, and digestive system connective tissue
- Ovoid cells with fine, regular basophilic granules
- Release histamine and vasoactive chemicals when exposed to allergens, causing immediate hypersensitivity allergic response
- Contain also weak anticoagulant heparin

Neutrophils

- Active phagocytes; engulf and destroy bacteria

Eosinophils

- Increase after parasitic infestation
- Phagocytize antigen–antibody complexes during allergic reactions

COLLAGEN FIBERS

- Type I most common and very strong; found in skin, tendons, ligaments, and bone
- Type II found in hyaline and elastic cartilage and the vitreous body of the eye; provide resistance to pressure
- Type III forms meshwork in liver, lymph node, spleen, and hematopoietic organs
- Type IV found in basal lamina of basement membrane; associated with hemidesmosomes

RETICULAR FIBERS

- Consist mainly of type III collagen; form delicate netlike framework in different organs
- Visible only when stained with silver stain

ELASTIC FIBERS

- Thin, branching fibers that allow stretch
- Composed of microfibrils and the protein elastin
- After stretching, return (recoil) to original size without deformation
- Found in the lungs, bladder, skin, and walls of large blood vessels
- In large blood vessel walls, smooth muscle synthesizes elastic fibers

GROUND SUBSTANCE AND CONNECTIVE TISSUE

- Consists of extracellular matrix, a semifluid gel with high water content
- Matrix binds, supports, and surrounds cells and fibers
- Contains polysaccharide chains of glycosaminoglycans, proteoglycans, and adhesive glycoproteins
- Hyaluronic acid is the main glycosaminoglycan
- Other glycosaminoglycans form proteoglycan aggregates, which attract water
- Facilitates diffusion of different substances between cells and blood vessels
- Acts as an efficient barrier to the spread of pathogens
- Bacteria can hydrolyze hyaluronic acid and reduce barrier viscosity
- Contains several adhesive glycoproteins, such as fibronectin, that bind cells to fibers
- Integrin protein binds collagen fibers to actin
- Laminin is a component of basement membrane and binds epithelial cells to basal lamina

Chapter 5 Review Questions

QUESTIONS

In the following multiple choice questions, choose the letter corresponding to the one best answer.

1. Brown fat has what following characterization?

    A. It is widely distributed in the body.
    B. It forms fat pads around organs and insulation under the skin.
    C. It stores lipid as a large, single droplet.
    D. It is a source of heat for hibernating animals and newborns.
    E. It influences appetite and food intake.

2. What increases carbohydrate and lipid metabolism and regulates food intake and appetite?

    A. Leptin hormone
    B. Norepinephrine
    C. Triglycerides
    D. Fatty acids
    E. Glycerol

3. What function does mesenchyme perform?

    A. It produces hormones that inhibit collagen synthesis.
    B. It is the source of type I collagen fibers.
    C. It is the source of all connective tissue.
    D. It secretes glycosaminoglycans, proteoglycans, and adhesive glycoproteins.
    E. It influences lipid metabolism in adipose tissues.

4. What serves as a barrier to the passage of large molecules and pathogens in the connective tissue?

    A. Collagen fibers
    B. Semifluid ground substance
    C. Fibroblasts
    D. Reticular fibers
    E. Dense connective tissue layers

5. What fibers form supporting meshworks in organs such as lymph nodes and the spleen?

    A. Elastic fibers
    B. Collagen fibers
    C. Reticular fibers
    D. Type I collagen fibers
    E. All connective tissue fibers

ANSWERS

1. **Correct Answer: D.** It is a source of heat for hibernating animals and newborns. During hibernation and in newborns, brown fat provides body heat as a protective measure.

2. **Correct Answer: A.** The hormone leptin. This hormone is produced by white adipose tissue cells and has an important role in food intake and appetite by acting on the cells in the hypothalamus of the central nervous system.

3. **Correct Answer: C.** It is the source of all connective tissue. The undifferentiated mesenchyme cells give rise to various other cells, including all connective tissue.

4. **Correct Answer: B.** Semifluid ground substance. Because of its viscosity, ground substance serves as an efficient barrier to large molecules and pathogens.

5. **Correct Answer: C.** Reticular fibers. These branching fibers are very thin and, in such organs as lymph nodes and the spleen, form a meshwork for filtering blood and lymph.

ADDITIONAL HISTOLOGIC IMAGES

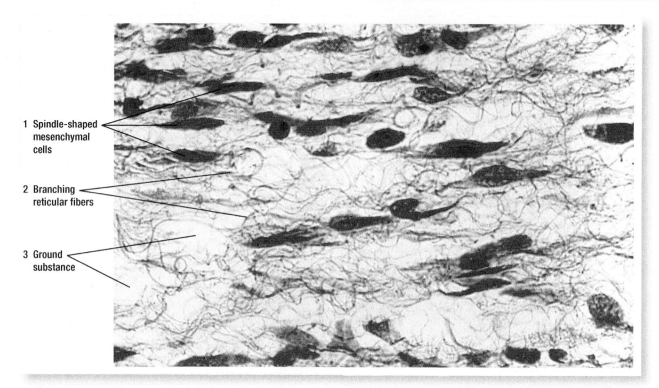

1 Spindle-shaped
  mesenchymal
  cells

2 Branching
  reticular fibers

3 Ground
  substance

FIGURE 5.14 ■ Mesenchymal tissue from a developing rodent fetus. Stain: hematoxylin and eosin. ×205.

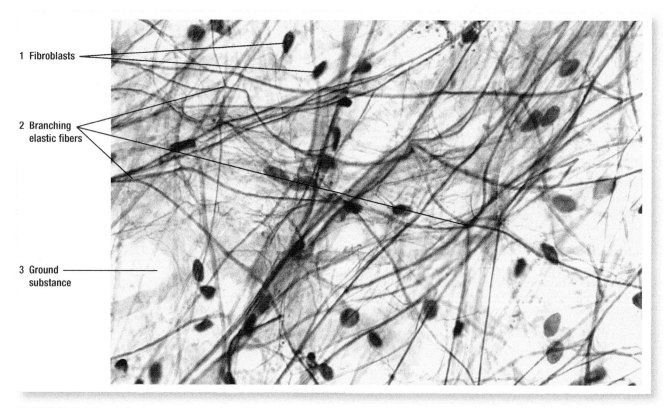

1 Fibroblasts

2 Branching
  elastic fibers

3 Ground
  substance

FIGURE 5.15 ■ Whole mount section through a mesentery illustrating the loose connective tissue, elastic fibers, fibroblasts, and the abundant surrounding ground substance. Stain: orcein. ×100.

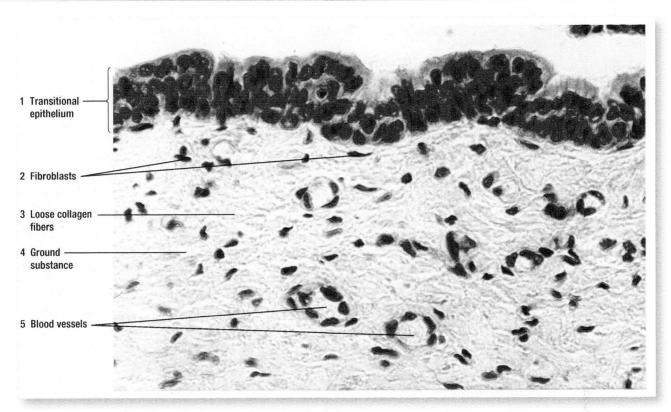

1 Transitional epithelium

2 Fibroblasts

3 Loose collagen fibers

4 Ground substance

5 Blood vessels

FIGURE 5.16 ■ Loose connective tissue below the transitional epithelium in a section from a primate urethra. Stain: hematoxylin and eosin. ×205.

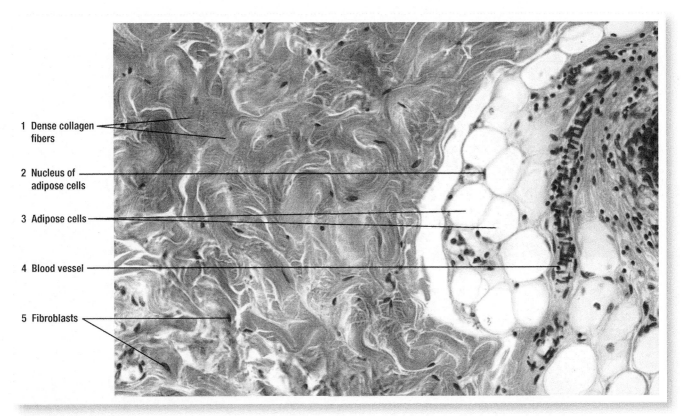

1 Dense collagen fibers

2 Nucleus of adipose cells

3 Adipose cells

4 Blood vessel

5 Fibroblasts

FIGURE 5.17 ■ Dense irregular connective tissue in a canine lip adjacent to white adipose cells (tissue). Stain: hematoxylin and eosin. ×64.

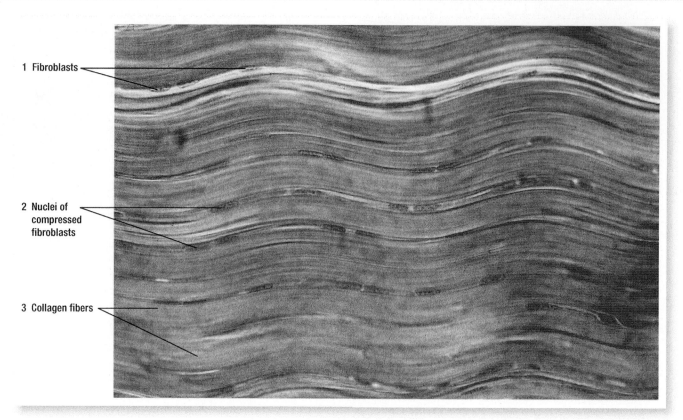

1 Fibroblasts

2 Nuclei of compressed fibroblasts

3 Collagen fibers

FIGURE 5.18 ■ Dense regular connective tissue from a primate tendon illustrating the dense arrangement of collagen fibers and the compressed fibroblasts. Stain: hematoxylin and eosin. ×64.

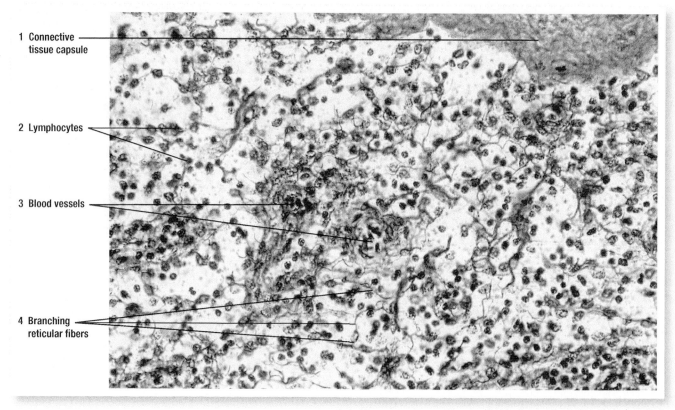

1 Connective tissue capsule

2 Lymphocytes

3 Blood vessels

4 Branching reticular fibers

FIGURE 5.19 ■ Reticular fiber meshwork in a primate lymph node. Silver impregnation. ×100.

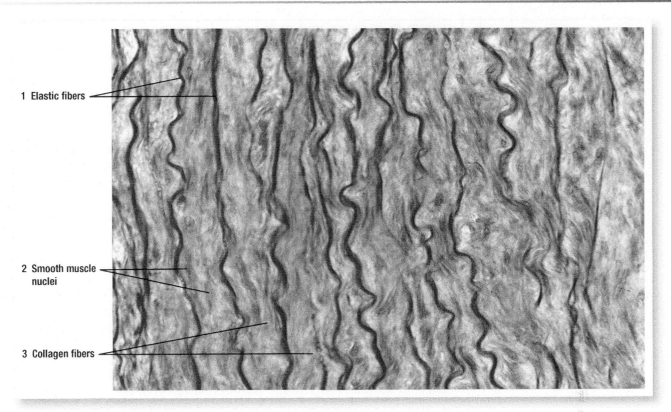

1 Elastic fibers

2 Smooth muscle nuclei

3 Collagen fibers

FIGURE 5.20 ■ A section of the wall from an aorta illustrating different connective tissue fibers and smooth muscle fibers. Stain: blue stain. ×130.

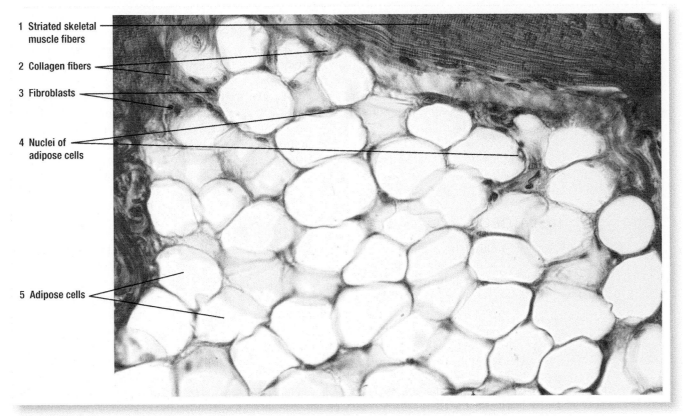

1 Striated skeletal muscle fibers

2 Collagen fibers

3 Fibroblasts

4 Nuclei of adipose cells

5 Adipose cells

FIGURE 5.21 ■ White adipose tissue (cells) adjacent to skeletal muscle fibers and dense irregular collagen fibers. Histologic preparation dissolved the lipids in the cell cytoplasm, showing only the nuclei. Stain: Mallory-Azan. ×130.

Hematopoietic Tissue

SECTION 1 Blood

Blood is a unique form of connective tissue in which its cells are suspended in a fluid component called **plasma**. The major cell types found in plasma are the **erythrocytes** (red blood cells [RBCs]) and **leukocytes** (white blood cells [WBCs]), which are divided into two categories **agranulocytes** and **granulocytes**. These cell types constitute the **formed elements** of the blood. Also, circulating in blood are cell fragments called **platelets** derived from large bone marrow cells, the **megakaryo-cytes.** Blood cells transport gases, nutrients, waste products, hormones, antibodies, various chemicals, ions, and other substances in plasma to and from different cells, tissues, and organs in the body. Blood cells have also a limited life span, and, as a result, they constantly wear out and are continuously replaced. The production of the formed elements of the blood is called hematopoiesis.

SITES OF HEMATOPOIESIS

Hematopoiesis occurs in different organs of the body, depending on the stage of development of the organism. In a developing **embryo**, hematopoiesis initially occurs in the **yolk sac** and later in the development in the liver, spleen, lymph nodes, and bone marrow. After birth, hematopoiesis continues almost exclusively in the **red marrow** of different bones. In the newborn individual, all bone marrow is red and functions in hematopoiesis.

The red bone marrow is a highly cellular structure and consists of hematopoietic **stem cells** and the precursors of different blood cells. Red marrow also contains a loose arrangement of fine reticular fibers that form an intricate connective tissue network. As the individual ages and reaches adulthood, the red marrow is primarily confined to the flat bones of the skull, sternum and ribs, vertebrae, and pelvic bones. The remaining long bones in the limbs of the body gradually accumulate fat, and their red marrow is replaced by fatty yellow marrow. Consequently, these sites lose the hematopoietic functions.

HEMATOPOIESIS

In this process, all blood cells originate from a **common stem cell** in the red bone marrow that is self-renewing. Because this stem cell type can produce all blood cell types, it is called the **pluripotential hematopoietic stem cell** (Fig. 6.1). Pluripotential stem cells, in turn, produce two major cell lineages that form the pluripotential **myeloid** stem cells and pluripotential **lymphoid** stem cells. Before maturation and release into the bloodstream, the stem cells from each lineage undergo numerous divisions and intermediate stages of differentiation before full maturation. Hematopoiesis is regulated by numerous **growth factors**, which activate and control blood cell formation. These growth factors influence different cell lineages and induce proliferation, differentiation, maturation and release the blood cells from the bone marrow into the blood. **Erythropoietin**, a protein substance produced by kidney cells, stimulates the proliferation and production of erythroid (RBC) progenitor cells. **Thrombopoietin**, also produced by kidneys, stimulates megakaryocyte differentiation and platelet formation. **Granulocyte-stimulating factor** and **monocyte-stimulating factor** stimulate the formation of the cells of granulocyte and

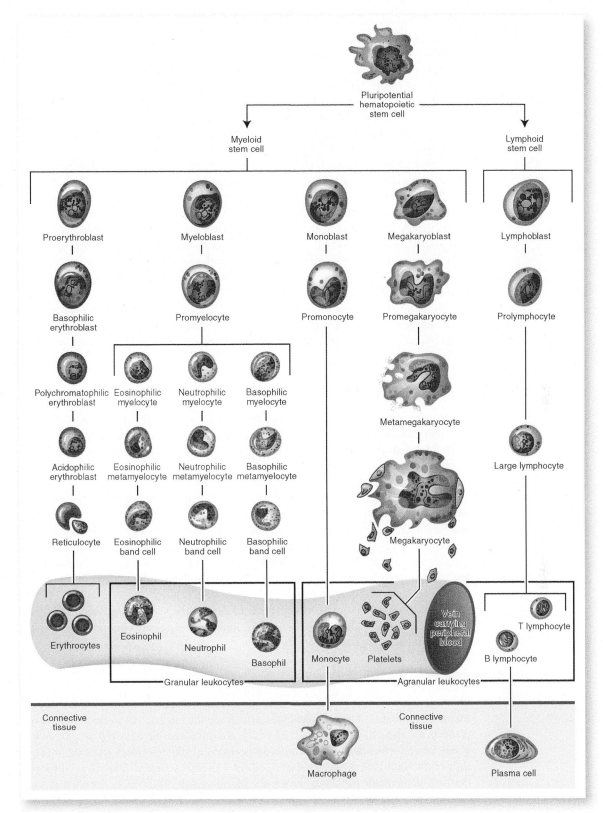

FIGURE 6.1 ■ Differentiation of myeloid and lymphoid stem cells into their mature forms and their distribution in the blood and connective tissue.

monocyte lineages. Different **interleukins** are responsible for development and function of B and T lymphocytes.

Myeloid stem cells develop in the red bone marrow and eventually give rise to **erythrocytes, eosinophils, neutrophils, basophils, monocytes,** and **megakaryocytes. Lymphoid stem cells** also develop in the red bone marrow. Some lymphoid cells remain in the bone marrow, proliferate, mature, and become **B lymphocytes.** Other lymphocytes leave the bone marrow and migrate via the bloodstream to **lymph nodes** and the **spleen,** where they proliferate and differentiate into B lymphocytes, after which they colonize peripheral lymphoid tissues (connective tissues, lymphoid tissues, and lymphoid organs).

Other undifferentiated lymphoid cells migrate to the **thymus gland,** where they proliferate and differentiate into immunocompetent **T lymphocytes.** Afterward, T lymphocytes enter the bloodstream and migrate to reside in the connective tissues and specific regions of peripheral lymphoid organs of the body. Both B and T lymphocytes reside in numerous peripheral lymphoid tissues, lymph nodes, and spleen. Here, they initiate immune responses when exposed to antigens. Although both the B and T lymphocytes are morphologically indistinguishable under a light microscope, their cell lines have separate pathways for growth, development, and function. Only the different protein markers on their cell surfaces allow these cells to be distinguished by immunohistochemical means.

Because all blood cells have a limited life span, the pluripotential hematopoietic stem cells continually divide and differentiate to produce new progeny of cells. When the blood cells become worn out and die, they are destroyed by macrophages in different lymphoid organs such as the spleen.

FORMED ELEMENTS: MAJOR BLOOD CELL TYPES

Microscopic examination of a stained blood smear reveals the major blood cell types. Mature **erythrocytes,** or RBCs, are nonnucleated cells and are the most numerous blood cells. During their final maturation process, the erythrocytes extrude their nuclei and assume a biconcave shape, and the mature blood cells enter the bloodstream. Erythrocytes remain in the blood and perform their major functions within the blood vessels.

In contrast, **leukocytes,** or WBCs, are nucleated and subdivided into **granulocytes** and **agranulocytes.** Granulocytes are the neutrophils, eosinophils, and basophils. Both eosinophils and basophils contain distinct stained granules in their cytoplasm, whereas neutrophils contain less obvious and smaller granules when viewed with the light microscope. Agranulocytes are the monocytes and lymphocytes. Leukocytes perform their major functions outside the blood vessels. They migrate out of the blood vessels through capillary walls and enter the connective tissue, lymphatic tissue, and bone marrow.

The primary function of leukocytes is to defend the body against bacterial invasion or the presence of foreign material. Consequently, most leukocytes are concentrated in the connective tissue of different organs.

PLATELETS

Platelets (thrombocytes) are the smallest, nonnucleated membrane-bound cytoplasmic **fragments** or remnants of **megakaryocytes,** which are the largest cells in the red bone marrow. The platelets are also called thrombocytes, which is a misnomer because platelets are not whole cells. Platelets are formed when small, uneven portions of the cytoplasm separate or fragment from the peripheries of the megakaryocytes and enter the bloodstream. Like the erythrocytes, platelets perform their major functions within the blood vessels. Their main function is to continually monitor the vascular system and detect any damage to the endothelial lining of the vessels. If the endothelial lining breaks, the platelets adhere to the damaged site and initiate a highly complex chemical process that produces a **blood clot.**

thePoint   Supplemental micrographic images are available at **www.thePoint.com/Eroschenko13e** under Blood Cells.

FUNCTIONAL CORRELATIONS 6.1 ■ Platelets

The platelets serve an important function. They repair minor tears in the walls of the blood vessels and promote blood clotting to prevent blood loss. Normally, intact endothelial cells of the blood vessels do not cause platelet aggregation to form the blood clot because laminin of the basement membrane and collagen fibers are not exposed. Instead, the endothelial cells produce **prostacyclin**, a chemical that inhibits platelet aggregation. Damage to the endothelial wall causes platelet aggregation and their adherence to exposed collagen and basement membrane proteins at the site of damage. This action activates the platelets to form a **platelet plug** to occlude the damaged vessel and to release **adhesive glycoproteins**, **adenosine diphosphate** (**ADP**), and **serotonin**. This increases the plug size by adhesion and attraction of other platelets. The damaged endothelial cells, in turn, release **tissue factor**, which initiates blood clotting, **von Willebrand** factor, which facilitates adhesion of platelets to laminin and collagen in the subendothelial tissue, and **endothelin**, which contracts the smooth muscle fibers in the damaged vessel. Surface receptors on platelets bind to **fibrinogen** in circulating plasma and the protein **thrombin** then converts fibrinogen into solid **fibrin** fibrils. Fibrin forms a loose meshwork of fibrils around the plug, trapping other platelets and blood cells to form and strengthen the blood clot, which enlarges until bleeding stops. After blood clot is formed and the bleeding stops, the aggregated platelets contribute to clot **retraction** by pulling the damaged edges of the blood vessels together. Following the vessel repair, the clot is removed by the proteolytic action of the enzyme **plasmin**, formed from the circulating plasma protein **plasminogen**.

FIGURE 6.2 | Human Blood Smear

A smear of human blood examined under lower magnification illustrates the formed elements. **Erythrocytes** (**1**) are the most abundant elements and the easiest to identify. Mature erythrocytes (RBCs) are anucleate (without a nucleus) and stain pink with eosin. They are uniform in size, have a biconcave shape, and measure about 7.5 μm in diameter, which is the approximate size of capillaries. In histological slides, the erythrocytes are often seen stacked or lined up in a single file in the lumen of the capillaries. Erythrocytes can be used as a size reference for other cell types.

Several leukocytes (WBCs) are visible in the blood smear. Leukocytes are subdivided into several categories according to the shape of their nuclei, the visibility of their cytoplasmic granules, and the staining affinities of the granules. Two **neutrophils** (**2**, **4**), one **eosinophil** (**7**) filled with red-pink granules, and one small **lymphocyte** (**5**) with a thin, bluish cytoplasm are visible. Scattered among the blood cells are small, blue-staining cellular fragments called **platelets** (**3**, **6**).

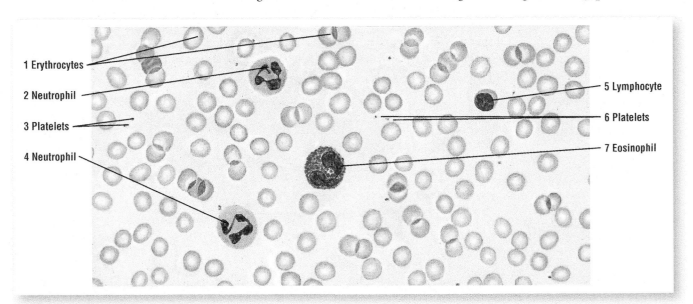

1 Erythrocytes
2 Neutrophil
3 Platelets
4 Neutrophil
5 Lymphocyte
6 Platelets
7 Eosinophil

FIGURE 6.2 ■ Human blood smear: erythrocytes, neutrophils, eosinophils, a lymphocyte, and platelets. Stain: Wright stain. High magnification.

FIGURE 6.3 | Human Blood Smear: RBCs, Neutrophils, Large Lymphocyte, and Platelets

A photomicrograph of a human blood smear shows different blood cell types. The most numerous blood cells are the **erythrocytes (RBCs)** (**1**). Also visible are two **neutrophils** (**2**, **4**), a large **lymphocyte** (**5**), and numerous **platelets** (**3**).

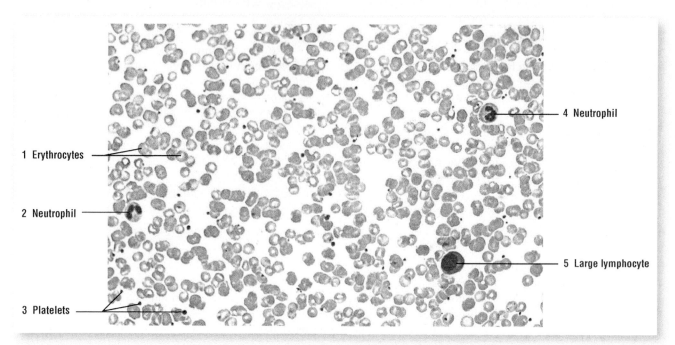

1 Erythrocytes

2 Neutrophil

3 Platelets

4 Neutrophil

5 Large lymphocyte

FIGURE 6.3 ■ Human blood smear: RBCs, neutrophils, a large lymphocyte, and platelets. Stain: Wright stain. ×205.

FIGURE 6.4 | Erythrocytes and Platelets

This illustration shows numerous **erythrocytes** (**1**) and **platelets** (**2**) that are usually seen in a blood smear. Blood platelets (2) are the smallest elements; they are nonnucleated cytoplasmic remnants of large-cell megakaryocytes, which are found only in the red bone marrow. Platelets (2) appear as irregular masses of the basophilic (blue) cytoplasm, and they tend to form clumps in blood smears. Each platelet exhibits a light blue peripheral zone and a dense central zone containing purple granules.

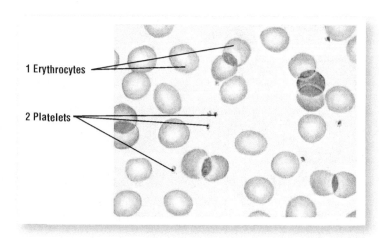

1 Erythrocytes

2 Platelets

FIGURE 6.4 ■ Erythrocytes and platelets in a blood smear. Stain: Wright stain. Oil immersion.

FIGURE 6.5 | Neutrophils

The leukocytes that contain cytoplasmic granules and lobulated nuclei are the polymorphonuclear granulocytes, of which the **neutrophils** (2) are the most abundant. The neutrophil cytoplasm (2) contains fine violet or pink granules that are difficult to see with a light microscope. As a result, the cytoplasm (2) of the neutrophils appears clear or neutral. The nucleus of the neutrophils (2) consists of **several lobes** connected by narrow chromatin strands. Immature neutrophils contain fewer nuclear lobes.

In human blood smears, an inactivated X chromosome of the female donor can be occasionally recognized as a **Barr body** (1) or a drumstick, which is a small extension of the chromatin next to one of the nuclear lobes. Numerous cells need to be examined in order to find the right orientation of the neutrophils to observe this extension or drumstick.

Neutrophils (1) constitute approximately 60% to 70% of blood leukocytes.

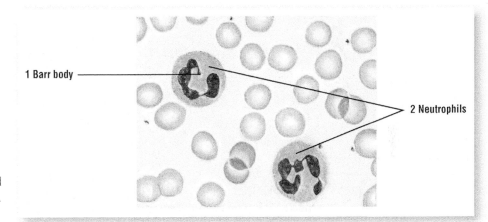

1 Barr body

2 Neutrophils

FIGURE 6.5 ■ Neutrophils and a Barr body. Stain: Wright stain. Oil immersion.

FUNCTIONAL CORRELATIONS 6.2 ■ Erythrocytes

Mature erythrocytes are specialized to transport **oxygen** and **carbon dioxide** because of the presence of the protein **hemoglobin** in their cytoplasm. Iron molecules in hemoglobin bind with oxygen molecules. As a result, most of the oxygen in the blood is carried in the combined form of **oxyhemoglobin**, which is responsible for the bright red color of arterial blood. Carbon dioxide diffuses from the cells and tissues into the blood vessels. It is carried to the lungs partly dissolved in the blood and partly in combination with hemoglobin in the erythrocytes as **carbaminohemo-globin**, which gives venous blood its bluish color.

During differentiation and maturation in the bone marrow, erythrocytes synthesize large amounts of hemoglobin. Before an erythrocyte is released into the systemic circulation, the nucleus is extruded from the cytoplasm, and the mature erythrocyte assumes a biconcave shape that provides more surface area for carrying respiratory gases. Thus, mature mammalian erythrocytes in the circulation are **nonnucleated** biconcave disks surrounded by a cell membrane and filled with hemoglobin and some enzymes.

The life span of erythrocytes is approximately 120 days, after which the worn-out cells are removed from the blood and phagocytosed by macrophages in the **spleen**, **liver**, and **bone marrow**.

FIGURE 6.6 | Eosinophil

Eosinophils (1) are identified in a blood smear by their cytoplasm that is filled with distinct, large, eosinophilic (bright pink) granules. The nucleus in eosinophils (1) is typically bilobed, but a small third lobe may be present.

Eosinophils (1) constitute approximately 2% to 4% of blood leukocytes.

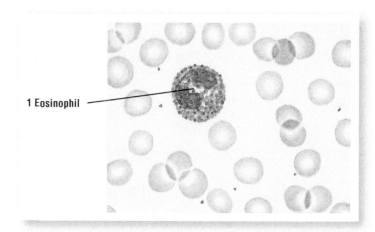

1 Eosinophil

FIGURE 6.6 ■ Eosinophil. Stain: Wright stain. Oil immersion.

FIGURE 6.7 | Lymphocytes

Agranular leukocytes contain few cytoplasmic granules and exhibit round to horseshoe-shaped nuclei. **Lymphocytes** (1, 2) vary in size from cells smaller than erythrocytes to cells almost twice as large. For a size comparison between lymphocytes and erythrocytes, this illustration of a human blood smear depicts a **large lymphocyte** (1) and a **small lymphocyte** (2) surrounded by the red-staining erythrocytes. In small lymphocytes (2), the densely stained nucleus occupies most of the cytoplasm, which appears as a thin basophilic rim around the nucleus. The cytoplasm in lymphocytes is usually agranular but may sometimes contain a few granules. In large lymphocytes (1), the basophilic cytoplasm is more abundant, and the larger and paler nucleus may contain one or two nucleoli.

Lymphocytes (1, 2) constitute approximately 20% to 30% of blood leukocytes. Most of the lymphocytes in the blood, about 90%, are the small lymphocytes. The large lymphocytes constitute about 3% of the circulating lymphocytes.

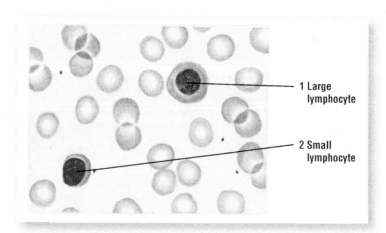

1 Large lymphocyte

2 Small lymphocyte

FIGURE 6.7 ■ Lymphocytes. Stain: Wright stain. Oil immersion.

FIGURE 6.8 | Monocyte

Monocytes (1) are the largest agranular leukocytes. The nucleus (1) varies from round or oval to indented or horseshoe shaped and stains lighter than the lymphocyte nucleus. The nuclear chromatin is finely dispersed in monocytes (1), and the abundant cytoplasm is lightly basophilic with few fine granules.

Monocytes (1) constitute approximately 3% to 8% of blood leukocytes.

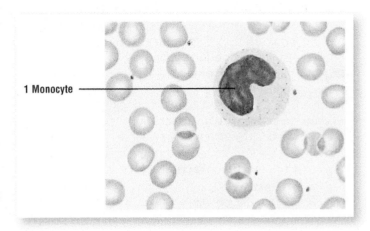

1 Monocyte

FIGURE 6.8 ■ Monocyte. Stain: Wright stain. Oil immersion.

FIGURE 6.9 | Basophil

The granules in **basophils** (1) are not as numerous as in eosinophils (see Fig. 6.5); however, they are more variable in size and less densely packed and stain dark blue or brown. Although the nucleus is not lobulated and stains palely basophilic, it is usually obscured by the density and number of granules.

The basophils (1) constitute less than 1% of blood leukocytes and are, therefore, the most difficult to find and identify in a blood smear.

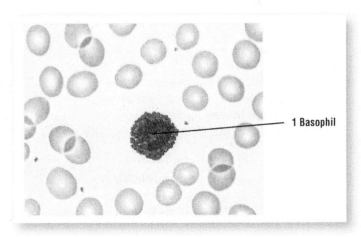

1 Basophil

FIGURE 6.9 ■ Basophil. Stain: Wright stain. Oil immersion.

FUNCTIONAL CORRELATIONS 6.3 ■ Leukocytes

Neutrophils have a short life span. They circulate in blood for some hours and then enter the connective tissue, where they can survive for another a couple of days. Although the cytoplasm of neutrophils appears neutral with normal blood stains, electron microscopy images show that neutrophils contain granules that are responsible for the cells' functions. The two main granules in the neutrophils are the larger azurophilic **primary granules** and the smaller specific **secondary granules**. The primary granules are the **lysosomes** that contain different lysosomal enzymes. The secondary granules exhibit diverse functions, including productions of various enzymes and enabling **antibacterial** functions of the neutrophils. Neutrophils are very active phagocytes that concentrate at the sites of infection. They are attracted by **chemotactic factors** (chemicals) produced by damaged or dead cells, tissues, or microorganisms, especially bacteria, which they first surround, phagocytose (ingest), fuse the phagocytized material with cytoplasmic (primary) granules, and quickly destroy the organism with their potent lysosomal enzymes.

Eosinophils also have a short life span and remain in blood for a period of time before migrating into the connective tissue. They are abundant in the connective tissue of the respiratory tract and intestinal organs. The cytoplasm of eosinophils is filled with large acidophilic granules that contain **major basic proteins**, which are powerful **hydrolytic enzymes** and toxins. One of the main functions of eosinophils is to defend the organism against helminthic **parasite** (worms) infestation. During such parasitic infestations, circulating eosinophils increase in number and combat the parasites by destroying them with the toxic hydrolytic enzymes. Eosinophils are also **phagocytic** cells. They phagocytize the parasites and the **antigen–antibody complexes** that are formed in tissues after allergic responses. The eosinophils also release enzyme **histaminase** that neutralizes or inactivates the vasoactive histamine released by basophils and mast cells and other mediators related to inflammatory allergic reactions.

Similar to eosinophils, **basophils** have also a short life span, and their function is similar to that of mast cells. They enter the connective tissue and increase in numbers in response to inflammatory conditions and allergic reactions. Their granules contain **histamine** and **heparin**. Basophils have surface receptors that bind to **immunoglobulin E** and, when activated by allergen binding, release histamine and other chemicals that effect and intensify inflammatory responses. These reactions cause severe allergic responses, vascular changes that lead to increased fluid leakage from blood vessels (tissue edema), and hypersensitivity and anaphylaxis.

All lymphocytes are produced in the bone marrow. Lymphocytes that mature in the bone marrow are the **B lymphocytes**, and those that mature in the thymus gland are the **T lymphocytes**. Other less abundant cells differentiate into **natural killer** (**NK**) **cells** in the bone marrow. Lymphocytes have a variable life span, from days to months, and show size variability. The difference between small and large lymphocytes has a functional significance. Small lymphocytes are the inactive cells, whereas large lymphocytes represent the cells that were **activated** by specific antigens and are considered as NK cells. Lymphocytes are essential for immunologic defense of the organism. Some lymphocytes (B lymphocytes), when stimulated by specific antigens, differentiate into **plasma cells** in the connective tissue and produce **antibodies** to counteract or destroy the invading organisms.

Monocytes can live in the blood for 2 to 3 days, after which they move into the connective tissue, where they become active and powerful **macrophages** (phagocytes) during inflammation in the tissue. Blood monocytes are precursors of the **mononuclear phagocyte system**. Although the cytoplasm appears agranular and pale under a light microscope, the cytoplasm is filled with small **lysosomes**. Once transformed into macrophages and with their cytoplasm filled with hydrolytic enzymes of the lysosomes, these cells destroy bacteria, cellular debris, and foreign matter. Monocytes are also antigen-presenting cells and play an important role in defense of the organism. They process antigens and present them to T lymphocytes to induce an appropriate immune response.

FIGURE 6.10 | Human Blood Smear: Basophil, Neutrophil, Erythrocytes, and Platelets

A high-magnification photomicrograph of a human blood smear shows **erythrocytes** (3), a **basophil** (1), a **neutrophil** (5), and **platelets** (4). The basophil (1) cytoplasm is filled with dense **basophilic granules** (2) that obscure the nucleus. In contrast, the neutrophil (5) cytoplasm does not show granules, and its **nucleus** is **multilobed** (6).

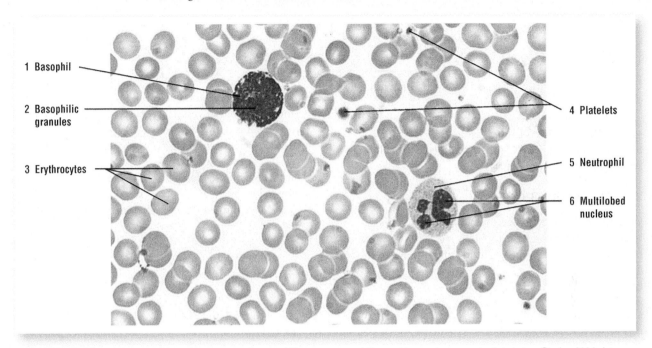

FIGURE 6.10 ■ Human blood smear: a basophil, a neutrophil, erythrocytes, and platelets. Stain: Wright stain. ×320.

FIGURE 6.11 | Human Blood Smear: Monocyte, Erythrocytes, and Platelets

A high-magnification photomicrograph shows numerous **erythrocytes** (1), **platelets** (2), and a large **monocyte** (3) with a characteristic kidney-shaped nucleus and nongranular cytoplasm.

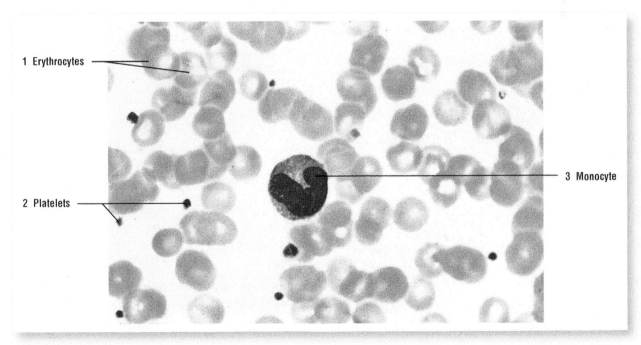

FIGURE 6.11 ■ Human blood smear: a monocyte, erythrocytes, and platelets. Stain: Wright stain. ×320.

Chapter 6 Summary

SECTION 1 • Blood

- Unique form of connective tissue in which cells are suspended in circulating fluid
- Consists of cells erythrocytes, leukocytes, and cell fragments platelets suspended in plasma
- Blood cells have limited life span and are continually replaced in the red bone marrow

SITES OF HEMATOPOIESIS

- Depend on the stage of development of the organism
- In embryo, the initial hematopoietic site is the yolk sac
- Later in development, liver, spleen, lymph nodes, and bone marrow form blood
- In adults, red marrow is limited to the skull, sternum, vertebrae, and pelvic bones
- Long bones become filled with fat, yellow marrow, and lose hematopoietic functions

HEMATOPOIESIS

- Common pluripotential stem cell forms pluripotential myeloid and lymphoid stem cells
- Myeloid stem cells give rise to erythrocytes, eosinophils, neutrophils, basophils, monocytes, and megakaryocytes
- Lymphoid stem cells give rise to B lymphocytes, T lymphocytes, and natural killer cells
- B lymphocytes mature in bone marrow; T lymphocytes mature in the thymus gland
- B lymphocytes and T lymphocytes have separate development paths
- B and T lymphocytes reside in peripheral lymphoid tissue, lymph nodes, and spleen

FORMED ELEMENTS: MAJOR BLOOD CELL TYPES

Erythrocytes

- Most numerous cells in blood
- Erythrocytes are nonnucleated cells that remain in blood
- Contain hemoglobin with iron molecules in the cytoplasm
- Carry oxygen as oxyhemoglobin and carbon dioxide as carbaminohemoglobin
- Biconcave shape increases the surface area to carry respiratory gases
- Life span is about 120 days, after which cells are phagocytosed in the spleen, liver, and bone marrow

Platelets

- Membrane-bound fragments of bone marrow megakaryocytes and are not blood cells
- Function in blood vessels to promote blood clotting when vessel wall is damaged
- In damaged vessels form a plug that increases with adhesive glycoproteins and fibrin
- Fibrin traps more platelets and blood cells and forms a blood clot
- Cause clot retraction and pull damaged edges of the blood vessel together
- Following vessel repair, the clot is removed by the proteolytic enzyme plasmin

Leukocytes

- Contain nuclei and are subdivided into granulocytes and agranulocytes
- Granulocytes with cytoplasmic granules are neutrophils, eosinophils, and basophils
- Agranulocytes without cytoplasmic granules are monocytes and lymphocytes

Granulocytes

Neutrophils

- Cytoplasm appears neutral under light microscope
- Under electron microscope, cytoplasmic primary granules are lysosomes
- Nucleus contains several lobes connected by thin chromatin strands
- Barr body or drumstick seen next to nuclear lobe indicates female blood
- Short life span in blood or connective tissue, ranging from hours to days
- Very active phagocytes that are attracted to foreign material by chemotactic factors
- Destroy phagocytosed (ingested) material with lysosomal enzymes
- Constitute about 60% to 70% of blood leukocytes

Eosinophils

- Cytoplasm filled with large pink or eosinophilic granules that contain major basic proteins
- Nucleus typically bilobed
- Short life span, in blood or connective tissue

- Increase in numbers to defend organism against and destroy parasitic infestations
- Phagocytic with affinity for antigen–antibody complexes
- Release a chemical histaminase that neutralizes histamine and other mediators of inflammatory reactions
- Constitute about 2% to 4% of blood leukocytes

Basophils

- Cytoplasm contains dark blue or brown granules and has a short life span
- Nucleus stains palely basophilic but is normally obscured by dense cytoplasmic granules
- Surface receptors bind to immunoglobulin E
- Activation by allergen release histamine from cytoplasmic granules
- Histamine causes intense inflammatory response in severe allergic reactions
- Constitute less than 1% of blood leukocytes

Agranulocytes

Lymphocytes

- Few visible granules in the cytoplasm are lysosomes
- Vary in size from small to large, depending on function

- Large lymphocytes are in the minority, about 3%, and represent activated cells by antigens
- There are B, T, and natural killer lymphocytes
- Dense-staining nucleus surrounded by a narrow cytoplasmic rim
- Life span is from days to months
- Essential in immunologic defense of organism
- When exposed to specific antigens, B lymphocytes become plasma cells in the connective tissue
- Plasma cells release antibodies to counteract or destroy invading organisms
- Constitute about 20% to 30% of blood leukocytes

Monocytes

- Largest agranular leukocyte characterized primarily by a kidney-shaped nucleus
- Small granules are lysosomes but not very visible with light microscope
- Live in connective tissue for months where they become powerful phagocytes
- Are part of the mononuclear phagocyte system
- Constitute about 3% to 8% of blood leukocytes

Chapter 6 Review Questions: Section 1

QUESTIONS

In the following multiple-choice questions, choose the letter corresponding to the one best answer.

1. **In the developing embryo, the first site of hematopoiesis occurs in the:**

   A. developing embryonic organs.
   B. red bone marrow.
   C. liver.
   D. yolk sac.
   E. spleen.

2. **In an adult organism, hematopoiesis occurs in:**

   A. bones with red marrow.
   B. all bones in the body.
   C. selected organs of the body.
   D. lymph nodes and the thymus gland.
   E. the heart and blood vessels.

3. **T lymphocytes proliferate and differentiate in:**

   A. sites of infection.
   B. red bone marrow.
   C. connective tissue.
   D. lymph nodes.
   E. the thymus gland.

4. **T lymphocytes and B lymphocytes can be distinguished in blood by:**

   A. their histological shape.
   B. their nuclear size.
   C. immunohistochemical means.
   D. cell size.
   E. cytoplasmic granules.

5. **Which blood cells perform their major functions in the blood?**

   A. Erythrocytes
   B. Neutrophils
   C. Monocytes
   D. Plasma cells
   E. All leukocytes

ANSWERS

1. **Correct answer: D.** Yolk sac. Early in development, blood cells arise from the yolk sac followed later by the other blood cells, forming organs.

2. **Correct answer: A.** Bones with red marrow. Bones such as the sternum, vertebrae, skull bones, and pelvic bones retain red marrow and are sites for blood cell formation.

3. **Correct answer: E.** The thymus gland. Blood lymphocytes arise in the red bone marrow and circulate to different organs. T lymphocytes enter the thymus gland where they mature and become immunocompetent.

4. **Correct answer: C.** Immunohistochemical means. Different immunocompetent lymphocytes cannot be distinguished with histological means because they have similar morphologies. Only immunochemical means can distinguish the different types of lymphocytes.

5. **Correct answer: A.** Erythrocytes. Erythrocytes, or red blood cells, remain in the blood and perform their functions in the blood, carrying oxygen and carbon dioxide for gaseous exchange.

SECTION 2 Bone Marrow

Although bones provide important structural support for the body, they also serve as important sites for blood cell formation. Bone marrow is a highly cellular tissue that is located in the medullary cavities of the bone. **Red bone marrow** is the principal site of blood cell formation or **hematopoiesis** located between the bony trabeculae of the bone. Red bone marrow consists of densely packed cords and islands of blood-forming (hematopoietic) stem cells. They are surrounded by numerous macrophages and abundant branching sinusoidal capillaries that open into the thin venous sinuses. These sinuses provide the main exit route through the openings in their endothelial lining for the newly differentiated blood cells to enter the systemic circulation. A connective tissue stroma of reticular cells and reticular fibers form a delicate **meshwork** that surrounds the islands of hematopoietic cells and provides support for the bone marrow.

The active red bone marrow in selected bones provides a steady rate of blood cell renewal to replace those that are worn out or lost. Also, the red bone marrow is the site where tissue macrophages engulf and phagocytose worn-out erythrocytes and store the iron recovered from the hemoglobin breakdown for the next generation of blood cells.

thePoint Supplemental micrographic images are available at **www.thePoint.com/Eroschenko13e** under Blood Cells.

FIGURE 6.12 | **Development of Different Blood Cells in Red Bone Marrow (Decalcified Section)**

In a section of the red bone marrow, all types of developing blood cells are difficult to distinguish. The cells are densely packed, and different cell types are intermixed. During the maturation process, hematopoietic cells become smaller and their nuclear chromatin more condensed. As the

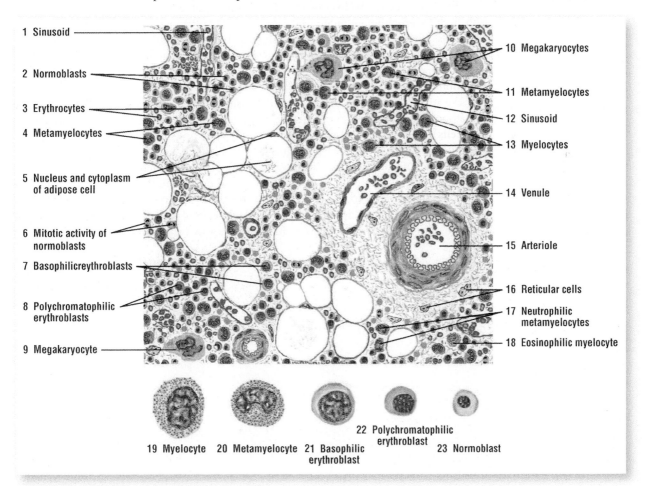

1 Sinusoid
2 Normoblasts
3 Erythrocytes
4 Metamyelocytes
5 Nucleus and cytoplasm of adipose cell
6 Mitotic activity of normoblasts
7 Basophilicreythroblasts
8 Polychromatophilic erythroblasts
9 Megakaryocyte

10 Megakaryocytes
11 Metamyelocytes
12 Sinusoid
13 Myelocytes
14 Venule
15 Arteriole
16 Reticular cells
17 Neutrophilic metamyelocytes
18 Eosinophilic myelocyte

19 Myelocyte 20 Metamyelocyte 21 Basophilic erythroblast 22 Polychromatophilic erythroblast 23 Normoblast

FIGURE 6.12 ■ Development of different blood cells in the red bone marrow (decalcified). Stain: hematoxylin and eosin. *Upper image*: high magnification; *lower image*: oil immersion.

blood cells pass through a series of developmental stages, they exhibit morphologic changes and become microscopically identifiable.

This section of bone marrow is stained with hematoxylin and eosin stain. At this magnification, little differentiation of cytoplasm is visible. In the erythrocytic line, early **basophilic erythroblasts (7, 21)** are recognized by a large but not very dense nucleus and basophilic cytoplasm. These cells give rise to the smaller **polychromatophilic erythroblasts (8, 22)** with a more condensed nuclear chromatin and a more variable color of the cytoplasm, with the cytoplasm becoming more eosinophilic. The most recognizable and most abundant cells of the erythrocytic line are **normoblasts (2, 23)**. They are characterized by small, dark-staining pyknotic nuclei and a reddish, or eosinophilic, cytoplasm. Early normoblasts (2, 23) exhibit **mitotic activity (6)** in the bone marrow. As normoblasts (2, 23) mature, the cells lose the ability to divide and extrude their densely staining pyknotic nuclei to become **erythrocytes (3)**. Cells of the erythrocytic lineage do not display any granules in their cytoplasm. Erythrocytes (3) are abundant in red bone marrow and are seen in the numerous **sinusoids (1, 12)**, **venule (14)**, and **arteriole (15)** as they are released into systemic circulation.

The early granulocytes initially exhibit numerous primary, or azurophilic, granules in their cytoplasm. As a result, the immature forms of neutrophils, eosinophils, and basophils are morphologically indistinguishable and become recognizable only in the myelocyte stage, when specific granules appear in recognizable quantities in their cytoplasm that can be stained for recognition. In neutrophilic cells, the specific granules are only faintly stained, and the cytoplasm appears clear or neutral. These granules are clearly recognized with electron microscope. In the eosinophilic line, the specific granules stain deep red, or eosinophilic. Basophilic granulocytes are rarely observed in the bone marrow because of their small numbers. The cytoplasm of mature basophils exhibits a bilobed nucleus and dense blue, or basophilic, granules.

The granulocytic **myelocytes (13, 19)** exhibit a large spherical nucleus and a cytoplasm with many azurophilic granules. The myelocytes (13, 19) give rise to **metamyelocytes (4, 11, 20)**, whose nuclei are bean or horseshoe shaped. The **neutrophilic metamyelocytes (17)** exhibit a deeply indented nuclei and cytoplasm with azurophilic granules and faintly stained specific granules. In contrast, a cell with bright-staining red (eosinophilic) granules in the cytoplasm is an **eosinophilic myelocyte (18)**.

The stroma of the reticular connective tissue in the bone marrow is almost obscured by hematopoietic cells. In less dense areas, the reticular connective tissue with the elongated **reticular cells (16)** is visible. Also, numerous thin-walled sinusoids (1, 12) and different types of blood vessels (14, 15) containing erythrocytes and leukocytes are present in the bone marrow. Also conspicuous are the large **adipose cells (5)** with large vacuoles (because of fat removal during section preparation) and a small, peripheral cytoplasm that surrounds the **nucleus (5)**. Other identifiable cells in the bone marrow are the very large **megakaryocytes (9, 10)** with varied nuclear lobulation. One of these megakaryocytes (10) is situated adjacent to a blood sinusoid, into which the fragments from its cytoplasmic extensions separate and discharged as platelets.

Selected blood cells from the red bone marrow are illustrated on the next page at a higher magnification.

FIGURE 6.13 | Bone Marrow Smear: Development of Different Cell Types

A bone marrow smear shows a few typical blood cells in different stages of development. In the erythrocytic series, the precursor cell **proerythroblast** (**3**) exhibits a thin rim of basophilic cytoplasm and a large, oval nucleus that occupies most of the cell. The chromatin is dispersed uniformly, and two or more nuclei may be present. Azurophilic granules are absent from the cytoplasm in all cells of the erythrocytic series. The proerythroblasts (**3**) divide to form the smaller **basophilic erythroblasts** (**8, 16**).

Basophilic erythroblasts (8, 16) are characterized by a rim of basophilic cytoplasm and a decreased cell and nuclear size. The nuclear chromatin is coarse and exhibits the characteristic "checkerboard" pattern. Nucleoli are either inconspicuous or absent. Basophilic erythroblasts (8, 16) give rise to the **polychromatophilic erythroblasts** (**12**), which are similar in size to basophilic erythroblasts (8, 16). The cytoplasm of the polychromatophilic erythroblast (12) becomes progressively less basophilic and more acidophilic as a result of increased hemoglobin accumulation. The nuclei of polychromatophilic erythroblasts (12) are smaller and exhibit a coarse checkerboard pattern.

When the polychromatophilic cells (12) acquire a more eosinophilic (pink) cytoplasm as a result of increased hemoglobin accumulation, their size decreases and they become **orthochromatophilic erythroblasts** (**late normoblasts**) (**1**). These cells are capable of **mitosis** (**2**). Initially, the nucleus of orthochromatophilic erythroblasts (1) exhibits a concentrated checkerboard chromatin pattern. Eventually, the nucleus decreases in size, becomes pyknotic, and is extruded from the cytoplasm, forming a biconcave-shaped cell with a bluish pink cytoplasm called a reticulocyte or young erythrocyte. With special supravital staining, a delicate reticulum is seen in the reticulocyte cytoplasm because of the remaining polyribosomes (see Fig. 6.14). After polyribosomes are lost from the cytoplasm, the cells become mature **erythrocytes** (**9**) and enter the systemic circulation via the numerous blood channels. Erythrocytes (9) are small cells with a homogeneous eosinophilic, or pink, cytoplasm.

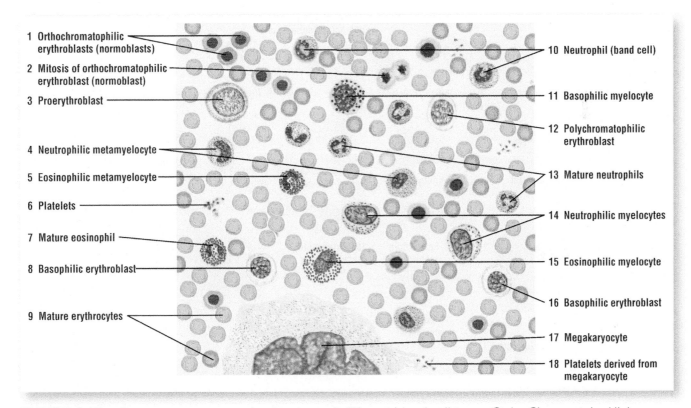

1 Orthochromatophilic erythroblasts (normoblasts)
2 Mitosis of orthochromatophilic erythroblast (normoblast)
3 Proerythroblast
4 Neutrophilic metamyelocyte
5 Eosinophilic metamyelocyte
6 Platelets
7 Mature eosinophil
8 Basophilic erythroblast
9 Mature erythrocytes

10 Neutrophil (band cell)
11 Basophilic myelocyte
12 Polychromatophilic erythroblast
13 Mature neutrophils
14 Neutrophilic myelocytes
15 Eosinophilic myelocyte
16 Basophilic erythroblast
17 Megakaryocyte
18 Platelets derived from megakaryocyte

FIGURE 6.13 ■ Bone marrow smear: development of different blood cell types. Stain: Giemsa stain. High magnification.

Also visible in the bone marrow smear are different types of myelocytes and metamyelocytes of the granulocytic cell line. Myelocytes exhibit an eccentric nucleus with condensed chromatin and a less basophilic cytoplasm with few azurophilic granules. Different types of myelocytes exhibit varying number of granules. More mature myelocytes, such as **neutrophilic myelocytes (14)**, an **eosinophilic myelocyte (15)**, and a rare **basophilic myelocyte (11)**, show an abundance of specific granules in their slightly acidophilic cytoplasm. The myelocyte is the last cell of the granulocytic line capable of mitosis, after which they mature into metamyelocytes.

The shape of the nucleus in the neutrophilic line changes from oval to one with indentation, as seen in **neutrophilic metamyelocytes (4)**. Before complete maturation and segmentation of the nucleus into distinct lobes, the neutrophils pass through a **band cell (10)** stage, in which the nucleus assumes a nearly uniform curved rod or band shape.

Mature neutrophils (13) with segmented nuclei are also present in the bone marrow smear, as well as a **mature eosinophil (7)** with specific pink granules filling its cytoplasm.

A section of a giant cell **megakaryocyte (17)** is visible. These cells measure approximately 50 to 100 μm in diameter and have a large, slightly acidophilic cytoplasm filled with fine azurophilic granules. Cytoplasmic fragments are shed from megakaryocytes as **platelets (18)**.

FIGURE 6.14 | Bone Marrow Smear: Selected Precursors of Different Blood Cells

This illustration shows at a higher magnification the selected precursor cells of different blood cells that develop and mature in the red bone marrow.

A common stem cell gives rise to different hematopoietic cell lines, from which arise erythrocytes, granulocytes, lymphocytes, and megakaryocytes. Because of its ability to differentiate into all blood cells, this cell is called the pluripotential hematopoietic stem cell.

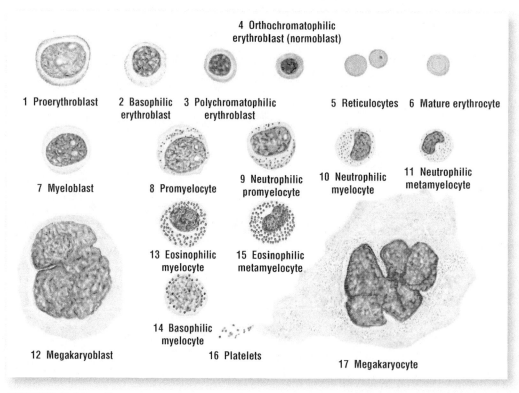

FIGURE 6.14 ■ Bone marrow smear: selected precursors of different blood cells. Stain: Giemsa stain. High magnification or oil immersion.

ERYTHROCYTE DEVELOPMENT

In the erythrocytic cell line, the **pluripotential stem cell** differentiates into a **proerythroblast** (**1**), a large cell with loose chromatin, one or two nucleoli, and a basophilic cytoplasm. The proerythroblast (**1**) divides to produce a smaller cell called a **basophilic erythroblast** (**2**) with a rim of basophilic cytoplasm and a more condensed nucleus without visible nucleoli. In the next stage, a smaller cell called the **polychromatophilic erythroblast** (**3**) is produced. These cells show a decrease in basophilic ribosomes and an increase in the acidophilic hemoglobin content of their cytoplasm. As a result, staining these cells produces several colors in their cytoplasm. As differentiation continues, there is a further reduction of the cell size, condensation of nuclear material, and a more uniform eosinophilic cytoplasm. At this stage, the cell is called an **orthochromatophilic erythroblast (normoblast)** (**4**). After extruding its nucleus, the orthochromatophilic erythroblast (**4**) becomes a **reticulocyte** (**5**) because a small number of ribosomes can be stained in its cytoplasm. After losing the ribosomes, the reticulocyte becomes a **mature erythrocyte** (**6**).

GRANULOCYTE DEVELOPMENT

The **myeloblast** (**7**) is the first recognizable precursor in the granulocytic cell line. The myeloblast (**7**) is a small cell with a large nucleus, dispersed chromatin, three or more nucleoli, and a basophilic cytoplasm rim that lacks specific granules. As development progresses, the cell enlarges, acquires azurophilic granules, and becomes a **promyelocyte** (**8, 9**). The chromatin in the oval nucleus is dispersed, and multiple nucleoli are evident. In more advanced promyelocytes, the cells become smaller, the nucleoli become inconspicuous, the number of azurophilic granules increases, and specific granules with different staining properties appear in the perinuclear region. Promyelocytes (**8, 9**) divide to form smaller **myelocytes** (**10, 13, 14**). The cytoplasm of myelocytes (**10, 13, 14**) is less basophilic and contains many azurophilic granules. Myelocytes differentiate into three kinds of granulocytes, which can be recognized only by the increased accumulation and staining properties of specific granules in their cytoplasm, as seen in the **eosinophilic myelocyte** (**13**) with red or eosinophilic granules and the rare **basophilic myelocyte** (**14**) with blue or basophilic granules. Myelocytes develop into metamyelocytes. The cytoplasm of a **neutrophilic metamyelocyte** (**11**) contains deep-staining azurophilic granules, lightly stained specific granules, and an indented, kidney-shaped nucleus. The **eosinophilic metamyelocytes** (**15**) are larger cells, and their specific cytoplasmic granules stain eosinophilic.

Megakaryoblasts (**12**) are large cells with a basophilic, homogeneous cytoplasm. The voluminous nucleus is ovoid or kidney shaped, contains numerous nucleoli, and exhibits a loose chromatin pattern. Platelets are not formed at this stage.

During differentiation, megakaryoblasts (**12**) become very large. Their nucleus becomes convoluted, with multiple, irregular lobes interconnected by constricted regions. The chromatin becomes condensed and coarse, and nucleoli are not visible. In mature **megakaryocytes** (**17**), the plasma membrane invaginates the cytoplasm and forms demarcation membranes that indicates the areas of the megakaryocyte cytoplasm that is shed into the blood as small cell fragments in the form of **platelets** (**16**).

Chapter 6 Summary

SECTION 2 • Bone Marrow

- Located in medullary cavities between bony trabeculae
- Red bone marrow is the principal site of hematopoiesis
- Consists of cords and islands of hematopoietic stem cells that replace lost cells
- A branching capillary network surrounds hematopoietic stem cells
- The site of macrophage breakdown of worn-out erythrocytes and storage of iron

DEVELOPING BLOOD CELLS

Development of Erythrocytes

- Precursor proerythroblast shows a rim of basophilic cytoplasm and a large nucleus
- Early basophilic erythroblasts are smaller and exhibit large nuclei and basophilic cytoplasm
- Polychromatophilic erythroblasts exhibit more condensed nuclei and more eosinophilic cytoplasm
- Increased hemoglobin accumulation, eosinophilic cytoplasm, and decreased size produce orthochromatophilic erythroblasts (late normoblasts)
- Most recognizable erythrocytic lines are normoblasts with early stages exhibiting mitosis
- Mature normoblasts lose the ability to divide, extrude their highly condensed pyknotic nuclei, and become eosinophilic erythrocytes

- Erythrocytes do not exhibit cytoplasmic granules as they enter systemic circulation

Development of Granulocytes

- Myeloblast, first recognizable granulocytic cell line, gives rise to promyelocyte
- Early granulocytes exhibit numerous azurophilic granules in the cytoplasm
- Promyelocytes divide and form myelocytes, which differentiate into three different kinds of granulocytes
- Myelocyte is the last stage of the granulocyte line that can divide
- Granulocyte cell lines are recognized in myelocytes as specific granules appear in the cytoplasm
- Myelocytes develop into metamyelocytes whose nuclei appear bean or kidney shaped
- Neutrophilic metamyelocytes show indented nuclei and faintly staining specific granules
- At maturation, neutrophils exhibit segmented nucleus into three lobes
- Eosinophilic metamyelocytes exhibit red or eosinophilic-specific granules in the cytoplasm
- Basophilic metamyelocytes exhibit dark or basophilic-specific granules in the cytoplasm

Chapter 6 Review Questions: Section 2

QUESTIONS

In the following multiple-choice questions, choose the letter corresponding to the one best answer.

1. **Before a mature erythrocyte enters the systemic circulation, what takes place?**

   A. The cell exhibits mitosis.
   B. The cytoplasm increases in size.
   C. The pyknotic nucleus is extruded.
   D. The cytoplasm is reduced in size.
   E. The nucleus exhibits a bean or kidney shape.

2. **Differentiation of myelocytes into the three types of granulocytes can be recognized primarily by:**

   A. accumulation of specific granules in their cytoplasm.
   B. increase in the size of the myelocyte.
   C. alteration of nuclear size.
   D. changes in the staining of the cytoplasm.
   E. lack or absence of granules in the cytoplasm.

3. **Which cells have an affinity for antigen–antibody complexes?**

   A. Plasma cells
   B. Eosinophils
   C. T lymphocytes
   D. Basophils
   E. Mast cells

4. **Under an electron microscope, the cytoplasm of neutrophils contains azurophilic primary granules. These granules contain:**

   A. crystals.
   B. phagocytic material.
   C. fatty acids.
   D. hormones.
   E. lysosomes.

5. **Which cells produce antibodies to fight off infections in the organism?**

   A. Lymphoblasts
   B. Plasma cells
   C. Eosinophils
   D. Basophils
   E. Pluropotential cells of bone marrow

ANSWERS

1. **Correct answer: C.** The pyknotic nucleus is extruded. In order to increase the area of the cytoplasm for gas-carrying capacity, the developing erythrocytes extrude their nuclei and enter the circulation.

2. **Correct answer: A.** Accumulation of specific granules in their cytoplasm. The accumulation of different granules in the cytoplasm of the myelocytes allows identification of differentiating myelocytes.

3. **Correct answer: B.** Eosinophils. These cells have affinity for and phagocytize the antigen–antibody complexes.

4. **Correct answer: E.** Lysosomes. With electron microscopic examination, the cytoplasm of neutrophils contains granules that have been shown to contain lysosomes.

5. **Correct answer: B.** Plasma cells. B lymphocytes differentiate into plasma cells when exposed to antigens, after which they produce antibodies to counteract invading or infectious organisms.

ADDITIONAL HISTOLOGIC IMAGES

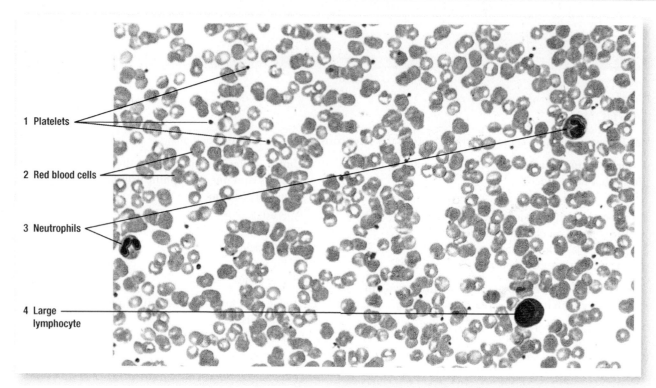

1 Platelets

2 Red blood cells

3 Neutrophils

4 Large lymphocyte

FIGURE 6.15 ■ Human blood smear showing different blood cells and cellular fragments, the platelets. Stain: Wright stain. ×165.

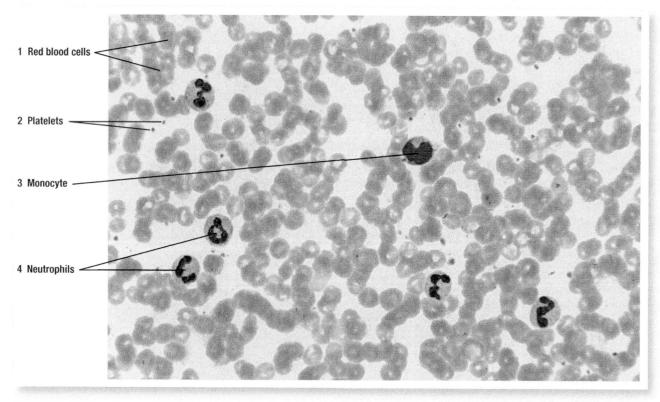

1 Red blood cells

2 Platelets

3 Monocyte

4 Neutrophils

FIGURE 6.16 ■ Human blood smear exhibiting different blood cells and cell fragments. Stain: Wright stain. ×165.

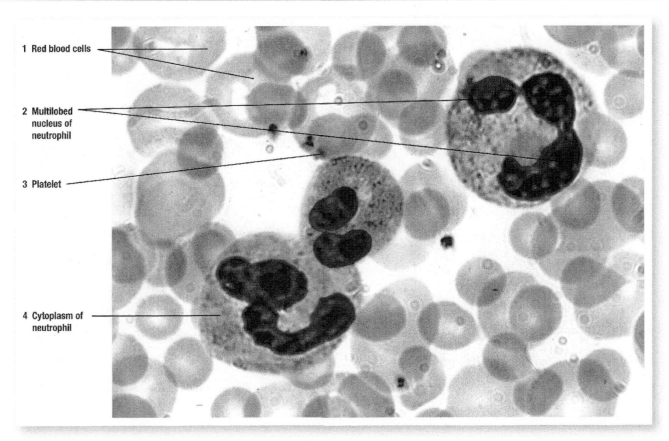

1 Red blood cells

2 Multilobed
   nucleus of
   neutrophil

3 Platelet

4 Cytoplasm of
   neutrophil

FIGURE 6.17 ■ High magnification of a human blood smear showing two neutrophils with multilobar nuclei and some light-staining cytoplasmic granules. Stain: Wright stain. ×320.

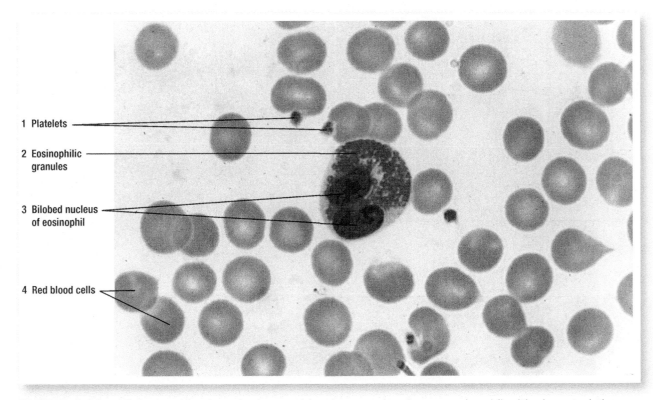

1 Platelets

2 Eosinophilic
   granules

3 Bilobed nucleus
   of eosinophil

4 Red blood cells

FIGURE 6.18 ■ High magnification of a human blood smear showing an eosinophil with characteristic pink-staining eosinophilic cytoplasmic granules and bilobed nucleus. Stain: Wright stain. ×320.

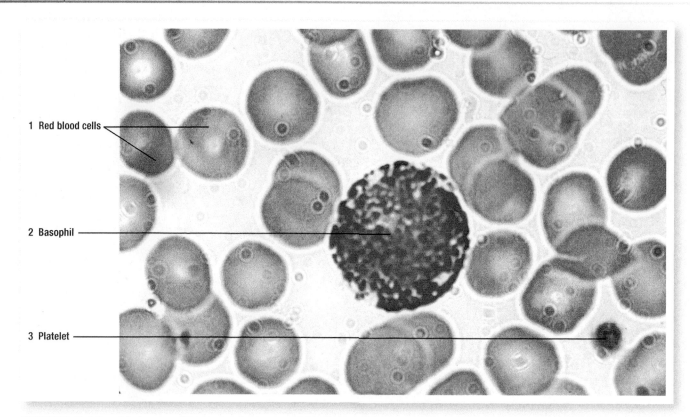

1 Red blood cells

2 Basophil

3 Platelet

FIGURE 6.19 ■ High magnification of a human blood smear showing a basophil with characteristic dark blue–staining cytoplasmic granules. Stain: Wright stain. ×350.

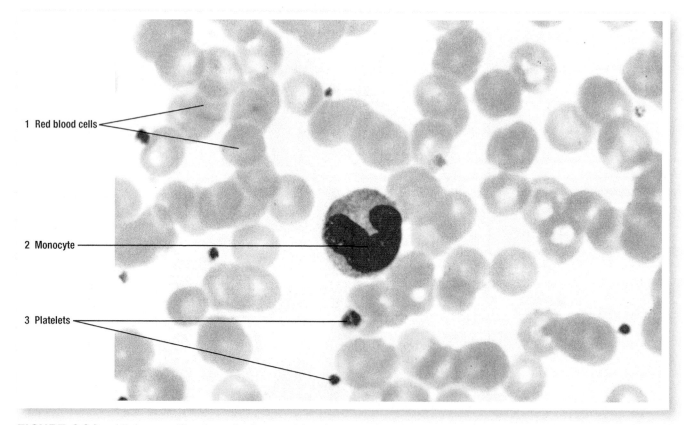

1 Red blood cells

2 Monocyte

3 Platelets

FIGURE 6.20 ■ High magnification of a human blood smear showing a large monocyte with characteristic "kidney-shaped" nucleus. Stain: Wright stain. ×350.

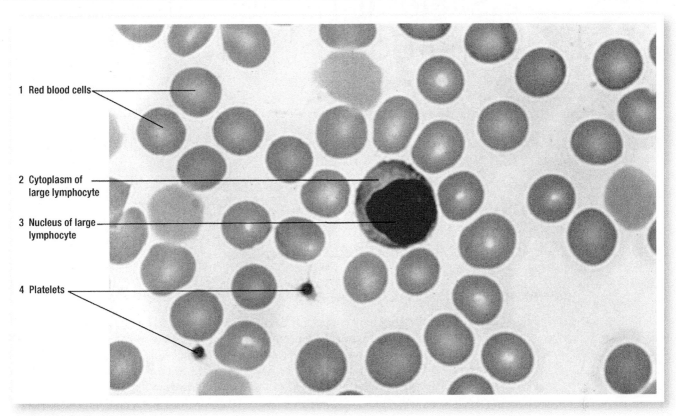

1 Red blood cells

2 Cytoplasm of large lymphocyte

3 Nucleus of large lymphocyte

4 Platelets

FIGURE 6.21 ■ High magnification of a human blood smear showing a seldom-seen large lymphocyte with a characteristic dense nucleus and a rim of visible, blue-staining cytoplasm. Stain: Wright stain. ×350.

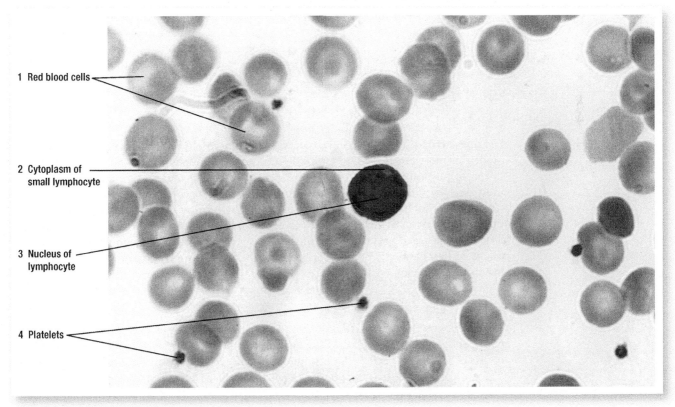

1 Red blood cells

2 Cytoplasm of small lymphocyte

3 Nucleus of lymphocyte

4 Platelets

FIGURE 6.22 ■ High magnification of a human blood smear showing a small lymphocyte with a dense blue nucleus occupying almost all of the cytoplasm. Stain: Wright stain. ×350.

Skeletal Tissue: Cartilage and Bone

SECTION 1 Cartilage

CHARACTERISTICS OF CARTILAGE

Cartilage is a special form of connective tissue that also develops from **embryonic mesenchymal cells**. Similar to other types of connective tissue, cartilage consists of cells and an **extracellular matrix** composed of connective tissue fibers and ground substance. In contrast to other connective tissue, however, cartilage does not have a direct blood supply; it is **nonvascular** (avascular). Because the extracellular cartilage matrix is **hydrated** (high water content), it receives its nutrition and eliminates its metabolic waste via **diffusion** through the extracellular matrix.

Cartilage exhibits tensile strength, provides firm structural support for soft tissues, allows flexibility without distortion, and is resilient to compression. Cartilage consists mainly of cells called **chondroblasts** and **chondrocytes** that synthesize the extensive extracellular matrix. This matrix contains **hyaluronic acid** and **glycosaminoglycans** that consist primarily of chondroitin sulfate and keratan sulfate. There are three main types of cartilage in the body: **hyaline**, **elastic**, and **fibrocartilage**. Their classification and histologic appearances are based on the amount and types of connective tissue fibers in the extracellular matrix.

CARTILAGE TYPES

Hyaline Cartilage

Hyaline cartilage is the most common type. In embryos, hyaline cartilage serves as a skeletal model for most bones. In developing bones of young individuals, hyaline cartilage persists in the **epiphyseal plates**, where its presence allows the bones to increase in length. As the individual ages, the cartilage model begins to calcify and be gradually replaced with bone (Fig. 7.1). In adults, epiphyseal plates fuse and the hyaline cartilage is replaced with bone, except on the articular surfaces of bones; at the ends of ribs (costal cartilage); and in the nose, larynx, trachea, and bronchi. Here, the hyaline cartilage persists throughout life and does not calcify to become bone. Bone is formed by either **endochondral ossification** or **intramembranous ossification**.

Elastic Cartilage

The histology of **elastic cartilage** is similar to hyaline cartilage, except for the presence of numerous branching, fine elastic fibers within its matrix. Elastic cartilage is highly flexible and occurs in the external ear; walls of the auditory tube; epiglottis; and a portion of the larynx, the cuneiform cartilage (thyroid). Similar to hyaline cartilage, chondroblasts synthesize the elastic fibers.

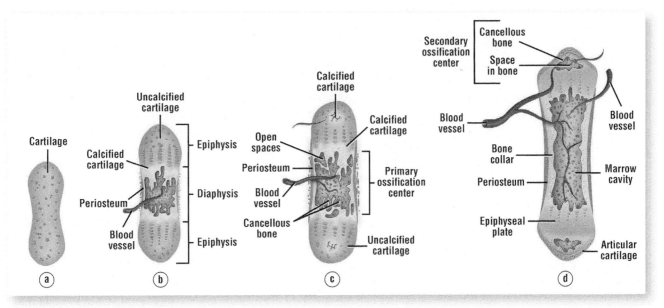

FIGURE 7.1 ■ Endochondral ossification illustrating the progressive stages of bone formation from a cartilage model of bone.

Fibrocartilage

Structurally, **fibrocartilage** exhibits a mixture of hyaline cartilage and dense bundles of coarse type I collagen fibers in its matrix. In contrast to hyaline and elastic cartilage, fibrocartilage consists of alternating layers of cartilage matrix and thick, strong, and dense layers of **type I collagen** fibers. The collagen fibers normally orient themselves in the direction of functional stress. In addition, the extracellular matrix is low on proteoglycans and water content. Fibrocartilage has a limited distribution in the body and is primarily found in the intervertebral disks, symphysis pubis, and certain joints.

PERICHONDRIUM

Most of the hyaline and elastic cartilage is surrounded by a peripheral layer of vascularized, dense, irregular connective tissue called the **perichondrium**. Its outer fibrous layer contains type I collagen fibers, fibroblasts, blood vessels, and nerves. The inner layer of perichondrium is cellular and contains undifferentiated **mesenchymal cells**, which differentiate into **chondroblasts** that secrete the external cartilage matrix. On the articulating surfaces of bones, however, hyaline cartilage is not lined or covered by perichondrium. Similarly, because fibrocartilage is always associated with dense connective tissue collagen fibers, it lacks the perichondrium seen in other cartilage.

CARTILAGE MATRIX

Cartilage matrix is produced and maintained by **chondrocytes** and **chondroblasts**. The collagen or elastic fibers give cartilage matrix its firmness and resilience. Similar to loose connective tissue, the extracellular **ground substance** of cartilage contains sulfated **glycosaminoglycans** and **hyaluronic acid** that bind with elastic and collagen fibers in the ground substance. Embedded within the cartilage matrix are collagen and elastic fibers, whose concentration determines whether the cartilage is hyaline, elastic, or fibrocartilage.

Hyaline cartilage matrix consists of the fine **type II collagen fibrils** embedded in a firm, amorphous hydrated matrix that is rich in proteoglycans and structural glycoproteins. Most proteoglycans in the cartilage matrix exist as large **proteoglycan aggregates** with sulfated glycosaminoglycans linked to core proteins and nonsulfated glycosaminoglycan hyaluronic acid.

The proteoglycan aggregates bind to the thin fibrils of the collagen matrix. The negatively charged glycosaminoglycan sulfated ions attract water molecules and hydrate the cartilage matrix. Hydrated cartilage matrix allows diffusion of molecules to and from the chondrocytes and allows cartilage to resist compression. Because of its hydration, cartilage can also act as a shock absorber in different parts of the body.

In addition to type II collagen fibrils and proteoglycans, cartilage matrix also contains an adhesive glycoprotein called **chondronectin**. These macromolecules bind to glycosaminoglycans and collagen fibers, providing adherence of chondroblasts and chondrocytes to collagen fibers of the surrounding matrix.

Although hyaline cartilage contains type II collagen fibers in its matrix, in routine histologic preparations, these collagen fibers are not seen because their reflective index is similar to that of the surrounding ground substance.

the**Point®** Supplemental micrographic images are available at **www.thePoint.com/Eroschenko13e** under Cartilage.

FIGURE 7.2 | Fetal Hyaline Cartilage

This figure illustrates hyaline cartilage in an early stage of development. **Superficial mesenchyme (1)** with cells and **blood vessels (5)** surrounds the nonvascular fetal cartilage. At this stage, lacunae around the **fetal chondroblasts (4, 7)** are not visible, and the chondroblasts (4, 7) resemble superficial mesenchymal cells (1). Fetal chondroblasts (4, 7) are randomly distributed without forming isogenous groups; they secrete the **intercellular cartilage matrix (8)**.

During fetal development, mesenchymal cells (1) concentrate on the periphery of the cartilage, and their nuclei become elongated. This region forms the **perichondrium (2, 6)**, a sheath of dense irregular connective tissue with fibroblasts (2, 6) that surrounds hyaline and elastic cartilage. The inner layer of the perichondrium (2, 6) becomes the **chondrogenic layer (3)** that gives rise to chondroblasts (4, 7).

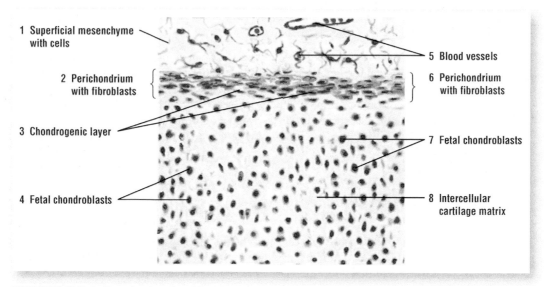

1 Superficial mesenchyme with cells

2 Perichondrium with fibroblasts

3 Chondrogenic layer

4 Fetal chondroblasts

5 Blood vessels

6 Perichondrium with fibroblasts

7 Fetal chondroblasts

8 Intercellular cartilage matrix

FIGURE 7.2 ■ Developing fetal hyaline cartilage. Stain: hematoxylin and eosin. Medium magnification.

FIGURE 7.3 | Hyaline Cartilage and Surrounding Structures: Trachea

This illustration depicts a hyaline cartilage plate from the trachea. The **perichondrium** (5) with **fibroblasts** (7) surrounds the cartilage. The inner **chondrogenic layer** (4) produces **chondroblasts** (8) that differentiate into chondrocytes. **Chondrocytes** in lacunae appear either single or in **isogenous groups** (3). Lacunae and chondrocytes (3) in the middle of the cartilage plate are large and spherical but become flatter toward the periphery, where these cells are differentiating into chondroblasts (8). The **interterritorial (intercellular) matrix** (1) stains lighter, whereas the **territorial matrix** (2) around the lacunae stains darker.

Vascular (9) **connective tissue** (10) and tracheal glands with grapelike secretory units called acini are near the cartilage. **Serous acini** (11) produce watery secretions, whereas mucous acini (12) secrete lubricating mucus. An **excretory duct** (6) delivers these secretions to the tracheal lumen.

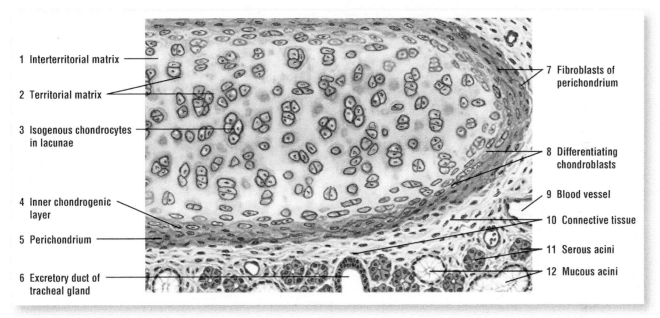

1 Interterritorial matrix

2 Territorial matrix

3 Isogenous chondrocytes in lacunae

4 Inner chondrogenic layer

5 Perichondrium

6 Excretory duct of tracheal gland

7 Fibroblasts of perichondrium

8 Differentiating chondroblasts

9 Blood vessel

10 Connective tissue

11 Serous acini

12 Mucous acini

FIGURE 7.3 ■ Hyaline cartilage and surrounding structures: trachea. Stain: hematoxylin and eosin. Medium magnification.

FUNCTIONAL CORRELATIONS 7.1 ■ Cartilage Cells

Cartilage develops from **mesenchymal cells** that differentiate into **chondroblasts**. These cells divide mitotically and synthesize the cartilage **matrix** and **extracellular material** around them. As the cartilage model grows, the individual chondroblasts become surrounded by the extracellular matrix and trapped in matrix compartments called **lacunae** (singular, lacuna). Lacunae contain mature cartilage cells called **chondrocytes**. The main function of chondrocytes is to maintain the components of the extracellular cartilage matrix. Some lacunae may contain more than one chondrocyte; these groups of chondrocytes are called **isogenous groups**.

Mesenchymal cells can also differentiate into fibroblasts that form the **perichondrium** around the cartilage. The inner cellular layer of the perichondrium contains chondrogenic cells that can differentiate into chondroblasts, secrete the cartilage matrix, and become trapped in lacunae as chondrocytes

FIGURE 7.4 | Cells and Matrix of Mature Hyaline Cartilage

Higher magnification illustrates an interior region of mature hyaline cartilage. Distributed throughout the homogeneous ground substance, the **matrix** (**4**, **5**), are ovoid spaces called **lacunae** (**3**) containing **mature chondrocytes** (**1**, **2**). In intact cartilage, chondrocytes fill the lacunae. Each chondrocyte has a granular cytoplasm and a **nucleus** (**1**). During histologic preparations, chondrocytes (**1**, **2**) shrink, and the lacunae (**3**) appear as clear spaces. Cartilage cells in the matrix are seen either singly or in isogenous groups.

Hyaline cartilage matrix (**4**, **5**) appears homogeneous and usually basophilic. The lighter-staining matrix between chondrocytes (**2**) is called **interterritorial matrix** (**5**). The more basophilic or darker matrix adjacent to the chondrocytes is the **territorial matrix** (**4**).

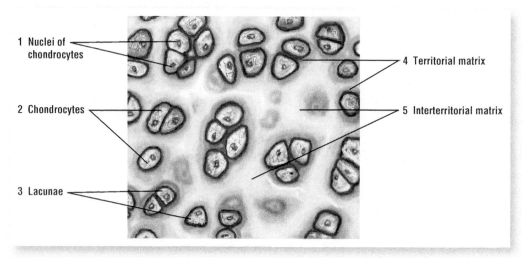

FIGURE 7.4 ■ Cells and matrix of mature hyaline cartilage. Stain: hematoxylin and eosin. High magnification.

FIGURE 7.5 | Hyaline Cartilage: Developing Bone

A photomicrograph of a section through a developing bone shows a portion of the hyaline cartilage and its homogenous **matrix** (**1**). Located within the matrix (**1**) are the mature hyaline cartilage cells, the **chondrocytes** (**3**) in their **lacunae** (**2**). Surrounding the hyaline cartilage is the

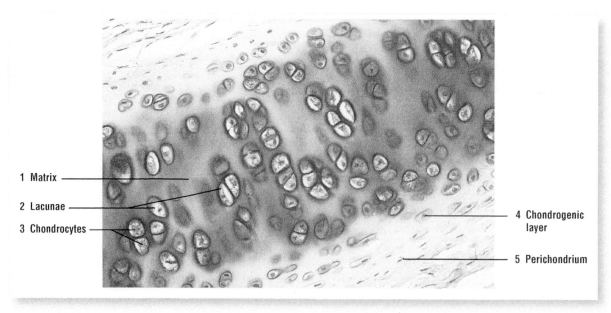

FIGURE 7.5 ■ Hyaline cartilage: developing bone. Stain: hematoxylin and eosin. ×80.

dense perichondrium (5). On the inner surface of the **perichondrium** (5) is the **chondrogenic layer** (4). The more central cells in the cartilage appear as rounded chondrocytes, whereas the peripheral cells are flattened and appear as typical chondroblasts.

FIGURE 7.6 | Elastic Cartilage: Epiglottis

Elastic cartilage differs from hyaline cartilage by the presence of numerous **elastic fibers** (4) in its **matrix** (7). Staining the cartilage of the epiglottis with silver reveals thin elastic fibers (4) that enter the cartilage matrix from the surrounding connective tissue **perichondrium** (1) and are distributed as branching and anastomosing fibers. The density of the fibers varies among elastic cartilages as well as among different areas of the same cartilage.

As in hyaline cartilage, larger **chondrocytes** in the **lacunae** (3, 8) are more prevalent in the interior of the plate. The smaller and flatter chondrocytes are located peripherally in the inner **chondrogenic layer** of the **perichondrium** (2), from which chondroblasts develop to synthesize the cartilage matrix. Also visible in the perichondrium (1) are the connective tissue **fibrocytes** (5) and a **venule** (6).

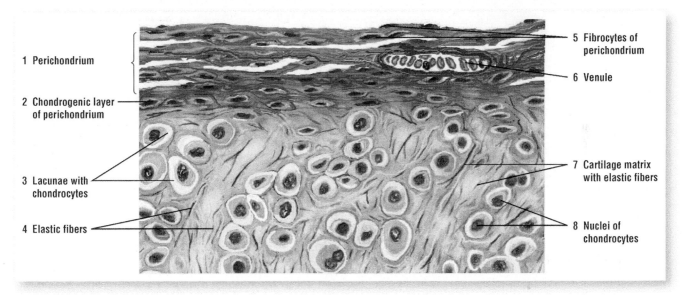

1 Perichondrium

2 Chondrogenic layer of perichondrium

3 Lacunae with chondrocytes

4 Elastic fibers

5 Fibrocytes of perichondrium

6 Venule

7 Cartilage matrix with elastic fibers

8 Nuclei of chondrocytes

FIGURE 7.6 ■ Elastic cartilage: epiglottis. Stain: silver. High magnification.

FUNCTIONAL CORRELATIONS 7.2 ■ Cartilage (Hyaline, Elastic, and Fibrocartilage)

Cartilage is nonvascular, but it is surrounded by vascular connective tissue, the **perichondrium**. Because of the high water (hydration) content in the cartilage, all nutrients enter and metabolites leave the cartilage by diffusing through the matrix. Also, the cartilage matrix is soft and pliable, not as hard or rigid as bone. As a result, cartilage can simultaneously grow by two different processes: interstitial growth and appositional growth.

Interstitial growth involves mitosis of chondroblasts within the matrix and deposition of new matrix between and around the new cells. This process increases cartilage growth and size from within. In contrast, **appositional growth** occurs on the periphery of the cartilage. Here, chondroblasts differentiate from the inner **chondrogenic** cellular layer of the perichondrium and deposit a layer of cartilage matrix

that is apposed to the existing cartilage layer. This growth process increases cartilage width.

Hyaline cartilage provides a firm structural and flexible support. Elastic cartilage with branching elastic fibers confers structural support as well as increased flexibility. In contrast to hyaline cartilage, which can calcify with aging, the matrix of elastic cartilage does not calcify, and the cartilage maintains its high flexibility.

Fibrocartilage is a tough, strong component that provides support for the body, especially in the vertebral column of the intervertebral disks. The main function of fibrocartilage is to provide tensile strength, bear weight, and resist stretch or compression. This cartilage type is always dense and filled with strong, thick type I collagen fibers and chondrocytes.

FIGURE 7.7 | Elastic Cartilage: Epiglottis

A photomicrograph of a section of an epiglottis shows the cartilage with fine, branching **elastic fibers** (2) in its **matrix** (5), in addition to distinct **chondrocytes** (3) and **lacunae** (4). The elastic fibers (2) gives this cartilage flexibility, in addition to support. Surrounding the elastic cartilage is the **perichondrium** (1).

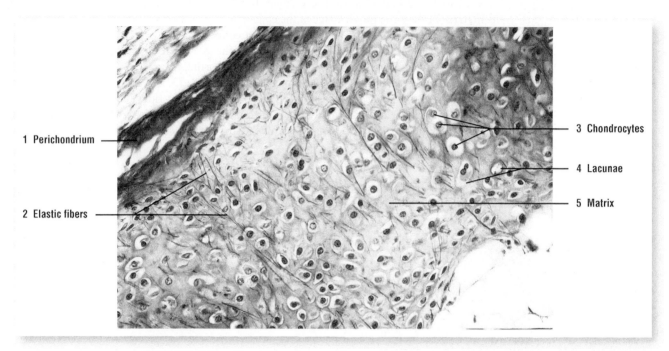

1 Perichondrium

2 Elastic fibers

3 Chondrocytes

4 Lacunae

5 Matrix

FIGURE 7.7 ■ Elastic cartilage: epiglottis. Stain: silver stain. ×80.

FIGURE 7.8 | Fibrocartilage: Intervertebral Disk

The fibrous cartilage **matrix** (5) is filled with dense **collagen fibers** (2, 6), which frequently exhibit parallel arrangement, as seen in tendons. Small **chondrocytes** (1, 4) in **lacunae** (3) are usually distributed in **rows** (4) within the fibrous cartilage matrix (5), rather than at random or in isogenous groups, as in hyaline or elastic cartilage. All chondrocytes and lacunae (1, 3, 4) are of similar size; there is no gradation from larger central chondrocytes to smaller and flatter peripheral cells.

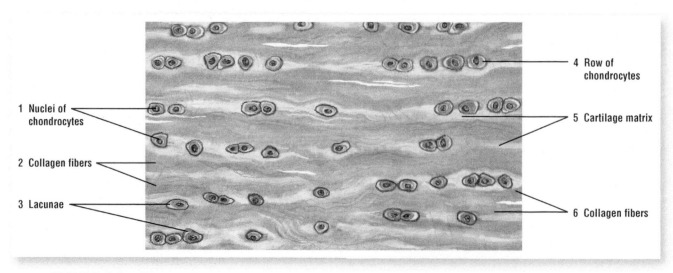

1 Nuclei of chondrocytes

2 Collagen fibers

3 Lacunae

4 Row of chondrocytes

5 Cartilage matrix

6 Collagen fibers

FIGURE 7.8 ■ Fibrocartilage: intervertebral disk. Stain: hematoxylin and eosin. High magnification.

A perichondrium is absent because fibrous cartilage usually forms a transitional area between hyaline cartilage and tendon or ligament.

The proportion of collagen fibers (2, 6) to cartilage matrix (5), the number of chondrocytes, and their arrangement in the matrix (5) vary. Collagen fibers (2, 6) may be so dense that the matrix (5) is invisible. In such case, chondrocytes and lacunae will appear flattened. Collagen fibers within a bundle are normally parallel, but collagen bundles may course in different directions.

FIGURE 7.9 | Fibrocartilage: Intervertebral Disk

This high-power photomicrograph from a section of an intervertebral disk illustrates the dense and compact composition of the fibrocartilage. Numerous **chondrocytes** in **lacunae** (**1**) are visible with dark **nuclei** (**3**). Some chondrocytes (1) are dispersed individually in the matrix or lined up in **rows** (**4, 5**) between the layers of dense **type I collagen fibers** (**2**) that course throughout the fibrous portion of the disk. The lighter-staining area between the collagen fibers (2) and the chondrocytes (1, 3, 4) is the **extracellular matrix** (**5**).

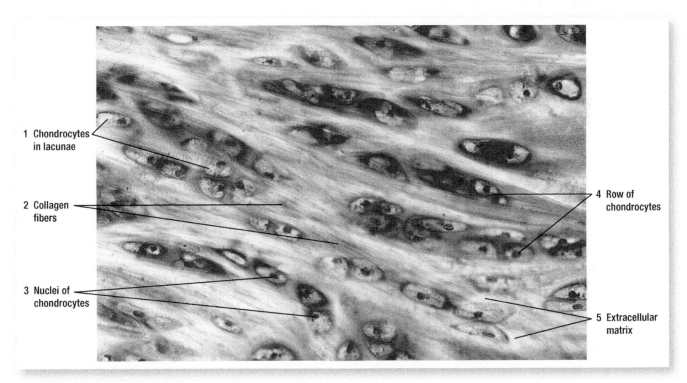

1 Chondrocytes in lacunae

2 Collagen fibers

3 Nuclei of chondrocytes

4 Row of chondrocytes

5 Extracellular matrix

FIGURE 7.9 ■ Dense fibrocartilage with chondrocytes and type I collagen fibers from a primate intervertebral disk. Stain: hematoxylin and eosin. ×205.

Chapter 7 Summary

SECTION 1 • Cartilage

CHARACTERISTICS OF CARTILAGE

- Develops from mesenchyme and consists of cells, connective tissue fibers, and ground substance
- Nonvascular, gets nutrients via diffusion through hydrated ground substance
- Performs numerous supportive functions
- Cells include chondroblasts and chondrocytes
- Three types of cartilage are hyaline, elastic, and fibrocartilage

HYALINE CARTILAGE

- Most common cartilage in the body and serves as a skeletal model for most bones
- In developing bones, cartilage present in epiphyseal plates allows bone growth in length
- Replaced by bone after calcification and endochondral ossification in certain areas
- Contains type II collagen fibrils, which are not seen in histologic sections due to a reflective index similar to that of ground substance
- In adults, perichondrium surrounds hyaline cartilage except on bone articulating surfaces
- Does not calcify on the articular surfaces of bones, ends of ribs (costal cartilage), the nose, larynx, trachea, and in bronchi

ELASTIC CARTILAGE

- Contains branching elastic fibers in matrix and is highly flexible
- Found in the external ear, auditory tube, epiglottis, and part of the larynx (cuneiform cartilage)

FIBROCARTILAGE

- Filled with dense of type I collagen fibers, extracellular matrix, and chondrocytes
- Provides tensile strength, bears weight, and resists compression in the vertebral column
- Found in intervertebral disks, symphysis pubis, and certain joints

PERICHONDRIUM

- Found on peripheries of hyaline and elastic cartilage
- Peripheral layer is dense vascular connective tissue with type I collagen
- Inner layer is chondrogenic and gives rise to chondroblasts that secrete cartilage matrix
- Articular hyaline cartilage of long bones and fibrocartilage not covered by perichondrium

CARTILAGE MATRIX

- Produced and maintained by chondrocytes and chondroblasts
- Contains large proteoglycan aggregates and is highly hydrated (high water content)
- Allows diffusion and is semirigid shock absorber
- Adhesive glycoprotein chondronectin binds cells and fibrils to the surrounding matrix
- Elastic cartilage provides structural support and increased flexibility without distortion

CARTILAGE CELLS

- Mesenchymal cells differentiate into chondroblasts that synthesize the matrix
- Mesenchyme also differentiates into fibroblasts in the perichondrium
- Mature cartilage cells, chondrocytes, become enclosed in lacunae
- Main function of chondrocytes is to maintain the cartilage matrix
- Inner layer of surrounding connective tissue perichondrium is chondrogenic
- Cartilage grows by both interstitial and appositional growth

Chapter 7 Review Questions: Section 1

QUESTIONS

In the following multiple choice questions, choose the letter corresponding to the one best answer.

1. What is responsible for the high water content in cartilage?

A. Proteoglycan aggregates
B. Collagen fibers
C. Perichondrium
D. Elastic fibers
E. Blood vessels

2. Type II collagen fibers are not seen histologically in hyaline cartilage because:

A. hyaline cartilage is devoid of any collagen fibers.
B. they are covered by chondrocytes and chondroblasts.
C. of the presence of type I collagen fibers.
D. of the increased density of the cartilage matrix.
E. their reflective index is similar to that of the ground substance.

3. What is located in the lacunae of the cartilage matrix?

A. Chondroblasts
B. Mesenchyme cells
C. Chondrocytes
D. Fibrocytes
E. Collagen fibers

4. Where are the chondrogenic cells located in a cartilage model?

A. In the cartilage matrix
B. On the inner layer of perichondrium
C. In the isogenic chondrocyte groups
D. Adjacent to the collagen fibers of the matrix
E. Outside of the perichondrium

5. What serves as a skeletal model for most bones?

A. Elastic cartilage
B. Perichondrium
C. Epiphyseal plate
D. Hyaline cartilage
E. Glycosaminoglycans

ANSWERS

1. **Correct Answer: A.** Proteoglycan aggregates. Water molecules are attracted to the negatively charged sulfate ions in the proteoglycan aggregates.

2. **Correct Answer: E.** Their reflective index is similar to that of the ground substance of hyaline cartilage.

3. **Correct Answer: C.** Chondrocytes. After synthesizing the matrix, chondroblasts become surrounded by cartilage matrix, stop dividing, and become chondrocytes.

4. **Correct Answer: B.** On the inner layer of the perichondrium. This layer contains mesenchymal cells that differentiate into chondrogenic cells, chondroblasts, that produce the cartilage matrix.

5. **Correct Answer: D.** Hyaline cartilage. This cartilage produces a bone model for most bones of the body. The hyaline cartilage in most bones eventually calcifies and transforms into a bony structure.

ADDITIONAL HISTOLOGIC IMAGES

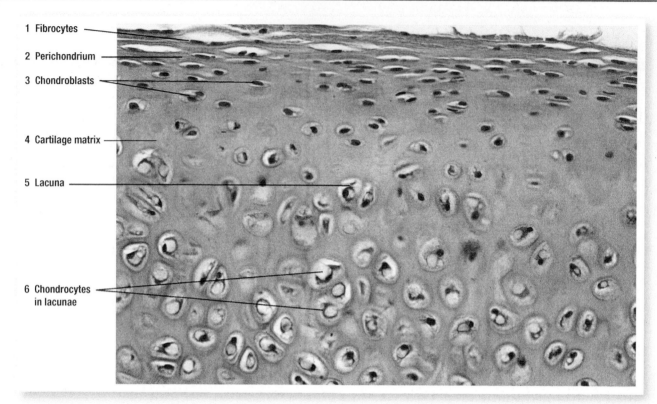

1 Fibrocytes
2 Perichondrium
3 Chondroblasts
4 Cartilage matrix
5 Lacuna
6 Chondrocytes in lacunae

FIGURE 7.10 ■ A peripheral section of hyaline cartilage showing the perichondrium and the cellular contents. Stain: hematoxylin and eosin. ×80.

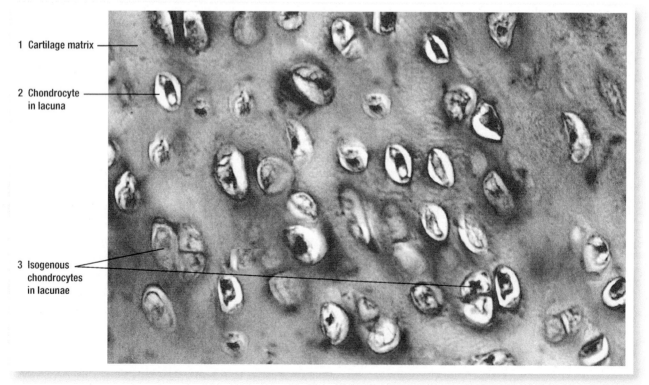

1 Cartilage matrix
2 Chondrocyte in lacuna
3 Isogenous chondrocytes in lacunae

FIGURE 7.11 ■ A higher magnification of the hyaline cartilage and its cellular contents. Stain: hematoxylin and eosin. ×130.

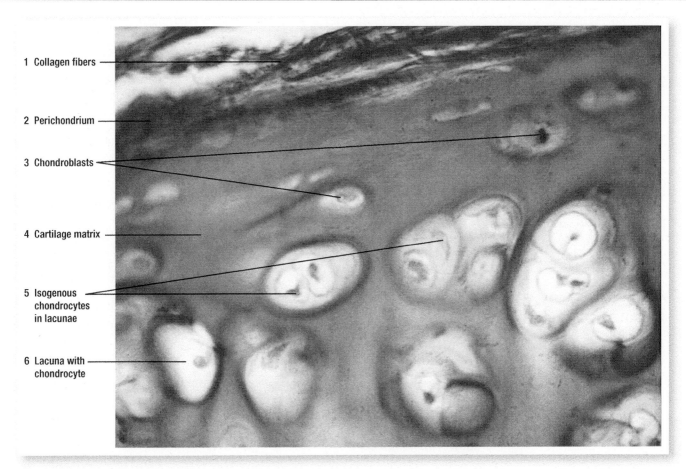

1 Collagen fibers
2 Perichondrium
3 Chondroblasts
4 Cartilage matrix
5 Isogenous chondrocytes in lacunae
6 Lacuna with chondrocyte

FIGURE 7.12 ■ A higher magnification of a peripheral section of hyaline cartilage with surrounding perichondrium. Stain: Mallory-Azan. ×205.

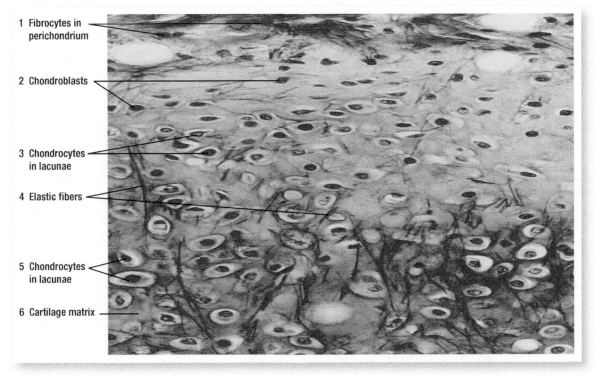

1 Fibrocytes in perichondrium
2 Chondroblasts
3 Chondrocytes in lacunae
4 Elastic fibers
5 Chondrocytes in lacunae
6 Cartilage matrix

FIGURE 7.13 ■ A section of an elastic cartilage showing the peripheral perichondrium and its contents. Stain: silver stain. ×80.

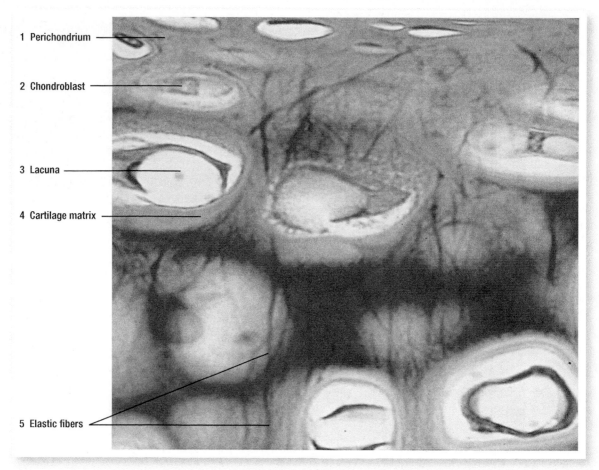

1 Perichondrium

2 Chondroblast

3 Lacuna

4 Cartilage matrix

5 Elastic fibers

FIGURE 7.14 ■ High magnification of elastic cartilage (peripheral section). Stain: blue stain. ×205.

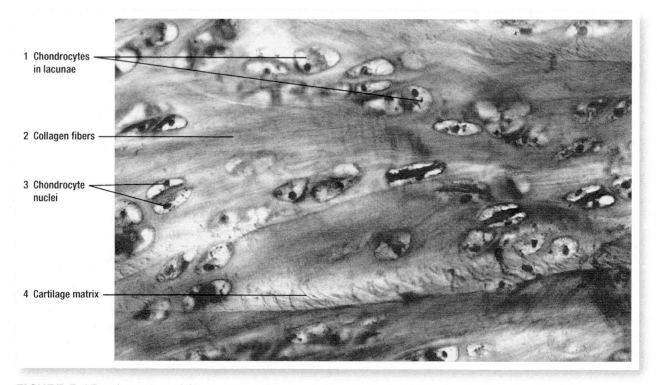

1 Chondrocytes
in lacunae

2 Collagen fibers

3 Chondrocyte
nuclei

4 Cartilage matrix

FIGURE 7.15 ■ A section of fibrocartilage from an intervertebral disk illustrating the density of the connective tissue. Stain: hematoxylin and eosin. ×205.

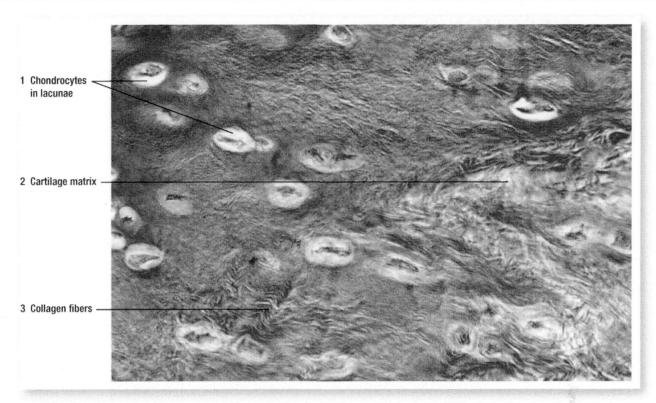

1 Chondrocytes in lacunae

2 Cartilage matrix

3 Collagen fibers

FIGURE 7.16 ■ A section of intervertebral disk showing the fibrocartilage cut at a different angle, the collagen fibers, and chondrocytes. Stain: blue stain. ×205.

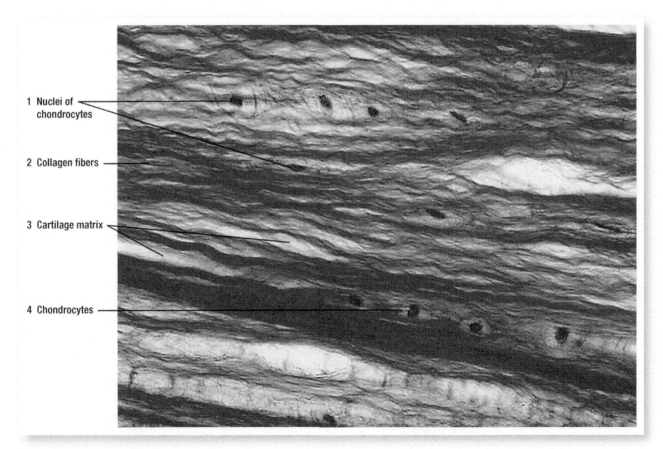

1 Nuclei of chondrocytes

2 Collagen fibers

3 Cartilage matrix

4 Chondrocytes

FIGURE 7.17 ■ Fibrocartilage from a different region of the intervertebral disk illustrating the dense collagen fibers and chondrocytes between the fibers. Stain: Mallory-Azan. ×205.

SECTION 2 Bone

CHARACTERISTICS OF BONE

Similar to cartilage, **bone** is also a special form of connective tissue consisting of **cells**, **connective tissue fibers**, and **extracellular matrix**. In contrast to cartilage, minerals accumulate and are deposited in the cartilage matrix causing calcification of the developing bones. Consequently, bones become hard and can bear more weight, serve as a rigid skeleton for the body, and provide attachment sites for muscles and organs.

Because of their strength, bones also protect the brain in the skull, the heart and lungs in the thorax, and the urinary and reproductive organs between the pelvic bones. In addition, adult bones with red marrow function in **hematopoiesis** (blood cell formation). Bones also serve as **reservoirs** for calcium, phosphate, and other essential minerals. Almost all (99%) of the calcium in the body is stored in bones, from which the body draws its daily calcium needs.

BONE MICROARCHITECTURE

All adult bones exhibit similar histology consisting of cells, bony matrix, and the neurovascular bundle (blood vessels, nerves, and lymphatics). Examination of bone in cross section shows two types: **compact bone** and **cancellous (spongy) bone** (Fig. 7.18). In long bones, the outer cylindrical part is the dense compact bone. The inner surface of the bone adjacent to the marrow cavity is the cancellous (spongy, not dense) bone with numerous interconnecting areas; however, both types of bone have a similar microscopic appearance. In newborns, the marrow cavities of long bones are red and produce blood cells. In adults, the marrow cavities of long bones are yellow and filled with adipose (fat) cells.

In compact bone, the collagen fibers are arranged in thin layers of bone called **lamellae** that are parallel to each other in the periphery or concentrically arranged around the blood vessels. In a long bone, the **outer circumferential lamellae** are deep to the surrounding connective tissue periosteum. **Inner circumferential lamellae** are located around the bone marrow cavity. **Concentric lamellae** surround the canals that contain an artery, vein, nerve, and loose connective tissue. Each concentric lamellar complex is called the **osteon (Haversian system)**. The space in the osteon that contains blood vessels and nerves is the **central (Haversian) canal**. Most of the compact bone consists of **osteons**, which are usually oriented along the long axis of the bone (see Fig. 7.18).

BONE TYPES

Distribution and orientation of the collagen fibers in the bone matrix indicate the bone type. The compact and cancellous adult bones exhibit a consistent structural pattern after maturation and mineralization. In contrast, **woven (immature or primary) bone** shows a random arrangement of collagen fibers; this type of arrangement is nonlamellar. The woven bone is encountered in the fetus during skeletal development and in repair of bone fractures. Also, the woven bone is **temporary** and is replaced by lamellar or mature bone as the individual ages.

The **lamellar (secondary or mature) bone** exhibits organized **lamellae** that are either multiple parallel or concentric layers of calcified matrix arranged around the central canals with the neurovascular bundle, or the osteons. Each lamella exhibits a parallel arrangement of collagen fibers that follow a helical course. Also, the bone cells, now called osteocytes, are in lacunae at regular intervals between the concentric layers of lamellae and are arranged circumferentially around the central canal. The matrix is more calcified in the lamellar bone than in the woven bone, and, as a result, the lamellar bone is stronger than the woven or immature bone.

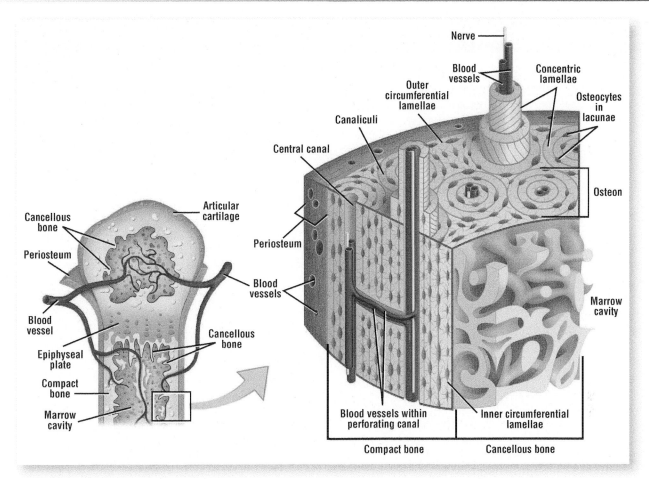

FIGURE 7.18 ■ Histology of a section of formed compact bone.

FUNCTIONAL CORRELATIONS 7.3 ■ Bone Cells and Their Function

All bones are lined on the internal and external surfaces by **osteogenic cells**. Developing and adult bones contain four cell types: osteoprogenitor cells, osteoblasts, osteocytes, and osteoclasts. Osteoprogenitor cells are undifferentiated, pluripotent stem cells derived from the connective tissue mesenchyme. Osteoprogenitor cells line the inner layer of the connective tissue that surrounds and contacts the bone, the **periosteum**, and in the thin, single layer of cells in the marrow cavities, the **endosteum**. Osteoprogenitor cells also line the osteons (Haversian system) and the perforating canals with blood vessels in the bone (see Fig. 7.18). The main functions of the periosteum and the endosteum are to provide nutrition for the bone and a continuous supply of new osteoblasts for growth, remodeling, and bone repair. During bone development, osteoprogenitor cells proliferate by mitosis and differentiate into osteoblasts, which secrete collagen fibers and the bony matrix.

Osteoblasts, derived from osteoprogenitor cells, are present on the inner surfaces of bone.

They synthesize, secrete, and deposit **osteoid**, the organic components of new bone matrix, which includes type I collagen fibers, several glycoproteins, and proteoglycans. Osteoid is initially uncalcified and does not contain any minerals; however, shortly after its deposition, it is rapidly mineralized and becomes hard bone. Osteoblasts initiate and regulate the mineralization of osteoid by releasing **matrix vesicles** that contain **alkaline phosphatase**, which increases phosphate ions that then combine with calcium ions. Increased concentrations of phosphate and calcium ions combine to form **hydroxyapatite crystals** and the initial centers of calcification. Further calcification surrounds these centers and embeds the collagen fibers and the glycoproteins.

Osteocytes are the mature osteoblasts that become surrounded by the mineralized bone matrix. They are also smaller than osteoblasts and are the principal cells of the bone. Like the chondrocytes in cartilage, osteocytes are trapped by the surrounding bone matrix in their **lacunae**. Osteocytes in

(continued)

FUNCTIONAL CORRELATIONS 7.3 ■ **Bone Cells and Their Function (*Continued*)**

the lacunae are very close to blood vessels. In contrast to cartilage, only one osteocyte is found per bony lacuna. Also, because mineralized bone matrix is harder than cartilage, nutrients and metabolites cannot diffuse through it to the osteocytes. Consequently, bone is highly vascular and possesses a unique system of channels or tiny canals called **canaliculi**, which open into the osteons.

Osteocytes exhibit numerous cytoplasmic extensions that enter the canaliculi and then radiate in all directions from each lacuna, and contact neighboring osteocytes via **gap junctions**, thus allowing the passage of ions and small molecules from cell to cell. The canaliculi contain extracellular fluid, and the gap junctions allow individual osteocytes to communicate with adjacent osteocytes and with materials in the blood vessels of the central canal. In this manner, the canaliculi form complex connections around the blood vessels in the osteons and constitute an efficient exchange mechanism: nutrients are brought to the osteocytes, gaseous exchange takes place between the blood and cells, and metabolic wastes are removed from the osteocytes. The canaliculi system keeps the osteocytes alive, and the osteocytes, in turn, maintain the homeostasis of the surrounding bone matrix and blood concentrations of calcium and phosphates. When an osteocyte dies, the surrounding bone matrix is reabsorbed by osteoclasts.

Osteoclasts are large, multinucleated cells found along bone surfaces where resorption (removal of bone), remodeling, and repair of bone take place.

Although osteoblasts and osteocytes arise from mesenchyme osteoprogenitor cell line, the osteoclasts are multinucleated cells that originate by fusion of blood or hematopoietic progenitor cells of the **mononuclear macrophage–monocyte cell line** of the red bone marrow. Osteoclasts are **phagocytic cells** that function in bone resorption during bone remodeling (renewal or restructuring) and are often located on the resorbed surfaces or in shallow depressions in the bone matrix called **Howship lacunae**. **Lysosomal enzymes** released by osteoclasts erode these depressions and demineralize the bony surface. During bone development, bone deposition by osteoblasts is closely coordinated with bone remodeling by the osteoclasts to maintain proper bone development and the bone mass.

Osteoclast activities are influenced by several hormones, including parathyroid hormone (PTH) from the parathyroid gland and calcitonin from the thyroid gland. Osteoblasts, activated by PTH, stimulate the development of osteoclasts by producing a molecule called **RANKL (receptor for activation of nuclear factor-kappa B ligand)**. This molecule in turn binds to **RANK receptors** on osteoclasts and stimulates the formation and activity of osteoclasts. Presence of membrane-bound proteins RANKL and **M-CSF (monocyte colony-stimulating factor)**, produced by surrounding stromal cells and osteoblasts, is needed for osteoclast formation. Activated osteoclasts increase the resorption of bone matrix and increase the levels of calcium in the blood.

BONE MATRIX

The bone matrix consists of **inorganic** (minerals), **organic** (collagen fibers) components, living cells, and extracellular material. Due to calcification or mineralization, the bone matrix is harder than cartilage, and no diffusion takes place. As a result, the bone matrix is highly vascularized. Blood vessels from the **periosteum** penetrate and enter the bone matrix via the perforating (**Volkmann) canals**. These canals run perpendicular to and join the vessels in the central canals of the osteon, which then supply all of the cellular components of the bone matrix.

The organic components enable bones to resist tension, whereas the mineral components resist compression. The major organic components of bone matrix are the coarse **type I collagen fibers**, the predominant proteins. The other organic components are sulfated glycosaminoglycans and hyaluronic acid that form larger proteoglycan aggregates. The glycoproteins **osteocalcin** and **osteopontin** bind tightly to calcium crystals and promote mineralization and calcification of the bone matrix. Another matrix protein, sialoprotein, binds osteoblasts to the extracellular matrix through the integrins of the plasma membrane proteins.

The inorganic component of bone matrix consists of the minerals calcium and phosphate in the form of hydroxyapatite crystals. The association of coarse collagen fibers with hydroxyapatite crystals provides the bone with its hardness, durability, and strength. In addition, as the need arises, actions of parathyroid hormone from the parathyroid gland and calcitonin from the thyroid gland on the bone adjust and maintain a proper mineral content in the blood.

PROCESS OF BONE FORMATION (OSSIFICATION)

Bone development begins in the embryo, the fetus, and continues after birth into adolescence. This development occurs by two processes: **endochondral ossification** and **intramembranous ossification**. Although the resulting bones are produced by two different methods, they exhibit the same histologic structure or morphology (see Fig. 7.1).

Endochondral Ossification

Most long bones, vertebrae, ribs, and the pelvis develop by **endochondral ossification** through replacement of the temporary hyaline cartilage models. This method allows the hyaline cartilage model to initially grow in length and width. Mesenchymal cells proliferate and differentiate into chondroblasts that produce the cartilage model for the bone. The cartilage model, surrounded by **perichondrium**, grows by both **interstitial** and **appositional** means, producing the short and long bones of the body. As the growth progresses, the chondroblasts divide, hypertrophy (enlarge), and mature, and the hyaline cartilage model begins to calcify. As calcification progresses, diffusion of nutrients and gases through the calcified cartilage matrix decreases. Consequently, chondrocytes degenerate and die, leaving a fragmented and porous calcified matrix as scaffolding for the deposition of bony material.

As the bony material is deposited around the calcifying cartilage, the inner perichondrial cells become osteogenic and form a thin bony collar around the midpoint of the shaft. The connective tissue around the new bone now becomes the **periosteum**, and the mesenchymal cells in the inner layer of periosteum differentiate into **osteoprogenitor** cells. Angiogenic factors produced by chondrocytes induce the formation of new blood vessels from the vascular periosteum. Osteoprogenitor cells and blood-forming cells invade the degenerating cartilage model with the blood vessels and differentiate into osteoblasts that proliferate, attach to the calcified cartilage remnants, and begin to deposit the bone matrix. Initially, the bone matrix is a soft collagenous **osteoid** that lacks minerals but is quickly mineralized into bone. The osteoblasts eventually become surrounded by bone in the lacunae and become osteocytes with one osteocyte per lacuna. Osteocytes establish a complex cell-to-cell connection through the canaliculi, which eventually open into central canals with blood vessels. In addition, osteoprogenitor cells also arise in **endosteum**, a single layer of cells that lines all internal cavities in the bone.

Mesenchymal tissue, osteoblasts, blood-forming cells, and blood vessels form the **primary ossification center** in the developing bone, which first appears in the **diaphysis** or the shaft of the long bone. This is followed by a **secondary ossification center** in the **epiphysis** or the articular surface of the expanded end of the bone. In all developing long bones, cartilage in the diaphysis and epiphysis is gradually replaced by bone, except in the **epiphyseal plate** region, located between the diaphysis and epiphysis. Interstitial cartilage growth in this region continues, lengthening the bone until bone growth stops. Expansion of the two ossification centers eventually replaces all cartilage with bone, including the epiphyseal plate, ending the bone growth in length. Hyaline cartilage is not replaced by bone on the free or **articulating** ends of long bones, where a layer of permanent hyaline cartilage covers the bone; this is the **articular cartilage**.

Intramembranous Ossification

In **intramembranous ossification**, bone development is not preceded by a hyaline cartilage model. Instead, bone develops directly from condensation of mesenchyme cells that produce **ossification centers**; flat bones develop by this method. The mesenchymal cells differentiate directly into osteoblasts that produce the surrounding osteoid matrix, which quickly calcifies. Numerous ossification centers are formed, anastomose, and produce a network of spongy bone that consists of thin rods, plates, and spines called **trabeculae**; this bone formation is by **appositional** growth. Located between the trabeculae is the hematopoietic tissue where the mesenchyme cells transform into blood-forming cells. In the bony matrix, osteoblasts also become surrounded by bone in the lacunae and become osteocytes. As in endochondral ossification, trapped osteocytes in the lacunae establish the cell-to-cell connection through the canaliculi.

The mandible, maxilla, clavicles, and most of the **flat bones** of the **skull** are formed by the intramembranous ossification. In the developing skull, the ossification centers grow radially, replace the connective tissue, and then fuse. In newborns, the **fontanelles** (soft spots) in the skull represent the membranous regions where intramembranous ossification of skull bones is still in the process of ossification. The surrounding mesenchymal tissue that does not ossify becomes the periosteum and endosteum of the new bones.

the Point® Supplemental micrographic images are available at **www.thePoint.com/Eroschenko13e** under Bone Development.

| FIGURE 7.19 | **Endochondral Ossification: Development of Long Bone (Panoramic View, Longitudinal Section)** |

During endochondral ossification, the bone is first formed as a model of embryonic hyaline cartilage. As bone development progresses, the cartilage is replaced by bone. The process of endochondral ossification can be followed by examining the upper part of the illustration and proceeding downward.

In the upper part, the hyaline cartilage is surrounded by the **perichondrium** (**13**). The **zone of reserve cartilage** (**1**) shows chondrocytes in their lacunae distributed singly or in small groups. Below this region is the **zone of proliferating chondrocytes** (**2**) where the chondrocytes divide and become arranged in vertical columns. **Chondrocytes in lacunae** (**14**) increase in size in the **zone of chondrocyte hypertrophy** (**3**) as a result of swelling of the nucleus and cytoplasm.

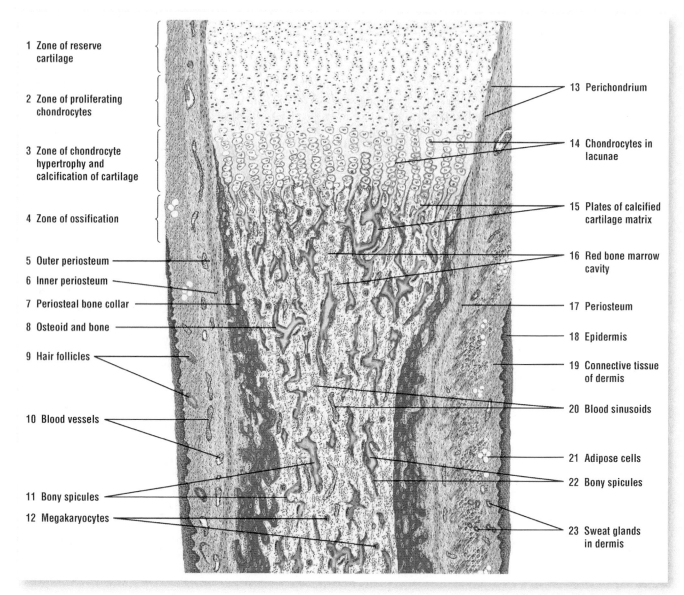

1 Zone of reserve cartilage

2 Zone of proliferating chondrocytes

3 Zone of chondrocyte hypertrophy and calcification of cartilage

4 Zone of ossification

5 Outer periosteum

6 Inner periosteum

7 Periosteal bone collar

8 Osteoid and bone

9 Hair follicles

10 Blood vessels

11 Bony spicules

12 Megakaryocytes

13 Perichondrium

14 Chondrocytes in lacunae

15 Plates of calcified cartilage matrix

16 Red bone marrow cavity

17 Periosteum

18 Epidermis

19 Connective tissue of dermis

20 Blood sinusoids

21 Adipose cells

22 Bony spicules

23 Sweat glands in dermis

FIGURE 7.19 ■ Endochondral ossification: development of a long bone (panoramic view, longitudinal section). Stain: hematoxylin and eosin. Low magnification.

The hypertrophied chondrocytes degenerate, forming thin **plates of calcified cartilage matrix (15)**. Below this region is the **zone of ossification (4)**, where a bony material is deposited on the plates of calcified cartilage matrix (15).

Blood sinusoids (20) or capillaries invade the calcifying cartilage. Lacunar walls and the calcified cartilage (15) are eroded, and the **red bone marrow cavity (16)** is formed. The connective tissue around the newly formed bone is now called **periosteum (5, 6, 17)** and is now the zone of ossification (4). In this illustration, bone is stained dark red. Osteoprogenitor cells from the **inner periosteum (6)** continue to differentiate into osteoblasts, deposit **osteoid** and **bone (8)** around the remaining plates of calcified cartilage (15), and form the **periosteal bone collar (7)**.

Formation of new periosteal bone (7) keeps pace with the formation of new endochondral bone. The bone collar (7) increases in thickness and compactness as development proceeds. The thickest portion of the bone collar (7) is in the central part of the developing bone called the diaphysis. The primary center of ossification is located in the diaphysis, where the initial periosteal bone collar (7) is formed.

Red bone marrow (16) fills the cavity of newly formed bone with hematopoietic (blood forming) cells. Fine reticular connective tissue fibers in the bone marrow (16) are obscured by masses of developing erythrocytes, granulocytes, **megakaryocytes (12)**, **bony spicules (11, 22)**, numerous blood sinusoids (20), capillaries, and blood vessels.

Surrounding the shaft of the developing bone are the soft tissues. The **epidermis (18)** of skin is lined by stratified squamous epithelium. Below the epidermis (18) is the subcutaneous **connective tissue of the dermis (19)**, in which are seen in **hair follicles (9)**, **blood vessels (10)**, **adipose cells (21)**, and **sweat glands (23)**.

FIGURE 7.20 | Endochondral Ossification: Zone of Ossification

This figure shows endochondral ossification at higher magnification and in greater detail and corresponds to the upper region of Figure 7.19.

Proliferating chondrocytes (1, 14) are arranged in distinct vertical columns. Below is the zone of **hypertrophied chondrocytes (2, 15)**. Chondrocytes and lacunae undergo

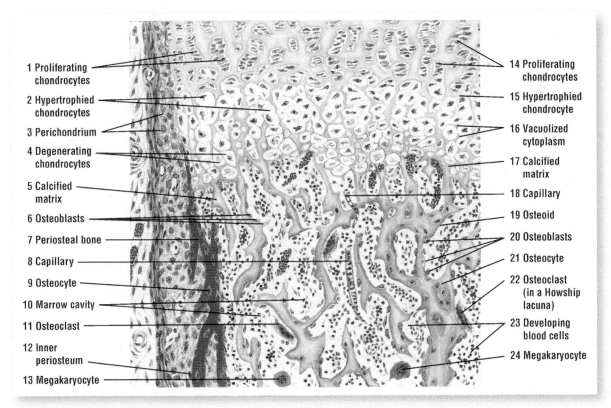

1 Proliferating chondrocytes
2 Hypertrophied chondrocytes
3 Perichondrium
4 Degenerating chondrocytes
5 Calcified matrix
6 Osteoblasts
7 Periosteal bone
8 Capillary
9 Osteocyte
10 Marrow cavity
11 Osteoclast
12 Inner periosteum
13 Megakaryocyte

14 Proliferating chondrocytes
15 Hypertrophied chondrocyte
16 Vacuolized cytoplasm
17 Calcified matrix
18 Capillary
19 Osteoid
20 Osteoblasts
21 Osteocyte
22 Osteoclast (in a Howship lacuna)
23 Developing blood cells
24 Megakaryocyte

FIGURE 7.20 ■ Endochondral ossification: zone of ossification. Stain: hematoxylin and eosin. Medium magnification.

hypertrophy as a result of increased glycogen and lipid accumulations in their cytoplasm and nuclear swelling. The cytoplasm of hypertrophied chondrocytes (2, 15) becomes **vacuolized** (16), the nuclei become pyknotic, and the thin cartilage plates become surrounded by **calcified matrix (5, 17)**.

Osteoblasts (6, 20) line up along remaining plates of calcified cartilage (5, 17) and lay down a layer of **osteoid (19)** and bone. Osteoblasts trapped in the osteoid or bone become **osteocytes (9, 21). Capillaries (8, 18)** from the **marrow cavity (10)** invade the newly ossified area.

The developing marrow cavity (10) contains numerous **megakaryocytes (13, 24)** and pluripotent stem cells that give rise to erythrocytic and granulocytic **blood cells (23)**. Multinucleated **osteoclasts (11, 22)** lie in shallow depressions called **Howship lacunae (11, 22)** and are adjacent to the bone that is being resorbed.

The left side of the illustration shows **periosteal bone** (7) with osteocytes (9) in their lacunae. The new bone is added peripherally by osteoblasts (6), which develop from osteoprogenitor cells of the **inner periosteum (12)**. The outer layer of connective tissues around the cartilage remains as the **perichondrium (3)**.

FIGURE 7.21 | Endochondral Ossification: Zone of Ossification

This photomicrograph illustrates the transformation of hyaline cartilage into bone through the process of endochondral ossification. The **hyaline cartilage matrix (6)** contains **proliferating chondrocytes (7)** and **hypertrophied chondrocytes (1)** with **vacuolated cytoplasm (2)**. Below these cells are plates or **spicules** of **calcified cartilage (3)** surrounded by **osteoblasts (4)**. As the cartilage calcifies, a **marrow cavity (5)** is formed with blood vessels, **hematopoietic tissue (10)**, osteoprogenitor cells, and osteoblasts (4). The hyaline cartilage is surrounded by the **perichondrium (8)**. The marrow cavity in the new bone is surrounded by the **periosteum (9)**.

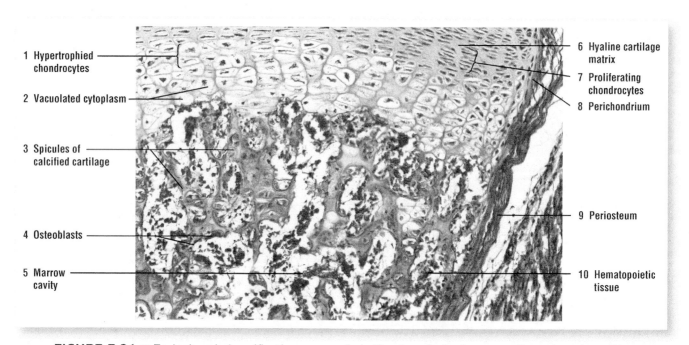

1 Hypertrophied chondrocytes
2 Vacuolated cytoplasm
3 Spicules of calcified cartilage
4 Osteoblasts
5 Marrow cavity
6 Hyaline cartilage matrix
7 Proliferating chondrocytes
8 Perichondrium
9 Periosteum
10 Hematopoietic tissue

FIGURE 7.21 ■ Endochondral ossification: zone of ossification. Stain: hematoxylin and eosin. ×50.

FIGURE 7.22 | Endochondral Ossification: Formation of Secondary (Epiphyseal) Centers of Ossification and Epiphyseal Plate in Long Bones (Longitudinal Section, Decalcified Bone)

The hyaline cartilage in the epiphyseal ends of two developing bones is illustrated. Both bones exhibit **secondary centers of ossification** (5, 11). Although cartilage is nonvascular, numerous **blood vessels** (1, 6), sectioned in a different plane, pass through the cartilage matrix to supply the osteoblasts and osteocytes in the secondary centers of ossification (5, 11). **Articular cartilage** (4, 12) covers both articulating ends of the future bone. A **synovial** or **joint cavity** (3) separates the two cartilage models. The inner synovial membrane of squamous cells lines the synovial cavity (3), except over the articular cartilages (4, 12). A synovial membrane, together with the connective tissue, may extend into the joint cavity as **synovial folds** (2, 13). The synovial cavity (3) is covered by a connective tissue capsule.

In the lower bone, an active **epiphyseal plate** (16) is seen between the secondary ossification center (5) and the developing shaft of the bone. A **zone** of **proliferating chondrocytes** (7) and a **zone** of **chondrocyte hypertrophy** and **calcification of cartilage** (8) are visible in the epiphyseal plate (16). Small **spicules of calcified cartilage** (9, 15) surrounded by red-stained bony material and **primitive bone marrow cavities** with **hematopoiesis** (14, 17) are seen in the shaft of the bone and the secondary center of ossification (5). A **megakaryocyte** (18) is also visible in the lower bone marrow cavity (17). **Periosteum** (19) surrounds the **compact bone** (10).

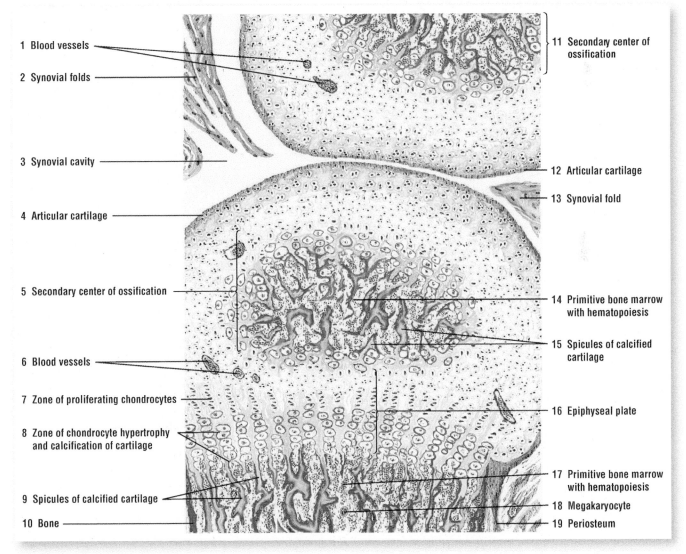

1 Blood vessels

2 Synovial folds

3 Synovial cavity

4 Articular cartilage

5 Secondary center of ossification

6 Blood vessels

7 Zone of proliferating chondrocytes

8 Zone of chondrocyte hypertrophy and calcification of cartilage

9 Spicules of calcified cartilage

10 Bone

11 Secondary center of ossification

12 Articular cartilage

13 Synovial fold

14 Primitive bone marrow with hematopoiesis

15 Spicules of calcified cartilage

16 Epiphyseal plate

17 Primitive bone marrow with hematopoiesis

18 Megakaryocyte

19 Periosteum

FIGURE 7.22 ■ Endochondral ossification: formation of secondary (epiphyseal) centers of ossification and the epiphyseal plate in a long bone (decalcified bone, longitudinal section). Stain: hematoxylin and eosin. Low magnification.

FIGURE 7.23 | Bone Formation: Development of Osteons (Haversian Systems; Transverse Section, Decalcified)

This illustration shows the **primitive bone marrow (15)** and developing osteons in a compact bone. Vascular tufts of connective tissue from the periosteum or endosteum invade and erode the bone and form primitive osteons. Bone reconstruction or remodeling will continue as the initial osteons, and then later ones, are broken down or eroded, followed by the formation of new osteons.

The new **bone matrix (11)** and **bone spicule (12)** of an immature compact bone are stained deep red with eosin due to the presence of collagen fibers. Numerous primitive osteons are visible in the transverse section, with large **central (Haversian) canals (2, 9)** surrounded by a few concentric **lamellae (9)** of bone and **osteocytes in lacunae (10)**. The central (Haversian) canals (2, 9) contain **primitive osteogenic connective tissue (13)** and **blood vessels (2)**. Bone deposition is continuing in some of the primitive osteons (2, 9), as indicated by the presence of **osteoblasts (1, 14)** around the central (Haversian) canals (2, 9) and the margin of the innermost bone lamella. In some osteons, the multinucleated **osteoclasts (6)** have formed and eroded shallow depressions called **Howship lacunae (5)** in the bone. Osteoclasts (6) continue to resorb and remodel the bone as it forms.

Primitive osteogenic connective tissue (13) passes through the bone, from which arise tufts of vascular connective tissue that give rise to new central (Haversian) canals (2, 9). Osteoblasts (1, 14) are located along the periphery of the developing central canals.

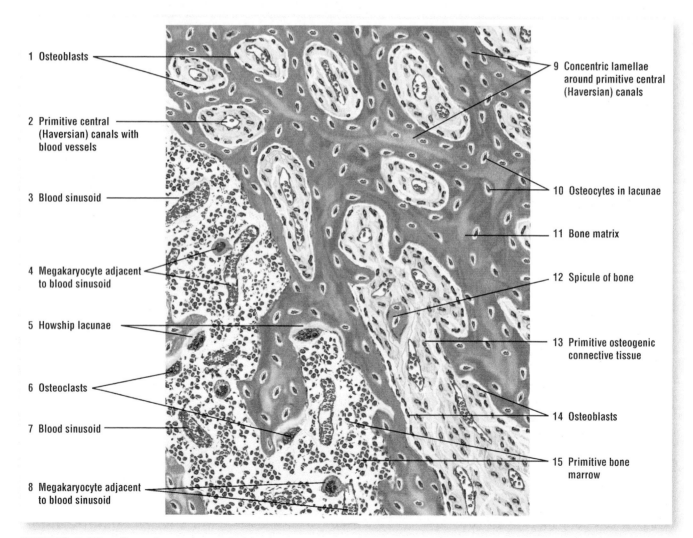

1 Osteoblasts

2 Primitive central (Haversian) canals with blood vessels

3 Blood sinusoid

4 Megakaryocyte adjacent to blood sinusoid

5 Howship lacunae

6 Osteoclasts

7 Blood sinusoid

8 Megakaryocyte adjacent to blood sinusoid

9 Concentric lamellae around primitive central (Haversian) canals

10 Osteocytes in lacunae

11 Bone matrix

12 Spicule of bone

13 Primitive osteogenic connective tissue

14 Osteoblasts

15 Primitive bone marrow

FIGURE 7.23 ■ Bone formation: primitive bone marrow and development of osteons (Haversian systems; decalcified bone, transverse section). Stain: hematoxylin and eosin. Medium magnification.

In the lower left corner of the figure is the primitive bone marrow (15), in which hematopoiesis (blood cell formation) is in progress; this is the red marrow. Also present in the bone marrow cavity (15) are developing erythrocytes and granulocytes, **megakaryocytes** (**4, 8**), **blood sinusoids (vessels)** (**3, 7**), and osteoclasts (6) in the eroded Howship lacunae (5). Some megakaryocytes (4, 8) are adjacent to the blood sinusoids. Their cytoplasmic processes protrude into these blood sinusoids, where they eventually fragment and enter the bloodstream as platelets.

FIGURE 7.24	**Intramembranous Ossification: Developing Mandible (Decalcified Bone, Transverse Section)**

This illustration depicts a section of mandible in the process of intramembranous ossification. External to the developing bone is the stratified squamous keratinized epithelium of the skin (1). Inferior to the **skin** (**1**), the embryonic mesenchyme has differentiated into the highly vascular primitive **connective tissue** (**2**) with **nerves and blood vessels** (**9**) and a denser **periosteum** (**3, 10**).

Below the periosteum (3, 10) is the developing bone. The cells in the periosteum (3, 10) have differentiated into **osteoblasts** (**6, 10**) and formed anastomosing **bone trabeculae** (**7, 11**) that surround the primitive **marrow cavities** (**8, 15**). In the marrow cavities (8, 15) are embryonic connective tissue cells and fibers, **blood vessels** (**4**), **arterioles** (**12**), and nerves. Peripherally, collagen fibers of the periosteum (3, 10) are in continuity with the fibers of the embryonic connective tissue of adjacent marrow cavities (3) and with collagen fibers within the trabeculae of bone (7, 11).

Osteoblasts (6, 10) deposit the bony matrix and are in linear arrangement along the developing trabeculae of bone (7, 11). **Osteoid** (**14**), the newly synthesized bony matrix, is seen on the margins of bony trabeculae. The **osteocytes** (**5**) are located in lacunae of the trabeculae (7, 11). The multinucleated **osteoclasts** (**13**) resorb and remodel bone during its formation.

Although collagen fibers in the bony matrix are obscured, the continuity with embryonic connective tissue fibers in the marrow cavities may be seen at the margins of numerous trabeculae (3).

Formation of new bone is not a continuous process. Inactive areas appear where ossification has temporarily ceased. Osteoid and osteoblasts are not present in these areas. In some primitive marrow cavities, fibroblasts differentiate into osteoblasts (3, 10).

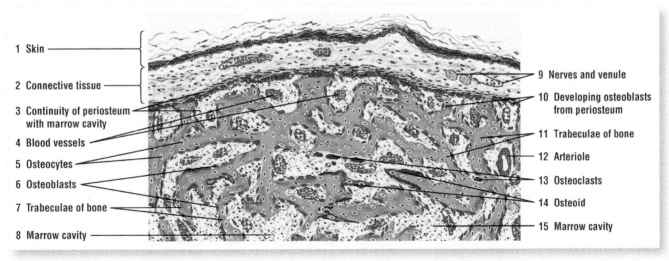

1 Skin
2 Connective tissue
3 Continuity of periosteum with marrow cavity
4 Blood vessels
5 Osteocytes
6 Osteoblasts
7 Trabeculae of bone
8 Marrow cavity

9 Nerves and venule
10 Developing osteoblasts from periosteum
11 Trabeculae of bone
12 Arteriole
13 Osteoclasts
14 Osteoid
15 Marrow cavity

FIGURE 7.24 ■ Intramembranous ossification: developing mandible (decalcified bone, transverse section). Stain: Mallory-Azan. Low magnification.

FIGURE 7.25 | Intramembranous Ossification: Developing Skull Bone

A higher-power photomicrograph illustrates the development of skull bone by the process of intramembranous ossification. The connective tissue **periosteum** (5) surrounds the developing bone and gives rise to the **osteoblasts** (1, 6) that form the **bone** (7). Osteoblasts (1, 6) are located along the developing **bony trabeculae** (3). Trapped within the formed bone (7) and the bony trabeculae (3) are the **osteocytes** (2) in their lacunae. Also associated with the bony trabeculae (3) are the multinuclear **osteoclasts** (8) that remodel the developing bone. A primitive **marrow cavity** (4) with **blood vessels** (9), **blood cells** (9), and hematopoietic tissue is located between the formed bony trabeculae (3).

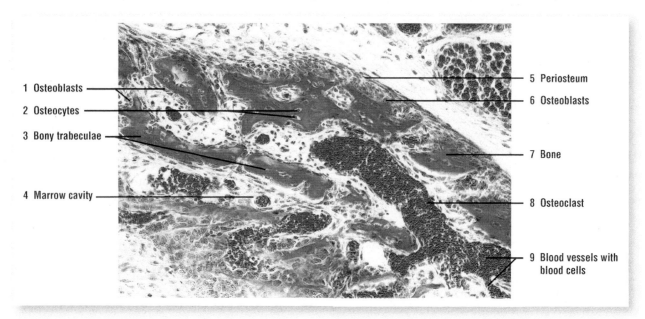

1 Osteoblasts
2 Osteocytes
3 Bony trabeculae
4 Marrow cavity

5 Periosteum
6 Osteoblasts
7 Bone
8 Osteoclast
9 Blood vessels with blood cells

FIGURE 7.25 ■ Intramembranous ossification: developing skull bone (decalcified bone; transverse section). Stain: Mallory-Azan. ×64.

FIGURE 7.26 | Cancellous Bone with Trabeculae and Marrow Cavities: Sternum (Transverse Section, Decalcified)

Cancellous bone consists of slender **bony trabeculae** (5) that ramify, anastomose, and enclose irregular **marrow cavities with blood vessels** (4). The **periosteum** (2, 7) that surrounds the trabeculae (5) of cancellous bone merges with adjacent dense irregular **connective tissue** with

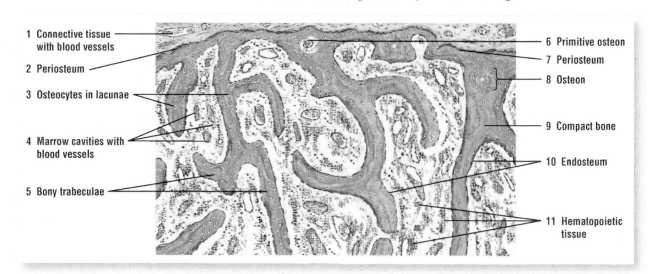

1 Connective tissue with blood vessels
2 Periosteum
3 Osteocytes in lacunae
4 Marrow cavities with blood vessels
5 Bony trabeculae

6 Primitive osteon
7 Periosteum
8 Osteon
9 Compact bone
10 Endosteum
11 Hematopoietic tissue

FIGURE 7.26 ■ Cancellous bone with trabeculae and bone marrow cavities: sternum (decalcified bone, transverse section). Stain: hematoxylin and eosin. Low magnification.

blood vessels (**1**). Inferior to the periosteum (**2, 7**), the bony trabeculae (**5**) merge with a thin layer of **compact bone** (**9**) that contains a forming or **primitive osteon** (**6**) and a **mature osteon (Haversian system)** (**8**) with concentric lamellae.

Except for concentric lamellae in the primitive osteon (**6**) and the mature osteon (**8**), the bone inferior to the periosteum (**2, 7**) and the bony trabeculae (**5**) exhibit parallel lamellae. **Osteocytes** (**3**) in lacunae are visible in trabeculae (**5**) and compact bone (**9**).

Between bony trabeculae (**5**) are the marrow cavities with blood vessels (**4**) and **hematopoietic tissue** (**11**) that gives rise to new blood cells. Because of the low magnification, individual red and white blood cells are not recognizable. Lining the bony trabeculae (**5**) in the marrow cavities (**4**) is a thin inner layer of cells called **endosteum** (**10**). Cells in the periosteum (**2, 7**) and in the endosteum (**10**) give rise to bone-forming osteoblasts.

FIGURE 7.27 | Cancellous Bone: Sternum (Transverse Section, Decalcified)

This photomicrograph shows a section of cancellous bone from the sternum. Cancellous bone is composed of numerous **bony trabeculae** (**1**) separated by the **marrow cavity** (**5**) with **blood vessels** (**7**) and different **blood cells** (**8**). Bony trabeculae (**1**) are lined by a thin inner layer of cells of the **endosteum** (**4, 6**). Osteoprogenitor cells in the endosteum (**4, 6**) give rise to osteoblasts. Formed bone matrix contains numerous **osteocytes** in **lacunae** (**2**). The large, multinuclear **osteoclasts** (**3**) are eroding or remodeling the formed bone matrix. Osteoclasts (**3**) erode part of the bone through enzymatic action and lie in Howship lacunae.

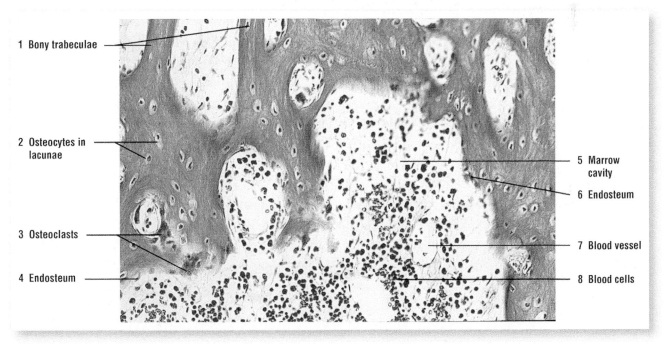

1 Bony trabeculae

2 Osteocytes in lacunae

3 Osteoclasts

4 Endosteum

5 Marrow cavity

6 Endosteum

7 Blood vessel

8 Blood cells

FIGURE 7.27 ■ Cancellous bone: sternum (decalcified bone, transverse section). Stain: hematoxylin and eosin. ×64.

FUNCTIONAL CORRELATIONS 7.4 ■ Bone

Bones are dynamic structures. They are continually renewed, or remodeled, in response to the mineral needs of the body, mechanical stress, thinning as a result of age or disease, and fracture healing. Calcium and phosphate are either stored in the bone matrix or released into the blood to maintain proper levels. Maintenance of normal blood calcium levels is critical to life, because calcium is essential for muscle contraction, blood coagulation, cell membrane permeability, transmission of nerve impulses, and numerous other functions.

Hormones regulate both the calcium release into the bloodstream and its deposition in the bones. When the calcium level falls below normal, **parathyroid hormone** (**PTH**), released from the parathyroid glands, indirectly promotes an increase in osteoclast proliferation and **osteoclast** activity by stimulating

osteoblasts to produce osteoclast-stimulating (differentiating) factors. This action induces increased breakdown of bone matrix by the osteoclasts and release of calcium. In addition, parathyroid hormone also increases calcium reabsorption in the kidneys and small intestine. These hormonal effects increase and/or maintain the calcium levels in the blood at normal levels. When the calcium level increases above normal, a hormone called **calcitonin**, released by **parafollicular cells or C cells** in the thyroid gland, decreases osteoclast activity, bone reabsorption, and blood calcium levels. In addition, the kidneys increase their excretion of both calcium and phosphate. These effects lower the circulating calcium levels in the body. The actions of both thyroid and parathyroid glands and their hormones are discussed in more detail in Chapter 19.

FIGURE 7.28 | Compact Bone, Dried (Transverse Section)

This illustration depicts a transverse section of a dried compact bone. The bone was ground to a thin section to show empty canals for blood vessels, lacunae for osteocytes, and the connecting canaliculi.

The structural units of a compact bone matrix are the **osteons** (**Haversian systems**) (**3, 10**). Each osteon (3, 10) consists of layers of concentric **lamellae** (**3b**) arranged around a **central** (**Haversian**) **canal** (**3a**). Central canals are shown in cross section (3a) and in oblique

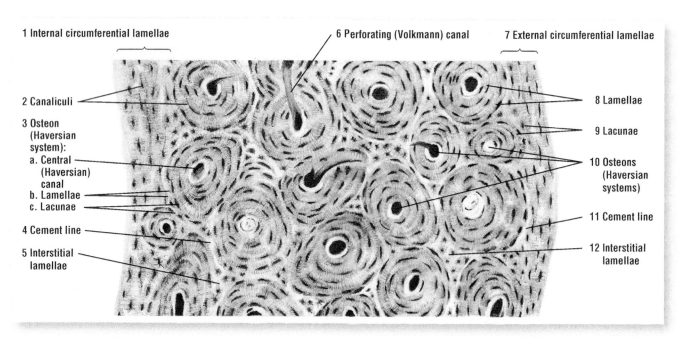

1 Internal circumferential lamellae
6 Perforating (Volkmann) canal
7 External circumferential lamellae
2 Canaliculi
3 Osteon (Haversian system):
a. Central (Haversian) canal
b. Lamellae
c. Lacunae
4 Cement line
5 Interstitial lamellae
8 Lamellae
9 Lacunae
10 Osteons (Haversian systems)
11 Cement line
12 Interstitial lamellae

FIGURE 7.28 ■ Dry, compact bone: ground, transverse section. Low magnification.

section (10, middle leader). Lamellae are thin plates of bone that contain osteocytes in almond-shaped spaces called **lacunae** (**3c**, **9**). Radiating from each lacuna in all directions are the **canaliculi** (**2**). Canaliculi (2) penetrate the lamellae (3b, 8), anastomose with canaliculi (2) from other lacunae (3c, 9), and form a network of communicating channels with other osteocytes. Some of the canaliculi (2) open directly into central (Haversian) canals (3a) of the osteon (3) and the marrow cavities of the bone. The small irregular areas of bone between osteons (3, 10) are the **interstitial lamellae** (**5**, **12**) that represent the remnants of eroded or remodeled osteons.

External **circumferential lamellae** (**7**) form the external wall of a compact bone (beneath the periosteum) and run parallel to each other and to the long axis of the bone. The internal wall of the bone (the endosteum along the marrow cavity) is lined by **internal circumferential lamellae** (**1**). Osteons (3, 10) are located between the internal circumferential lamellae (1) and the external circumferential lamellae (7).

In a living bone, the lacunae of each osteon (3c, 9) house osteocytes. The central canals (3a) contain reticular connective tissue, blood vessels, and nerves. The boundary between each osteon (3, 10) is outlined by a refractile line of modified bone matrix called the **cement line** (**4**, **11**). Anastomoses between central canals (3a) are called **perforating (Volkmann) canals** (**6**).

FIGURE 7.29	**Compact Bone, Dried (Longitudinal Section)**

This figure represents a small area of a dried compact bone, ground in a longitudinal plane. Because **central canals** (**1**, **9**) course longitudinally, each central canal is seen as a vertical tube that shows branching. Central canals (1, 9) are surrounded by **lamellae** (**2**, **6**) with **lacunae** (**4**) and radiating **canaliculi** (**5**). The lamellae (2, 6), lacunae (4), and the osteon boundaries, the **cement lines** (**3**, **8**), course parallel to the central canals (1, 9) in the compact bone.

Other canals that extend in either a transverse or oblique direction are the **perforating (Volkmann) canals** (**7**). Perforating canals (7) join the central canals (1, 9) of osteons with the marrow cavity. The perforating canals (7) do not have concentric lamellae. Instead, they penetrate directly through the lamellae (2, 6).

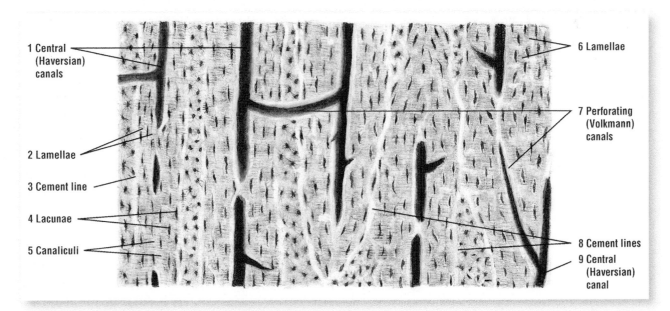

1 Central (Haversian) canals
2 Lamellae
3 Cement line
4 Lacunae
5 Canaliculi
6 Lamellae
7 Perforating (Volkmann) canals
8 Cement lines
9 Central (Haversian) canal

FIGURE 7.29 ■ Dry, compact bone: ground, longitudinal section. Low magnification.

FIGURE 7.30 | Compact Bone, Dried: Osteon (Transverse Section)

A higher magnification illustrates the details of one osteon and portions of adjacent osteons. Located in the center of the osteon is the dark-staining **central (Haversian) canal** (3) surrounded by the concentric **lamellae** (4). Between adjacent osteons are the **interstitial lamellae** (5). The dark, almond-shaped structures between the lamellae (4) are the **lacunae** (1, 7) that house osteocytes in living bone.

Tiny **canaliculi** (2) radiate from individual lacuna (1, 7) to adjacent lacunae and form a system of communicating canaliculi (2) throughout the bony matrix and within the central canal (3). The canaliculi (2) contain tiny cytoplasmic extensions of the osteocytes. In this manner, osteocytes around the osteon communicate with each other and blood vessels in the central canals. The outer boundary of the osteon is separated by a **cement line** (6).

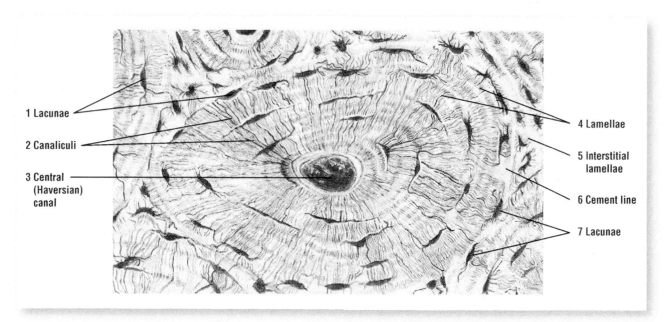

1 Lacunae
2 Canaliculi
3 Central (Haversian) canal
4 Lamellae
5 Interstitial lamellae
6 Cement line
7 Lacunae

FIGURE 7.30 ■ Dry, compact bone: an osteon, transverse section. High magnification.

Chapter 7 Summary

SECTION 2 • Bone

CHARACTERISTICS OF BONE

- Consists of cells, connective tissue fibers, and extracellular material
- Mineral deposits in the bone matrix produce a hard structure for protecting various organs
- Functions in hematopoiesis and as reservoir for calcium and minerals

BONE MICROARCHITECTURE

- All bones exhibit similar histology; there are two types of bones
- Compact bone is the outer cylindrical part of long bone
- Inner bone adjacent to bone marrow is the cancellous (spongy) bone
- In newborn bones, marrow is red and hematopoietic; in adults, the marrow of long bone is yellow and does not function in hematopoiesis
- Outer circumferential lamellae are located deep to the periosteum
- Inner circumferential lamellae are located around the bone marrow
- Concentric lamellae form osteons in compact bone and surround the central canal
- Most osteons are oriented in the long axis of the bone

BONE TYPES

- Orientation of collagen fibers indicates bone type
- Compact and cancellous bones show similar microscopic structure
- Woven (immature) bone has a random orientation of collagen fibers and is nonlamellar
- Woven bone is seen during fetal bone development and bone repair
- Lamellar (mature) bone with concentric lamellae around the central canal is in adults
- In lamellar bone, collagen fibers exhibit parallel arrangements that follow a helical course
- Osteocytes in lamellar bone are arranged around the central canal

BONE CELLS AND THEIR FUNCTION

Osteoprogenitor Cells

- Osteoprogenitor cells are derived from mesenchyme and are located in the inner layer of periosteum, endosteum, osteons, and perforating canals
- Osteoprogenitor cells differentiate into osteoblasts

Osteoblasts

- Osteoblasts are on the bone surfaces and synthesize the osteoid matrix with collagen fibers and different glycoproteins
- Osteoblasts release matrix vesicles that form hydroxyapatite and calcification of osteoid
- Osteoblasts produce RANKL (receptor for activation of nuclear factor-kappa B ligand)
- M-CSF (monocyte colony–stimulating factor) produced by osteoblasts is needed for osteoclast formation

Osteocytes

- Osteocytes are mature osteoblasts, are located in lacunae, and use canaliculi for communication and exchange of metabolic products and nutrients
- Osteocytes maintain homeostasis of bone and blood concentrations of calcium and phosphate

Osteoclasts

- Osteoclasts are multinucleated phagocytic cells responsible for resorption, remodeling, and bone repair
- Belong to the mononuclear macrophage–monocyte cell line and are found in enzyme-eroded depressions (Howship lacunae)
- Activity influenced by parathyroid hormone and calcitonin
- RANKL molecule binds to RANK receptors on osteoclasts and stimulates osteoclast activity

BONE MATRIX

- Highly vascularized with blood vessels from periosteum to aid diffusion through calcified matrix
- Organic components of bone resist tension, whereas mineral components resist compression
- Major organic component is coarse type I collagen fibers

- Glycoprotein components bind to calcium crystals during mineralization
- Inorganic components are calcium and phosphate in the form of hydroxyapatite crystals
- Hormones from the parathyroid gland (parathyroid hormone) and the thyroid gland (calcitonin) are responsible for maintaining the proper mineral content of blood

PROCESS OF BONE FORMATION (OSSIFICATION)

Endochondral Ossification

- Most bones develop by this process, with a hyaline cartilage model preceding bone
- Hyaline cartilage model grows in length and width, then calcifies, and chondrocytes die
- Mesenchymal cells in the periosteum differentiate into osteoprogenitor cells and form osteoblasts
- Osteoblasts synthesize the osteoid matrix, which calcifies and traps osteoblasts in lacunae as osteocytes
- Osteocytes establish cell-to-cell communication via canaliculi that open into blood channels
- Primary ossification center forms in the diaphysis and secondary center of ossification in the epiphysis
- Epiphyseal plate between the diaphysis and epiphysis allows for growth in bone length
- Eventually, all cartilage is replaced by bone except the articular cartilage

Intramembranous Ossification

- Mesenchymal cells differentiate directly into osteoblasts
- Osteoblasts produce the osteoid matrix that quickly calcifies

- Osteoblasts initially form spongy bone that consists of trabeculae and trap osteocytes
- Mandible, maxilla, clavicle, and flat skull bones are formed by this process
- Fontanelles in newborn skulls represent intramembranous ossification in progress

BONE TYPES

- In long bones, the outer part is compact bone, and the inner surface is cancellous bone
- Both bone types have the same microscopic appearance
- In compact bones, collagen fibers arranged in lamellae
- Lamellae deep to the periosteum are outer circumferential lamellae
- Lamellae surrounding the bone marrow are inner circumferential lamellae
- Lamellae surrounding the blood vessels, nerves, and loose connective tissue are osteons
- Within an osteon is the central canal, which is found in most compact bone

FUNCTIONAL CORRELATIONS OF BONE

- Continually remodeled in response to mineral needs, mechanical stress, thinning, or disease
- Maintain normal calcium levels in blood; critical to functions of numerous organs and life
- Parathyroid hormone increases calcium levels by indirectly stimulating osteoclasts to resorb bone as well as reabsorb calcium in the kidney and small intestine
- Hormones from the thyroid gland parafollicular (C) cells counteract parathyroid hormone
- Calcitonin inhibits osteoclasts, decreases calcium reabsorption, and increases calcium excretion in kidneys

Chapter 7 Review Questions: Section 2

QUESTIONS

In the following multiple choice questions, choose the letter corresponding to the one best answer.

1. During the process of endochondral ossification:

A. chondroblasts originate from periosteum that surrounds the model.

B. the cartilage model grows by interstitial and appositional means.

C. the cartilage bone model is supplied by newly formed blood vessels.

D. chondrocytes calcify the cartilage matrix and lacunae.

E. osteoprogenitor cells synthesize cartilage matrix.

2. What forms between the primary and secondary centers of ossification?

A. Epiphyseal plate

B. Bone marrow

C. Numerous blood vessels

D. Osteoprogenitor center

E. Calcified cartilage

3. In intramembranous ossification, bone cells originate from:

A. bone marrow.

B. perichondrium.

C. connective tissue mesenchyme.

D. connective tissue fibroblasts.

E. osteoid matrix.

4. Parathyroid hormone eventually affects the function and activity of which cells?

A. Osteoblasts

B. Osteoprogenitor cells

C. Osteocytes

D. Fibrocytes

E. Osteoclasts

5. What function does the hormone calcitonin perform?

A. It activates osteoclast activity.

B. It decreases bone resorption and decreases calcium levels.

C. It stimulates osteoid and bone matrix formation.

D. It increases calcium absorption and raises calcium levels.

E. It stimulates parathyroid hormone production.

ANSWERS

1. **Correct Answer: B.** The cartilage model grows by interstitial and appositional means. Because the cartilage matrix is soft, cartilage during endochondral ossification can grow in length and width by interstitial and appositional growth methods.

2. **Correct Answer: A.** Epiphyseal plate. This soft plate allows the cartilage cells to grow and lengthen the bone.

3. **Correct Answer: C.** Connective tissue mesenchyme. These cells form ossification centers where the mesenchyme cells differentiate into osteoblasts to form the bone.

4. **Correct Answer: E.** Osteoclasts. Parathyroid hormone indirectly influences osteoclasts by acting first on the osteoblasts.

5. **Correct Answer: B.** It decreases bone resorption and decreases calcium levels. Calcitonin counteracts the effect of parathyroid hormone, by decreasing osteoclast activity and calcium resorption.

ADDITIONAL HISTOLOGIC IMAGES

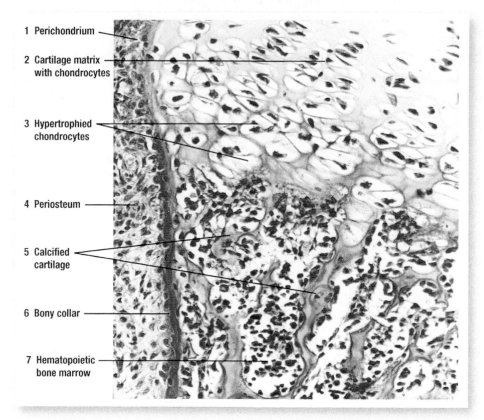

1 Perichondrium
2 Cartilage matrix with chondrocytes
3 Hypertrophied chondrocytes
4 Periosteum
5 Calcified cartilage
6 Bony collar
7 Hematopoietic bone marrow

FIGURE 7.31 ■ Endochondral ossification illustrating the hyaline cartilage matrix, calcified cartilage, and formation of the bony collar. Stain: hematoxylin and eosin. ×50.

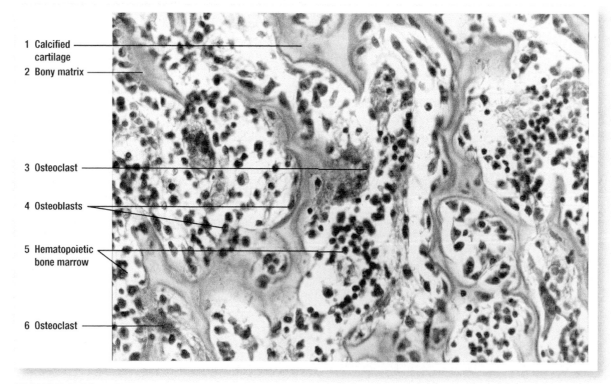

1 Calcified cartilage
2 Bony matrix
3 Osteoclast
4 Osteoblasts
5 Hematopoietic bone marrow
6 Osteoclast

FIGURE 7.32 ■ Endochondral ossification showing calcified cartilage with bony layers and the developing bone marrow. Stain: hematoxylin and eosin. ×165.

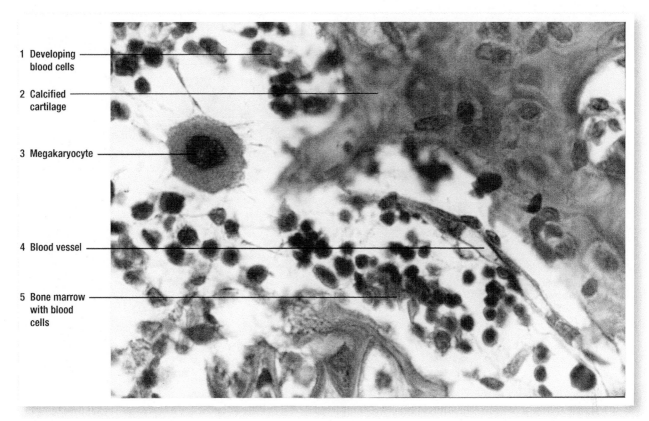

1 Developing blood cells

2 Calcified cartilage

3 Megakaryocyte

4 Blood vessel

5 Bone marrow with blood cells

FIGURE 7.33 ■ A section of the calcified cartilage in endochondral ossification with bone marrow cells. Stain: hematoxylin and eosin. ×205.

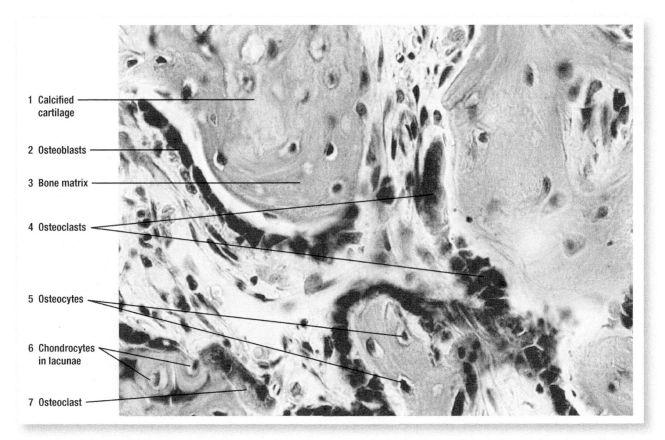

1 Calcified cartilage

2 Osteoblasts

3 Bone matrix

4 Osteoclasts

5 Osteocytes

6 Chondrocytes in lacunae

7 Osteoclast

FIGURE 7.34 ■ Endochondral ossification with calcified cartilage, bone matrix, and bone-forming cells. Stain: hematoxylin and eosin. ×205.

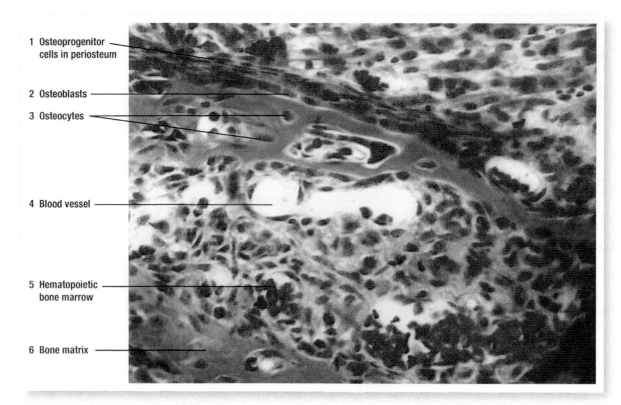

1 Osteoprogenitor cells in periosteum

2 Osteoblasts

3 Osteocytes

4 Blood vessel

5 Hematopoietic bone marrow

6 Bone matrix

FIGURE 7.35 ■ Intramembranous ossification showing the bone-forming cells and the developing bone marrow. Stain: Mallory-Azan. ×205.

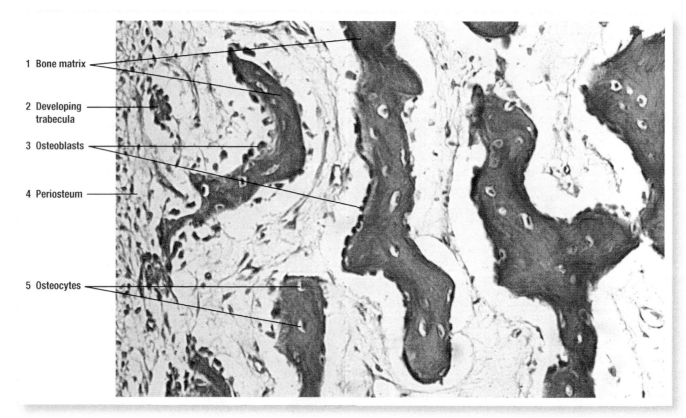

1 Bone matrix

2 Developing trabecula

3 Osteoblasts

4 Periosteum

5 Osteocytes

FIGURE 7.36 ■ Bone trabeculae undergoing development by intramembranous ossification. Stain: hematoxylin and eosin. ×35.

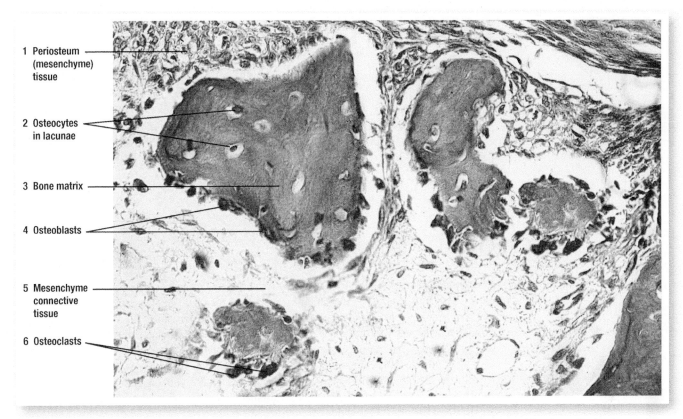

1 Periosteum (mesenchyme) tissue

2 Osteocytes in lacunae

3 Bone matrix

4 Osteoblasts

5 Mesenchyme connective tissue

6 Osteoclasts

FIGURE 7.37 ■ Higher-magnification bony trabeculae undergoing intramembranous ossification. Stain: hematoxylin and eosin. ×165.

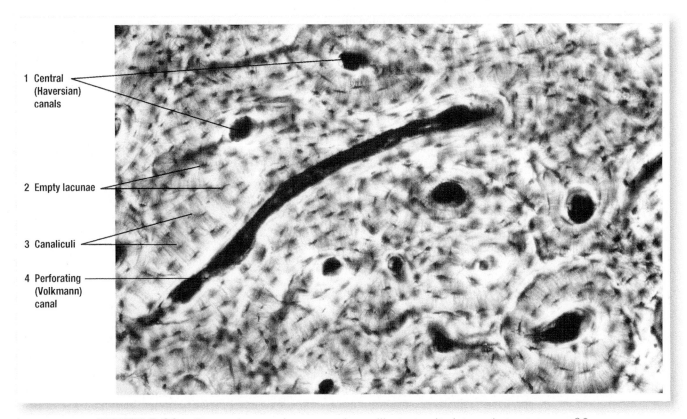

1 Central (Haversian) canals

2 Empty lacunae

3 Canaliculi

4 Perforating (Volkmann) canal

FIGURE 7.38 ■ Dry and ground compact bone illustrates its internal structures. ×30.

Muscle Tissue

SECTION 1   Skeletal Muscle

There are three types of muscle tissues in the body: **skeletal muscle**, **cardiac muscle**, and **smooth muscle**. These muscles can be identified by their structure and function, with each muscle type showing morphologic and functional similarities as well as differences. All muscle tissues consist of elongated cells called **fibers**. The cytoplasm of muscle cells is called **sarcoplasm**, and the surrounding cell membrane or plasmalemma is called **sarcolemma**.

Skeletal muscle fibers are long, cylindrical, **multinucleated cells**, with peripheral nuclei because of the fusion of numerous mesenchymal cells called **myoblasts** during embryonic development. Each muscle fiber is composed of smaller subunits called **myofibrils** that extend the entire length of the fiber. The myofibrils, in turn, are composed of tiny **myofilament** units formed by the contractile thin protein actin and the thick protein **myosin**.

In the sarcoplasm of each skeletal muscle, the arrangement of actin and myosin filaments is very regular, forming the distinct **cross-striation** patterns seen under a light microscope as lighter-staining **I bands** and dark-staining **A bands**. Because of these cross-striations, skeletal muscle is also called **striated muscle**. Transmission electron microscopy illustrates the internal organization of the contractile proteins in each myofibril. These high-resolution images show that each light I band is bisected by a dense transverse **Z line** (disc or band). Between the two adjacent Z lines is found the smallest structural and functional contractile unit of the muscle, the **sarcomere**. Sarcomeres are the repeating contractile units seen along the entire length of each myofibril and are highly characteristic features of the sarcoplasm of skeletal and cardiac muscle fibers.

The center and the dark-staining part of each sarcomere contains the thick (myosin) filaments, which form the A band. The peripheries and the light-staining portion of the sarcomere contain the light-staining, thin actin filaments. Actin and myosin filaments are precisely aligned and stabilized within individual myofibrils and sarcomeres by accessory proteins. The thin actin filaments are bound to the protein **α-actinin**, which binds them to the dense Z line (band, disc). The thick myosin filaments are anchored to the Z line by the very large protein called **titin** that positions and centers the myosin filaments on the Z line. Titin acts like a spring between the end of the myosin filament and the Z line. Another large protein, **nebulin**, extends the length of the thin filaments actin, anchors them to the Z line, and functions in regulating the length of the actin filament. Further support is provided by the protein **desmin** that extends from Z line of one myofibril to the adjacent myofibril, linking them together and attaching them to the sarcolemma (cell membrane). This stabilizes the position of muscle myofibrils within the sarcoplasm.

Skeletal muscles are surrounded by a dense, irregular connective tissue layer called **epimysium**. From the epimysium, a less dense and thinner irregular connective tissue layer called **perimysium** extends into the muscle and divides the muscle mass into smaller bundles of muscle fibers, the **fascicles**, and surrounds them. An even thinner layer of reticular connective tissue fibers, called **endomysium**, invests individual muscle fibers. Located in all connective tissue sheaths are blood vessels, nerves, and lymphatics, with a rich capillary plexus as illustrated in Figure 8.1.

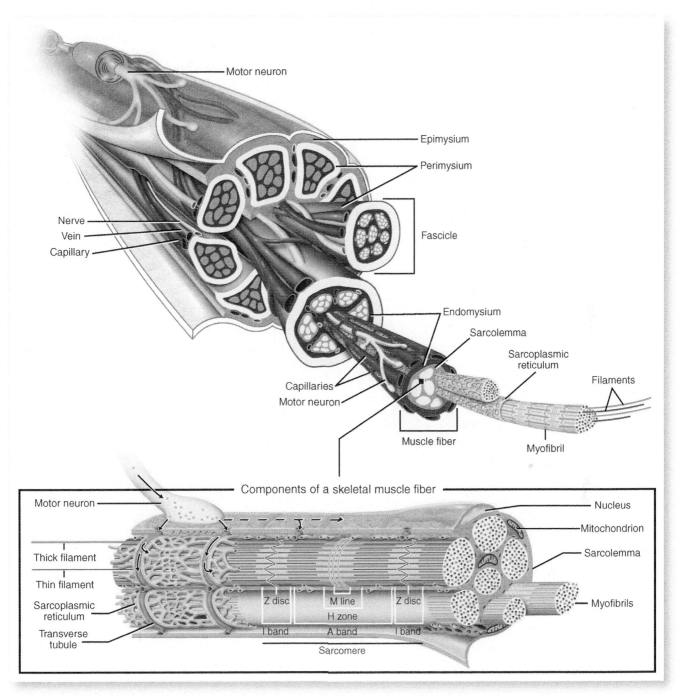

FIGURE 8.1 ■ Diagrammatic representation of the microscopic appearance of skeletal muscle.

thePoint· Supplemental micrographic images are available at **www.thePoint.com/Eroschenko13e** under Muscle Tissue.

FIGURE 8.2 | Longitudinal and Transverse Sections of Skeletal (Striated) Muscles: Tongue

In the tongue, skeletal muscle fibers are arranged in bundles that course in different directions. This image illustrates the tongue muscle fibers in both the longitudinal (*upper region*) and transverse (*lower region*) sections.

Each **skeletal muscle fiber** (**9**, **transverse section**; **11**, **longitudinal section**) is multinucleated. The **nuclei** (**1**, **6**) are situated peripherally and below the sarcolemma of each muscle fiber. (The sarcolemma is not visible in the figure.) Also, each skeletal muscle fiber shows **cross-striations** (**3**) that are visible as alternating dark **A bands** (**3a**) and light **I bands** (**3b**). With higher magnification and transmission electron microscopy, additional details of the cross-striations are visible (see Figs. 8.5 and 8.6).

Skeletal muscle fibers are aggregated into bundles or **fascicles** (**15**), surrounded by fibers of **connective tissue** (**5**) sheath around each muscle fascicle (**15**) called the perimysium (**12**). From each **perimysium** (**12**), thin partitions of connective tissue extend into each muscle fascicle (**15**) and invest individual muscle fibers (**9**, **11**) with a connective tissue layer called the **endomysium** (**4**, **7**). Small **blood vessels** (**8**) and **capillaries** (**2**, **14**) are present in the connective tissue (**5**) around each muscle fiber (**9**, **11**).

The skeletal muscle fibers that were sectioned longitudinally (**11**) show light and dark cross-striations (**3a**, **3b**). The muscle fibers that were sectioned transversely (**9**) exhibit cross sections of **myofibrils** (**13**) and peripheral nuclei (**6**).

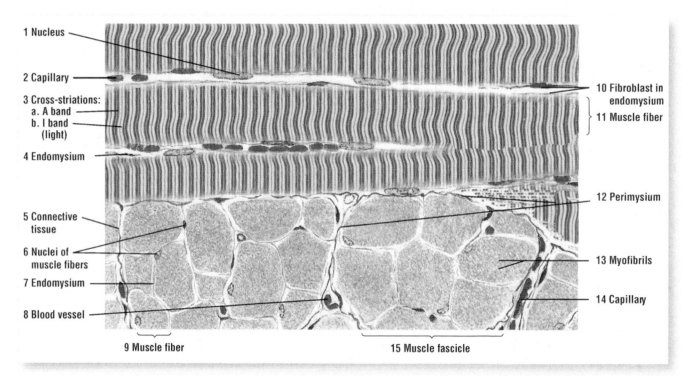

1 Nucleus
2 Capillary
3 Cross-striations:
 a. A band
 b. I band (light)
4 Endomysium
5 Connective tissue
6 Nuclei of muscle fibers
7 Endomysium
8 Blood vessel
9 Muscle fiber
10 Fibroblast in endomysium
11 Muscle fiber
12 Perimysium
13 Myofibrils
14 Capillary
15 Muscle fascicle

FIGURE 8.2 ■ Longitudinal and transverse sections of skeletal (striated) muscles of the tongue. Stain: hematoxylin and eosin. High magnification.

FIGURE 8.3 | Skeletal (Striated) Muscles: Tongue (Longitudinal Section and Cross Section)

A higher-magnification photomicrograph of the tongue illustrates individual **skeletal muscle fibers** (**3, 9**) in both cross section (**3**) and longitudinal section (**9**). In each, the muscle fibers are visible as tiny **myofibrils** (**4**). In the longitudinal section of the muscle fiber (**9**), the multiple **cross-striations** (**10**) are visible with peripheral **nuclei** (**5, 9**). Surrounding each skeletal muscle fiber (**3, 9**) is a thin layer of connective tissue **endomysium** (**2, 6**), seen both in cross section (**2**) and in longitudinal section (**6**). The thicker connective tissue layer **perimysium** (**1, 7**) surrounds a group of individual muscle fibers called fascicles. Visible in the perimysium (**7**) are tiny **capillaries** with flattened **erythrocytes** (**8**).

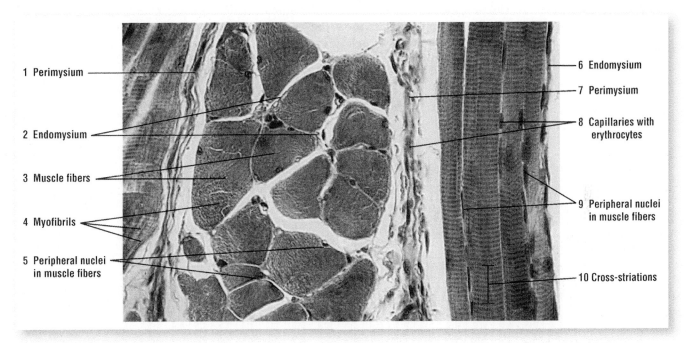

1 Perimysium

2 Endomysium

3 Muscle fibers

4 Myofibrils

5 Peripheral nuclei in muscle fibers

6 Endomysium

7 Perimysium

8 Capillaries with erythrocytes

9 Peripheral nuclei in muscle fibers

10 Cross-striations

FIGURE 8.3 ■ Skeletal (striated) muscles of the tongue (longitudinal and transverse section). Stain: Masson trichrome. ×130.

FIGURE 8.4 | Skeletal Muscle Fibers (Longitudinal Section)

A higher-magnification illustrates greater detail of individual skeletal muscle fibers and the cross-striations. A cell membrane, or **sarcolemma** (4), surrounds each skeletal **muscle fiber** (2). The flattened muscle fiber **nuclei** (1, 10) are in the periphery. Adjacent to the nuclei (1, 10) is the thin cytoplasm or **sarcoplasm** (5) with its organelles. Each muscle fiber (2) consists of **individual myofibrils** (8) that are arranged longitudinally. Myofibrils (8) are best seen in cross sections of the skeletal muscle fibers in Figure 8.3. Surrounding each skeletal muscle fiber (2) is a thin connective tissue **endomysium** (9), with **fibrocytes** (3, 6), and **capillaries** (7) with blood cells.

The cross-striations of skeletal muscle fibers are the light-staining **I bands** and dark-staining **A bands**. Each A band is bisected by the lighter H band and the darker **M band**. Crossing the central region of each I band is a distinct, narrow **Z line**. The filamentous and cellular segments between the Z lines represent a **sarcomere**, the structural and functional unit of striated muscles (skeletal and cardiac). When the myofibrils (8) are separated from the muscle fiber (2), the A, I, and Z lines remain visible. The close longitudinal arrangement of parallel myofibrils gives the skeletal muscle fibers their characteristic striated appearance. A direct comparison with the ultrastructural image of the myofibrils is presented in the next figure.

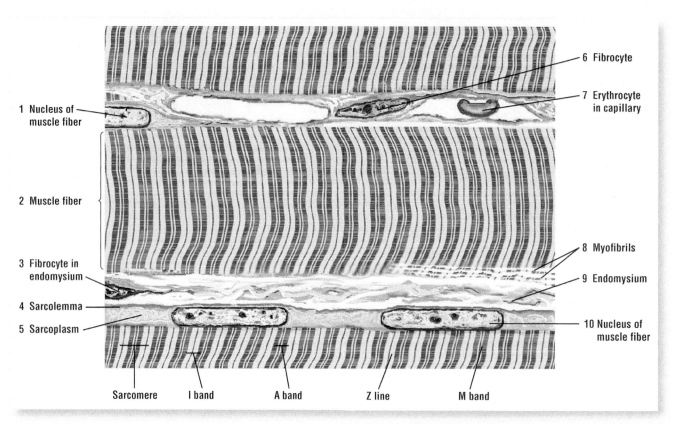

1 Nucleus of muscle fiber

2 Muscle fiber

3 Fibrocyte in endomysium

4 Sarcolemma

5 Sarcoplasm

6 Fibrocyte

7 Erythrocyte in capillary

8 Myofibrils

9 Endomysium

10 Nucleus of muscle fiber

Sarcomere   I band   A band   Z line   M band

FIGURE 8.4 ■ Skeletal muscle fibers (longitudinal section). Stain: hematoxylin and eosin. Plastic section. High magnification.

FIGURE 8.5 | Ultrastructure of Myofibrils in Skeletal Muscle

To compare the light microscope illustration of Figure 8.4, an ultrastructure section of the skeletal muscle is shown. This transmission electron micrograph illustrates the organization of the myofibrils and myofilaments in a partially contracted skeletal muscle. Each myofibril consists of repeating units called sarcomeres, the contractile elements in striated muscles. A **sarcomere** (5) is located between two electron-dense **Z lines**. Located in each sarcomere (5) are the light-staining thin actin and the dark-staining thick myosin myofilaments. The thin actin filaments extend from the Z lines and form the light-staining **I bands**. In the center of each sarcomere (5) is the dark-staining **A band** composed mainly of the thick myosin filaments overlapping the thin actin filaments. Each A band is bisected by a denser **M band** where the adjacent myosin filaments are linked. On each side of the M band are smaller lighter **H bands** (2, 3) that consist only of myosin filaments. Surrounding each sarcomere are the tubules of the **sarcoplasmic reticulum** (4) and **mitochondria** (1). During muscle contraction, the length of the thick and thin filaments remains unchanged, whereas the size of each sarcomere (5) decreases (see Fig. 8.6).

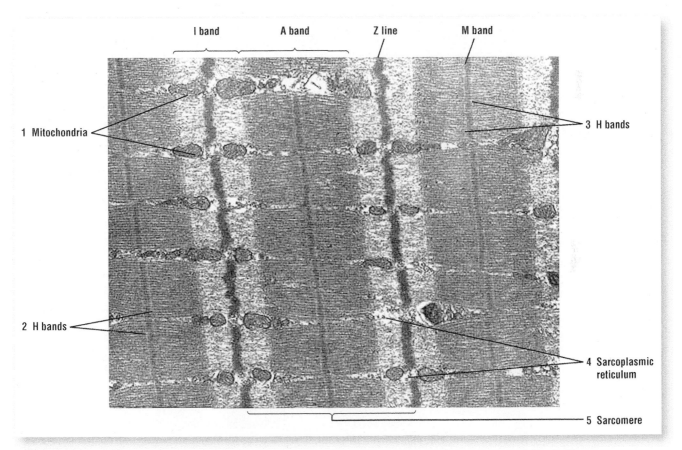

FIGURE 8.5 ■ Ultrastructure of myofibrils in skeletal muscle. Courtesy of Carter Rowley, Ft. Collins, CO. ×33,500.

FIGURE 8.6 | Ultrastructure of Sarcomeres, Tubules, and Triads in Skeletal Muscle

A higher magnification with the transmission electron micrograph illustrates the sarcomeres in a contracted skeletal muscle. During muscle contraction, the sarcomere shortens, the **Z lines** (**2, 6**) are drawn closer together, and the thick and thin filaments slide past each other. This action narrows the **I bands** (**7**) and **H bands** (**8**), whereas the **A band** (**1**) remains unchanged. In the middle of the sarcomere is the dense-staining **M band** (**4**). The tubules or the cisternae of the sarcoplasmic reticulum surround each sarcomere of every myofibril (see Fig. 8.5). At the A band (1) and I band (7) junction (A–I junctions), the sarcoplasmic reticulum tubules expand into terminal cisternae. To allow synchronous stimulation and contraction of all sarcomeres, tiny tubular invaginations of the sarcolemma, called the **T tubules** (**3**), penetrate every myofibril, and are located at the A–I junctions (1, 7). Here, one T tubule (3) is surrounded on each side by the expanded terminal cisternae of the sarcoplasmic reticulum and forms a **triad** (**5**). In mammalian skeletal muscles, the triads (5) are located at the A–I junctions. The stimulus for muscle contraction, delivered via a nerve, is then disseminated to each sarcomere of each myofibril through the T tubules (3) in the triads (5).

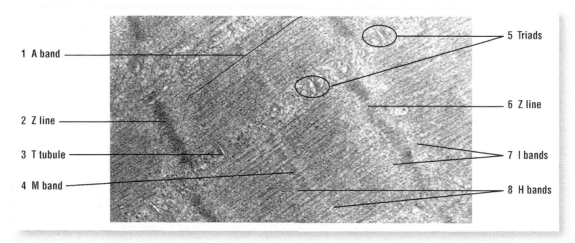

FIGURE 8.6 ■ Ultrastructure of sarcomeres, T tubules, and triads in skeletal muscle. Courtesy of Carter Rowley, Ft. Collins, CO. ×50,000.

FIGURE 8.7 | Skeletal Muscles, Nerves, and Motor Endplates

A group of **skeletal muscle fibers** (**6, 7**) have been teased apart and stained to illustrate nerve terminations or myoneural junctions on individual muscle fibers. The characteristic **cross-striations** (**2, 8**) are visible in each muscle fiber (6, 7). The dark-stained, stringlike structures between the

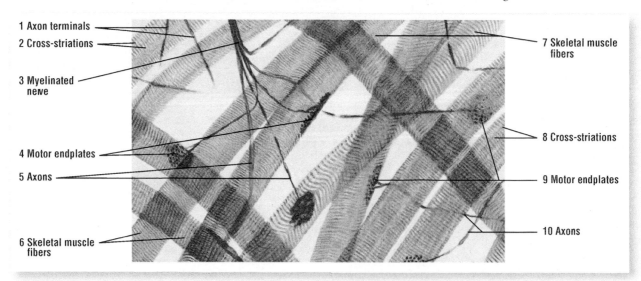

FIGURE 8.7 ■ Skeletal muscles, nerves, axons, and motor endplates. Stain: silver. High magnification.

separated muscle fibers (6, 7) are the **myelinated motor nerves** (3) and their branches, the **axons** (1, 5, 10). The motor nerve (3) courses within the muscle, branches, and distributes its axons (1, 5, 10) to the individual muscle fibers (6, 7). The axons (1, 5, 10) terminate on individual muscle fibers as specialized junctional regions called **motor endplates** (4, 9). The small, dark, round structures seen in each motor endplate (4, 9) are the terminal expansion of the axons (1, 5, 10). Some axons (1) are also seen without motor endplates as a result of tissue preparation.

FUNCTIONAL CORRELATIONS 8.1 ■ Skeletal Muscles

SKELETAL MUSCLE AND MOTOR ENDPLATES

Skeletal muscles are **voluntary** because the stimulation for their contraction and relaxation is under conscious control. Large motor nerves or axons innervate skeletal muscles. Near the skeletal muscle, the motor nerve branches, and a smaller axon branch individually innervates a single muscle fiber. As a result, skeletal muscle fibers contract only when stimulated by an axon. Also, each skeletal muscle fiber exhibits a specialized site where the axon terminates. This **neuromuscular junction**, or **motor endplate**, is the site where the impulse from the axon is transmitted to the skeletal muscle fiber.

The terminal end of each efferent (motor) axon contains numerous small **vesicles** that contain the neurotransmitter **acetylcholine**. Arrival of a nerve impulse, or **action potential**, at the axon terminal causes the synaptic vesicles to fuse with the plasma membrane of the axon and release the acetylcholine into the **synaptic cleft**, a small gap between the axon terminal and cell membrane (sarcolemma) of the muscle fiber. The neurotransmitter then diffuses across the synaptic cleft, combines with **acetylcholine receptors** on the cell membrane of the muscle fiber, and stimulates the muscle to contract. An enzyme called **acetylcholinesterase**, located in the basal lamina of the synaptic cleft, inactivates or neutralizes the released and excess acetylcholine. Inactivation of acetylcholine is necessary in order to prevent further muscle stimulation and muscle contraction until the next impulse arrives at the axon terminal.

CONTRACTION OF SKELETAL MUSCLES

Before the arrival of the nerve stimulus to the muscle, the muscle is relaxed, and **calcium ions** are stored in the cisternae of the **sarcoplasmic reticulum** bound to protein **calsequestrin**. Muscle contractions depend on the availability of calcium ions. After the arrival of the nerve stimulus and the release of the neurotransmitter at the motor endplates, the sarcolemma is depolarized, or activated. The stimulus signal (action potential) is propagated along the entire length of the sarcolemma and rapidly transmitted deep to every myofiber by the network of the **T tubules** that surround each sarcomere at the **A–I junction**. Expanded terminal cisternae of the sarcoplasmic reticulum and T tubules form **triads**. At each triad, the action potential is transmitted from the T tubules to every myofiber and myofibril as well as the sarcoplasmic reticulum membrane. After stimulation, cisternae of the sarcoplasmic reticulum in each myofibril release calcium ions into the individual sarcomeres and the overlapping thick and thin myofilaments of the myofibril. Calcium ions activate binding between actin and myosin, which results in their sliding past each other, causing muscle contraction and muscle shortening. When the stimulus subsides and the membrane is no longer stimulated, calcium ions are actively transported back into and stored in the cisternae of the sarcoplasmic reticulum, causing muscle relaxation.

Nearly all skeletal muscles contain sensitive stretch receptors called **neuromuscular spindles**. These spindles consist of a connective tissue **capsule** that contains modified muscle fibers called **intrafusal fibers** and numerous **nerve endings**, surrounded by a fluid-filled space. The muscles surrounding the neuromuscular spindles are called the **extrafusal fibers**. The neuromuscular spindles monitor the changes (distension) in muscle length and activate complex reflexes to regulate muscle activity. When skeletal muscles are stretched, the neuromuscular spindles initiate a reflex contraction and shortening of the muscle.

FIGURE 8.8 | Skeletal Muscle with Muscle Spindle (Transverse Section)

Skeletal muscles contain sensory stretch receptors called muscle spindles that are surrounded by connective tissue capsules. A transverse section of an extraocular skeletal muscle shows individual **muscle fibers (2)** surrounded by connective tissue, the **endomysium (6)**. The muscle fibers (2), in turn, are grouped into **fascicles (1)** and surrounded by interfascicular connective tissue **perimysium (4)**. Located within the muscle fascicles (1) is a cross section of a **muscle spindle (3)**. Surrounding the muscle spindle (3) and the skeletal muscle fibers (2) are **arterioles (5)** in the perimysium (4).

The connective tissue **capsule (8)** surrounding the muscle spindle (3) extends from the adjacent **perimysium (11)** and encloses several components of the spindle. The specialized muscle fibers located in the spindle and surrounded by the capsule (8) are called **intrafusal fibers (10)**, in contrast to the extrafusal **skeletal muscle fibers (7)** located outside of the spindle capsule (8). Small nerve fibers associated with the muscle spindles (3) are the myelinated and terminal unmyelinated **nerve fibers (axons) (9)** surrounded by the supportive Schwann cells. Small blood vessels and an **arteriole (12)** from the perimysium (11) are found in and around the capsule of the muscle spindle (3).

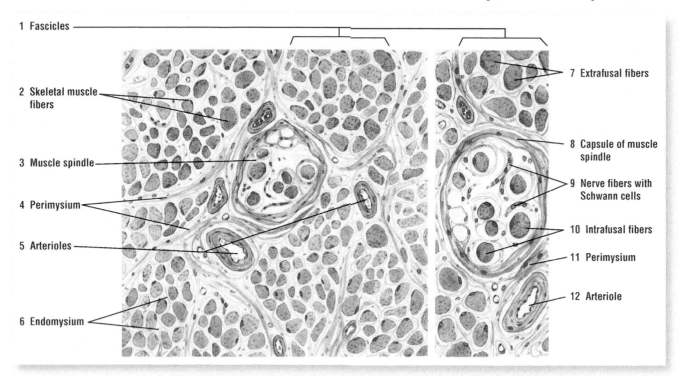

FIGURE 8.8 ■ Skeletal muscle with a muscle spindle (transverse section). Frozen section stained with modified Van Gieson method (hematoxylin, picric acid–ponceau stain). *Left*, medium magnification; *right*, high magnification. Courtesy of Dr. Mark DeSantis, Professor Emeritus, WWAMI Medical Program, University of Idaho, Moscow, ID.

FUNCTIONAL CORRELATIONS 8.2 ■ Muscle Spindles

Muscle spindles are specialized **stretch receptors** located parallel to muscle fibers in nearly all skeletal muscles. Their main function is to detect changes in the length of the muscle fibers. An increase in the length of muscle fibers stimulates the muscle spindle and sends **impulses** via the afferent (sensory) axons into the spinal cord. These impulses result in a **stretch reflex** that immediately causes **contraction** of the **extrafusal muscle fibers**, thereby shortening the stretched muscle and producing movement.

A decrease in skeletal muscle length stops the stimulation of the muscle spindle fibers and the conduction of its impulses to the spinal cord.

The simple **stretch reflex arc** illustrates the function of these receptors. Gently tapping the patellar tendon on the knee with a rubber mallet stretches the skeletal muscle and stimulates the muscle spindle. This action results in rapid muscle contraction of the stretched muscle and produces an involuntary knee-jerk response, or stretch reflex.

SECTION 2   Cardiac Muscle

Cardiac muscle fibers are also cylindrical. They are primarily located in the walls and septa of the **heart** and in the walls of the large vessels attached to the heart (the aorta and pulmonary trunk). Similar to skeletal muscle, cardiac muscle fibers exhibit distinct **cross-striations** because of regular arrangements of actin and myosin filaments in the sarcomeres. Transmission electron microscopy reveals similar A bands, I bands, Z lines, and the repeating sarcomere units. In contrast to skeletal muscles, however, the cardiac muscle fibers exhibit some important differences. The cardiac muscles develop by joining the cells end to end through anchoring cell junctions called the **intercalated discs** that form the distinguishing characteristic features of cardiac muscles. These dense-staining discs are special attachment sites that cross the cardiac cells in a stepwise fashion at irregular intervals. Cardiac muscles cells also exhibit only one or two **central nuclei**, are shorter than the skeletal muscles, and exhibit **branching** (Fig. 8.9).

the**Point** Supplemental micrographic images are available at **www.thePoint.com/Eroschenko13e** under Muscle Tissue.

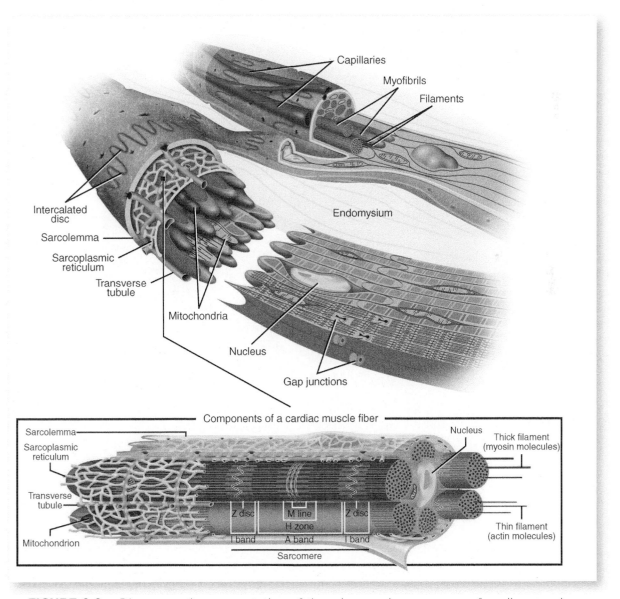

FIGURE 8.9 ■ Diagrammatic representation of the microscopic appearance of cardiac muscle.

FIGURE 8.10 | Longitudinal and Transverse Sections of Cardiac Muscle

Cardiac muscle fibers exhibit similar features that are seen in skeletal muscle fibers. This figure illustrates a section of a cardiac muscle cut in both longitudinal (*upper portion*) and transverse (*lower portion*) planes. The **cross-striations** (2) in the cardiac muscle fibers closely resemble those of skeletal muscles. In contrast, the cardiac muscle fibers show **branching** (5, 10) without much change in their diameters. Also, cardiac muscle fibers are shorter than a skeletal muscle fiber with a single, centrally located **nucleus** (3, 7). **Binucleate** (two nuclei) **muscle fibers** (8) are also occasionally seen. The nuclei (7) are visible in the center of each muscle fiber when cut in a transverse section. Around these central nuclei (3, 7, 8) are the clear zones of nonfibrillar **perinuclear sarcoplasm** (1, 13). In transverse sections, the perinuclear sarcoplasm (13) appears as a clear space if the section is not through the nucleus. Also visible in transverse sections are individual **myofibrils** (14) of cardiac muscle fibers.

Highly characteristic features of cardiac muscle fibers are the **intercalated discs** (4, 9). These dark-staining structures are found at irregular intervals and represent the specialized junctional complexes between cardiac muscle fibers.

Cardiac muscle has a vast blood supply. Numerous small blood vessels and **capillaries** (6) are found in the **connective tissue** (11) septa and the delicate, indistinct **endomysium** (12) between individual muscle fibers.

Other examples of cardiac muscles are seen in Chapter 10.

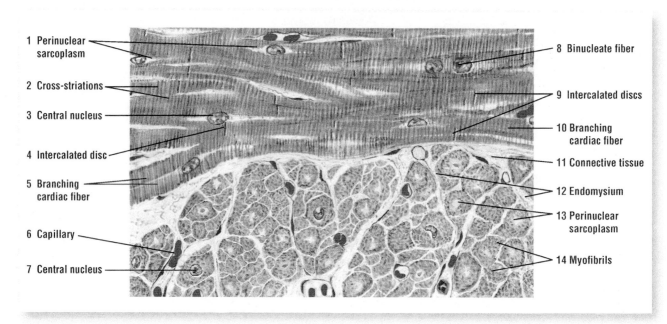

FIGURE 8.10 ■ Longitudinal and transverse sections of cardiac muscle. Stain: hematoxylin and eosin. High magnification.

FIGURE 8.11 | Cardiac Muscle (Longitudinal Section)

A high-magnification photomicrograph illustrates a section of the cardiac muscle cut in a longitudinal plane. **Cardiac muscle fibers** (1) exhibit **cross-striations** (3), **branching fibers** (8), and a single central **nucleus** (6). The dark-staining **intercalated discs** (2) connect individual cardiac muscle fibers (1). Small **myofibrils** (4) are visible within each cardiac muscle fiber (1). The flattened and fusiform cells surrounding the cardiac muscle fibers (1) represent the **fibrocytes of the endomysium** (5). Although not visible in this illustration, delicate strands of connective tissue endomysium surround the individual cardiac muscle fibers.

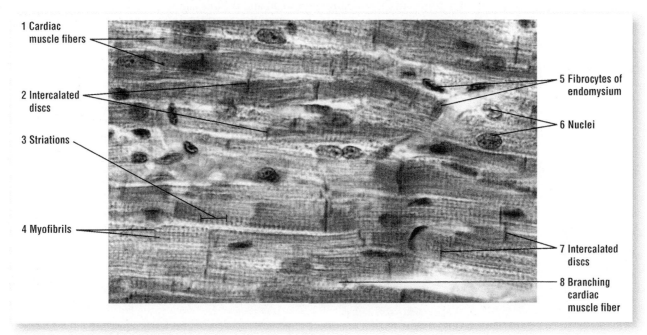

1 Cardiac muscle fibers
2 Intercalated discs
3 Striations
4 Myofibrils
5 Fibrocytes of endomysium
6 Nuclei
7 Intercalated discs
8 Branching cardiac muscle fiber

FIGURE 8.11 ■ Cardiac muscle (longitudinal section). Stain: Masson trichrome. ×130.

FIGURE 8.12 | Cardiac Muscle in Longitudinal Section

Comparison of the cardiac muscle fibers with skeletal muscles at higher magnification and with the same stain (Fig. 8.4) illustrates the similarities and differences between the two types of muscle tissue.

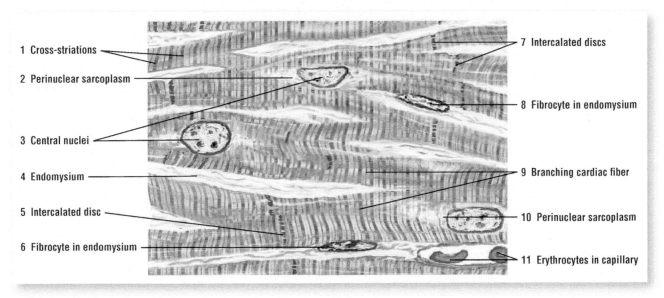

1 Cross-striations
2 Perinuclear sarcoplasm
3 Central nuclei
4 Endomysium
5 Intercalated disc
6 Fibrocyte in endomysium
7 Intercalated discs
8 Fibrocyte in endomysium
9 Branching cardiac fiber
10 Perinuclear sarcoplasm
11 Erythrocytes in capillary

FIGURE 8.12 ■ Cardiac muscle in longitudinal section. Stain: hematoxylin and eosin. High magnification.

The cross-striations (1) are similar in both the skeletal and cardiac muscle types but are less prominent in cardiac muscle fibers. The branching **cardiac fibers** (9) are in contrast to the individual, elongated fibers of the skeletal muscle. The characteristic **intercalated discs** (5, 7) of cardiac muscle fibers and their irregular structure are more prominent at higher magnification. The intercalated discs (5, 7) appear as either straight bands (5) or staggered (7) across individual fibers.

The large, oval **nuclei** (3), usually one per cell, are centrally located in cardiac fibers, in contrast to the multiple flattened and peripheral nuclei in skeletal muscle fibers. Surrounding the nucleus of a cardiac muscle fiber is a prominent **perinuclear sarcoplasm** (2, 10) that is devoid of cross-striations and myofibrils.

The connective tissue **fibrocytes** (6, 8) and the fine connective tissue fibers of **endomysium** (4) surround the cardiac muscle fibers. **Capillaries** with **erythrocytes** (11) are normally seen in the endomysium (4, 6, 8).

FIGURE 8.13 | **Ultrastructure of Cardiac Muscle in Longitudinal Section**

This ultrastructure image illustrates the internal structures of cardiac muscle fiber. A distinct **sarcomere** (1) with regular arrangements of thin actin and thick myosin filaments is located between the dense-staining **Z lines** (3). Visible in the sarcomere (1) is the denser **A band** (2) containing both actin and myosin filaments and the light-staining **I band** (8) with actin filaments that are bisected by the Z lines (3). Located between the myofibrils are the large **mitochondria** (4) that are characteristic of cardiac muscle. In contrast to skeletal muscle, the **sarcoplasmic reticulum** (5) is not as well organized and exhibits only small terminal cisternae. Also, cardiac muscles exhibit only one **T tubule** (9) per sarcomere, seen at the level of the Z line (3). In the middle of the sarcomere (1) are darker **M bands** (7) bands that represent the linkages of the thick myosin filaments.

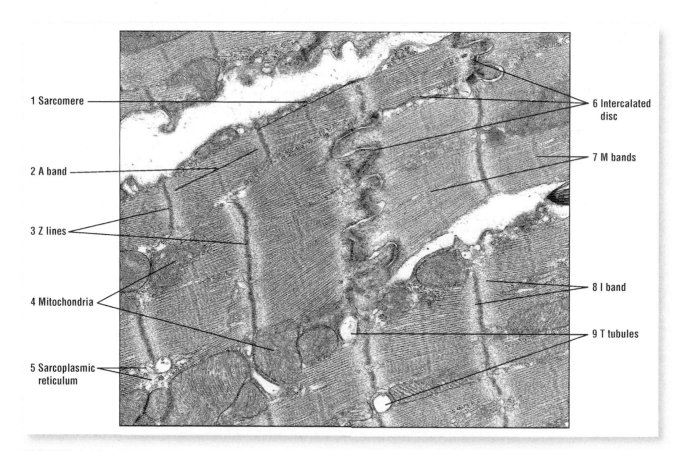

FIGURE 8.13 Ultrastructure of cardiac muscle in longitudinal section. ×24,800. Used with permission from Cui D. *Atlas of Histology with Functional and Clinical Correlations*. Baltimore, MD: Wolters Kluwer/ Lippincott Williams and Wilkins; 2011.

A highly characteristic feature of the cardiac muscle fibers is the dense-staining **intercalated disc** (**6**) with its irregular, zigzag pattern that crosses the cardiac muscle fibers. These discs represent important attachment sites between individual cardiac muscle fibers. The clear spaces between the myofibrils represent the branching features of different cardiac muscle fibers.

FUNCTIONAL CORRELATIONS 8.3 ■ Cardiac Muscle

Although the organization of the contractile proteins (actin and myosin) in cardiac myofibers and their arrangement in sarcomeres is essentially the same as in skeletal muscles, there are important differences. The **T tubules** are located at the Z lines and are much larger than those in skeletal muscles. Furthermore, the sarcoplasmic reticulum is less developed. Also, the mitochondria are larger and more abundant in the cardiac cells indicating the increased metabolic demands on the cardiac muscle fibers for continuous function.

Cardiac cells are joined end to end by specialized, interdigitating **intercalated discs** composed of fascia adherens, desmosomes, and **gap junctions**. The gap junctions couple all cardiac muscle fibers and allow a very rapid spread of stimuli throughout the entire cardiac muscle mass. Conduction of excitatory impulses to the cardiac sarcomeres is through the T tubules and the sarcoplasmic reticulum. Diffusion of ions through the pores in gap junctions between individual cardiac muscle fibers coordinates heart function and allows the cardiac muscle to act as a **functional syncytium**, allowing the stimuli for contraction to pass through the entire cardiac musculature.

As in the skeletal muscle, calcium is essential for cardiac muscle contractions. In cardiac muscles, however, the sarcoplasmic reticulum is less well developed and does not store sufficient amounts of calcium for uninterrupted contractions. As a result, during muscle stimulation and contraction, calcium is imported from outside the cardiac muscle cells into the sarcoplasm as well as from the sparse sarcoplasmic reticulum. At the end of the stimulus, this calcium movement is reversed.

Cardiac muscle fibers exhibit **autorhythmicity**, an ability to spontaneously generate stimuli. Both the **parasympathetic** and **sympathetic divisions** of the autonomic nervous system innervate the heart. Nerve fibers from the parasympathetic division, by way of the vagus nerve, slow the heart and decrease blood pressure. Nerve fibers from the sympathetic division produce the opposite effect and increase heart rate and blood pressure.

Additional information on cardiac muscle histology, the heart pacemaker, Purkinje fibers, and heart hormones is presented in more detail in Chapter 10.

SECTION 3 Smooth Muscle

Smooth muscles have a wide distribution in the body and predominantly line the **visceral hollow organs** and **blood vessels**. In digestive tract organs, the uterus, ureters, and other hollow organs, smooth muscles occur in large sheets or layers. In the dermis of the skin, smooth muscles are associated with hair follicles. Zonula adherens bind the cells, and the numerous **gap junctions** provide functional coupling between individual smooth muscle cells.

Under a light microscope, smooth muscle appears as elongated individual fibers with fusiform shapes of slender fascicle bundles. Individual muscle fibers are also shorter than the skeletal muscles and exhibit a single central nucleus. Connective tissue surrounds individual muscle fibers as well as muscle layers. In the blood vessels, smooth muscle fibers are arranged in a circular pattern, where they control blood pressure by altering luminal diameters. In intestines, smooth muscles are arranged in concentric layers around the organs.

Individual smooth muscle fibers contain contractile **actin** and **myosin** filaments; however, they are not arranged in the regular, cross-striated patterns that are visible in both the skeletal and cardiac muscle fibers (Fig. 8.14). Instead, actin and myosin course obliquely throughout the cell in the form of a lattice network that crisscrosses the sarcoplasm. As a result of the irregular distribution of contractile elements, these muscle fibers appear **smooth**, or **nonstriated**. The actin filaments attach to **dense bodies**, structures that are unique to smooth muscles. The dense bodies are either scattered throughout the cytoplasm or attached to the cytoplasmic side of the

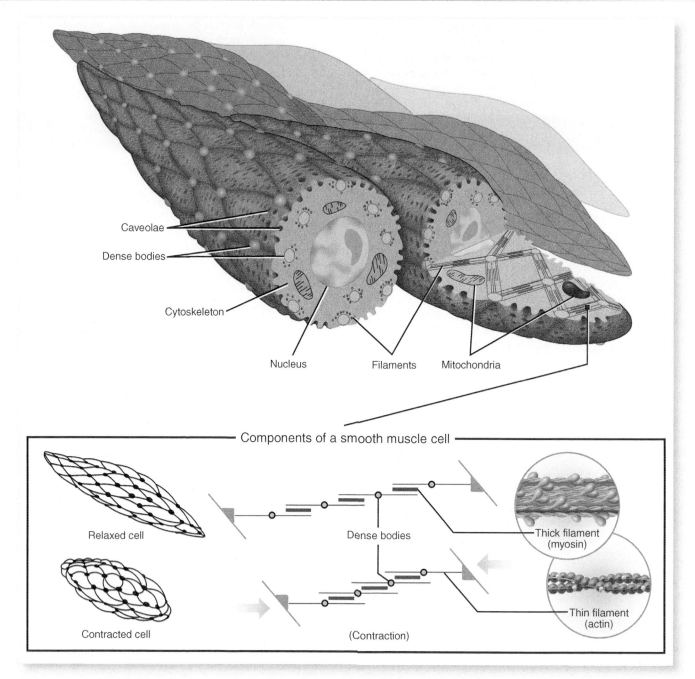

Caveolae

Dense bodies

Cytoskeleton

Nucleus   Filaments   Mitochondria

Components of a smooth muscle cell

Relaxed cell

Contracted cell

Dense bodies

(Contraction)

Thick filament (myosin)

Thin filament (actin)

FIGURE 8.14 ■ Diagrammatic representation of the microscopic appearance of smooth muscle.

cell membrane. The intermediate and actin filaments attach to the dense bodies in the cytoplasm and the dense bodies in the cell membrane. The dense bodies also contain **α-actinin** and other accessory Z-disc proteins such as desmin that are similar to the Z discs of the skeletal and cardiac muscles. Another characteristic feature of smooth muscle fibers is the presence of numerous vesicular invaginations of the cell membrane that look like the endocytotic or pinocytotic vesicles in other cells. These are the caveolae and are believed to function like the T tubules of skeletal muscles that transmit the stimulatory signals to the interior of the muscle fibers for contraction.

thePoint   Supplemental micrographic images are available at **www.thePoint.com/Eroschenko13e** under Muscle Tissue.

FIGURE 8.15 | Longitudinal and Transverse Section of Smooth Muscle: Wall of Small Intestine

In the small intestine, smooth muscle fibers that surround the lumen are arranged in two concentric layers: an inner circular layer and an outer longitudinal layer. Here, the muscle fibers of one layer are arranged at right angles to the fibers of the adjacent layer.

The upper smooth muscle fibers of the inner circular layer are cut in longitudinal section. **Smooth muscle fibers** (**1**) are spindle-shaped cells with tapered ends. The cytoplasm (sarcoplasm) of each muscle fiber stains dark. An elongated or ovoid single **nucleus** (**7**) is present in the center of each smooth muscle fiber.

The muscles of the adjacent longitudinal layer are cut in transverse section. Because the spindle-shaped muscle fibers are sectioned at different places along their length, their central nuclei exhibit different shapes and sizes. Large **nuclei** (**5**) are seen in **smooth muscle fibers** (**5**) that have been sectioned through their center. Muscle fibers not sectioned through the center appear only as deeply stained areas of clear **cytoplasm (sarcoplasm)** (**3**, upper leader; **9**, lower leader) or exhibit only a small portion of their cytoplasm with a section of their nuclei (**3**, lower leader; **9**, upper leader).

In the small intestine, the smooth muscle layers are close to each other with only a minimal amount of **connective tissue fibers** and **fibrocytes** (**4, 8, 10**) present between the two layers. Smooth muscle also has a rich blood supply, evidenced by the numerous **capillaries** (**6, 11**) between individual fibers and layers. Between the inner circular muscle layer and the outer longitudinal muscle layer are found numerous **neurons** of the **myenteric nerve plexus** (**2**).

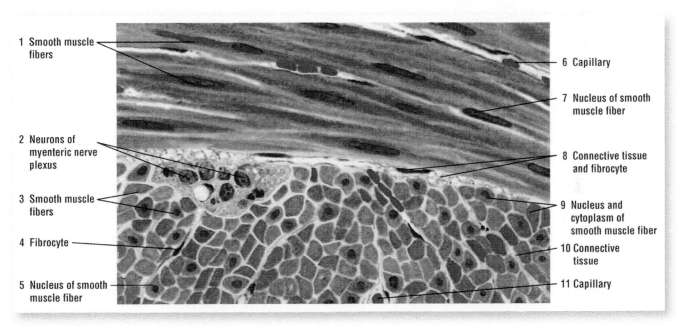

FIGURE 8.15 ■ Longitudinal and transverse section of smooth muscle in the wall of the small intestine. Stain: hematoxylin and eosin. High magnification.

FIGURE 8.16 | Smooth Muscle: Wall of Small Intestine (Transverse and Longitudinal Section)

A photomicrograph of the small intestine illustrates its muscular outer wall. The smooth muscle fibers are arranged in two layers: an **inner circular layer** (7) and an **outer longitudinal layer** (8). In the inner circular layer (7), a single **nucleus** (1) is visible in the center of the **cytoplasm** (2) of different fibers. In the outer longitudinal layer (8), cut in transverse section, the **cytoplasm** (5) appears empty, and single **nuclei** (6) of individual muscle fibers are visible if the plane of section passes through them. Located between the two smooth muscle layers is a group of autonomic **neurons** of the **myenteric nerve plexus** (3). Small **blood vessels** (4) are seen between individual muscle fibers and muscle layers.

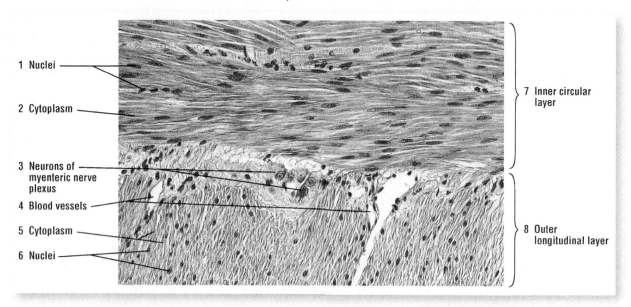

FIGURE 8.16 ■ Smooth muscle: wall of the small intestine (transverse and longitudinal section). Stain: hematoxylin and eosin. ×80.

FIGURE 8.17 | Ultrastructure of Smooth Muscle Fibers from Section of Intestinal Wall

In comparing the ultrastructure of the skeletal (see Figs. 8.5 and 8.6) and cardiac (see Fig. 8.13) muscle fibers with smooth muscle fibers, there is a significant difference in their internal morphology. The orderly arrangement of actin and myosin that gave skeletal and cardiac muscles a

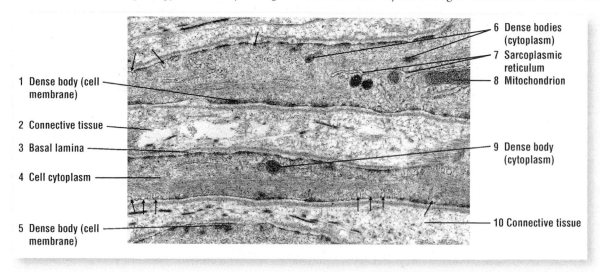

FIGURE 8.17 ■ Ultrastructure of smooth muscle fibers from a section of an intestinal wall. Courtesy of Dr. Rex A. Hess, Professor Emeritus Comparative Biosciences, College of Veterinary Medicine, University of Illinois, Urbana, IL. Approximately ×10,500.

striated appearance is absent. Although individual filaments are visible in the **cell cytoplasm** (**4**), their arrangement is random. The thin actin filaments attach to the **dense bodies** (**1, 5**) at the **cell membrane** (**1, 5**) or to **dense bodies** (**6, 9**) scattered in the cytoplasm (**4**) of smooth muscle cell (**4**). The dense bodies (**1, 5, 6, 9**) are functionally similar to the Z discs of the skeletal and cardiac muscles. The numerous invaginations along muscle cell membranes are the **caveolae** (arrows). Within the cell cytoplasm (**4**) are also seen a **mitochondrion** (**8**) and remnants of the **sarcoplasmic reticulum** (**7**). Smooth muscle cytoplasm (**4**) is surrounded by **basal lamina** (**3**), and between individual smooth muscle fibers, there are collagen fibers of the **connective tissue** (**2, 10**).

FUNCTIONAL CORRELATIONS 8.4 ■ Smooth Muscle

Unlike in skeletal and cardiac muscle, there are no T tubules in smooth muscle, and the sarcoplasmic reticulum is not well developed for storing much calcium. In addition, smooth muscles exhibit numerous vesicular invaginations of the cell membrane called **caveolae**. These caveolae appear to have similar functions of the T tubules of striated muscles by controlling calcium release into the cells following stimulation. During stimulation and contraction of the smooth muscle, calcium enters the sarcoplasm from the sarcoplasmic reticulum and from the cell membrane caveolae, where it binds to a protein called **calmodulin**, a calcium-binding protein that stimulates the interaction of actin and myosin, inducing them to slide past each other. Both actin and myosin contract by a sliding filament mechanism that is similar to that in skeletal muscles. The contraction of the filaments pulls **dense bodies** closer together, producing contraction and shortening of the smooth muscle. Because the dense bodies of the neighboring smooth muscle cells are connected, the force of contraction is transmitted to all connected smooth muscle cells, allowing the smooth muscles to function as a unit.

Smooth muscle exhibits spontaneous wavelike activity that passes in a slow, sustained contraction throughout the entire muscle, producing a continuous contraction of low force that maintains **tonus** in hollow structures. In ureters, the uterus, and digestive organs, contraction of smooth muscle produces **peristaltic contractions**, which propel the contents along the lengths of these organs. In arteries and other blood vessels, smooth muscles regulate the luminal diameters.

Smooth muscle fibers are also in close contacts with each other via **gap junctions**. These gap junctions allow rapid ionic communications between the smooth muscle fibers, producing coordinated activity in smooth muscle sheets or layers. Smooth muscles are also **involuntary** muscles. They are innervated and regulated by nerves from postganglionic neurons of the **sympathetic** and **parasympathetic divisions** of the **autonomic nervous system**. These innervations influence the rate and force of contractility. In addition, smooth muscle fibers contract and relax in response to nonneural stimulation, such as **stretching** or exposure to **different hormones**.

Chapter 8 Summary

Muscle Tissue

- Three muscle types are skeletal muscle, cardiac muscle, and smooth muscle
- All muscles show similarities and differences
- All muscles are composed of elongated cells called fibers
- Muscle cytoplasm is sarcoplasm, and muscle cell membrane is sarcolemma
- Muscle fibers contain myofibrils made of contractile proteins actin and myosin

SKELETAL MUSCLE

- Fibers are multinucleated with peripheral nuclei
- Multiple nuclei are because of the fusion of mesenchyme myoblasts during embryonic development
- Each muscle fiber is composed of myofibrils and myofilaments
- Actin and myosin filaments form distinct cross-striation patterns
- Light I bands contain thin actin, and dark A bands contain thick myosin filaments
- Dense Z line bisects I bands; between Z lines is the contractile unit, the sarcomere
- Accessory proteins align and stabilize actin and myosin filaments
- Titin protein anchors myosin filaments, and α-actinin binds actin filaments to Z lines
- Titin centers, positions, and acts like a spring between myosin and Z lines
- The protein nebulin anchors thin filaments to Z lines and regulates actin filament length
- The protein desmin links myofibrils at Z lines and attaches them to the sarcolemma
- Muscle is surrounded by connective tissue epimysium
- Muscle fascicles are surrounded by connective tissue perimysium
- Each muscle fiber is surrounded by connective tissue endomysium
- Voluntary muscles are under conscious control
- Neuromuscular spindles are specialized stretch receptors in almost all skeletal muscles
- Intrafusal fibers and nerve endings are found in spindle capsules
- Stretching of muscle produces a stretch reflex and movement to shorten muscle

Transmission Electron Microscopy of Skeletal Muscle

- Light bands are I bands and are formed by thin actin filaments
- I bands are crossed by dense Z lines
- Between Z lines is the smallest contractile unit of muscle, the sarcomere
- Dark bands are A bands and are located in the middle of sarcomere
- A bands are formed by overlapping actin and myosin filaments
- M bands in the middle of A bands represent linkage of myosin filaments
- H bands on each side of M bands contain only myosin filaments
- The sarcoplasmic reticulum and mitochondria surround each sarcomere

Functional Correlations of Skeletal Muscles

- Skeletal muscles are voluntary, are under conscious control, and contract only when stimulated
- Motor endplates are the sites of nerve innervations and transmission of stimuli to muscle
- Axon terminals of motor endplates contain vesicles with the neurotransmitter acetylcholine
- Action potential releases acetylcholine into synaptic cleft
- Acetylcholine combines with its receptors on muscle membrane
- Acetylcholinesterase neutralizes acetylcholine and prevents further contraction
- Before arrival of impulse, calcium is stored in the sarcoplasmic reticulum bound to the protein calsequestrin
- Sarcolemma invaginations into each myofiber form T tubules
- Expanded terminal cisternae of the sarcoplasmic reticulum and T tubules form triads
- Triads are located at A–I junctions in mammalian skeletal muscles
- Stimulus for muscle contraction is carried by T tubules to every myofiber, myofibril, and sarcoplasmic reticulum membrane
- After stimulation, the sarcoplasmic reticulum releases calcium ions into sarcomeres

- Calcium activates the binding of actin and myosin, causing muscle contraction and shortening
- After the end of the stimulus, calcium is actively transported and stored in the sarcoplasmic reticulum
- When muscle contracts, I and H bands shorten, whereas A bands stay the same
- Muscle contraction and shortening draw Z lines closer together and shorten sarcomere

CARDIAC MUSCLE

- Located in the heart and large vessels attached to the heart
- Cross-striations of actin and myosin form similar I bands, A bands, and Z lines as in skeletal muscle
- Characterized by dense junctional complexes called intercalated discs that contain gap junctions
- Contain one or two central nuclei; fibers are shorter and show branching
- T tubules are located at Z lines and are larger in skeletal muscle
- The sarcoplasmic reticulum is less well developed than in skeletal muscles
- Mitochondria are larger and more abundant in cardiac fibers
- Gap junctions couple all fibers for rhythmic contraction and form the functional syncytium
- For contraction, calcium is imported from outside the cell and from the sarcoplasmic reticulum
- Exhibit autorhythmicity and spontaneously generate stimuli
- The autonomic nervous system innervates the heart and influences heart rate and blood pressure

SMOOTH MUSCLE

- Found in hollow organs and blood vessels
- Zonula adherens binds muscle cells, whereas gap junctions provide functional coupling
- Contain actin and myosin filaments without cross-striation patterns
- Fibers are fusiform in shape and contain single central nuclei
- In intestines, muscles are arranged in concentric layers and in blood vessels in a circular pattern
- Actin and myosin filaments are present, but they do not show regular arrangement or striations
- Actin and myosin form lattice network, and they insert into dense bodies in sarcoplasm and cytoplasm
- Dense bodies contain α-actinin and other Z-disc proteins
- The sarcoplasmic reticulum is not well developed for calcium storage
- Sarcolemma contains invaginations called caveolae
- Caveolae may control influx of calcium into the cell after stimulation
- Following stimulation, calcium enters sarcoplasm from the caveolae and sarcoplasmic reticulum
- Calmodulin, a calcium-binding protein, stimulates actin and myosin interaction
- Actin and myosin contract muscle by a sliding mechanism similar to skeletal muscle
- Connection of dense bodies with adjacent cells transmits force of contraction to all cells
- Exhibit spontaneous activity and maintain tonus in hollow organs
- Peristaltic contractions propel contents in the organs
- Gap junctions couple muscles and allow ionic communication between all fibers
- Innervated by postganglionic neurons of sympathetic and parasympathetic divisions
- Involuntary muscles regulated by autonomic nervous system, hormones, and stretching

Chapter 8 Review Questions

QUESTIONS

In the following multiple-choice questions, choose the letter corresponding to the one best answer.

1. **What is the difference between T tubules in skeletal and cardiac muscles?**

   A. There is no difference in T tubules between the different striated muscles.
   B. T tubules are larger and store more calcium in skeletal muscles.
   C. T tubules in cardiac muscles are branched.
   D. T tubules are larger in cardiac muscles than in the skeletal muscle.
   E. T tubules in skeletal muscle are located over the Z lines.

2. **Calcium is essential for muscle contraction. In cardiac muscles, calcium ions enter the sarcomere from:**

   A. the sarcoplasmic reticulum cisternae.
   B. T tubules and sarcoplasmic storage sites.
   C. outside of the muscle fibers and from the sarcoplasmic reticulum.
   D. interstitial fluid outside of the muscle fibers and the T tubules.
   E. T tubules and the triads.

3. **The dense bodies of the smooth muscle are similar to:**

   A. Z lines in the striated muscles.
   B. myosin myofilaments.
   C. actin myofilaments.
   D. T tubules and the sarcoplasmic reticulum.
   E. T tubules and triads.

4. **The caveolae in the smooth muscle are located in the:**

   A. dense bodies.
   B. actin and myosin myofilaments.
   C. cisternae of the sarcoplasmic reticulum.
   D. sarcoplasm (cell interior).
   E. cell membrane.

5. **The caveolae in smooth muscle perform what function?**

   A. They bind calcium in the sarcoplasm.
   B. They attach to actin and myosin during smooth muscle contraction.
   C. They control the influx of calcium into the smooth muscle fibers.
   D. They conduct stimulatory impulses to the dense bodies.
   E. They transmit contracting force to neighboring cells.

ANSWERS

1. **Correct Answer: B.** T tubules are larger and store more calcium in skeletal muscles. The T tubules in cardiac muscles are less well developed, and for proper muscular contraction, some calcium must be imported from outside of the cell into the sarcoplasm.

2. **Correct Answer: C.** In cardiac muscles, calcium ions enter the sarcomere from outside of the muscle fibers and from the sarcoplasmic reticulum, which is less well developed than in the skeletal muscle.

3. **Correct Answer: A.** Z lines in the striated muscles. The dense bodies contain similar proteins found in the Z lines of striated muscles.

4. **Correct Answer: E.** Cell membrane. The caveolae appear to have similar functions to those of the T tubules in striated muscles.

5. **Correct Answer: C.** Caveolae in smooth muscle control the influx of calcium into the smooth muscle fibers in a way that is similar to the T tubules of striated muscles.

ADDITIONAL HISTOLOGIC IMAGES

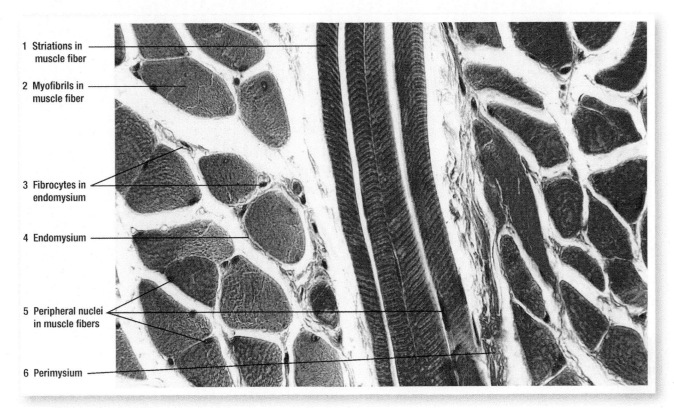

1 Striations in muscle fiber

2 Myofibrils in muscle fiber

3 Fibrocytes in endomysium

4 Endomysium

5 Peripheral nuclei in muscle fibers

6 Perimysium

FIGURE 8.18 ■ Cross and longitudinal section of skeletal muscle fibers from a primate tongue. Stain: Mallory-Azan. ×70.

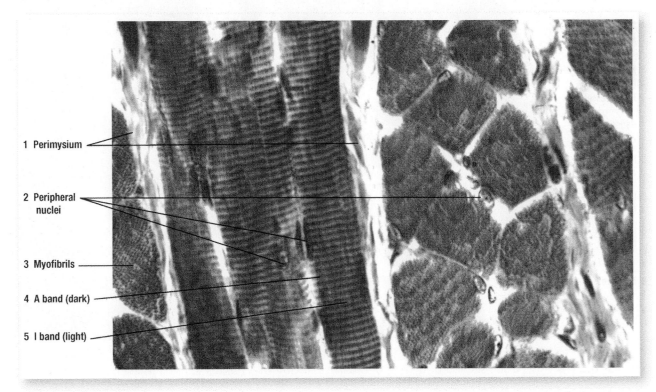

1 Perimysium

2 Peripheral nuclei

3 Myofibrils

4 A band (dark)

5 I band (light)

FIGURE 8.19 ■ Higher magnification of skeletal muscle from the tongue sectioned in longitudinal and transverse planes. Stain: Mallory-Azan. ×205.

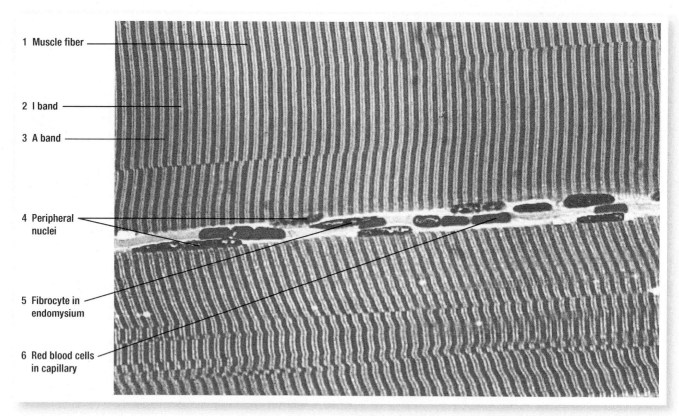

1 Muscle fiber

2 I band

3 A band

4 Peripheral nuclei

5 Fibrocyte in endomysium

6 Red blood cells in capillary

FIGURE 8.20 ■ High magnification of a plastic section showing skeletal muscle striations, peripheral nuclei, and the surrounding connective tissue. Stain: hematoxylin and eosin. ×405.

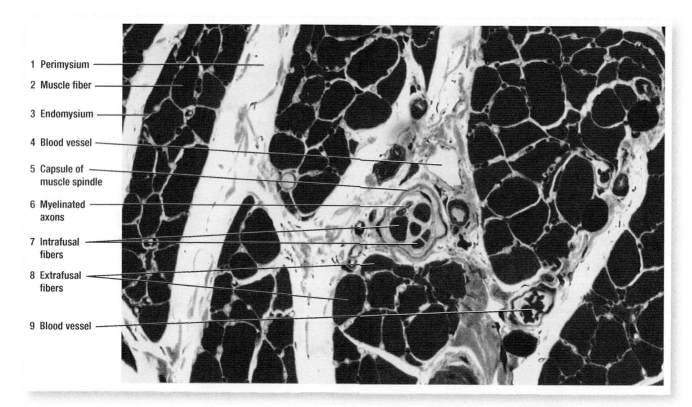

1 Perimysium

2 Muscle fiber

3 Endomysium

4 Blood vessel

5 Capsule of muscle spindle

6 Myelinated axons

7 Intrafusal fibers

8 Extrafusal fibers

9 Blood vessel

FIGURE 8.21 ■ Thin plastic section of a skeletal muscle showing the muscle spindle, its contents, and the surrounding muscle fibers. Stain: toluidine blue. ×40. Courtesy of Dr. Mark DeSantis, Professor Emeritus, WWAMI Medical Program, University of Idaho, Moscow, ID.

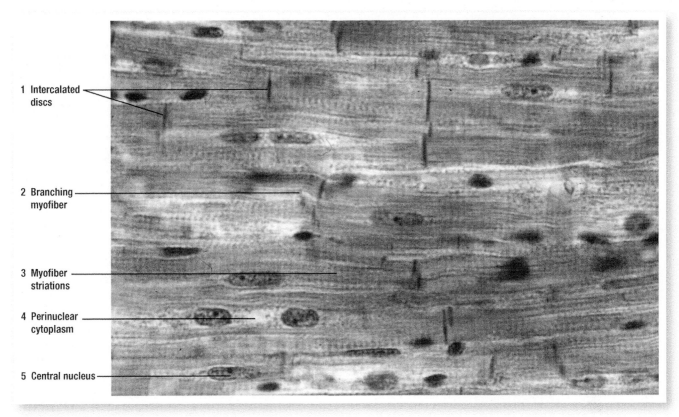

1 Intercalated discs

2 Branching myofiber

3 Myofiber striations

4 Perinuclear cytoplasm

5 Central nucleus

FIGURE 8.22 ■ High magnification of a section of primate cardiac muscle showing the central nuclei and intercalated discs. Stain: hematoxylin and eosin. ×165.

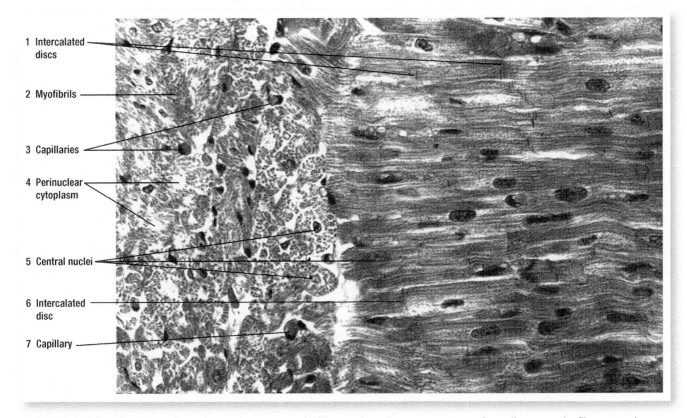

1 Intercalated discs

2 Myofibrils

3 Capillaries

4 Perinuclear cytoplasm

5 Central nuclei

6 Intercalated disc

7 Capillary

FIGURE 8.23 ■ Section of a primate heart muscle illustrating the appearance of cardiac muscle fibers cut in different planes. Stain: hematoxylin and eosin. ×165.

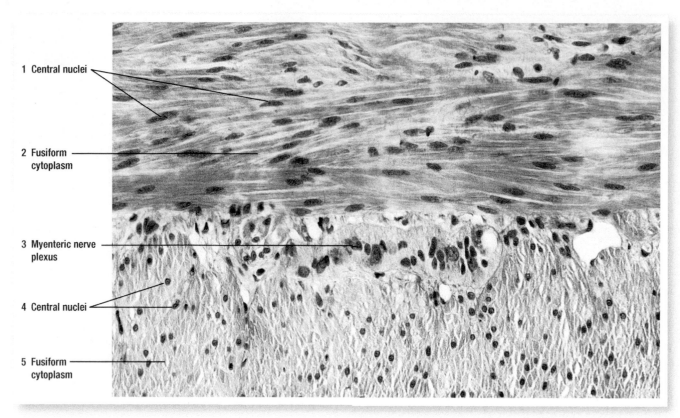

1 Central nuclei

2 Fusiform
cytoplasm

3 Myenteric nerve
plexus

4 Central nuclei

5 Fusiform
cytoplasm

FIGURE 8.24 ■ A cross section of a small intestine wall showing the circular (*upper*) and longitudinal (*lower*) smooth muscle layers. Stain: hematoxylin and eosin. ×165.

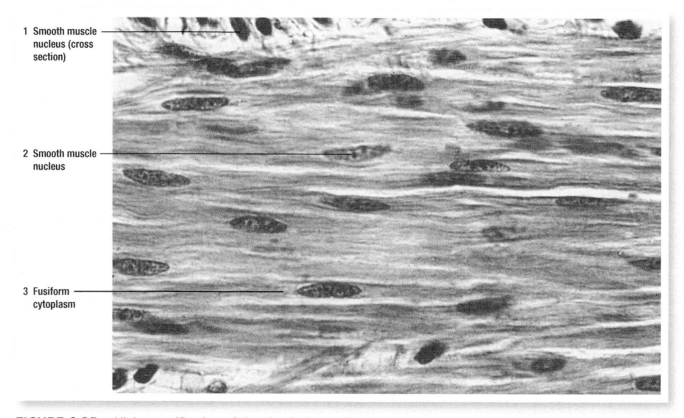

1 Smooth muscle
nucleus (cross
section)

2 Smooth muscle
nucleus

3 Fusiform
cytoplasm

FIGURE 8.25 ■ High magnification of the circular layer of the smooth muscle in the wall of a primate small intestine. Stain: hematoxylin and eosin. ×205.

Nervous Tissue

SECTION 1 Central Nervous System: Brain and Spinal Cord

INTRODUCTION

The mammalian nervous system is the most complex system in the body. It is divided into two major parts: the **central nervous system** (**CNS**) consists of the **brain** and **spinal cord** that are surrounded and protected by the cranium and vertebral bones, respectively, and the **peripheral nervous system** (**PNS**) located outside of the CNS and consists of cranial, spinal, and peripheral nerves that conduct information to (afferent or sensory) and from (efferent or motor) the CNS.

PROTECTIVE LAYERS OF THE CENTRAL NERVOUS SYSTEM

Nervous tissue is very delicate. Bones, connective tissue layers, and a watery cerebrospinal fluid (CSF) surround and protect the brain and the spinal cord. Deep to the cranial bones in the skull and the vertebral foramen are the meninges, a connective tissue that consists of three distinct layers: the dura mater, arachnoid mater, and pia mater (Fig. 9.1).

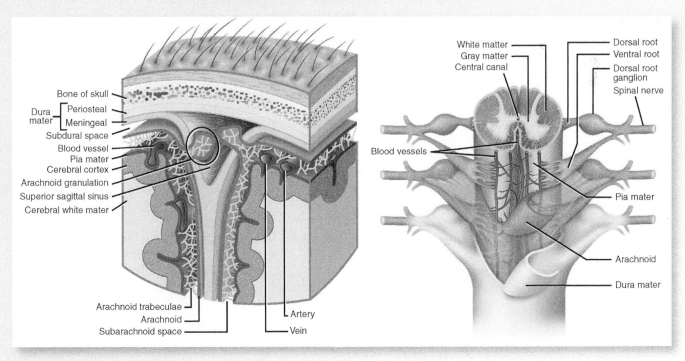

FIGURE 9.1 ■ Central nervous system (CNS). The CNS is composed of the brain and spinal cord. A section of the brain and spinal cord is illustrated with their protective connective tissue layers called meninges (dura mater, arachnoid mater, and pia mater).

The outermost meningeal layer is the **dura mater**, a tough, strong, and thick layer of dense connective tissue fibers. Deep to the dura mater is a more delicate connective tissue, the **arachnoid mater**. The dura mater and arachnoid mater surround the brain and spinal cord on their external surfaces. The innermost meningeal layer is the delicate connective tissue **pia mater**. This layer contains numerous blood vessels and adheres directly to the surfaces of the brain and spinal cord.

Between the arachnoid mater and the pia mater is the **subarachnoid space**. Delicate, web-like strands of collagen and elastic fibers attach the arachnoid mater to the pia mater. Filling and circulating in the subarachnoid space is the CSF that bathes and protects both the brain and spinal cord from shock and injury.

CEREBROSPINAL FLUID

The **CSF** is a clear, colorless fluid that cushions the brain and spinal cord and provides protective buoyancy from physical injuries. CSF is continually produced by the **choroid plexuses** in the lateral, third, and fourth ventricles or cavities of the brain, with the majority of the fluid produced in the lateral ventricles. Choroid plexuses are small, vascular extensions of dilated and fenestrated capillaries that penetrate the interior of brain ventricles. Blood that is selectively filtered through the cells of the choroids plexus forms the CSF, a clear, colorless fluid with Na^+, K^+, and Cl^- ions that are needed for neuronal functions. The CSF circulates through the ventricles and around the outer surfaces of the brain and spinal cord in the subarachnoid space and in the central canal of the spinal cord.

CSF is important for homeostasis and brain metabolism. It brings nutrients to nourish brain cells, removes metabolites that enter the CSF from the brain cells, and provides an optimal chemical environment for neuronal functions and impulse conduction. After circulation, CSF is reabsorbed from the arachnoid space via the **arachnoid villi** into venous blood, mainly at the superior sagittal sinus—a major vein that drains the brain. Arachnoid villi are small, thin-walled arachnoid extensions that penetrate the dura mater and project into the venous sinuses located between the periosteal and meningeal layers of dura mater.

MORPHOLOGY OF A TYPICAL NEURON

The nervous system contains complex intercommunicating networks of nerve cells that receive and conduct **impulses** along their neural pathways or axons to the CNS for analysis, integration, interpretation, and response. The appropriate response to a stimulus from the neurons of the CNS is the activation of muscle (skeletal, smooth, or cardiac) functions or glandular secretions (endocrine or exocrine).

The structural and functional cells of the nervous tissue are the **neurons** (Fig. 9.2). Although neurons vary in size and shape, they share common features. Each neuron consists

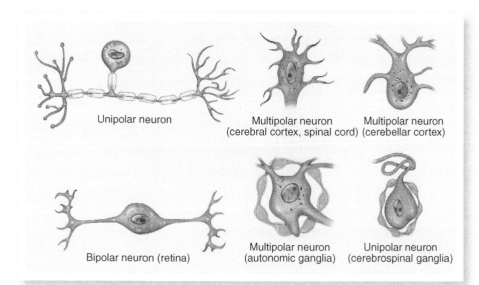

FIGURE 9.2 ■ Examples of different types of neurons located in various ganglia and organs outside the CNS.

Unipolar neuron

Multipolar neuron (cerebral cortex, spinal cord)

Multipolar neuron (cerebellar cortex)

Bipolar neuron (retina)

Multipolar neuron (autonomic ganglia)

Unipolar neuron (cerebrospinal ganglia)

of **soma or cell body**, numerous **dendrites**, and a single **axon**. The cell body contains the nucleus, nucleolus, numerous different organelles, and the surrounding cytoplasm or perikaryon. Projecting from the cell body are numerous cytoplasmic extensions called dendrites that form a dendritic tree.

Surrounding the neurons are the smaller and more numerous supportive cells collectively called **neuroglia**. These cells form the nonneural components of the CNS.

TYPES OF NEURONS IN THE CENTRAL NERVOUS SYSTEM

The three major types of neurons in the nervous system are multipolar, bipolar, and unipolar. This anatomic classification is based on the number of dendrites and axons that originate from the cell body.

- **Multipolar neurons**. These are the most common type in the CNS and include all **motor neurons** and **interneurons** of the brain, cerebellum, and spinal cord. Projecting from one side of the neuron cell body are numerous branched dendrites in contrast to a single axon on the opposite site.

- **Bipolar neurons**. These are less common and are purely **sensory neurons**. In bipolar neurons, a single dendrite and a single axon are associated with the cell body. Bipolar neurons are found in the retina of the eye, in hearing and equilibrium region organs of the inner ear, and in the olfactory epithelium of the nose (the latter two are found in the PNS).

- **Unipolar neurons**. Most neurons in the adult organism that exhibit only one process leaving the cell body were initially bipolar during embryonic development. The two neuronal processes fuse during later development and form one axon process. This process then divides close to the cell body into two long axonal branches. One of these branches continues to the CNS, whereas the other branch extends to the peripheral organ. The unipolar neurons (formerly called pseudounipolar neurons) are also **sensory**. The cell bodies of unipolar neurons are found in numerous dorsal root ganglia of spinal nerves and cranial nerve ganglia. The ganglia represent a collection of neurons surrounded by their supportive cells and can be either sensory or motor.

MYELIN SHEATH AND MYELINATION OF AXONS

Specialized cells in both the CNS and the PNS surround and wrap around the axon multiple times. This process builds up successive layers of modified cell membrane and forms a lipid-rich, insulating sheath around the axon called the **myelin sheath**. As the wrapping around the axon continues, the cells' cytoplasm is gradually forced or squeezed out from between the membranes of the concentric layers. Along the myelin sheath are small islands of Schwann cell cytoplasm between the myelin membranes that were not squeezed out during the myelination process. These are **Schmidt-Lanterman incisures or clefts** seen best with electron microscopy as they pass obliquely across the width of the myelin sheath.

The myelin sheath extends from the initial segments of the axon to the terminal branches. Interspersed along the length of a myelinated axon are small gaps or spaces in the myelin sheath because the myelin sheath is formed by numerous cells. Where the myelinating cells meet is a tiny area that is devoid of myelin. These gaps in myelin sheath are called **nodes of Ranvier**. Axons in both the CNS and the PNS can be either myelinated or unmyelinated.

In the PNS, all axons are surrounded by **Schwann cells** that either myelinate the axons or envelope the unmyelinated axons with their cytoplasm. Schwann cells myelinate individual peripheral axons and extend along their entire length, from their origin at the cell body to their termination in the muscle or gland. In contrast, each Schwann cell cytoplasm can envelope numerous unmyelinated axons. Unmyelinated axons enveloped by Schwann cells do not show nodes of Ranvier. Smaller axons in the peripheral nerves, such as those in the autonomic nervous system (ANS), are unmyelinated and surrounded only by the Schwann cell cytoplasm.

There are no Schwann cells in the CNS. Instead, neuroglial cells called **oligodendrocytes** myelinate the axons in the CNS. Oligodendrocytes differ from Schwann cells in that the cytoplasmic branching processes extend radially from one oligodendrocyte and myelinate numerous adjacent axons.

GRAY AND WHITE MATTER

The brain and the spinal cord contain gray matter and white matter. The **gray matter** of the CNS consists of neurons, their dendrites, and the supportive cells called **neuroglia**. This region also represents the site of connections or **synapses** between a multitude of neurons and dendrites. Gray matter forms the outer surface of the brain (cerebrum) and cerebellum. The size, shape, and mode of branching of these neurons are highly variable and depend on which region of the CNS is examined.

The gray matter also contains a meshwork of neural tissues such as axonal, dendritic, and glial processes that are packed very tightly together and that fill the interneural spaces. This associated meshwork of neural processes in the gray matter is called the **neuropil**. **White matter** in the CNS is devoid of neuronal cell bodies and consists primarily of myelinated axons, some unmyelinated axons, the supportive neuroglial oligodendrocytes, and blood vessels. The myelin sheaths around the axons impart a white color to this region of the CNS.

SYNAPSES

Synapses are specialized sites for chemical or electrical transmission for communication between neurons, interneurons, and effector cells, such as the muscle fibers or glands. Synapses are too small to be visible with routine histologic preparations but can be seen ultrastructurally with transmission electron microscopy. The transmission of an impulse at the synapse is from one **presynaptic** cell to a **postsynaptic** cell and is always unidirectional. Synapses that occur between axons and dendrites are classified as **axodendritic**, between an axon and the neuron cell body as **axosomatic**, and between axons as **axoaxonic**. A typical synapse in the CNS consists of a presynaptic component with a **presynaptic membrane**, a **synaptic cleft**, and a **postsynaptic membrane**. The synaptic cleft separates the presynaptic and postsynaptic membranes.

SUPPORTING CELLS IN THE CENTRAL NERVOUS SYSTEM: NEUROGLIA

Neuroglia are the highly branched, supportive, nonneuronal cells in the CNS that surround the neurons, their axons, and dendrites. These cells do not become stimulated or conduct impulses and are morphologically and functionally different from the neurons. Neuroglial cells can be distinguished by their much smaller size and dark-staining nuclei. The CNS contains approximately 10-fold more neuroglial cells than neurons. The four types of neuroglial cells are **astrocytes**, **oligodendrocytes**, **microglia**, and **ependymal cells**.

the**Point**⁺   Supplemental micrographic images are available at **www.thePoint.com/Eroschenko13e** under Nervous Tissue.

FIGURE 9.3 | Spinal Cord: Midthoracic Region (Transverse Section)

The transverse section of a spinal cord cut in the midthoracic region and stained with hematoxylin and eosin is illustrated. Although a basic structural pattern is seen throughout the spinal cord, the shape and structure of the cord vary at different levels (cervical, thoracic, lumbar, and sacral).

The thoracic region of the spinal cord differs from the cervical region illustrated in Figure 9.5. The thoracic spinal cord exhibits slender **posterior gray horns (6)** and smaller **anterior gray horns (10, 20)** with fewer **motor neurons (10, 20)**. The **lateral gray horns (8, 19)** are well developed in the thoracic region and contain the **motor neurons (8, 19)** of the sympathetic division of the ANS.

The remaining structures in the midthoracic region of the spinal cord correspond to the structures illustrated in the cervical cord region in Figure 9.5. These are the **posterior median sulcus (15)**, **anterior median fissure (22)**, **fasciculus gracilis (16)** and **fasciculus cuneatus (17)** (seen in the mid-to-upper-thoracic region of the spinal cord) of the **posterior white column (16, 17)**, **lateral white column (7)**, **central canal (9)**, and the **gray commissure (18)**. Associated with the posterior gray horns (6) are axons of the **posterior roots (5)**, and leaving the anterior gray horns (10, 20) are the **axons (11, 21)** of the **anterior roots (11)**.

Surrounding the spinal cord are the connective tissue layers of the meninges. These are the thick and fibrous outer **dura mater (2)**, the thinner and middle **arachnoid mater (3)**, and the delicate inner pia mater (4), which closely adheres to the surface of the spinal cord. Located in the **pia mater (4)** are numerous anterior and posterior **spinal blood vessels (1, 12)**. Between the arachnoid (3) and the pia mater (4) is the **subarachnoid space (14)**. Fine trabeculae located in the subarachnoid space (14) connect the pia mater (4) with the arachnoid mater (3). In life, the subarachnoid space (14) is filled with circulating CSF. Between the arachnoid mater (3) and the dura mater (2) is the **subdural space (13)**. In this preparation, the subdural space (13) appears unusually large because of the artifactual retraction of the arachnoid during the specimen preparation.

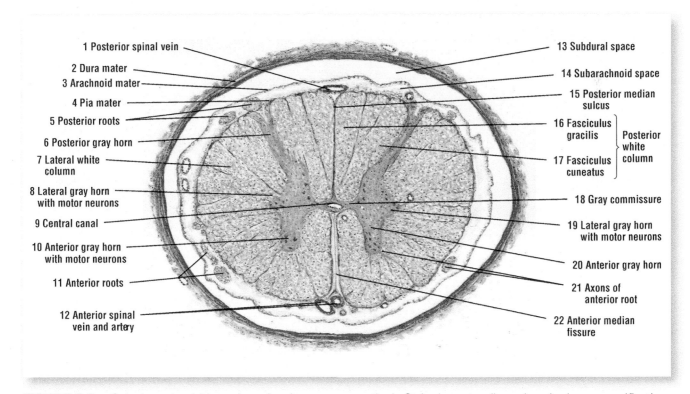

FIGURE 9.3 ■ Spinal cord: midthoracic region (transverse section). Stain: hematoxylin and eosin. Low magnification.

FIGURE 9.4 | Spinal Cord: Anterior Gray Horn, Motor Neurons, and Adjacent Anterior White Matter

A higher magnification of a small section of the anterior horn of the thoracic region of the spinal cord illustrates the **white matter**, **gray matter**, neurons, **neuroglia**, and axons stained with hematoxylin and eosin. The cells in this region are **multipolar motor neurons** (**2, 7, 10**). The cytoplasm is characterized by a prominent vesicular **nucleus** (**10**), a distinct **nucleolus** (**10**), and coarse clumps of basophilic material called the **Nissl substance** (**3**). The Nissl substance extends into the dendrites but not into the axons. Two of the neurons exhibit the axons and their **axon hillocks** (**4, 9**), which is devoid of the Nissl substance; this feature characterizes the axon hillock. In certain **multipolar neurons** (**7**), the plane of section missed the nucleus, and, as a result, the cytoplasm appears enucleated (without a nucleus) and exhibits only the Nissl substance in the cytoplasm.

The nonneural supportive neuroglia (**8**), seen as basophilic nuclei, are small in comparison to the multipolar neurons (**2, 7, 10**). The neuroglia (**8**) occupy the spaces between the neurons. The anterior white matter of the spinal cord contains myelinated axons of various sizes. Because of the use solvent chemicals (xylene) in preparation of this section, the myelin sheaths were lost or washed out and appear as clear spaces around the dark-staining central **axons** (**5**). Also visible in the image are capillaries, venules, and an **arteriole** (**6**).

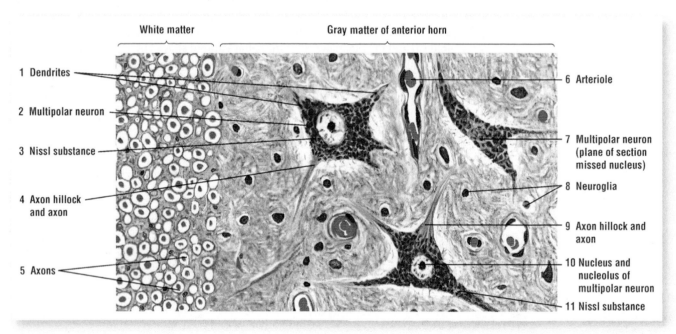

FIGURE 9.4 ■ Spinal cord: anterior gray horn, motor neuron, and adjacent white matter. Stain: hematoxylin and eosin. Medium magnification.

FIGURE 9.5 | **Spinal Cord: Midcervical Region (Transverse Section)**

A cross section of the spinal cord was prepared with the silver impregnation technique to illustrate the **white matter** and the **gray matter**. After staining, the dark brown, outer white matter (**3**) and the light-staining, inner gray matter (**4, 14**) are visible. The white matter (**3**) consists primarily of ascending and descending myelinated nerve fibers or axons. By contrast, the gray matter contains neurons and interneurons. The gray matter also exhibits a symmetrical H-shape, with the two sides connected across the midline of the spinal cord by the **gray commissure** (**15**). In the center of the gray commissure is the **central canal** (**16**) of the spinal cord.

The anterior **horns** (**6**) of the gray matter are more prominent than the **posterior horns** (**2, 13**) and contain the cell bodies of the large **motor neurons** (**7, 17**). Some **axons** (**8, 20**) from these motor neurons cross the white matter and exit from the spinal cord as **anterior roots** (**9, 21**) of the peripheral nerves. The posterior horns (**2, 13**) are the sensory areas and contain cell bodies of smaller neurons.

The spinal cord is surrounded by connective tissue meninges, consisting of an outer dura mater, a middle **arachnoid mater** (**5**), and an inner **pia mater** (**18**). The spinal cord is also partially divided into right and left halves by a narrow, posterior (dorsal) groove—the posterior

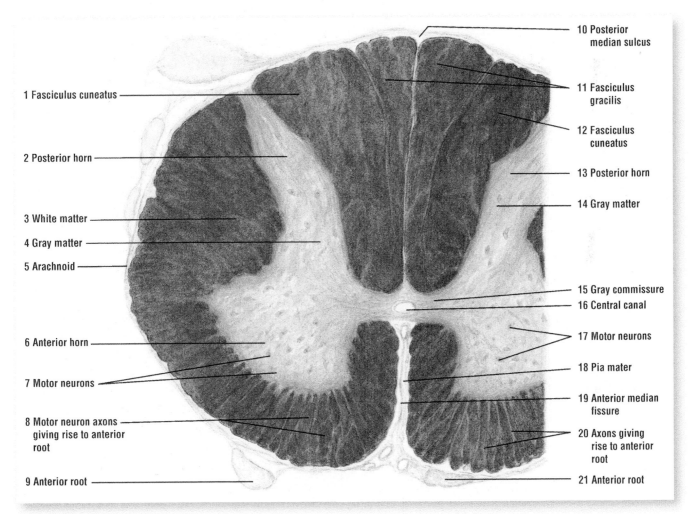

1 Fasciculus cuneatus

2 Posterior horn

3 White matter

4 Gray matter

5 Arachnoid

6 Anterior horn

7 Motor neurons

8 Motor neuron axons giving rise to anterior root

9 Anterior root

10 Posterior median sulcus

11 Fasciculus gracilis

12 Fasciculus cuneatus

13 Posterior horn

14 Gray matter

15 Gray commissure

16 Central canal

17 Motor neurons

18 Pia mater

19 Anterior median fissure

20 Axons giving rise to anterior root

21 Anterior root

FIGURE 9.5 ■ Spinal cord: midcervical region (transverse section). Stain: silver impregnation (Cajal method). Low magnification.

median sulcus (**10**)—and a deep, anterior (ventral) cleft—the anterior median fissure (**19**). In this illustration, pia mater (**18**) is best seen in the **anterior median fissure** (**19**).

Between the posterior median sulcus (**10**) and the posterior horns (**2, 13**) of the gray matter are the posterior columns of the white matter. In the midcervical region of the spinal cord, each dorsal column is subdivided into two fascicles, the posteromedial column—the **fasciculus gracilis** (**11**)—and the posterolateral column—the **fasciculus cuneatus** (**1, 12**).

FIGURE 9.6 | Spinal Cord: Anterior Gray Horn, Motor Neurons, and Adjacent Anterior White Matter

A section of the white matter and the gray matter of the anterior horn of the spinal cord is illustrated at a higher magnification. The gray matter contains large, **multipolar motor neurons** (**2, 3**). These are characterized by numerous **dendrites** (**5, 6**) that extend in different directions from the perikaryon (cell bodies). In some neurons, the **nucleus** (**8**) is visible with its prominent **nucleolus** (**8**). In other neurons, the plane of section missed the nucleus and the perikaryon appears empty (**2**). Surrounding the motor neurons are the small, light-staining, supportive cells, the **neuroglia** (**7**).

The white matter contains closely packed myelinated axons. In cross sections, the **axons** (**1**) appear dark-stained and surrounded by clear spaces that are the remnants of the lost myelin sheaths. The axons in the white matter represent the ascending and descending neural pathways of the spinal cord. The **axons** (**4**) of the anterior horn motor neurons aggregate into groups, pass through the white matter, and exit the spinal cord as the anterior (ventral) root fibers (see Fig. 9.5).

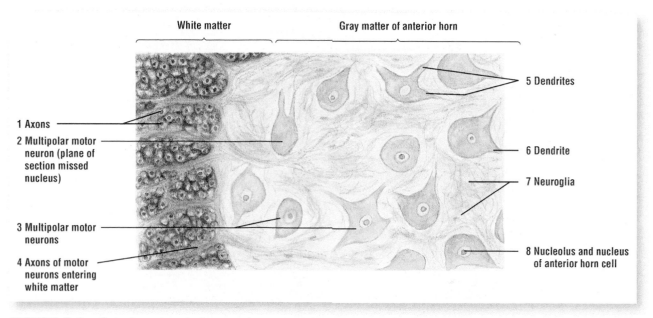

FIGURE 9.6 ■ Spinal cord: anterior gray horn, motor neurons, and adjacent anterior white matter. Stain: silver impregnation (Cajal method). Medium magnification.

FIGURE 9.7 | Ultrastructure of Typical Axodendritic Synapses in the CNS

It is not possible to see synapses in the CNS with routine hematoxylin and eosin preparations. This high-magnification transmission electron micrograph shows two typical axodendritic synapses (2, 4) in the CNS. The terminal end of the presynaptic component (1, 3) is expanded and contains numerous small **neurotransmitter vesicles** (1, 3). A small intercellular space, called the **synaptic cleft** (2, 4), is located between and separates the **presynaptic membrane** (2, 4) from the **postsynaptic membranes** (8). The postsynaptic membranes (8) appear thicker and denser than the presynaptic membrane (2, 4). In the center of the image is a section of a **dendrite** (7) with **neurofilaments, microtubules,** and large **mitochondria** (7). Located around the dendrite (7) are smaller **myelinated axons** (5) with a dense, thick **myelin sheath** (9). In the upper region of the figure are numerous **unmyelinated axons** (6). Both the myelinated axons (5) and the unmyelinated axons (6, 7) contain dark-staining, oval **mitochondria** (6) with shelf-like cristae.

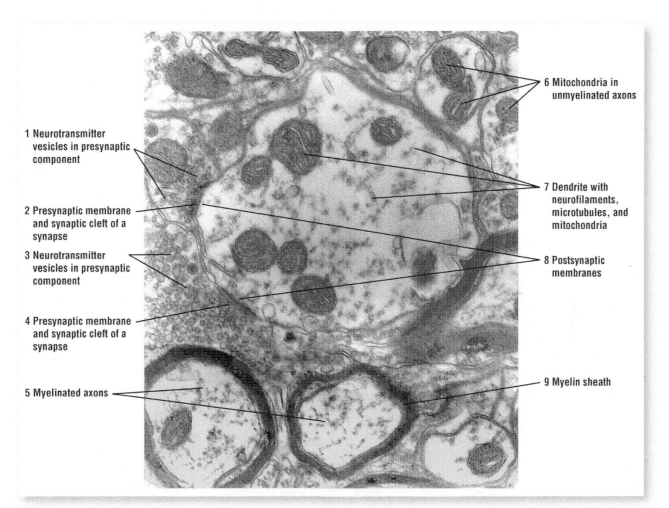

1 Neurotransmitter vesicles in presynaptic component

2 Presynaptic membrane and synaptic cleft of a synapse

3 Neurotransmitter vesicles in presynaptic component

4 Presynaptic membrane and synaptic cleft of a synapse

5 Myelinated axons

6 Mitochondria in unmyelinated axons

7 Dendrite with neurofilaments, microtubules, and mitochondria

8 Postsynaptic membranes

9 Myelin sheath

FIGURE 9.7 ■ Ultrastructure of typical axodendritic synapses in the CNS. Transmission electron micrograph. Courtesy of Dr. Mark Desantis, Professor Emeritus, WWAMI Medical Program, University of Idaho, Moscow, ID. ×75,000.

FUNCTIONAL CORRELATIONS 9.1 ■ Synapses

Synapses are specialized membrane junctions where transmissions of nerve impulses are conveyed unidirectionally from a **presynaptic** neuron to a **postsynaptic** membrane of a neuron; effector cells, such as muscle fibers; or gland cells. The synapses process and convert an impulse from the presynaptic cell into a signal that affects the postsynaptic cell membranes and initiates stimulatory neuronal activities. Most synapses in mammals release **chemical neurotransmitters** from the presynaptic portion of one axon or dendrite to the postsynaptic membrane of another cell. Numerous neurotransmitters exist, including amino acids such as glutamate, catecholamines, acetylcholamine, and others. Neurotransmitter chemicals first cross the **synaptic cleft**, bind to specific **neurotransmitter receptors** on the postsynaptic membrane, and produce either an **excitatory** response or an **inhibitory** response at the postsynaptic membrane. The final generation of nerve impulse in a postsynaptic cell depends on the summation of excitatory or inhibitory effects of many synapses on the target cell allowing a more precise regulation of responses from postsynaptic neurons, muscles, or glands. Thus, the synapses regulate neuronal activity in the nervous system by inducing either excitatory or inhibitory effects on the target cells after which the neurotransmitters are rapidly removed from the synaptic cleft by enzymes, diffusion, or endocytosis.

FIGURE 9.8 | Motor Neurons: Anterior Horn of Spinal Cord

The large, multipolar **motor neurons** (**7**) of the CNS have a large central **nucleus** (**11**), a prominent **nucleolus** (**12**), and several radiating cell processes—the **dendrites** (**10, 16**). A single, thin **axon** (**5, 14**) arises from a cone-shaped, clear area of the neuron; this is the **axon hillock** (**13**). The axons (**5, 14**) that leave the motor neurons (**7**) are thinner and much longer than the thicker and shorter dendrites (**10, 16**).

The cytoplasm, or perikaryon, of the neuron is characterized by coarse granules (basophilic masses). These are the **Nissl bodies** (**4, 8**), and they represent the granular endoplasmic

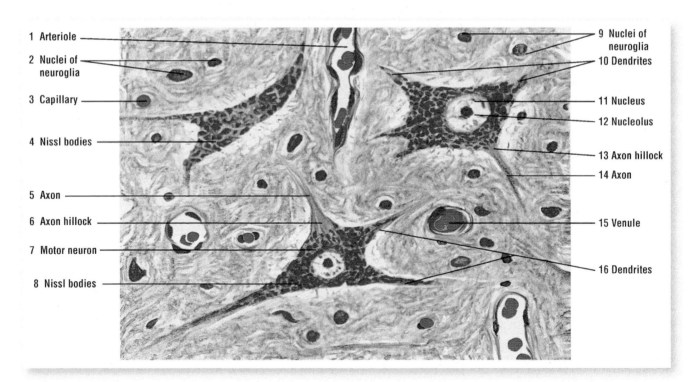

1 Arteriole
2 Nuclei of neuroglia
3 Capillary
4 Nissl bodies
5 Axon
6 Axon hillock
7 Motor neuron
8 Nissl bodies

9 Nuclei of neuroglia
10 Dendrites
11 Nucleus
12 Nucleolus
13 Axon hillock
14 Axon
15 Venule
16 Dendrites

FIGURE 9.8 ■ Motor neurons: anterior horn of the spinal cord. Stain: hematoxylin and eosin. High magnification.

reticulum of the neuron. When the plane of section misses the nucleus (4), only the dark-staining Nissl bodies (4) are seen in the perikaryon of the neuron. The Nissl bodies (4, 8) extend into the dendrites (10, 16) but not into the axon hillock (6, 13) or into the axon (5, 14). This feature distinguishes the axons (5, 14) from the dendrites (10, 16). The nucleus of the neuron stains light because of the uniform dispersion of the chromatin, whereas the nucleolus (12) is prominent, dense, and stains dark. The nuclei (2, 9) of the surrounding **neuroglia** (**2, 9**) are stained prominently, whereas their small cytoplasm remains unstained. The neuroglia (2, 9) are nonneural cells of the CNS; they provide the structural and metabolic support for the neurons (7).

Surrounding the neurons (7) and the neuroglia (2, 9) are numerous **blood vessels** (**1, 3, 15**) of various sizes.

FUNCTIONAL CORRELATIONS 9.2 ■ Neurons, Interneurons, Axons, and Dendrites

Functionally, neurons are classified as **afferent** (sensory), **efferent** (motor), or **interneurons**. Sensory or afferent neurons conduct impulses from receptors in the internal organs or from the external environment to the CNS. **Somatic afferent** fibers conduct impulses from the body surface and body organs, such as muscles, tendons, and joints. **Visceral afferent** fibers conduct impulses from internal organs, glands, and blood vessels. Motor, or efferent, fibers convey impulses from the CNS to the effector muscles or glands in the peripheries. Interneurons constitute the majority of the neurons in the CNS. They serve as intermediaries or integrators of nerve impulses and connect neuronal circuits between sensory neurons, motor neurons, and other interneurons in the CNS.

Neurons are specialized for **irritability, conductivity**, and production or **synthesis of neurotransmitters** and **neurohormones**. After a mechanical or chemical stimulus, these neurons react (irritability) to the stimulus and transmit (conductivity) the information via axons to other neurons or interneurons in different regions of the nervous system. Strong stimuli create a wave of excitation, or nerve impulse (action potential), which is then propagated along the entire length of the axon (nerve fiber).

Extending from the neurons are dendrites that divide in a treelike fashion allowing the dendrites to connect with and receive stimuli from axon terminals of other neurons. The surface of the dendrites is covered by **dendritic spines** that connect (synapse) with axon terminals from other neurons. The surface membranes of the neurons and the dendrites are specialized to receive and to integrate information from other dendrites, neurons, or axons. The axons, in turn, conduct the received information from the neuron to an interneuron,

another neuron, or to an effector organ, such as a muscle or gland.

Axons arise from the funnel-shaped region of the cell body called the **axon hillock**. The **initial segment** of the axon is located between the axon hillock and where myelination starts. It is at the initial segment that the stimuli, whether inhibitory or stimulatory, are summed and nerve stimuli are generated. The rate of conduction of the stimulus is dependent on the size of the axon and myelination. Myelinated axons conduct at a much faster rate (velocity) than the unmyelinated axons of the same size. To initiate a nerve impulse, neurotransmitters are released at different synapses.

In addition to impulse conduction, axons also exhibit a **bidirectional transport** of chemical substances, organelles, or membrane-bound neurotransmitters between the neuron and the axon terminals. Materials that are synthesized in the neurons are transported in tiny **microtubules** to the region where the axon terminates or **synapses** with other dendrites, a cell body, or other axons. This movement in axons is called **anterograde transport**. Similarly, material carried from the axon terminals and dendrites toward the neurons is called **retrograde transport**. Transport by microtubules in either direction requires energy, which is used by microtubule-associated motor proteins. The mechanism for anterograde transport involves **kinesin**, a microtubule-associated motor protein that moves substances along the axonal microtubules away from the neuron. The retrograde transport in axons toward the neurons is mediated by microtubule-associated motor protein called **dynein**.

In addition, microtubules and microfilaments serve a role in the growth of axons during development and their regeneration following an injury.

FIGURE 9.9 | Neurofibrils and Motor Neurons in Gray Matter of Anterior Horn of Spinal Cord

The anterior horn of the spinal cord was prepared by silver impregnation (the Cajal method) to demonstrate **neurofibrils** in both the **gray matter** and **motor neurons**. Fine neurofibrils (2, 4) are distributed throughout the **cytoplasm (perikaryon)** (4) and **dendrites** (2, 9) of the motor neurons (1, 10, 11).

The nuclei of the **motor neurons** (1, 11) appear yellow stained and their **nucleoli** (5, 10) dark stained. Not all motor neurons were sectioned through the middle. As a result, some motor neurons show only a nucleus (1) without a nucleolus, whereas others show only the **peripheral cytoplasm** (8) without a nucleus.

There are also many neurofibrils in the gray matter (3), some of which belong to the axons of anterior horn neurons (1, 11) or the adjacent **neuroglia** (7), whose **nuclei** (7) are visible throughout the gray matter (3) (see also Fig. 9.10).

The clear spaces around the neurons and their processes are artifacts caused by the chemical preparations of the nervous tissue.

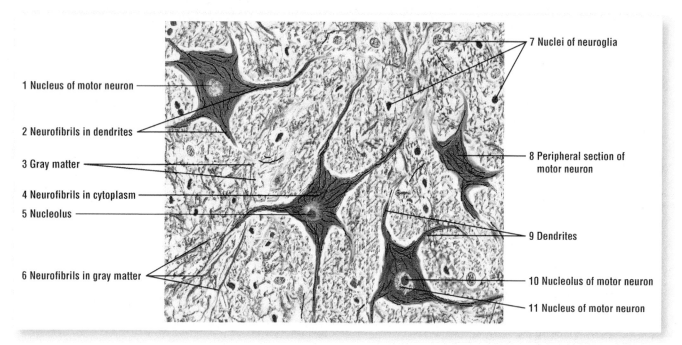

1 Nucleus of motor neuron

2 Neurofibrils in dendrites

3 Gray matter

4 Neurofibrils in cytoplasm

5 Nucleolus

6 Neurofibrils in gray matter

7 Nuclei of neuroglia

8 Peripheral section of motor neuron

9 Dendrites

10 Nucleolus of motor neuron

11 Nucleus of motor neuron

FIGURE 9.9 ■ Neurofibrils and motor neurons in the gray matter of the anterior horn of the spinal cord. Stain: silver impregnation (Cajal method). High magnification.

FIGURE 9.10 | Anterior Gray Horn of Spinal Cord: Multipolar Motor Neurons, Axons, and Neuroglial Cells

This medium-magnification photomicrograph of the anterior gray horn of the spinal cord was prepared with silver stain to show the neurons and **axons** of the CNS. The large multipolar **motor neurons** (1) exhibit numerous **dendrites** (4). Each motor neuron (1) contains a **nucleus** (5) and a **nucleolus** (6). Within the cytoplasm of the motor neurons (1) is the cytoskeleton consisting of numerous **neurofibrils** (3) that course through the cell body and extend into the dendrites (4) and axons (8). Visible also are numerous axons of a size different from other nerve cells in the spinal cord. Surrounding the motor neurons (1) are **nuclei** of **neuroglial cells** (2), a **blood vessel** (7) with blood cells and a meshwork of neural processes, the **neuropil** (9).

Similar to Figure 9.8, the clear spaces around the neurons and their processes are artifacts caused by tissue shrinkage during the preparation of the spinal cord.

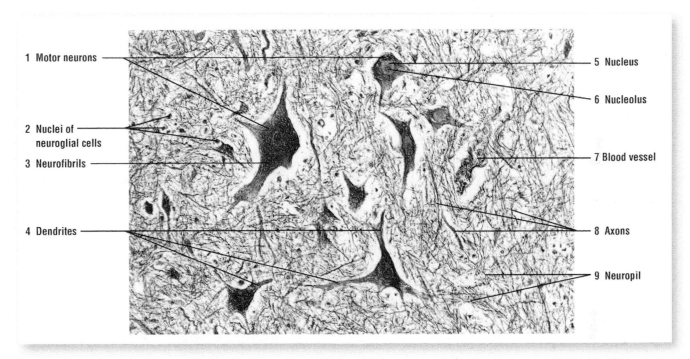

FIGURE 9.10 ■ Anterior gray horn of the spinal cord: multipolar neurons, axons, and neuroglial cells. Stain: silver impregnation (Cajal method). ×80.

FIGURE 9.11 | Cerebral Cortex: Gray Matter

Cell types that constitute the gray matter of the cerebral cortex are distributed in six layers, with one or more cell types predominant in each layer. Although there are variations in the arrangement of cells in the cerebral cortex, distinct layers are recognized in most regions. Horizontal and radial axons associated with neuronal cells in different layers give the cerebral cortex a laminated appearance. These layers are labeled with Roman numerals on the right side of the figure.

The most superficial is the **molecular layer** (**I**). Overlying the molecular cell layer (I) is the delicate connective tissue of the brain, the **pia mater** (**1**). The peripheral portion of molecular layer (I) is composed predominantly of **neuroglial cells** (**2**) and horizontal cells of Cajal. Their axons contribute to the horizontal fibers that are seen in the molecular layer (I).

The external **granular layer** (**II**) contains different types of neuroglial cells and **small pyramidal cells** (**3**). The pyramidal cells get progressively larger in successively deeper layers of the cortex. The **apical dendrites** of the **pyramidal cells** (**4, 7**) are directed toward the periphery of the cortex, whereas their axons extend from the cell bases (see Fig. 9.12 [4, 10]). In the **external pyramidal layer** (**III**), **medium-sized pyramidal cells** (**5**) predominate.

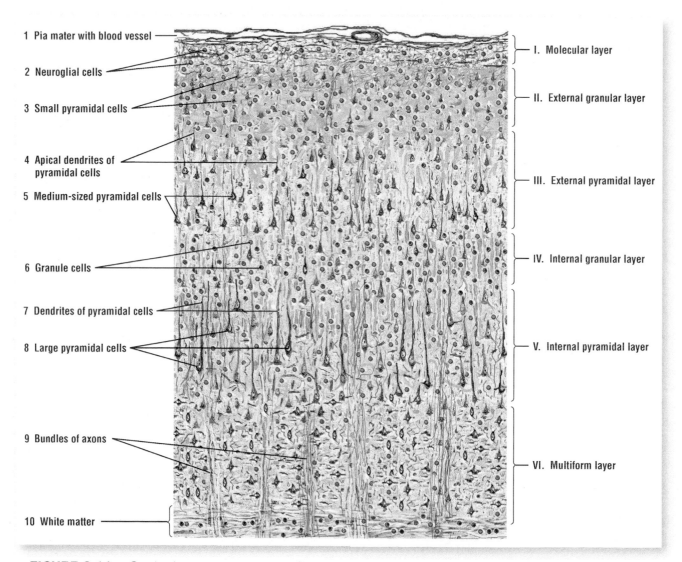

1 Pia mater with blood vessel

2 Neuroglial cells

3 Small pyramidal cells

4 Apical dendrites of pyramidal cells

5 Medium-sized pyramidal cells

6 Granule cells

7 Dendrites of pyramidal cells

8 Large pyramidal cells

9 Bundles of axons

10 White matter

I. Molecular layer

II. External granular layer

III. External pyramidal layer

IV. Internal granular layer

V. Internal pyramidal layer

VI. Multiform layer

FIGURE 9.11 ■ Cerebral cortex: gray matter: Stain: silver impregnation (Cajal method). Low magnification.

The **internal granular layer** (**IV**) is a thin layer and contains mainly small **granule cells** (**6**), some pyramidal cells, and neuroglia that form complex connections with the pyramidal cells. The **internal pyramidal layer** (**V**) contains neuroglial cells and the largest **pyramidal cells** (**8**), especially in the motor area of the cerebral cortex. The deepest layer is the **multiform layer** (**VI**) that is adjacent to the **white matter** (**10**) of the cerebral cortex. The multiform layer (VI) contains intermixed cells of varying shapes and sizes, such as the fusiform cells, granule cells, stellate cells, and cells of Martinotti. **Bundles of axons** (**9**) enter and leave the white matter (**10**).

FIGURE 9.12 | Layer V of Cerebral Cortex

A higher magnification of layer V of the cerebral cortex illustrates the large **pyramidal cells** (**3**). Note the l large vesicular **nucleus** (**3**) with its **nucleolus** (**3**). The silver stain also shows numerous **neurofibrils** (**9**) in the pyramidal cells (**3**). The most prominent cell processes are the **apical dendrites** (**1, 7**) of the pyramidal cells (**3**), which are directed toward the surface of the cortex. The **axons** (**4, 10**) of the pyramidal cells (**3**) arise from the base of the cell body and pass into the white matter (see Fig. 9.11 [10]).

The intercellular area is occupied by **neuroglial cells** (**2, 8**) in the cortex, small astrocytes, and blood vessels—**venule** (**5**) and **capillary** (**6**).

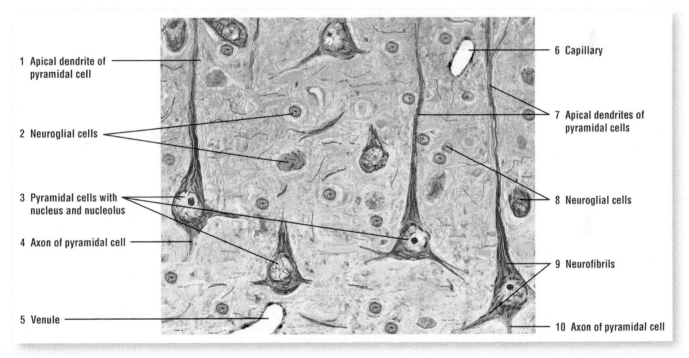

1 Apical dendrite of pyramidal cell

2 Neuroglial cells

3 Pyramidal cells with nucleus and nucleolus

4 Axon of pyramidal cell

5 Venule

6 Capillary

7 Apical dendrites of pyramidal cells

8 Neuroglial cells

9 Neurofibrils

10 Axon of pyramidal cell

FIGURE 9.12 ■ Layer V of the cerebral cortex. Stain: silver impregnation (Cajal method). High magnification.

FIGURE 9.13 | Cerebellum (Transverse Section)

The **cerebellar cortex** (**1**, **10**) exhibits numerous deeply convoluted folds called **cerebellar folia** (**6**) (singular: folium) separated by **sulci** (**9**). The cerebellar folia (6) are covered by the thin connective tissue, the pia mater (7), which follows the surface of each folium (6) into the adjacent sulci (9). The detachment of the **pia mater** (**7**) from the cerebellar cortex (1, 10) is an artifact caused by tissue fixation and preparation.

The cerebellum (1, 10) consists of an outer **gray matter or cortex** (**1**, **10**) and an inner **white matter** (**5**, **8**). Three distinct cell layers are distinguished in the cerebellar cortex (1, 10): an outer **molecular layer** (**2**) with few and small neuronal cell bodies and fibers that extend parallel to the length of the folium, a central or middle **Purkinje cell layer** (**3**), and an inner **granular layer** (**4**) with small neurons that exhibit stained nuclei. The Purkinje cells (3) are pyriform, or pyramidal, in shape with ramified dendrites that extend into the molecular layer (2).

The white matter (5, 8) forms the core of each cerebellar folium (6) and consists of myelinated nerve fibers, or axons. The axons are the afferent and efferent fibers of the cerebellar cortex.

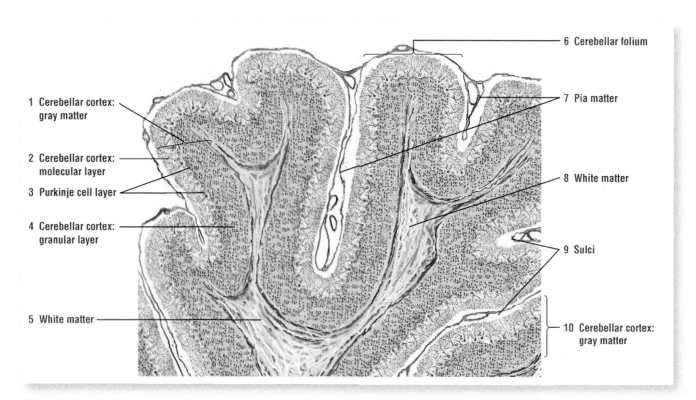

1 Cerebellar cortex: gray matter
2 Cerebellar cortex: molecular layer
3 Purkinje cell layer
4 Cerebellar cortex: granular layer
5 White matter
6 Cerebellar folium
7 Pia matter
8 White matter
9 Sulci
10 Cerebellar cortex: gray matter

FIGURE 9.13 ■ Cerebellum (transverse section). Stain: silver impregnation (Cajal method). Low magnification.

FIGURE 9.14 | Cerebellar Cortex: Molecular Layer, Purkinje Cell Layer, and Granular Cell Layer

This illustration shows a small section of the cerebellar cortex above the white matter at a higher magnification. The **Purkinje cells** (**3**) form the **Purkinje cell layer** (**7**), with their prominent nuclei and nucleoli, and are arranged in a single row between the **molecular cell layer** (**6**) and the **granular cell layer** (**4**). The large "flask-shaped" bodies of the Purkinje cells (**3, 7**) exhibit thick **dendrites** (**2**) that branch throughout the molecular cell layer (**6**) to the cerebellar surface. Thin axons (not shown) leave the base of the Purkinje cells, pass through the granular cell layer (**4**), become myelinated, and enter the **white matter** (**5, 11**).

The molecular cell layer (**6**) contains **basket cells** (**1**) with unmyelinated axons that course horizontally. Descending collaterals of more deeply placed basket cells (**1**) arborize around the Purkinje cells (**3, 7**). Axons of the **granule cells** (**9**) in the granular cell layer (**4**) extend into the molecular layer (**6**) and also course horizontally as unmyelinated axons.

The granular cell layer (**4**) contains small granule cells (**9**) with dark-staining nuclei and little cytoplasm and larger **Golgi type II cells** (**8**) with vesicular nuclei and more cytoplasm. Throughout the granular layer are small, irregularly dispersed, clear spaces called the **glomeruli** (**10**) that contain only synaptic complexes.

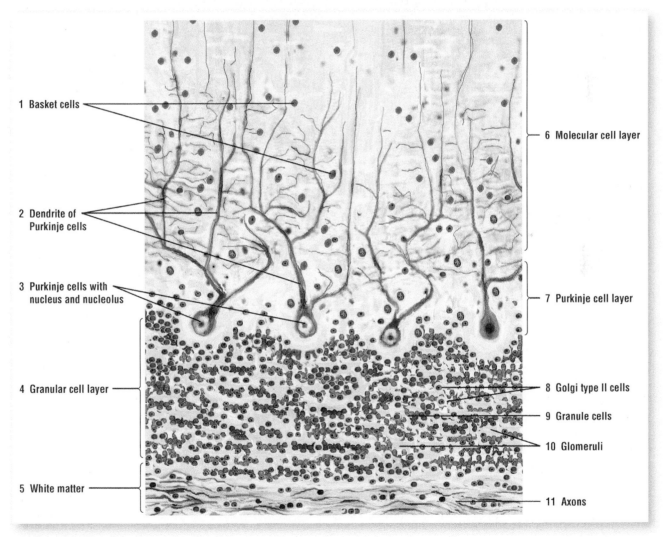

1 Basket cells

2 Dendrite of Purkinje cells

3 Purkinje cells with nucleus and nucleolus

4 Granular cell layer

5 White matter

6 Molecular cell layer

7 Purkinje cell layer

8 Golgi type II cells

9 Granule cells

10 Glomeruli

11 Axons

FIGURE 9.14 ■ Cerebellar cortex: molecular, Purkinje cell, and granular cell layers. Stain: silver impregnation (Cajal method). High magnification.

FIGURE 9.15 | **Fibrous Astrocytes of Brain**

A section of the brain prepared by the Cajal method demonstrates the supportive **neuroglial** cells called astrocytes. The **fibrous astrocytes (2, 5)** exhibit a small **cell body (5)**, a large oval **nucleus (5)**, and a **dark-stained nucleolus (5)**. Extending from the cell body are long, thin, and smooth radiating **processes (4, 6)** found between the neurons and blood vessels. A **perivascular fibrous astrocyte (2)** surrounds a **capillary (8)** with red blood cells (erythrocytes). From other fibrous astrocytes **(2, 5)**, the long processes **(4, 6)** extend to and terminate on the capillary **(8)** as **perivascular endfeet (3, 7)**.

Also seen in the illustration are nuclei of different neuroglial **(1)** cells of the brain.

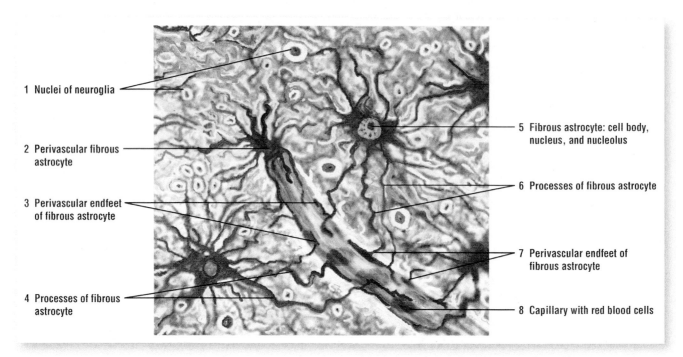

1 Nuclei of neuroglia

2 Perivascular fibrous astrocyte

3 Perivascular endfeet of fibrous astrocyte

4 Processes of fibrous astrocyte

5 Fibrous astrocyte: cell body, nucleus, and nucleolus

6 Processes of fibrous astrocyte

7 Perivascular endfeet of fibrous astrocyte

8 Capillary with red blood cells

FIGURE 9.15 ■ Fibrous astrocytes and capillary in the brain. Stain: silver impregnation (Cajal method). High magnification.

FIGURE 9.16 | Ultrastructure of CNS Capillary and Perivascular Endfeet of Astrocytes

This transmission electron micrograph shows a cross section of a continuous type of capillary in the CNS. Lining the **capillary lumen** is a thin endothelial layer and the nucleus of an **endothelial cell** (**2**). Attached externally to the **capillary wall** (**5**) are numerous **perivascular endfeet of astrocytes** (**3, 4**) that completely envelop the capillary wall (**5**) to form part of the blood–brain barrier. Surrounding the capillary wall (**5**) and the endfeet of astrocytes (**3, 4**) is the **CNS neuropil** (**1**), a dense meshwork of fibers from axons, dendrites, and various glial cells that fill the spaces in the CNS. Located below the capillary are **myelinated axons** (**6**) that were myelinated in the CNS by oligodendrocytes (not illustrated).

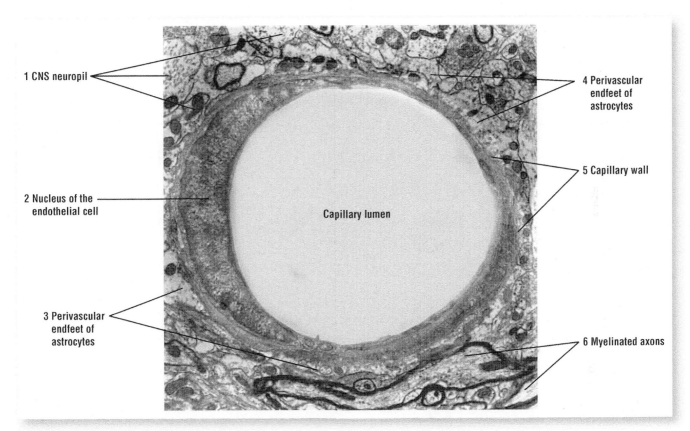

1 CNS neuropil

2 Nucleus of the endothelial cell

3 Perivascular endfeet of astrocytes

Capillary lumen

4 Perivascular endfeet of astrocytes

5 Capillary wall

6 Myelinated axons

FIGURE 9.16 ■ Ultrastructure of a capillary in the CNS and the perivascular endfeet of astrocytes. Transmission electron micrograph. Courtesy of Dr. Mark DeSantis, Professor Emeritus, WWAMI. Medical Program, University of Idaho, Moscow, ID. ×20,000.

FIGURE 9.17 | Oligodendrocytes of Brain

This brain section was also prepared with the Cajal method to show the supportive neuroglial cells called **oligodendrocytes** (**1, 4, 7**). In comparison to a **fibrous astrocyte** (**3**), the oligodendrocytes (1, 4, 7) are smaller and exhibit few, thin, short processes without excessive branching.

The oligodendrocytes (1, 4, 7) are found in both the gray and white matter of the CNS. In the white matter, the oligodendrocytes form myelin sheaths around numerous axons and are analogous to the Schwann cells that myelinate individual axons in the PNS.

Two **neurons** (**2, 6**) are also illustrated to contrast their size with those of a fibrous astrocyte (3) and the oligodendrocytes (1, 4, 7). A **capillary** (**5**) passes between the different cells.

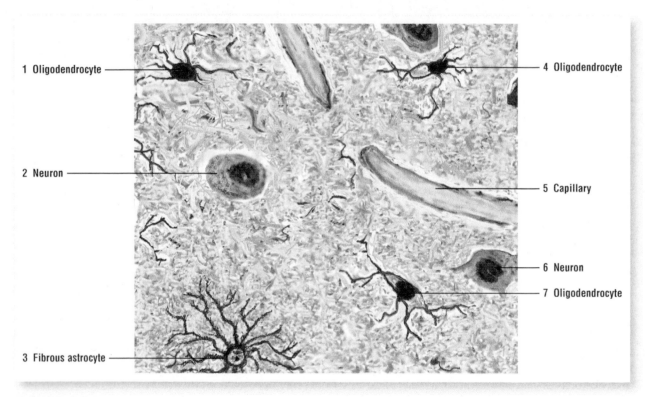

1 Oligodendrocyte

2 Neuron

3 Fibrous astrocyte

4 Oligodendrocyte

5 Capillary

6 Neuron

7 Oligodendrocyte

FIGURE 9.17 ■ Oligodendrocytes of the brain. Stain: silver impregnation (Cajal method). High magnification.

FIGURE 9.18 | Ultrastructure of CNS Oligodendrocyte with Myelinated Axons

This transmission electron micrograph illustrates internal morphology of the **oligodendrocyte** (**2**), the myelin-producing cell of the CNS. The cytoplasm exhibits a well-developed **granular endoplasmic reticulum** (**3, 5**), a **Golgi apparatus** (**6**), and numerous free ribosomes around the organelles. Numerous **myelinated axons** (**1, 4, 8**), cut in cross and longitudinal sections, are surrounded with **myelin sheaths** (**7**) that are associated with the cytoplasm of the oligodendrocyte. Located in the myelinated axons (**1, 4**) are oval, dark-staining **mitochondria** (**4**) and numerous **neurofilaments** (**8**).

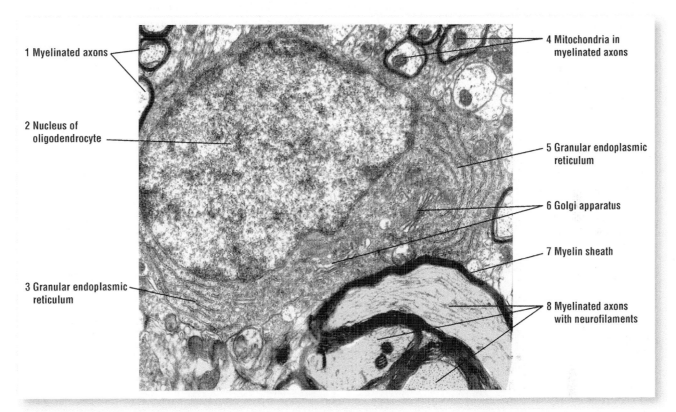

1 Myelinated axons

2 Nucleus of oligodendrocyte

3 Granular endoplasmic reticulum

4 Mitochondria in myelinated axons

5 Granular endoplasmic reticulum

6 Golgi apparatus

7 Myelin sheath

8 Myelinated axons with neurofilaments

FIGURE 9.18 ■ Ultrastructure of an oligodendrocyte in the CNS with myelinated axons. Transmission electron micrograph. Courtesy of Dr. Mark DeSantis, Professor Emeritus, WWAMI Medical Program, University of Idaho, Mascow, ID. ×25,000.

FIGURE 9.19 | Ultrastructure of CNS Myelinated Axons with Node of Ranvier

A transmission electron micrograph shows a **myelinated axon** (7) sectioned in a longitudinal plane and a cross section of a **myelinated axon** (2) in close associated with the cytoplasm and the organelles of the myelinating cell, the oligodendrocyte. Because the **myelin sheath** is not continuous along the entire axon length, there is a small nodal gap called the node of **Ranvier** (4). This region is located where myelin sheaths (5, 6) are absent, and the axon is surrounded by the processes or loops containing the **cellular cytoplasm** (3, 8) of the oligodendrocyte that covers and contacts the axon. At the node of Ranvier (4), the oligodendrocyte cell cytoplasm (3, 8) was not completely displaced during the wrapping of the cell around the axon and formation of the myelin sheath (5, 6). Located in the myelinated axons (2) are numerous **neurofilaments** (2, 7) and dark-staining **mitochondria** (1). Located near the myelinated axon (7) are cross sections of **unmyelinated axons** (9) and the **cytoplasm** (10) of an adjacent cell.

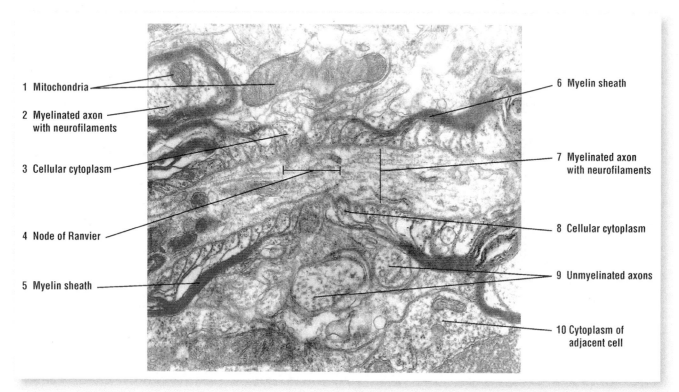

1 Mitochondria

2 Myelinated axon with neurofilaments

3 Cellular cytoplasm

4 Node of Ranvier

5 Myelin sheath

6 Myelin sheath

7 Myelinated axon with neurofilaments

8 Cellular cytoplasm

9 Unmyelinated axons

10 Cytoplasm of adjacent cell

FIGURE 9.19 ■ Ultrastructure of myelinated axons in the CNS with a node of Ranvier. Transmission electron micrograph. Courtesy of Dr. Mark DeSantis, Professor Emeritus, WWAMI Medical Program, University of Idaho, Moscow, ID. Approximately ×55,000.

FIGURE 9.20 | Microglia of Brain

This section of the brain was prepared with the Hortega method to show the smallest neuroglial cells called **microglia** (**2, 3**). The microglia (2, 3) vary in shape and often exhibit irregular contours, and the small, deeply stained nucleus almost fills the entire cell. The cell processes of the microglia (2, 3) are few, short, and slender. Both the cell body and the processes of microglia (2, 3) are covered with small spines. Two **neurons** (**1**) and a **capillary** with **red blood cells** (**erythrocytes**) (**4**) provide a size comparison with the microglia (2, 3).

Microglia are found in both the white and gray matter of the CNS and are the main phagocytes of the CNS.

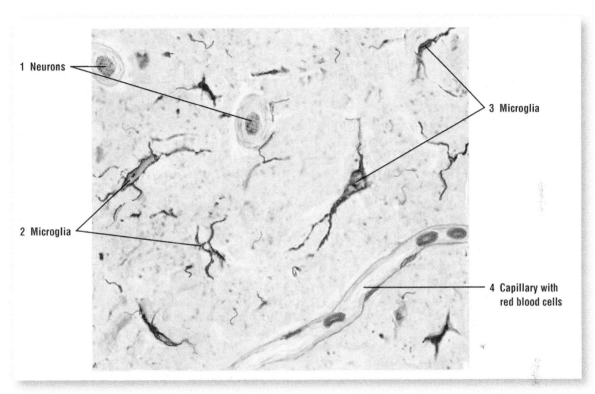

FIGURE 9.20 ■ Microglia of the brain. Stain: Hortega method. Medium magnification.

FUNCTIONAL CORRELATIONS 9.3 ■ Neuroglia

There are four types of neuroglial cells in the CNS: astrocytes, oligodendrocytes, microglia, and ependymal cells.

Astrocytes are the largest and most abundant neuroglia cells in the gray matter and consist of two types: fibrous astrocytes and protoplasmic astrocytes. In the CNS, both types of astrocytes attach to the surfaces of **capillaries** and **neurons**. Their perivascular endfeet surround the capillary basement membrane, form the tight junctions around the capillaries, and form part of the **blood–brain barrier**. The blood–brain barrier is a physiologic barrier that regulates the passage of substances from blood to brain. This allows for a stable and balanced ionic composition in the interstitial neuronal environment and protects the cells from potentially harmful substances. The branched processes of astrocytes also extend to the basal lamina of the pia mater to form an impermeable barrier, the **glia limitans**, or glial limiting membrane, which surrounds the brain and spinal cord. They support **metabolic exchange** between the neurons and capillaries of the CNS. In addition, the astrocytes control the **chemical environment** around neurons by clearing intercellular spaces of increased **potassium ions** and released **neurotransmitters**, such as **glutamate**, at active synaptic sites to maintain a proper ionic environment for their function. If these metabolic chemicals are not removed from these sites, they can interfere with neuronal functions. Astrocytes inactivate glutamate and convert it to glutamine, which is returned to the neurons. Astrocytes also contain reserves of glycogen that they release as glucose, contributing to the energy metabolism of the CNS. Also, with the presence of gap junctions, the astrocytes form a structural syncytium and a communicating network in the CNS. In response to brain injury, the astrocytes divide, proliferate, and form a scar.

Oligodendrocytes are smaller than astrocytes with fewer cytoplasmic processes. Oligodendrocytes produce and **myelinate** the axons in the CNS for insulation. Because of several cytoplasmic processes, a single oligodendrocyte surrounds and myelinates several axons. As a result, oligodendrocytes do not surround multiple unmyelinated axons. During myelination, the plasma membrane of the oligodendrocyte is wrapped around the adjacent axons and at intervals exhibits the **nodes of Ranvier**. In the PNS, **Schwann cells** myelinate the axons, and in contrast to oligodendrocytes, a Schwann cell myelinates only a single axon.

Microglia are the smallest neuroglial cells and are considered to be part of the **mononuclear phagocyte system** of the CNS derived from the circulating monocytes that originate in the bone marrow. Microglia enter the CNS through the vascular system, and their main function is similar to that of the **macrophages** of the connective tissue. During nervous tissue injury or damage, microglia migrate to the region, proliferate, become phagocytic, and remove dead or foreign tissue. Microglia constitute the brain's major immune system and, when activated, function as antigen-presenting cells and secrete immunoregulatory cytokines.

Ependymal cells are simple cuboidal or low columnar epithelial cells that line the ventricles of the brain and the central canal in the spinal cord. Their apices contain cilia and microvilli. Cilia facilitate the movement of the CSF through the central canal of the spinal cord, whereas microvilli may have some absorptive functions.

Chapter 9 Summary

SECTION 1 • Central Nervous System: Brain and Spinal Cord

MAMMALIAN NERVOUS SYSTEM

- CNS consists of the brain and spinal cord
- PNS consists of cranial, spinal, and peripheral nerves
- Afferent nerves conduct to and efferent nerves conduct from the CNS

PROTECTIVE LAYERS OF THE CENTRAL NERVOUS SYSTEM

- Surrounded by bones, connective tissue, and cerebrospinal fluid (CSF)
- Dura mater is the tough outermost connective tissue layer around the CNS
- Delicate arachnoid mater is located below the dura mater
- Innermost pia mater adheres directly to the surface of the brain and spinal cord
- Between pia mater and arachnoid mater is subarachnoid space that is filled with CSF

CEREBROSPINAL FLUID (CSF)

- Clear, colorless fluid that cushions and protects the brain and spinal cord
- Continually produced by choroid plexuses in brain ventricles, with most in the lateral ventricles
- CSF is important for homeostasis, brain metabolism, and optimal neuronal environment
- CSF is reabsorbed into venous blood (superior sagittal sinus) via the arachnoid villi

MORPHOLOGY AND TYPES OF NEURONS IN THE CENTRAL NERVOUS SYSTEM (CNS)

- Neurons are structural and functional units of the CNS that receive and conduct impulses
- Consist of soma (cell body), dendrites, and axons
- Three main neuron types are multipolar, bipolar, and unipolar
- Multipolar are most common and include all motor neurons and interneurons of the CNS
- Multipolar neurons contain numerous dendrites and a single axon
- Bipolar neurons are sensory and found in the eyes, nose, and ears

- Bipolar neurons contain a single dendrite and a single axon
- Unipolar neurons are found in sensory ganglia and dorsal root ganglia of spinal and cranial nerves
- Unipolar neurons exhibit one process from the cell body that divides into two axonal branches
- One unipolar branch continues to the CNS, the other to the peripheries
- Interneurons found in the CNS integrate and coordinate stimuli between sensory, motor, and other interneurons

MYELIN SHEATH AND MYELINATION OF AXONS

- Specialized cells wrap around axons to form lipid-rich, insulating myelin sheath
- Myelin sheath extends along the length of the axon to its terminal branches
- Gaps between myelin sheaths are nodes of Ranvier
- In the PNS, Schwann cells myelinate individual axons and envelope unmyelinated axons
- Islands of Schwann cell cytoplasm form Schmidt-Lanterman incisures or clefts
- Unmyelinated axons do not show nodes of Ranvier
- In the CNS, processes from single neuroglial oligodendrocyte cells extend and myelinate numerous axons

GRAY AND WHITE MATTER

- Gray matter contains neurons, dendrites, and neuroglia
- Gray matter is the site of connections or synapses between neurons and dendrites
- Posterior horns of the spinal cord are associated with axons of posterior roots
- Anterior horns of the spinal cord are associated with axons of anterior roots
- White matter contains only myelinated axons, unmyelinated axons, and neuroglia

SYNAPSES

- Specialized sites for the transmission of chemical/electrical communication
- Transmission is unidirectional from presynaptic to postsynaptic neurons
- The three main synapses are axodendritic, axosomatic, and axoaxonic
- Consist of presynaptic component, synaptic cleft, and postsynaptic membrane

- Transmit nerve impulses from presynaptic to postsynaptic cells
- Convert impulses into signals to affect postsynaptic cell activities
- Most synapses contain chemical neurotransmitters in presynaptic regions
- Neurotransmitters cross synaptic cleft and bind with receptors on the postsynaptic membrane
- Neurotransmitters produce either excitatory or inhibitory responses
- Summation of excitatory or inhibitory effects on the target regulates the effects of stimulus
- After release, the neurotransmitters are quickly removed from synaptic clefts

SPINAL CORD

- Thoracic region of spinal cord contains anterior, posterior, and lateral gray horns
- Lateral horns contain motor neurons of sympathetic division of autonomic nervous system
- Anterior horns of gray matter contain motor neurons
- Axons from anterior horns form anterior roots of spinal nerves
- White matter contains closely packed ascending and descending axons
- Posterior columns of white matter contain fasciculus gracilis and fasciculus cuneatus
- Gray matter inside the spinal cord is H-shaped and contains neurons and interneurons
- Gray commissure connects two sides of the gray matter and contains the central canal

NEURONS, AXONS, AND DENDRITES

- Classified as afferent (sensory), efferent (motor), or interneurons
- Somatic afferent fibers conduct impulses from body surface and body organs to the CNS
- Visceral afferent fibers conduct impulses from internal organs, glands, and blood vessels to the CNS
- Efferent fibers conduct from the CNS to the effector organs in the peripheries
- Interneurons act as intermediaries between different neuron types
- Neuron cell body and dendrites contain Nissl substance (granular endoplasmic reticulum)
- Neurofibrils in the neuron cell body extend into dendrites and axons
- Axons arise from a funnel-shaped region called an axon hillock
- Axons and axon hillocks are devoid of Nissl substance
- Neurons show irritability and conductivity and synthesize various products
- Neurons synthesize neurotransmitters and neurohormones in the cell body

- Axons transport neurotransmitters in microtubules to synapses
- Stimuli cause conduction of nerve impulse (action potential) along the axons
- Initial segment of an axon is the site where stimuli are summated and nerve impulse is generated
- Rate of impulse conduction dependent on axon size and myelination
- Dendrites are covered with dendritic spines for connections (synapses) with other neurons
- Dendrites receive and integrate information from dendrites, neurons, or axons
- Axons also exhibit bidirectional transport of chemicals, organelles, and neurotransmitters
- Anterograde transport is via microtubules in axons to axon terminals or synapses
- Retrograde transport is via microtubules from axon terminals and dendrites to neurons
- Axonal transport requires microtubule-associated motor proteins kinesin and dynein

SUPPORTIVE CELLS IN CNS: NEUROGLIA

- Supportive, nonneural cells that surround neurons, axons, and dendrites
- Small cells that do not conduct impulses
- Ten times more numerous than neurons
- Four types: astrocytes, oligodendrocytes, microglia, and ependymal cells

Astrocytes

- Are the largest and most numerous in gray matter
- Consist of two types: fibrous astrocytes and protoplasmic astrocytes
- Both types abut on capillaries and form tight junctions and blood–brain barrier
- Form glial limiting membrane that surrounds the brain and the spinal cord
- Support metabolic exchange and contribute to the energy metabolism of the CNS
- Control the chemical environment around neurons by clearing increased potassium ions and neurotransmitters such as glutamate
- Gap junctions form structural syncytia in the CNS and the communication network in the brain
- In response to injury, cells divide and form scar tissue

Oligodendrocytes

- Surround and myelinate numerous axons at one time, in contrast to Schwann cells
- Do not surround multiple and unmyelinated axons

Microglia

- Part of the mononuclear phagocyte system and found throughout the CNS

- Phagocytic cells in the CNS, function similar to that of connective tissue macrophages
- In response to injury, proliferate and become phagocytic
- Are brain's major immune system and function as antigen-presenting cells

Ependymal Cells

- Line the ventricles in the brain and central canal of the spinal cord
- Ciliated cells move the CSF through the central canal of the spinal cord

CEREBRAL CORTEX: GRAY MATTER (LAYERS I TO IV)

- Molecular layer (I): most superficial and covered by pia mater and contains neuroglial cells and horizontal cells of Cajal
- External granular layer (II): contains neuroglial cells and small pyramidal cells

- External pyramidal layer (III): medium-sized pyramidal cells predominant type
- Internal granular layer (IV): thin layer with small granule, pyramidal cells, and neuroglia
- Internal pyramidal layer (V): contains neuroglial cells and largest pyramidal cells
- Multiform layer (VI): deepest layer, adjacent to white matter with various cell types

CEREBELLAR CORTEX

- Deep folds in the cortex called cerebellar folia separated by sulci
- Outer molecular layer contains small neurons and fibers
- Middle Purkinje layer contains large Purkinje cells whose dendrites branch in molecular layer
- Granule cell layer contains small granule cells, Golgi type II cells, and empty spaces called glomeruli

Chapter 9 Review Questions: Section 1

QUESTIONS

In the following multiple choice questions, choose the letter corresponding to the one best answer.

1. The cerebrospinal (CSF) fluid circulates:

A. between the dura mater layers.
B. between the pia mater and the brain surface.
C. in the subarachnoid space.
D. between the dura mater and arachnoid mater.
E. above the dura mater.

2. What is the function of arachnoid villi?

A. Produce cerebrospinal fluid
B. Absorb cerebrospinal fluid
C. Circulate cerebrospinal fluid
D. Support the choroid plexus
E. Line the choroid plexus

3. Unipolar neurons are primarily found in the:

A. spinal and cranial nerve ganglia.
B. cerebellum.
C. eyes and ears.
D. spinal cord.
E. cerebrum.

4. Multipolar neurons can be described as:

A. containing a single dendrite and single axon.
B. the least common type of neuron in the central nervous system.
C. sensory.
D. having a single axon that divides near the cell body.
E. motor.

5. The main function of Schwann cells and oligodendrocytes is to:

A. provide protection to the brain and spinal cord.
B. produce cerebrospinal fluid.
C. surround the axons with a myelin sheath.
D. surround capillaries and form a protective blood–brain barrier.
E. perform phagocytic functions around axons and nerves.

ANSWERS

1. **Correct Answer: C.** Subarachnoid space. From the ventricles in the brain, CSF circulates around the brain and the spinal cord in the subarachnoid space.

2. **Correct Answer: B.** Absorb cerebrospinal fluid (CSF). The arachnoid villi penetrate the venous sinuses in the brain into which they deliver the absorbed CSF.

3. **Correct Answer: A.** Spinal and cranial nerve ganglia. These neurons have a single axon and are surrounded by capsule cells in the ganglia.

4. **Correct Answer: E.** Motor. Multipolar neurons in the spinal cord and brain are considered motor neurons in that their action initiates responses in muscles or glands.

5. **Correct Answer: C.** Surround the axons with myelin sheath. Schwann cells surround single axons in the PNS, whereas oligodendrocytes surround numerous axons in the CNS.

SECTION 2 Peripheral Nervous System (PNS)

The **PNS** consists of neurons, supportive cells, nerves, and axons that are located outside of the CNS (Fig. 9.21). These include **cranial nerves** from the brain and **spinal nerves** from the spinal cord along with their associated **ganglia**. Ganglia (singular, ganglion) are small accumulations of neurons and their supportive glial cells surrounded by a connective tissue capsule. The nerves of the PNS contain both sensory and motor axons. These axons transmit information between the peripheral organs and the CNS. The neurons of the peripheral nerves are located either within the CNS or outside of the CNS in different ganglia. Nerves, arteries, veins, and lymphatic vessels that course together form the **neurovascular bundle**.

CONNECTIVE TISSUE LAYERS IN THE PERIPHERAL NERVOUS SYSTEM

A peripheral nerve is composed of axons of various sizes surrounded by layers of connective tissue that partition the nerve into several nerve (axon) bundles or **fascicles**. The outermost connective tissue layer is the strong fibrous sheath, the **epineurium** that binds all fascicles together. It consists of dense irregular connective tissue that completely surrounds the peripheral nerve.

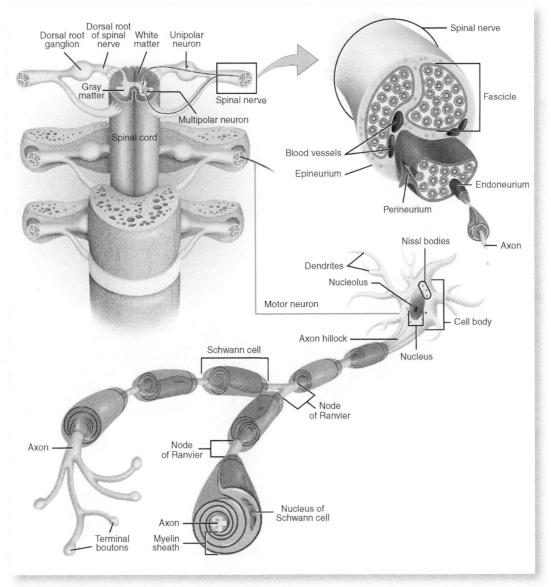

FIGURE 9.21 ■ Peripheral nervous system (PNS). The PNS is composed of the cranial and spinal nerves. A cross section of the spinal cord is illustrated with the characteristic features of the motor neuron and a cross section of a peripheral nerve.

A thinner connective tissue layer, the **perineurium**, extends into the nerve, subdivides, and surrounds one or more nerve fascicles. The cells in the perineurium are joined together by **tight junctions**, and the perineurium serves as a selective metabolically active diffusion barrier that forms the **blood–nerve barrier**. This barrier restricts passage to many macromolecules and functions in maintaining the proper internal microenvironment and protection of the axons. Within each fascicle are individual axons and their supporting cells, the **Schwann cells**. Each myelinated axon or a cluster of unmyelinated axons associated with a Schwann cell is surrounded by a loose vascular connective tissue layer of thin reticular fibers, called the **endoneurium**.

thePoint Supplemental micrographic images are available at **www.thePoint.com/Eroschenko13e** under Nervous Tissue.

FIGURE 9.22 | Peripheral Nerves and Blood Vessels (Transverse Section)

Bundles of nerve **axons** (fibers) or **nerve fascicles** (**1**) with blood vessels have been sectioned in the transverse plane. Each nerve fascicle (**1**) is surrounded by a sheath of connective tissue **perineurium** (**5**) that merges with surrounding **interfascicular connective tissue** (**9**). Delicate connective tissue strands from the perineurium (**5**) surround individual nerve axons (fibers) in a fascicle and form the innermost layer endoneurium (not visible in this figure and at this magnification).

Most nuclei seen between individual nerve axons (fibers) in the nerve fascicles (**1**) are the **nuclei of Schwann cells** (**2**) that surround and myelinate the axons. The myelin sheaths surrounding the axons (**3**) appear as empty spaces because the chemicals used in preparation of the tissue washed out the myelin. Other nuclei in the nerve fascicles (**1**) are the **fibrocytes** (**4**) of the endoneurium (see Fig. 9.25).

The arterial blood vessels in the interfascicular connective tissue (**9**) send branches into each nerve fascicle (**1**) where they branch into capillaries in the endoneurium. Different size **arterioles** (**7, 12**) and **venules** (**11**) in the interfascicular connective tissue (**9**) surround the nerve fascicles (**1**). The larger arteriole (**7**) contains blood cells, an **internal elastic membrane** (**8**), and a muscular **tunica media** (**6**). **Adipose cells** (**10**) are also present in the interfascicular connective tissue (**9**).

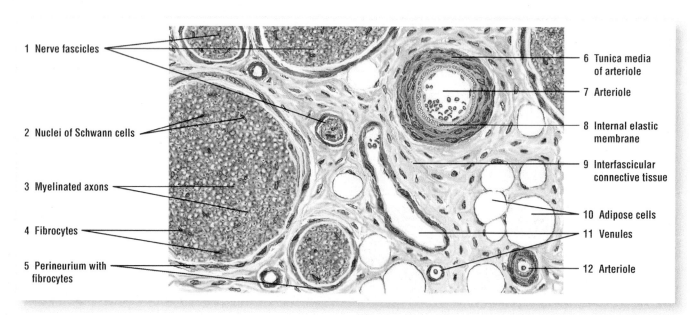

1 Nerve fascicles

2 Nuclei of Schwann cells

3 Myelinated axons

4 Fibrocytes

5 Perineurium with fibrocytes

6 Tunica media of arteriole

7 Arteriole

8 Internal elastic membrane

9 Interfascicular connective tissue

10 Adipose cells

11 Venules

12 Arteriole

FIGURE 9.22 ■ Peripheral nerves and blood vessels (transverse section). Stain: hematoxylin and eosin. Medium magnification.

FIGURE 9.23 | Myelinated Nerve Fibers in Longitudinal and Transverse Sections

Schwann cells surround the axons in peripheral nerves and form a myelin sheath. To illustrate the myelin sheaths, nerve fibers are fixed in osmium tetroxide; this preparation stains the lipid in the myelin sheath black. In this illustration, a peripheral nerve has been prepared in a longitudinal section (*upper figure*) and in a cross section (*lower figure*).

In the longitudinal section, the **myelin sheath** (**1**) is a thick, black band surrounding a lighter, central **axon** (**2**). The length of an axon myelinated by one Schwann cell is the nodal or internodal segment. Between the internodal segments, which can be a few millimeters in length, the myelin sheath exhibits discontinuity that represent the **nodes of Ranvier** (**4**), which can span approximately 1 or 2 micrometers (μm).

A group of nerve fibers or fascicle is surrounded by a light-appearing connective tissue layer, the **perineurium** (**3, 5, 8**). In turn, each individual nerve fiber or axon is surrounded by a thin layer of connective tissue, the **endoneurium** (**7, 10**). In the transverse plane (*lower figure*), different diameters of myelinated axons are seen. The **myelin sheath** (**9**) appears as a thick, black ring around the light, unstained **axon** (**12**) that is in the center.

The connective tissue surrounding individual nerve fibers, or the fascicle, exhibits a rich supply of **blood vessels** (**6, 11**) of different sizes.

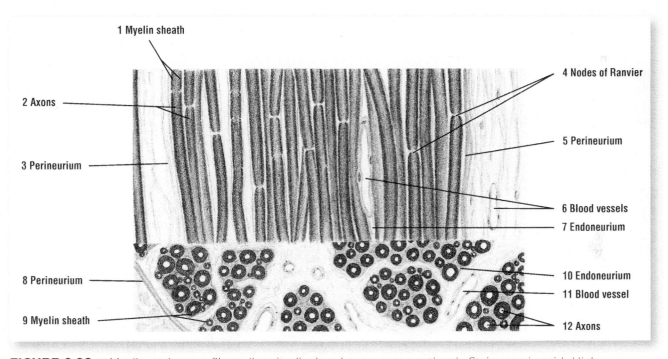

FIGURE 9.23 ■ Myelinated nerve fibers (longitudinal and transverse sections). Stain: osmic acid. High magnification.

FUNCTIONAL CORRELATIONS 9.4 ■ Axon Myelination and Supporting Cells in the PNS

The supportive cells in the PNS are the **Schwann cells**. Their main function is to surround and form the insulating, lipid-rich **myelin sheaths** around the larger axons. The myelin sheaths protect axons and maintain proper ionic environment for impulse conduction and propagation. Each Schwann cell myelinates a portion of a single axon. However, a single Schwann cell can surround its cytoplasm with numerous unmyelinated axons. The function of Schwann cells in the PNS is similar to that of the **oligodendrocytes** in the **CNS**, except that the cytoplasmic processes of a single oligodendrocyte can myelinate numerous axons. Myelin sheaths are not continuous, solid sheets along the entire axon; rather, they exhibit small nodal gaps called **nodes of Ranvier** that are located between the myelin sheaths produced by the myelinating cells. The length of the axon covered by the myelin sheath of one Schwann cell is called the **internode** or **internodal segment**. The size of the internodes varies with the size of the axon. The node of Ranvier measures between 1 and 2 μm, whereas the internodes can be a few millimeters, depending on the size of the axon. At the nodes of Ranvier, the axons are not insulated by myelin sheaths. As a result, these nodes significantly accelerate the conduction of **nerve impulses** (**action potentials**) along the axons.

In large, myelinated axons, the nerve impulse or action potential jumps from node to node, resulting in a more efficient and faster conduction of the impulse. This type of fast impulse propagation along the myelinated axons is called **saltatory conduction**.

Small unmyelinated axons conduct nerve impulses at a much slower rate than larger, myelinated axons. In unmyelinated axons, even though they are surrounded by the cytoplasm of the Schwann cell, the impulse travels along the entire length of the axon; as a result, conduction efficiency of the impulse and velocity is reduced. Thus, the larger, myelinated axons have the highest velocity of impulse conduction. Also, the rate of impulse conduction depends directly on the axon size and the myelin sheath.

The **satellite cells** are small, flat cells that surround the neurons of PNS ganglia. Ganglia are collections of neurons that are located outside of the CNS. Peripheral ganglia are located parallel to the vertebral column near the junction of the dorsal and ventral roots of the spinal nerves and near visceral organs. Satellite cells provide **structural support** for the neurons, insulate them, and regulate the exchange of different metabolic substances between the neurons and the interstitial fluid.

FIGURE 9.24 | Sciatic Nerve (Longitudinal Section)

A longitudinal section of a sciatic nerve is illustrated at a low magnification. A portion of the **epineurium** (1) that surrounds the entire nerve is visible with numerous **blood vessels** (5) and **adipose cells** (6).

The connective tissue sheath inferior to the epineurium (1) around the bundles of nerve fibers or **nerve fascicles** (3) is the **perineurium** (2). Epineurium (1) with **blood vessels** (4) between the nerve fascicles (3) forms the **interfascicular connective tissue** (7).

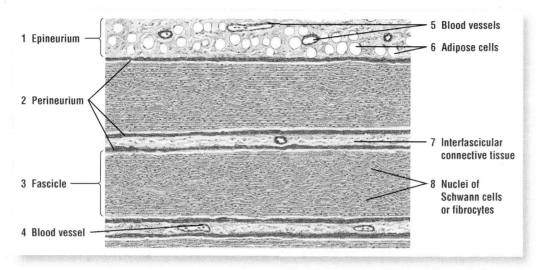

- 1 Epineurium
- 2 Perineurium
- 3 Fascicle
- 4 Blood vessel
- 5 Blood vessels
- 6 Adipose cells
- 7 Interfascicular connective tissue
- 8 Nuclei of Schwann cells or fibrocytes

FIGURE 9.24 ■ Sciatic nerve (longitudinal section). Stain: hematoxylin and eosin. Low magnification.

In a longitudinal section, the individual axons follow a characteristic wavy pattern. Located among the wavy axons in the nerve fascicle (3) are **nuclei** (8) of the Schwann cells and fibrocytes of the endoneurium connective tissue. Schwann cells and fibrocytes cannot be differentiated at this magnification.

FIGURE 9.25 | Sciatic Nerve (Longitudinal Section)

A portion of the sciatic nerve, illustrated in Figure 9.24, is presented at a higher magnification. The central **axons** (1) appear as slender threads stained lightly with hematoxylin and eosin. The surrounding myelin sheath has been washed out or lost due to chemicals used in histologic preparation, leaving a **protein network** (6) in its place. **Schwann cells** (4) are not always distinguishable from the connective tissue **endoneurium** (5) that surrounds each axon. At the **node of Ranvier** (2), the Schwann cell membrane (4) is a thin, peripheral boundary that descends toward the axon.

Two **Schwann cell nuclei** (4), cut in different planes, are around the periphery of the myelinated axons (1). The **fibrocytes** of the **endoneurium** (3a) and **perineurium** (3b) are seen in the illustration. The fibrocyte of the endoneurium (3a) is outside of the myelin sheath, in contrast to the Schwann cells (4) that myelinate or surround the axons (1). It is often difficult to distinguish between the nuclei of Schwann cells (4) and the fibrocytes (3) of the endoneurium.

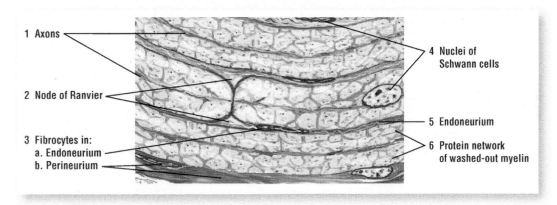

FIGURE 9.25 ■ Sciatic nerve (longitudinal section). Stain: hematoxylin and eosin. High magnification (oil immersion).

FIGURE 9.26 | Sciatic Nerve (Transverse Section)

A higher magnification of a transverse section of the sciatic nerve illustrated in Figure 9.24 shows the myelinated nerve fibers. The **axons** (5) are thin, dark central structures, surrounded by the washed-out remnants of myelin, the **protein network** (2) with peripheral radial lines.

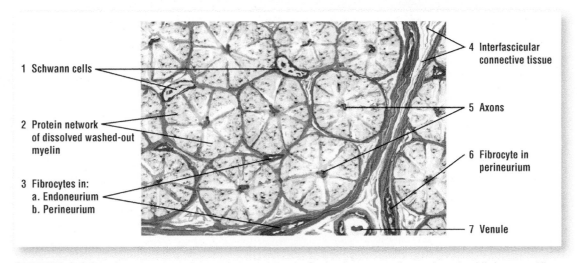

FIGURE 9.26 ■ Sciatic nerve (transverse section). Stain: hematoxylin and eosin. High magnification (oil immersion).

The nuclei and cell membranes of the **Schwann cells** (1) are peripheral to the myelinated axon (5). The crescent shape of the Schwann cells (1) that encircle the axons allows their identification.

The collagen fibers of the endoneurium are faintly distinguishable, whereas the **fibrocytes** (**3a**) in the endoneurium and **perineurium** (**3b, 6**) are clearly seen. Located in the **interfascicular connective tissue** (4) is a small **venule** (7).

FIGURE 9.27 | Peripheral Nerve: Nodes of Ranvier and Axons

A medium-magnification photomicrograph of a peripheral nerve sectioned in a longitudinal plane is shown. The myelin sheaths that surround the **axons** (**2, 8**) have been lost or washed out in this preparation, and only **myelin spaces** (7) with protein network are seen. A centrally located axon (2, 8) is seen in some of the nerve fibers that exhibited myelin sheaths. At regular intervals along the axon are indentations or in the myelin sheaths. These represent the **nodes of Ranvier** (**1, 9**). These sites indicate the edges of two different myelin sheaths that enclose the axon. A possible **Schwann cell nucleus** (3) is seen with one of the axons (2, 8) and a thin, blue connective tissue layer **endoneurium** (6) around some of the axons (2, 8). Outside of the axons (2, 8) are **capillary** (4) with blood cells and **fibrocytes** (5) of the connective tissue.

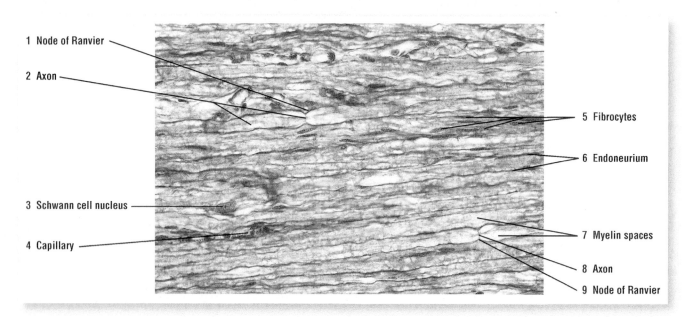

1 Node of Ranvier
2 Axon
3 Schwann cell nucleus
4 Capillary
5 Fibrocytes
6 Endoneurium
7 Myelin spaces
8 Axon
9 Node of Ranvier

FIGURE 9.27 ■ Peripheral nerve: nodes of Ranvier and axons. Stain: Masson trichrome. ×100.

FIGURE 9.28 | **Ultrastructure of Peripheral Nerve Fascicle in PNS Cut in Transverse Plane**

A transmission electron micrograph of a nerve fascicle sectioned in a transverse plane shows two large **myelinated axons** (**3**) on the left side and small **unmyelinated axons** (**7**) on the right side. In contrast to the CNS, the Schwann cells only form **myelin sheaths** (**2**) around a section of one axon. A thin rim of **Schwann cell cytoplasm** (**5**) surrounds the myelinated axon, which is invested by an outer thin layer of basal lamina (**6**). Within the axons are oval-shaped, dense-staining mitochondria (**4**). On the right side are Schwann cells that surround numerous unmyelinated axons (**7**) that are embedded in the **Schwann cell cytoplasm** (**8**). A thin **basal lamina** (**10**) also surrounds the Schwann cell cytoplasm (**8**) that encloses the unmyelinated axons (**7**). Similar oval-shaped **mitochondria** (**9**) and neurofilaments are found in the unmyelinated axons (**7**). Enclosing the nerve fascicle is a thin layer of connective tissue **perineurium** (**12**). On the peripheries of the fascicle are cells with developed rough endoplasmic reticulum that are most likely the **fibroblasts** (**1, 11**).

A transmission electron micrograph of Figure 9.19 illustrates the node of Ranvier from the CNS. Except for a few ultrastructural differences, the structures of the nodes of Ranvier in the PNS and the CNS are similar. The nodes in the PNS are covered by the **basal lamina**, whereas the nodes in the CNS lack an overlying basal lamina.

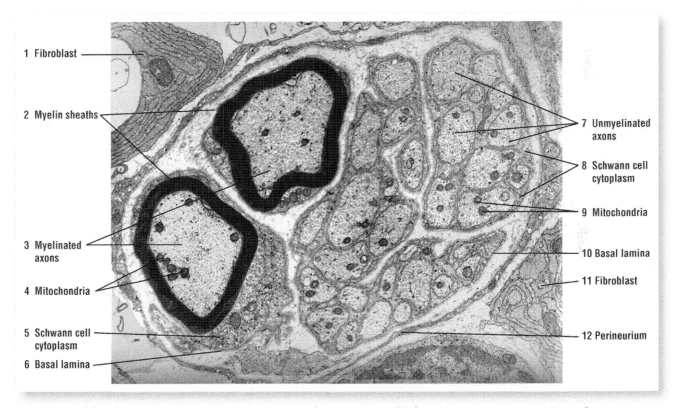

1 Fibroblast

2 Myelin sheaths

3 Myelinated axons

4 Mitochondria

5 Schwann cell cytoplasm

6 Basal lamina

7 Unmyelinated axons

8 Schwann cell cytoplasm

9 Mitochondria

10 Basal lamina

11 Fibroblast

12 Perineurium

FIGURE 9.28 ■ Ultrastructure of peripheral nerve fascicle in the PNS cut in the transverse plane. Courtesy of Dr. Mark DeSantis, Professor Emeritus, WWAMI Medical Program, University of Idaho, Moscow, ID. Approximately ×25,000.

FIGURE 9.29 | Dorsal Root Ganglion with Dorsal and Ventral Roots and Spinal Nerve (Longitudinal Section)

The dorsal root ganglia are aggregations of neuron cell bodies that are located outside the CNS. The **dorsal (posterior) root ganglion** (**7**) is situated on the **dorsal (posterior) nerve root** (**9**), which joins the spinal cord. Numerous round (pseudo-) **unipolar neurons** (**2**), or sensory neurons, constitute the majority of the ganglion. Fascicles of **nerve fibers** (**3**) pass between the unipolar neurons (2) and course either in the dorsal nerve root (9) or the **spinal nerve** (**5**). The nerve fibers (3) represent the peripheral processes that are formed by the bifurcation of a single axon that emerges from each unipolar neuron (2).

Each dorsal root ganglion (7) is enclosed by an **irregular connective tissue layer** (**1**) that contains adipose cells, **nerves** (**6**), and **blood vessels** (**6**). The connective tissue (1, 6) around the ganglion (7) merges with the **epineurium** (**4**) of the peripheral spinal nerve (5). The nerve fibers in the **ventral (anterior) root** (**11**) join the nerve fibers that emerge from the ganglion (7) to form the spinal nerve (5). The spinal nerve (5) is formed when the dorsal nerve root (9) and the ventral (anterior) root (11) unite.

On emerging from the spinal cord, the dorsal (9) and ventral roots (11) are surrounded by pia mater and an **arachnoid sheath** (**8, 10**). These become continuous with the epineurium (4) of the spinal nerve (5). The perineurium around the nerve fascicles (3) and the endoneurium around individual nerve fibers in the spinal nerve (5) or in the ganglion (7) are not distinguishable at this magnification.

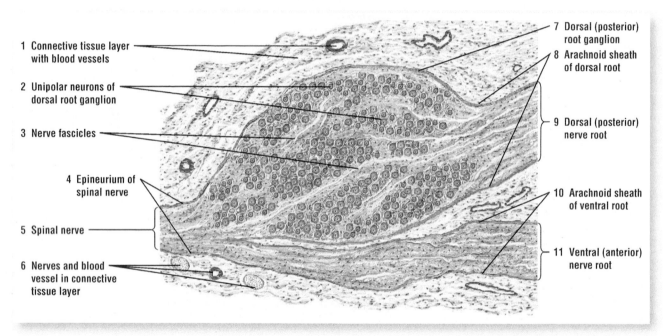

1 Connective tissue layer with blood vessels
2 Unipolar neurons of dorsal root ganglion
3 Nerve fascicles
4 Epineurium of spinal nerve
5 Spinal nerve
6 Nerves and blood vessel in connective tissue layer
7 Dorsal (posterior) root ganglion
8 Arachnoid sheath of dorsal root
9 Dorsal (posterior) nerve root
10 Arachnoid sheath of ventral root
11 Ventral (anterior) nerve root

FIGURE 9.29 ■ Dorsal root ganglion, with dorsal and ventral roots, spinal nerve (longitudinal section). Stain: hematoxylin and eosin. Low magnification.

FIGURE 9.30 | Cells and Unipolar Neurons of Dorsal Root Ganglion

The unipolar **neurons** (**1, 6**) of a dorsal (posterior) root ganglion are illustrated at higher magnification. When the plane of section passes through the middle of a neuron (**1, 6**), a pink-staining **cytoplasm** (**1b, 4**) and a round **nucleus** (**1a**) is visible with its characteristic, dark-staining **nucleolus** (**1a**). Some of the unipolar neurons (**1, 6**) contain small clumps of brownish **lipofuscin pigment** (**9**) in their cytoplasm (see also Fig. 9.21).

The cell body of each unipolar neuron (**1, 6**) is surrounded by two cellular capsules. The inner cell layer is within the perineuronal space and closely surrounds the unipolar neurons (**1, 6**). These are the smaller, flat epithelium-like **satellite cells** (**3, 8**) that exhibit spherical nuclei, are of neuroectodermal origin, and are continuous with similar **Schwann cells** (**11**) that surround the unmyelinated and **myelinated axons** (**5, 10**). The satellite cells (**3, 8**), in turn, are surrounded by an outer layer of **capsule cells** (**7**) of the connective tissue. Between the unipolar neurons (**1, 6**) are **fibrocytes** (**2**) randomly arranged in the connective tissue and continue into the endoneurium between the axons (**5**).

With hematoxylin and eosin stain, small axons and individual connective tissue fibers are not defined. Large myelinated axons (**5**) are recognizable when sectioned longitudinally.

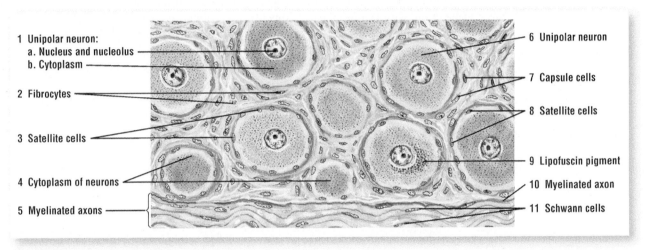

1 Unipolar neuron:
  a. Nucleus and nucleolus
  b. Cytoplasm

2 Fibrocytes

3 Satellite cells

4 Cytoplasm of neurons

5 Myelinated axons

6 Unipolar neuron

7 Capsule cells

8 Satellite cells

9 Lipofuscin pigment

10 Myelinated axon

11 Schwann cells

FIGURE 9.30 ■ Cells and unipolar neurons of a dorsal root ganglion. Stain: hematoxylin and eosin. High magnification.

FIGURE 9.31 | Multipolar Neurons, Surrounding Cells, and Nerve Fibers of Sympathetic Ganglion

In contrast to the neurons of the dorsal root ganglion (Fig. 9.30), the **neurons** (**3, 9**) of the sympathetic trunk are multipolar, smaller, and more uniform in size. As a result, the outlines of the

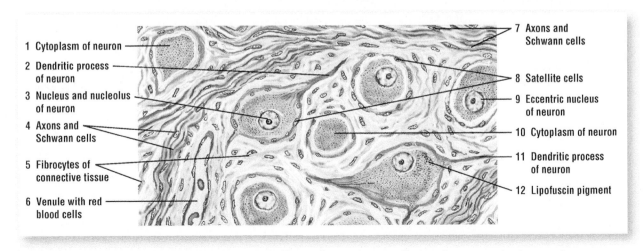

1 Cytoplasm of neuron

2 Dendritic process of neuron

3 Nucleus and nucleolus of neuron

4 Axons and Schwann cells

5 Fibrocytes of connective tissue

6 Venule with red blood cells

7 Axons and Schwann cells

8 Satellite cells

9 Eccentric nucleus of neuron

10 Cytoplasm of neuron

11 Dendritic process of neuron

12 Lipofuscin pigment

FIGURE 9.31 ■ Multipolar neurons, surrounding cells, and nerve fibers of a sympathetic ganglion. Stain: hematoxylin and eosin. High magnification.

neurons (3, 9) and their **dendritic processes** (2, 11) appear irregular. Also, if the plane of section does not pass through the middle of the neuron, only the **cytoplasm** (1, 10) is visible. The sympathetic neurons (3, 9) also often exhibit **eccentric nuclei** (9), and binucleated cells are not uncommon. In older individuals, a brownish **lipofuscin pigment** (12) accumulates in the cytoplasm of neurons (1, 10, 12).

The **satellite cells** (8) surround the multipolar neurons (3, 9) but are less numerous than around the neurons in the dorsal root ganglion. Also, the connective tissue capsule with its capsule cells may not be well defined. Surrounding the neurons (3, 9) are **fibrocytes** (5) of the intercellular connective tissue and blood vessels such as a venule with **blood cells** (6). Unmyelinated and myelinated nerve **axons** (4, 7) aggregate into bundles and course through the sympathetic ganglion. The flattened nuclei on the peripheries of the myelinated axons (4, 7) are the **Schwann cells** (4, 7). These nerve fibers represent the preganglionic axons, postganglionic visceral efferent axons, and visceral afferent axons.

FIGURE 9.32 | Dorsal Root Ganglion: Unipolar Neurons and Surrounding Cells

A medium-magnification photomicrograph of the dorsal root ganglion illustrates the spherical shape of the sensory **unipolar neurons** (2). The cytoplasm contains a central **nucleus** (6) and a prominent dense **nucleolus** (5). Surrounding the unipolar neurons (2) are the smaller **satellite cells** (1). Cells outside the satellite cells are the connective tissue **fibrocytes** (3). Coursing through the dorsal root ganglion between the unipolar neurons (2) are numerous **bundles of sensory axons** (4) from the periphery.

The clear space around the neurons and the surrounding cells is an artifact caused by the tissue shrinkage during the chemical preparation of the dorsal root ganglion.

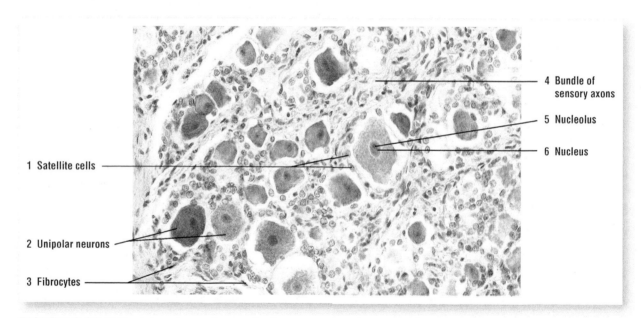

FIGURE 9.32 ■ Dorsal root ganglion: unipolar neurons and surrounding cells. Stain: hematoxylin and eosin. ×100.

Chapter 9 Summary

SECTION 2 • Peripheral Nervous System

PERIPHERAL NERVOUS SYSTEM

- Consists of neurons, neuroglia, nerves, and axons outside the CNS
- Cranial nerves arise from the brain and spinal nerves from the spinal cord
- Ganglia are accumulations of neurons and are covered by connective tissue
- Contains both sensory and motor nerves
- Neurons of peripheral nerves can be located in the CNS or in ganglia

CONNECTIVE TISSUE LAYERS IN PERIPHERAL NERVES

- Peripheral nerves are partitioned by layers of connective tissue into fascicles
- Outermost connective tissue around the nerve is the epineurium
- Perineurium surrounds one or more nerve fascicles and forms a blood–nerve barrier
- Vascular connective tissue layer endoneurium surrounds individual axons

PERIPHERAL NERVES

- Nuclei seen between individual axons are Schwann cells and fibrocytes
- Schwann cells myelinate and surround individual axons or enclose unmyelinated axons
- Between individual Schwann cells in myelinated axons are the nodes of Ranvier
- Conduction along a myelinated axon is called saltatory conduction
- Small satellite cells surround the neurons of PNS ganglia
- Satellite cells provide structural support, insulate, and regulate metabolic exchanges

DORSAL ROOT GANGLIA AND UNIPOLAR NEURONS OF PNS

- Situated on dorsal nerve roots that join the spinal cord
- Sensory (round) unipolar neurons constitute the ganglia
- Bundles of sensory nerve fibers or axons pass between the unipolar neurons
- Connective tissue capsule encloses the ganglia and merges with the epineurium of the peripheral nerve
- Unipolar neurons are surrounded by satellite cells, which are enclosed by connective tissue capsule cells

Chapter 9 Review Questions: Section 2

QUESTIONS

In the following multiple choice questions, choose the letter corresponding to the one best answer.

1. **The blood–nerve barrier in the peripheral nervous system is formed by:**
   A. endoneurium.
   B. epineurium.
   C. perineurium.
   D. myelin sheath.
   E. Schwann cells.

2. **The nodes of Ranvier represent:**
   A. gaps or spaces in the myelin sheath.
   B. intervals between myelinating cells.
   C. the length or segment of an axon covered by the myelin sheath.
   D. sites of axonal synapses.
   E. sites of neurotransmitter location.

3. **Saltatory conduction indicates:**
   A. a normal impulse conduction in all axons.
   B. passage of impulses across the synapses in myelinated axons.
   C. a rapid impulse conduction in unmyelinated axons.
   D. a rapid impulse conduction in large myelinated axons.
   E. a slow impulse conduction in large myelinated axons.

4. **The sensory neurons for the peripheral nerves of the spinal cord are located in the:**
   A. dorsal root ganglia.
   B. spinal cord.
   C. cerebrum.
   D. cerebellum.
   E. peripheral organs.

5. **Satellite cells:**
   A. surround the Schwann cells.
   B. enclose the oligodendrocytes.
   C. are sensory neurons in ganglia.
   D. surround sensory neurons in different ganglia.
   E. surround the peripheral axons.

ANSWERS

1. **Correct Answer: C.** Perineurium. Connective tissue cells are joined by tight junctions to form a blood–nerve barrier.

2. **Correct Answer: B.** Intervals between myelinating cells. The nodes of Ranvier are the intermodal segments and represent the length in the neuron covered by the myelinating cell.

3. **Correct Answer: D.** A rapid impulse conduction in large myelinated axons. In saltatory conduction, the impulse jumps from node to node, resulting in fast transmission of an impulse.

4. **Correct Answer: A.** Dorsal root ganglia. These are located on each side of the spinal cord.

5. **Correct Answer: D.** Surround sensory neurons in different ganglia. Satellite cells provide structural support for the neurons.

ADDITIONAL HISTOLOGIC IMAGES

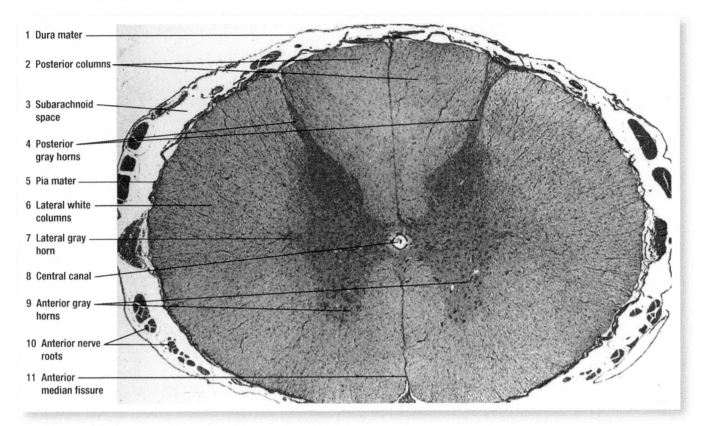

1 Dura mater
2 Posterior columns
3 Subarachnoid space
4 Posterior gray horns
5 Pia mater
6 Lateral white columns
7 Lateral gray horn
8 Central canal
9 Anterior gray horns
10 Anterior nerve roots
11 Anterior median fissure

FIGURE 9.33 ■ Transverse section of a spinal cord through the midthoracic region. Stain: hematoxylin and eosin. ×2.5.

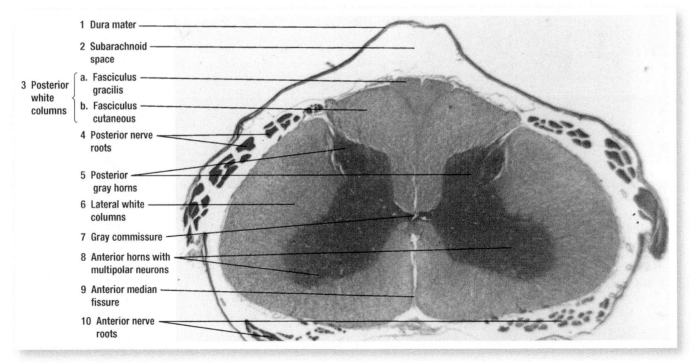

1 Dura mater
2 Subarachnoid space
3 Posterior white columns
  a. Fasciculus gracilis
  b. Fasciculus cutaneous
4 Posterior nerve roots
5 Posterior gray horns
6 Lateral white columns
7 Gray commissure
8 Anterior horns with multipolar neurons
9 Anterior median fissure
10 Anterior nerve roots

FIGURE 9.34 ■ Transverse section of a spinal cord through the lumbar region. Stain: hematoxylin and eosin. ×2.5.

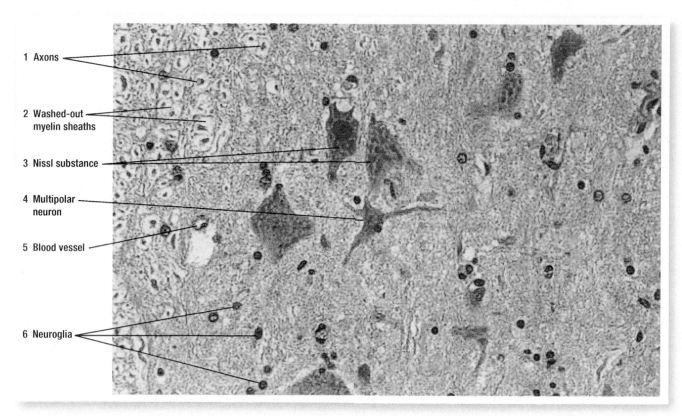

1 Axons

2 Washed-out myelin sheaths

3 Nissl substance

4 Multipolar neuron

5 Blood vessel

6 Neuroglia

FIGURE 9.35 ■ A section of the anterior horn of spinal cord illustrating multipolar motor neurons and the adjacent myelinated axons. Stain: hematoxylin and eosin. ×80.

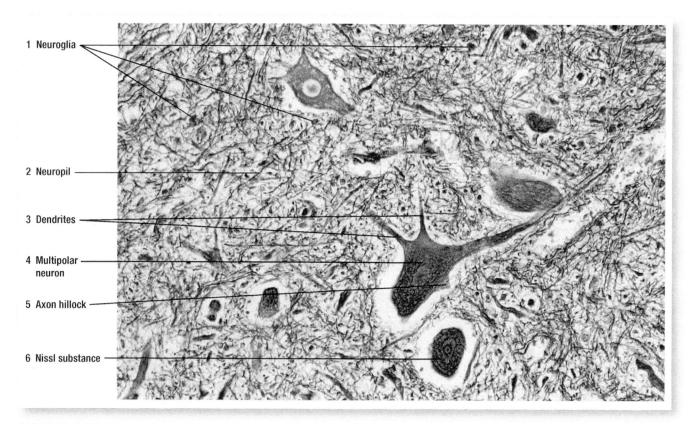

1 Neuroglia

2 Neuropil

3 Dendrites

4 Multipolar neuron

5 Axon hillock

6 Nissl substance

FIGURE 9.36 ■ A section of an anterior horn of the spinal cord illustrating the cellular and fibrillar components of the cord. Silver impregnation (Cajal method). ×80.

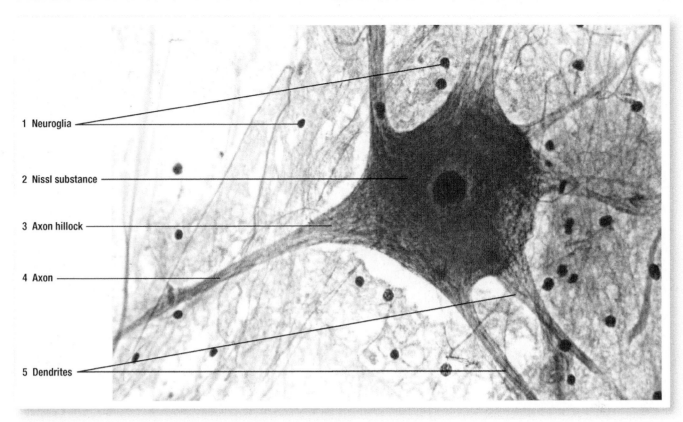

1 Neuroglia

2 Nissl substance

3 Axon hillock

4 Axon

5 Dendrites

FIGURE 9.37 ■ Spinal cord spread showing a multipolar motor neuron in the anterior horn. Stain: hematoxylin and eosin. ×205.

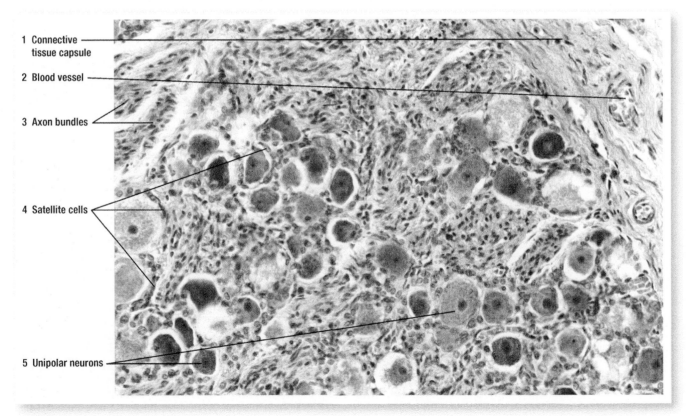

1 Connective tissue capsule

2 Blood vessel

3 Axon bundles

4 Satellite cells

5 Unipolar neurons

FIGURE 9.38 ■ A section of sensory dorsal root ganglion with its unipolar neurons, axons bundles, and the surrounding connective tissue capsule. Stain: hematoxylin and eosin. ×100.

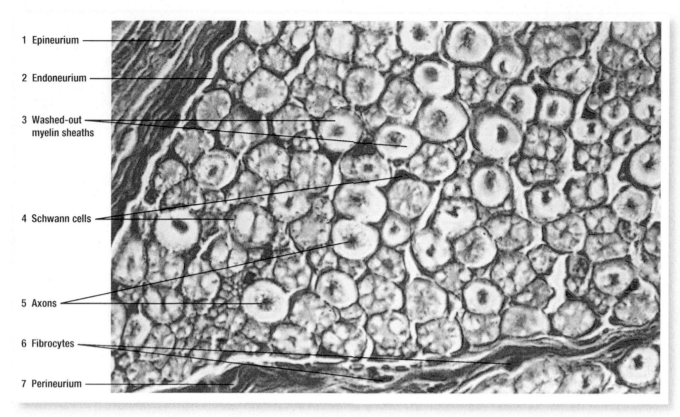

1 Epineurium
2 Endoneurium
3 Washed-out myelin sheaths
4 Schwann cells
5 Axons
6 Fibrocytes
7 Perineurium

FIGURE 9.39 ■ A transverse section of a nerve illustrating individual cells, axons, and the surrounding connective tissue. Stain: hematoxylin and eosin. Masson stain. ×100.

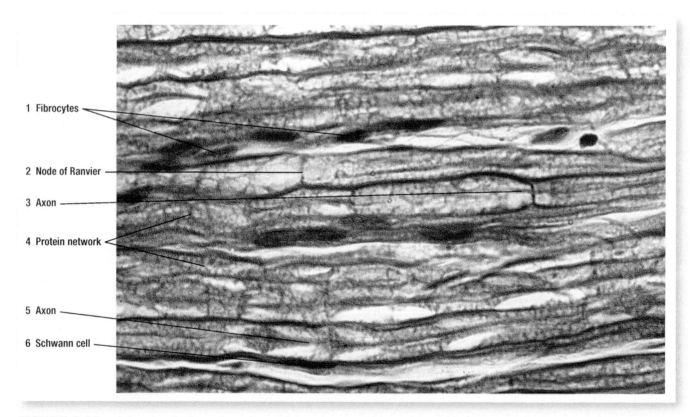

1 Fibrocytes
2 Node of Ranvier
3 Axon
4 Protein network
5 Axon
6 Schwann cell

FIGURE 9.40 ■ A longitudinal section of a peripheral nerve with nodes of Ranvier, axons, and the protein network in the washed-out myelin sheaths. Masson trichrome. ×165.

PART IV

Systems

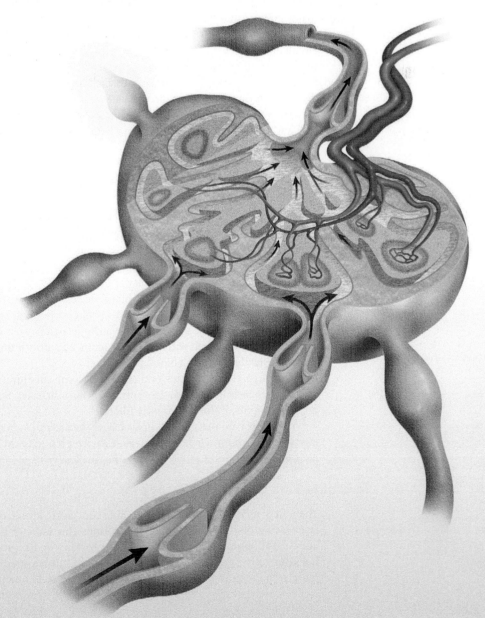

Circulatory System

The mammalian circulatory system comprises two major systems: the cardiovascular system and the lymphatic vascular system.

CARDIOVASCULAR SYSTEM

The **cardiovascular system** consists of the heart, major arteries, arterioles, capillaries, venules, and veins that form a closed system of blood vessels that carry blood. Within this system are two major circuits that distribute blood, the **systemic circulation** and the **pulmonary circulation**. Both circuits depend on the pumping action of the heart for blood distribution. The systemic circulation carries the blood from the heart to all organs, tissues, and cells via arterial vessels and then back to the heart via the venous vessels. The pulmonary system carries deoxygenated blood from the heart to the lungs for gaseous exchange and the oxygenated blood back to the heart for distribution via the systemic circulation.

The main functions of the blood vascular system are gaseous exchange; temperature control; and transport of oxygen, carbon dioxide, nutrients, hormones, metabolic products, cells of immune defense system, and many other essential products. The histology of the heart muscle has been described in detail in Chapter 8 as one of the four main tissues. In this chapter, heart histology is illustrated only as part of the cardiovascular system.

Types of Arteries

There are three types of arteries in an organism: elastic arteries, muscular arteries, and arterioles. Arteries that leave the heart with the oxygenated blood become smaller as they exhibit progressive branching. With each branching, the luminal diameters of the arteries gradually decrease until the smallest vessel, the capillary, is formed.

Elastic arteries are the largest blood vessels and include the **pulmonary trunk** and **aorta** with their major branches, the brachiocephalic, common carotid, subclavian, vertebral, pulmonary, and common iliac arteries. The walls of elastic vessels are composed of elastic connective tissue fibers interspersed with circularly arranged **smooth muscle fibers** that provide great resilience and flexibility during blood flow.

The large elastic arteries branch and become medium-sized **muscular arteries**, the most numerous vessels in the body. In contrast to elastic arteries, the walls of muscular arteries contain greater amounts of **smooth muscle fibers**.

Arterioles are the smallest branches of the arterial system. Their walls consist of one to five layers of smooth muscle fibers. Arterioles deliver blood to the smallest blood vessels, the capillaries; capillaries connect arterioles with the smallest veins or venules.

Structural Plan of Arteries

The wall of a typical artery contains three concentric layers, or **tunics** (Fig. 10.1). The innermost layer facing the lumen is the **tunica intima**. This layer consists of a simple squamous epithelium, called **endothelium** in the vascular system, and a thin underlying layer of **subendothelial connective tissue**. The middle layer is the **tunica media**, composed primarily of smooth muscle fibers. Interspersed among the smooth muscle fibers are elastic and reticular fibers. In

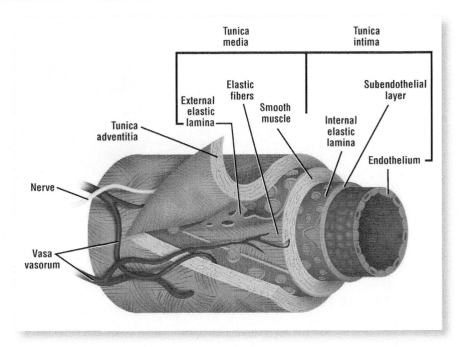

FIGURE 10.1 ■ Muscular artery.

the muscular and elastic arteries, smooth muscle fibers produce the **elastic fibers**, some **collagen fibers**, and extracellular elements. The collagen fibers provide tensile strength to the arterial walls, whereas the elastic fibers allow for the distention and recoil of the vessel walls during heart contraction and blood ejection. The outermost layer is the **tunica adventitia**, composed primarily of longitudinally oriented collagen fibers and elastic connective tissue fibers; adventitia consists primarily of **collagen type I fibers**.

The walls of some muscular arteries also exhibit two thin, wavy bands of elastic fibers. The **internal elastic lamina** (IEL) is located between the tunica intima and the tunica media. This lamina exhibits elastin sheets that contain numerous openings or **fenestrations** that allow diffusion of nutrients through the lamina to cells that are deep within the vessel walls. IEL is not seen in smaller arteries.

The **external elastic lamina** (EEL) is peripheral to the muscular tunica media and is primarily seen in large muscular arteries. This lamina separates the tunica media from the collagenous tunica adventitia.

Structural Plan of Veins

Capillaries unite to form larger blood vessels called **venules** that usually accompany arterioles. Venous blood initially flows into smaller **postcapillary venules** and then into veins of increasing size. The veins are arbitrarily classified as small, medium, and large. Compared with arteries, veins are more numerous and have thinner walls, larger diameters, and greater structural variation. Blood that enters the veins is under low pressure. Small-sized and medium-sized veins, particularly veins in the extremities (arms and legs) and those that convey blood against gravity, have **valves**. Because of the low blood pressure in the veins, blood flow to the heart in the veins is slow and can even back up. The presence of valves in veins assists venous blood flow toward the heart by preventing backflow. When blood flows toward the heart, pressure in the veins forces the valves to open. As the blood begins to flow backward, the valve flaps close the lumen and prevent backflow of blood. Venous blood between the valves in the extremities flows toward the heart because of the contraction of surrounding muscles, contractions between muscles, or contractions of organs that have some muscle such as the spleen. However, valves are absent in veins of the central nervous system (CNS), the inferior and superior venae cavae, and the viscera.

The walls of the veins, like the arteries, also exhibit three layers or tunics; however, the muscular layer is much thinner and less prominent. The **tunica intima** in veins exhibits an endothelium

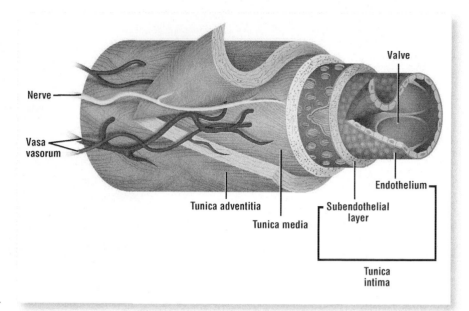

FIGURE 10.2 ■ Large vein.

and subendothelial connective tissue. In contrast to arteries, the muscular **tunica media** is thin in the veins, and the smooth muscles intermix with connective tissue fibers. The **tunica adventitia** is the thickest and best-developed layer of the three tunics. Longitudinal bundles of smooth muscle fibers are common in the connective tissue of this layer (Fig. 10.2). The structure of the venous walls allows flexibility and the accommodation of a large blood volume. As a result, veins contain most of the blood in the body.

Vasa Vasorum

The walls of medium and large arteries and veins are too thick to provide nourishment to the cells by direct diffusion from their lumina. As a result, these walls are supplied by their own small blood vessels from adjacent small arteries called the **vasa vasorum** (blood vessels of the larger blood vessel). The vasa vasorum allows for the exchange of nutrients and metabolites with cells in the tunica adventitia and the deeper tunica media. The vessels of vasa vasorum are much more extensive in the walls of the veins than in the arteries because of the poor oxygen content of venous blood.

Types of Capillaries

Capillaries are the smallest blood vessels. Their average diameter is about **8 μm**, which is about the size of an **erythrocyte** (red blood cell [RBC]). Each capillary consists of a thin endothelium, an underlying basal lamina, and a few randomly scattered **pericytes**. These cells surround the capillaries with branching cytoplasm and are enclosed by a basal lamina that also encloses the capillary endothelium. There are three types of capillaries: continuous capillaries, fenestrated capillaries, and sinusoids (Fig. 10.3). These structural variations in capillaries allow for different types of metabolic exchange between blood and the surrounding tissues.

Continuous capillaries are the most common. They are found in muscle, connective tissue, nervous tissue, skin, respiratory organs, and exocrine glands. In these capillaries, the **endothelial cells** are joined and form an uninterrupted, solid endothelial lining. Tight junctions, desmosomes, and gap junctions are seen in these capillaries.

Fenestrated capillaries are characterized by openings or **fenestrations** (pores) in the cytoplasm of endothelial cells designed for rapid exchange of molecules between blood and tissues. Fenestrated capillaries are found in those organs/tissues where enhanced exchange of substances

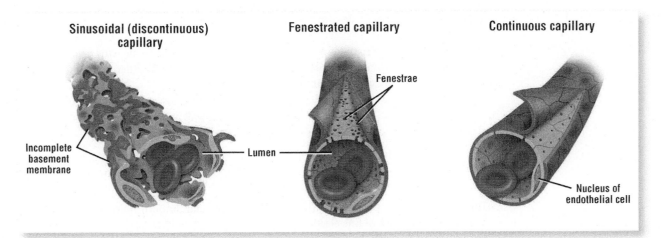

Sinusoidal (discontinuous) capillary

Incomplete basement membrane

Lumen

Fenestrated capillary

Fenestrae

Continuous capillary

Nucleus of endothelial cell

FIGURE 10.3 ■ Three types of capillaries (transverse sections).

occurs between tissues and blood. Endocrine tissues and glands, the small intestine, the kidney glomeruli, and the choroid plexus in the brain ventricles are organs that exhibit fenestrated capillaries.

Sinusoidal (discontinuous) capillaries are blood vessels that exhibit irregular, tortuous paths. Their much wider diameters slow down the flow of blood. Endothelial cell junctions are rare in sinusoidal capillaries, and wide gaps exist between individual endothelial cells. Also, because a **basement membrane** underlying the endothelium is either incomplete or absent, direct exchange of molecules occurs between blood contents and cells. Sinusoidal capillaries are found in the liver, spleen, and bone marrow.

LYMPHATIC VASCULAR SYSTEM

The lymphatic vascular system is closely associated with the circulatory system. It is composed of vascular channels that drain extracellular fluid called **lymph** from the tissues. The **lymphatic system** consists of lymph capillaries and lymph vessels that originate as blind-ending tubules or lymphatic capillaries in the connective tissue of organs. The lymph capillaries lie close to the blood capillaries and collect the excess **interstitial fluid (lymph)** from the tissues. The collected lymph is returned to the venous blood via the large **lymph vessels**, the thoracic duct, and the right lymphatic duct after it is filtered through numerous lymph nodes located throughout the body. Also, the walls of lymph vessels show more permeability than the walls of blood capillaries because the **endothelium** in lymph capillaries is extremely thin. The structure of larger lymph vessels is similar to that of veins except that their walls are much thinner.

Lymph movement in the lymphatic vessels is similar to that of venous blood. In larger lymph vessels, the contraction of smooth muscles in their walls moves the lymph forward. In addition, external factors such as the contractions of surrounding skeletal muscles, arterial pulsations, and compression of tissues also assist in the lymph flow. Similar to the veins, numerous **valves** in the lymph vessels prevent backflow of the collected lymph. Lymph vessels are found in all tissues except in the CNS, cartilage, bone and bone marrow, thymus, placenta, and teeth. Lymph capillaries also take up and deliver the absorbed lipids from the intestines into the bloodstream.

thePoint®   Supplemental micrographic images are available at **www.thePoint.com/Eroschenko13e** under Blood Vessels.

FIGURE 10.4 | Different Blood and Lymphatic Vessels in Connective Tissue

This composite figure illustrates a section of irregular connective tissue with nerve fibers, blood and lymphatic vessels, and adipose tissue. To illustrate structural differences, the vessels have been sectioned in transverse, longitudinal, or oblique planes.

A **small artery** (3) with its wall structure is shown in the lower left corner of the illustration. In contrast to veins (11), an artery has a relatively thick wall and a small lumen. In cross section, the wall of a small artery (3) exhibits the following layers:

- **Tunica intima** (4) is the innermost layer. It is composed of **endothelium** (4a), a **subendothelial** (4b) connective tissue, and an **IEL (membrane)** (4c), which separates the tunica intima (4) from the **tunica media** (5).
- Tunica media (5) is predominantly composed of circular smooth muscle fibers with a loose, interspersed network of fine elastic fibers.
- **Tunica adventitia** (6) is the connective tissue layer around the vessel that contains small nerves and blood vessels. In tunica adventitia (6), the blood vessels are collectively called **vasa vasorum** (7), or "blood vessels of the blood vessel."

Arteries with about 25 or more layers of smooth muscle fibers in the tunica media are called muscular or distributing arteries. Elastic fibers become more numerous in the tunica media as thin fibers and networks.

A **venule** (9) and small vein (11) are also illustrated with a thin wall and a large lumen. The thin wall, however, appears to have many cell layers when the vein is sectioned in an **oblique plane** (9). In cross section, the wall of the vein exhibits the following layers:

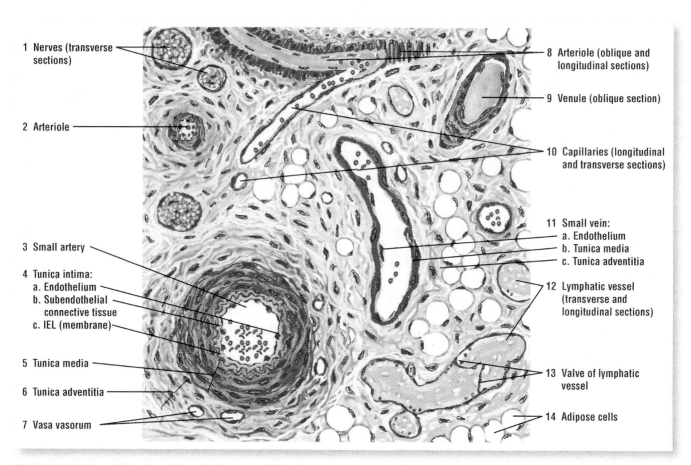

1 Nerves (transverse sections)

2 Arteriole

3 Small artery

4 Tunica intima:
  a. Endothelium
  b. Subendothelial connective tissue
  c. IEL (membrane)

5 Tunica media

6 Tunica adventitia

7 Vasa vasorum

8 Arteriole (oblique and longitudinal sections)

9 Venule (oblique section)

10 Capillaries (longitudinal and transverse sections)

11 Small vein:
  a. Endothelium
  b. Tunica media
  c. Tunica adventitia

12 Lymphatic vessel (transverse and longitudinal sections)

13 Valve of lymphatic vessel

14 Adipose cells

FIGURE 10.4 ■ Blood and lymphatic vessels in the connective tissue. Stain: hematoxylin and eosin. Low magnification.

- Tunica intima composed of **endothelium** (**11a**) and an extremely thin layer of fine collagen and elastic fibers that blend with the connective tissue of the **tunica media** (**11b**).

- Tunica media (11b) consists of a thin layer of circularly arranged smooth muscle embedded in connective tissue. Tunica media (11b) is much thinner in veins than in arteries (5).

- **Tunica adventitia** (**11c**) exhibits a wide layer of connective tissue, and in veins, the tunica adventitia (11c) layer is thicker than the tunica media (11b).

Two **arterioles** (**2, 8**) are cut in different planes. The arterioles (2, 8) have a thin IEL and a layer of smooth muscle fibers in the tunica media. One **arteriole** (**8**) is shown cut in longitudinal plane with a branching **capillary** (**10**). An arteriole (8) cut at an oblique angle shown only the circular smooth muscle layer of the tunica media. Also visible are capillaries (10) sectioned in longitudinal and oblique planes and small **nerves** (**1**) in transverse planes.

The **lymphatic vessels** (**12, 13**) exhibit the thinnest walls. When cut in a longitudinal plane, the flaps of a **valve** (**13**) are seen in the lumen of the lymphatic vessel. Many veins in the arms and legs have similar valves in their lumina.

Numerous **adipose cells** (**14**) are found in the surrounding connective tissue.

FIGURE 10.5 | Capillaries Sectioned in Transverse and Longitudinal Planes in Mesentery of Small Intestine

This high-magnification photomicrograph of the mesentery connective tissue shows the **capillaries** (**1, 3, 4, 5**) sectioned in both transverse (1, 5) and longitudinal planes (3, 4). The lumen of the capillaries (1, 3, 4, 5) is about the size of an RBC. In the transverse plane (1, 5), the RBCs fill the lumina of the capillaries (1, 5), and in the longitudinal plane (3, 4), the RBCs are lined up in a row. Surrounding the capillaries (1, 3, 4, 5) are the **adipose cells** (**2**) of the intestinal mesentery, which appear empty because of the chemicals used for the preparation of this slide. Blue-staining collagen fibers of the **connective tissue** (**6**) surround the adipose cells (2) and the capillaries (1, 3, 4, 5).

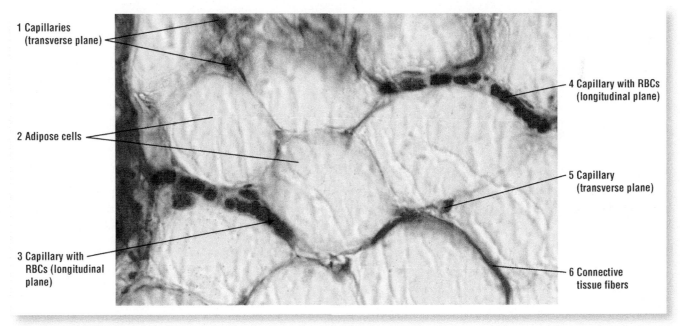

1 Capillaries (transverse plane)

4 Capillary with RBCs (longitudinal plane)

2 Adipose cells

5 Capillary (transverse plane)

3 Capillary with RBCs (longitudinal plane)

6 Connective tissue fibers

FIGURE 10.5 ■ Capillaries sectioned in transverse and longitudinal planes in the mesentery of a small intestine. Stain: Mallory-Azan. ×205.

FIGURE 10.6 | Ultrastructure of Continuous Capillary Sectioned in Transverse Plane

This ultrastructure micrograph shows a capillary in the CNS, sectioned in a transverse plane. A layer of **continuous endothelium of the capillary** (6) surrounds the **capillary lumen**. Also visible on the left side of the capillary are the **nucleus of the endothelial cell** (3) and a section of a **pericyte process** (5) closely attached to the capillary wall. The capillary endothelium (6), the **nucleus of the endothelial cell** (3), and the section of the pericyte process (5) are surrounded by a **basal lamina** (2, 7). Adjacent to the capillary wall is a section of a **myelinated axon** (8) and a dense meshwork of fibers from axons, dendrites, and astrocytic endfeet of glial cells. This neural meshwork that fills the spaces in the CNS is called **neuropil** (1, 4).

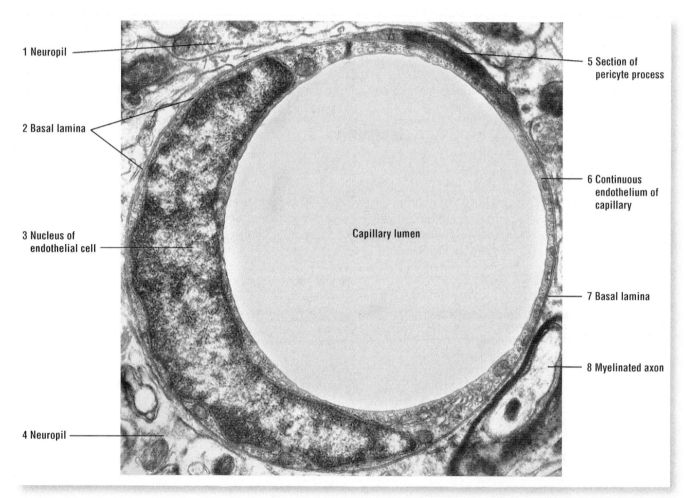

1 Neuropil

2 Basal lamina

3 Nucleus of endothelial cell

4 Neuropil

Capillary lumen

5 Section of pericyte process

6 Continuous endothelium of capillary

7 Basal lamina

8 Myelinated axon

FIGURE 10.6 ■ Ultrastructure of a continuous capillary sectioned in the transverse plane in the CNS. Courtesy of Dr. Mark DeSantis, Professor Emeritus, WWAMI medical Program, University of Idaho, Moscow, ID. ×25,000.

FIGURE 10.7 | **Ultrastructure of Fenestrated Capillary Sectioned in Transverse Plane in Choroid Plexus of CNS Ventricle**

The ultrastructure of a fenestrated capillary exhibits a different type of endothelium that is seen in a continuous capillary (see Fig. 10.6). This capillary **endothelium** (3) exhibits numerous opening or **fenestrations** (*arrows*) (3) around the entire periphery of the **capillary lumen** (5) that are closed by thin diaphragms (*arrows*) (3). On the right side of the capillary is the **cytoplasm of an endothelia cell** (7) with organelles. Located in the center and completely filling the capillary lumen is a section of a densely stained **RBC** (2) with its characteristic biconcave shape (see Fig. 10.5 for comparison). Surrounding the fenestrated endothelium (3) and the cytoplasm of the endothelial cell (7) is a **basal lamina** (4, 6). Surrounding the capillary and the basal lamina (4, 6) are the sections of the **ependymal cell cytoplasm** (1, 8) of the choroid plexus.

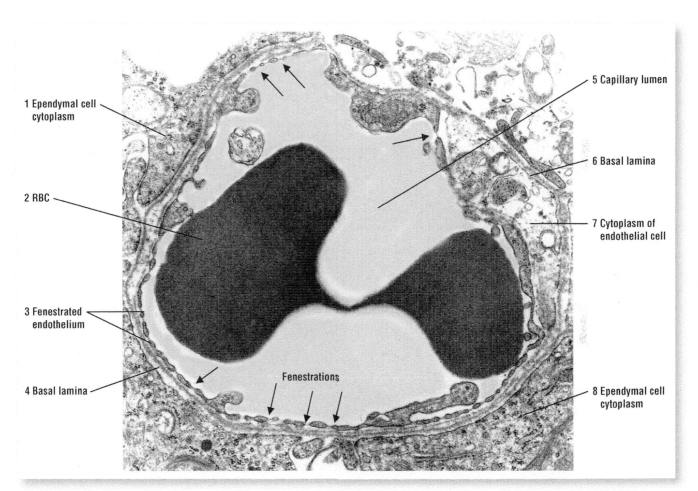

FIGURE 10.7 ■ Ultrastructure of a fenestrated capillary sectioned in the transverse plane in the choroid plexus of a CNS ventricle. ×25,000.

FIGURE 10.8 | Muscular Artery and Vein (Transverse Section)

The walls of blood vessels contain elastic tissue that allows them to expand and contract. In this illustration, a muscular **artery** (**1**) and **vein** (**4**) have been cut in the transverse plane and prepared with a plastic stain to illustrate the distribution of elastic fibers in their walls. The elastic fibers stain black, and the collagen fibers stain light yellow.

The wall of the artery (**1**) is thicker and contains more smooth muscle fibers than the wall of the vein (**4**). The innermost layer tunica intima of the artery (**1**) is stained dark because of the thick **IEL** (**1a**). The thick middle layer of the muscular artery, the **tunica media** (**1b**), contains several layers of smooth muscle fibers, arranged in a circular pattern, and thin dark strands of **elastic fibers** (**1b**). On the periphery of the tunica media (**1b**) is the less conspicuous **EEL** (**1c**). Surrounding the artery is the connective tissue **tunica adventitia** (**1d**), which contains both the light-staining **collagen fibers** (**2**) and the dark-staining **elastic fibers** (**3**).

The wall of the vein (**4**) also contains the layers **tunica intima** (**4a**), **tunica media** (**4b**), and **tunica adventitia** (**4c**). However, these three layers in the vein (**4**) are not as thick as those in the wall of the artery (**1**).

Surrounding both vessels are the **capillary** (**5**), **arteriole** (**7**), **venule** (**6**), and cells of the **adipose tissue** (**8**). Present in the lumina of both vessels (**1**, **4**) are numerous erythrocytes and leukocytes.

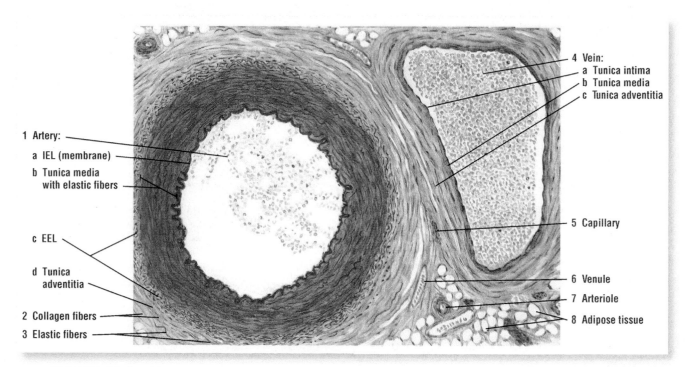

FIGURE 10.8 ■ Muscular artery and vein (transverse section). Stain: elastic stain. Low magnification.

FIGURE 10.9 | Artery and Vein in Dense Irregular Connective Tissue of Vas Deferens

This photomicrograph illustrates the differences between a **small artery** (**1**) and a small **vein** (**6**) in dense irregular **connective tissue** (**5**). The small artery (**1**) has a thick muscular wall and a small lumen. The arterial wall consists of the **tunica intima** (**2**), composed of an inner layer of **endothelium** (**2a**), a **subendothelial** (**2b**) connective tissue, and an **IEL** (**membrane**) (**2c**). This membrane (**2c**) separates the tunica intima (**2**) from the layer of circular smooth muscle fibers of the **tunica media** (**3**). Surrounding the tunica media (**3**) is the connective tissue layer of **tunica adventitia** (**4**).

Adjacent to the small artery (**1**) is a small vein (**6**) with a larger lumen that is filled with blood cells. The wall of the vein (**6**) is thinner in comparison to that of the artery (**1**) but also consists of **tunica intima** (**7**) composed of **endothelium** (**7a**), a thin layer of circular smooth muscle **tunica media** (**8**), and the layer of connective tissue **tunica adventitia** (**9**).

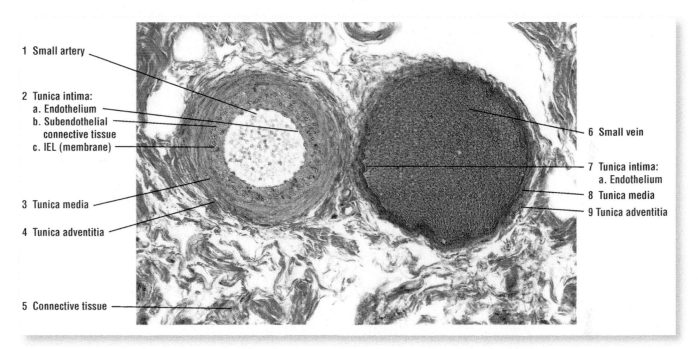

1 Small artery

2 Tunica intima:
   a. Endothelium
   b. Subendothelial
      connective tissue
   c. IEL (membrane)

3 Tunica media

4 Tunica adventitia

5 Connective tissue

6 Small vein

7 Tunica intima:
   a. Endothelium
8 Tunica media
9 Tunica adventitia

FIGURE 10.9 ■ Artery and vein in the dense irregular connective tissue of the vas deferens. Stain: iron hematoxylin and Alcian blue. ×64.

FIGURE 10.10 | Wall of Elastic Artery: Aorta (Transverse Section)

The wall of the aorta is similar in morphology to that of the artery illustrated in Figure 10.9. Instead of smooth muscle fibers, the **elastic fibers** (4) constitute the bulk of the **tunica media** (6), with **smooth muscle fibers** (10) less abundant than in the muscular arteries. The arrangement of the elastic fibers (4) in the tunica media (6) are demonstrated with the elastic stain. Fine elastic fibers and smooth muscle fibers (10) are either lightly stained or remain colorless.

The simple squamous **endothelium** (1) and the **subendothelial connective tissue** (2) in the **tunica intima** (5) are indicated but remain unstained. The first visible elastic membrane is the dark-stained **IEL** (**membrane**) (3).

The **tunica adventitia** (7), less stained with elastic stain, is a narrow, peripheral zone of connective tissue. A **venule** (9a) and an **arteriole** (9b) of the **vasa vasorum** (9) supply the tunica adventitia (7). In such large blood vessels as the aorta and the pulmonary arteries, tunica media (6) occupies most of the vessel wall, whereas tunica adventitia (7) is reduced, as illustrated in this figure.

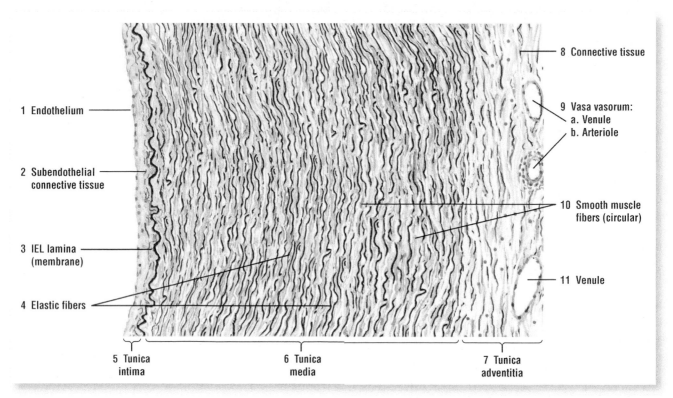

1 Endothelium

2 Subendothelial connective tissue

3 IEL lamina (membrane)

4 Elastic fibers

8 Connective tissue

9 Vasa vasorum:
a. Venule
b. Arteriole

10 Smooth muscle fibers (circular)

11 Venule

5 Tunica intima

6 Tunica media

7 Tunica adventitia

FIGURE 10.10 ■ Wall of a large elastic artery: aorta (transverse section). Stain: elastic stain. Low magnification.

FIGURE 10.11 | Wall of Large Vein: Portal Vein (Transverse Section)

In contrast to the wall of a large artery (Fig. 10.10), the wall of a large vein is characterized by thick, muscular **tunica adventitia (6)** in which the **smooth muscle fibers (7)** show a longitudinal orientation. In the transverse section of the portal vein, the smooth muscle fibers (7) are segregated into bundles and are seen in cross section, surrounded by the connective tissue of the tunica adventitia (6). An **arteriole (8a)**, two **venules (8b)**, and a **capillary (8c)** in a longitudinal section of the **vasa vasorum (8)** are visible in the tunica adventitia (6).

In contrast to the thick tunica adventitia (6), the **tunica media (5)** is thinner. The **smooth muscle fibers (3)** exhibit a circular orientation. In other large veins, the tunica media (5) may be extremely thin and compact.

The **tunica intima (4)** is part of the **endothelium (1)** and is supported by a small amount of **subendothelial connective tissue (2)**. In addition, large veins may exhibit an IEL that is not as well developed as in the arteries.

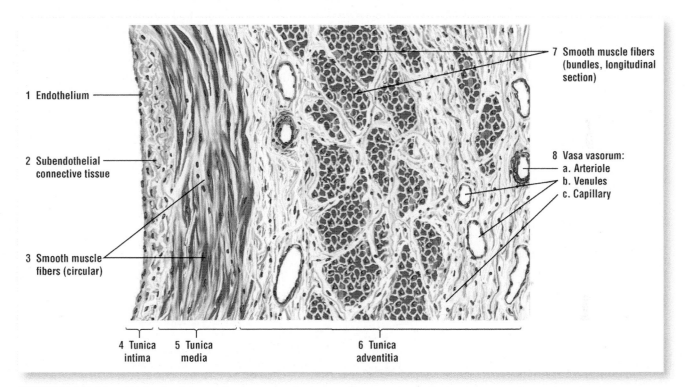

FIGURE 10.11 ■ Wall of a large vein: portal vein (transverse section). Stain: hematoxylin and eosin. Low magnification.

FIGURE 10.12 | Heart: Left Atrium, Atrioventricular Valve, and Left Ventricle (Longitudinal Section)

The wall of the heart consists of three layers: an inner **endocardium**, a middle **myocardium**, and an outer **epicardium**. The endocardium consists of a simple squamous endothelium and a thin subendothelial connective tissue. Deeper to the endocardium is the **subendocardial layer of connective tissue**. Here are found small blood vessels and Purkinje fibers. The subendocardial layer attaches to the connective tissue endomysium of the cardiac muscle fibers. The myocardium is the thickest layer and consists of cardiac muscle fibers. The epicardium consists of a simple squamous mesothelium and an underlying **subepicardial layer** of connective tissue. The subepicardial layer contains **coronary blood vessels**, nerves, and **adipose tissue**.

A longitudinal section through the left side of the heart illustrates a portion of the **atrium** (**1**), the **cusps of the atrioventricular (mitral) valve** (**5**), and a section of the **ventricle** (**19**). The endocardium (1, 9) lines the cavities of the atrium and the ventricle. Below the endocardium (1, 9) is the subendocardial connective tissue (2). The myocardium (3, 19) in both the atrium (3) and the ventricle (19) consists of cardiac muscle fibers.

The outer epicardium (13, 16) of the atrium (13) and the ventricle (16) is continuous and covers the heart externally with mesothelium. A subepicardial layer (17) contains connective tissue, adipose tissue (15), and numerous coronary blood vessels (15). The epicardium (13, 16) also extends into the coronary (atrioventricular [AV]) sulcus and the interventricular sulcus of the heart.

Between the atrium (1) and the ventricle (19) is a layer of dense fibrous connective tissue called the **annulus fibrosus** (**4**). A bicuspid (mitral) AV valve separates the atrium (1) from the ventricle (19). The cusps of the AV (mitral) valve (5) are formed by a double membrane of the **endocardium** (**6**) and a dense **connective tissue core** (**7**) that is continuous with the annulus fibrosus (4). On the ventral surface of each cusp (5) are the insertions of the connective tissue cords, the **chordae tendineae** (**8**), which extend from the cusps of the valve (5) and attach to the **papillary muscles** (**11**) that project from the ventricle wall. The inner surface of the ventricle also

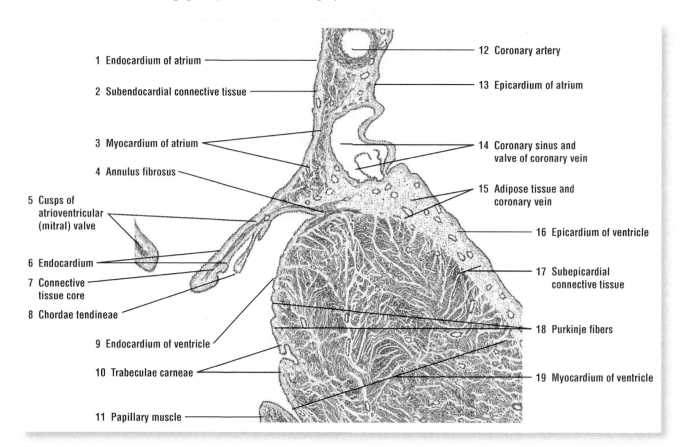

1 Endocardium of atrium
2 Subendocardial connective tissue
3 Myocardium of atrium
4 Annulus fibrosus
5 Cusps of atrioventricular (mitral) valve
6 Endocardium
7 Connective tissue core
8 Chordae tendineae
9 Endocardium of ventricle
10 Trabeculae carneae
11 Papillary muscle

12 Coronary artery
13 Epicardium of atrium
14 Coronary sinus and valve of coronary vein
15 Adipose tissue and coronary vein
16 Epicardium of ventricle
17 Subepicardial connective tissue
18 Purkinje fibers
19 Myocardium of ventricle

FIGURE 10.12 ■ Heart: a section of the left atrium, atrioventricular valve, and left ventricle (longitudinal section). Stain: hematoxylin and eosin. Low magnification.

contains prominent muscular (myocardial) ridges called **trabeculae carneae** (**10**) that give rise to the papillary muscles (11). The papillary muscles (11) via the chordae tendineae (8) hold and stabilize the cusps in the AV valves of the right and left ventricles during ventricular contractions.

The **Purkinje fibers** (**18**), or impulse-conducting fibers, are located beneath the thin endocardium in the subendocardial connective tissue (2). They are distinguished from cardiac muscle fibers by their larger size and lighter-staining properties. The Purkinje fibers are illustrated in greater detail and higher magnification in Figures 10.14 and 10.15.

The large **coronary artery** (**12**) is found in the subepicardial connective tissue (17). Below the coronary artery is the **coronary sinus** (**14**), a blood vessel that drains the heart. Entering the coronary sinus (14) is a **coronary vein** (**14**) with its valve. Smaller coronary blood vessels (15) are in the subepicardial connective tissue (17) and in the connective tissue septa of the myocardium (19).

FIGURE 10.13 | Heart: Right Ventricle, Pulmonary Trunk, and Pulmonary Valve (Longitudinal Section)

A section of the right ventricle and a lower portion of the **pulmonary trunk** (**5**) are illustrated. As in other blood vessels, the pulmonary trunk (5) is lined by the endothelium of the **tunica intima** (**5a**). The **tunica media** (**5b**) constitutes the thickest portion of the wall of the pulmonary trunk (5); however, its thick, elastic laminae are not seen at this magnification. The thin connective tissue **tunica adventitia** (**5c**) merges with the surrounding **subepicardial connective tissue** (**2**), with **adipose tissue**, **coronary arterioles**, and **venules** (**3**).

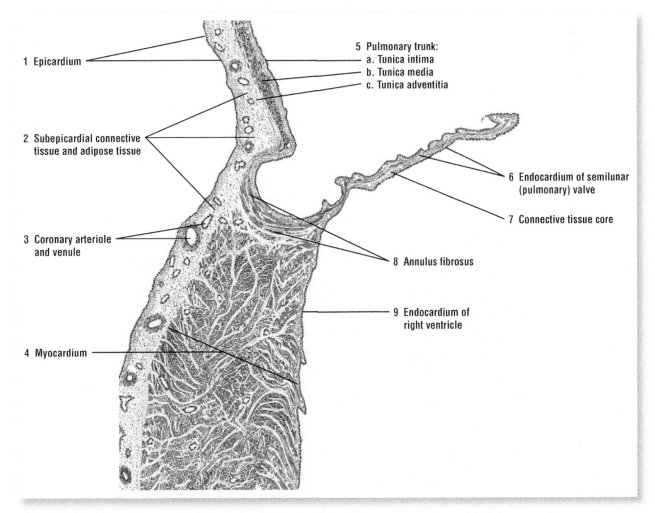

1 Epicardium

2 Subepicardial connective tissue and adipose tissue

3 Coronary arteriole and venule

4 Myocardium

5 Pulmonary trunk:
a. Tunica intima
b. Tunica media
c. Tunica adventitia

6 Endocardium of semilunar (pulmonary) valve

7 Connective tissue core

8 Annulus fibrosus

9 Endocardium of right ventricle

FIGURE 10.13 ■ Heart: a section of the right ventricle, pulmonary trunk, and pulmonary valve (longitudinal section). Stain: hematoxylin and eosin. Low magnification.

The pulmonary trunk (5) arises from the **annulus fibrosus** (8). One cusp of its **semilunar (pulmonary) valve** (6) is illustrated. Similar to the AV valve (see Fig. 10.12), the semilunar valve (6) of the pulmonary trunk (5) is covered with **endocardium** (6). A **connective tissue cor**e (7) from the annulus fibrosus (8) extends into the base of the semilunar valve (6) and forms its central core.

The thick **myocardium** (4) of the right ventricle is lined internally by the **endocardium** (9). The endocardium (9) extends over the pulmonary valve (6) and the annulus fibrosus (8) and blends in with the tunica intima (5a) of the pulmonary trunk (5).

The pulmonary trunk (5) is lined by the subepicardial connective tissue and adipose tissue (2), which, in turn, is covered by the **epicardium** (1). Both of these layers cover the external surface of the right ventricle. Coronary arterioles and venules (3) are found in the subepicardial connective tissue (2).

FIGURE 10.14 | Heart: Contracting Cardiac Muscle Fibers and Impulse-Conducting Purkinje Fibers

This figure illustrates a section of the heart stained with Mallory-Azan stain. The blue-stained collagen fibers accentuate the **subendocardial connective tissue** (9) that surrounds the **Purkinje fibers** (6, 10). The characteristic features of Purkinje fibers (6, 10) are visible in both longitudinal and transverse planes. In transverse plane (6), the Purkinje fibers exhibit fewer peripheral myofibrils leaving a perinuclear zone of comparatively clear sarcoplasm. A central nucleus is seen in some transverse sections; in others, a central area of clear sarcoplasm is seen, with the plane of section bypassing the nucleus.

The Purkinje fibers (6, 10) are located inferior to the **endocardium** (7), which represents the endothelium of the heart cavities. The Purkinje fibers (6, 10) are different from typical **cardiac muscle fibers** (1, 3) in that the Purkinje fibers (6, 10) are larger and show less intense staining.

The cardiac muscle fibers (1, 3) are connected to each other via the prominent **intercalated discs** (4). The intercalated discs (4) are not observed in the Purkinje fibers (6, 10). Instead, the Purkinje fibers (6, 10) are connected to each other via desmosomes and gap junctions and eventually merge with cardiac muscle fibers (1, 3).

The heart musculature has a rich blood supply; visible are a **capillary** (8), **arteriole** (5), and **venule** (2).

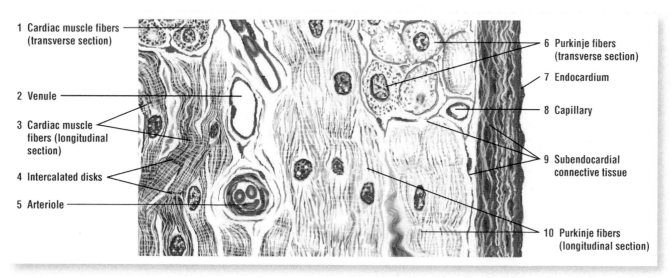

1 Cardiac muscle fibers (transverse section)

2 Venule

3 Cardiac muscle fibers (longitudinal section)

4 Intercalated disks

5 Arteriole

6 Purkinje fibers (transverse section)

7 Endocardium

8 Capillary

9 Subendocardial connective tissue

10 Purkinje fibers (longitudinal section)

FIGURE 10.14 ■ Heart: contracting cardiac muscle fibers and impulse-conducting Purkinje fibers. Stain: Mallory-Azan. High magnification.

FIGURE 10.15 | Heart Wall: Purkinje Fibers

A photomicrograph of the ventricular heart wall illustrates the **endocardium** (3), **subendocardial connective tissue** (4), and the underlying **Purkinje fibers** (5). In comparison with red-stained **cardiac muscle fibers** (1), the Purkinje fibers (5) are larger and exhibit less intense staining. Also, the Purkinje fibers (5) exhibit fewer myofibrils, which are peripherally distributed, and a perinuclear zone of clear sarcoplasm. Purkinje fibers (5) gradually merge with the cardiac muscle fibers (1). Surrounding both the Purkinje fibers (5) and the cardiac muscle fibers (1) are **connective tissue fibers** (2).

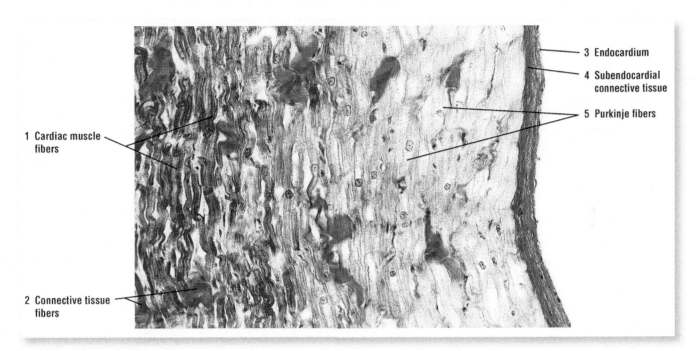

FIGURE 10.15 ■ A section of heart wall: Purkinje fibers. Stain: Mallory-Azan. ×64.

FUNCTIONAL CORRELATIONS 10.1 ■ Circulatory System

BLOOD VESSELS

The **elastic arteries** transport the ejected blood from the heart and move it along the systemic vascular path. The presence of **elastic fibers** in their walls allows the elastic arteries to greatly expand in diameter during **systole** (heart contraction), when a large volume of blood is forcefully ejected from the ventricles into their lumina. During **diastole** (heart relaxation), the expanded elastic walls recoil upon the volume of blood in their lumina and force the blood to move forward through the vascular channels. As a result, a less variable systemic blood pressure is maintained, and blood flows evenly through the body during heartbeats.

In contrast, the **muscular arteries** control blood flow and blood pressure through **vasoconstriction** (narrowing) or **vasodilation** (expanding) of their lumina. Vasoconstriction and vasodilation are controlled by unmyelinated axons of the **sympathetic division** of the **autonomic nervous system** (**ANS**). Similarly, by autonomic constriction or dilation of their lumina, the **smooth muscle fibers** in smaller muscular arteries or arterioles regulate blood flow into the capillary beds.

Terminal arterioles give rise to the smallest blood vessels, the **capillaries**. Because of their very thin walls, capillaries are sites for the exchange of gases, metabolites, nutrients, and waste products between blood and interstitial tissues.

LYMPHATIC VESSELS

The main function of the **lymphatic vascular system** is to collect excess tissue fluid and proteins, called **lymph**, from the intercellular spaces of the connective tissue and return it into the venous blood vascular system. Lymph is a clear fluid and an **ultrafiltrate** of the blood plasma. Numerous lymph nodes are located along the route of the lymph vessels. In the maze of lymph node channels, the collected lymph is filtered of cells and particulate matter. Lymph that flows through the lymph nodes is also exposed to the numerous macrophages that reside here. These engulf foreign microorganisms and other suspended matter. The lymph vessels also bring to the systemic bloodstream **lymphocytes**, **fatty acids** absorbed through the capillary lymph vessels called **lacteals** in the small intestine, and **immunoglobulins** (antibodies) produced in the lymph nodes. Thus, the lymphatic vessels serve as an important component of the immune system of the body.

ENDOTHELIUM

The endothelium lining the lumina of blood vessels performs numerous physiologic, metabolic, and secretory functions. The endothelial cells form a **semipermeable barrier** between blood and the interstitial tissue. The cells are anchored to the basal lamina and attached to each other by adhesion junctions. The presence of **pinocytotic** vesicles in the endothelial cells indicates a bidirectional movement of molecules between blood and tissues. The smooth lining of the endothelium in the blood vessels and the secretion of **anticoagulants** by the endothelial cells prevent blood clotting. The endothelium surface is also lined by **glycocalyx** protein. In addition, endothelial cells secrete **prostacyclin**, an antithrombotic substance that prevents platelet adhesion in the blood vessels and blood clot formation.

Endothelial cells also produce vasoactive chemicals **nitrous oxide** and its related compounds to induce **vasodilation** and increase blood flow. Conversely, the secretion of **endothelin proteins** by endothelial cells counteracts the nitrous oxide effects by causing vasoconstriction and decreased blood flow. The endothelium also converts **angiotensin I** to **angiotensin II**, a powerful vasoconstrictor that increases blood pressure. Endothelium changes prostaglandins, bradykinin, and serotonin to biologically inactive compounds, degrades lipoproteins, and produces growth factors for fibroblasts, blood cell colonies, and platelets. The arterial endothelial cytoplasm contains small membrane-bound, electron-dense structures called **Weibel-Palade bodies** that store the procoagulant glycoprotein **von Willebrand factor**. When the endothelium is damaged, von Willebrand factor is released into the bloodstream to induce platelets adhesion, blood coagulation, and **blood clot formation**.

HEART WALL

Pacemaker of the Heart

Cardiac muscle is **involuntary** and contracts rhythmically and automatically. The **impulse-generating** and **impulse-conducting** portions of the heart are specialized or modified **cardiac muscle fibers** located in the **sinoatrial** (**SA**) **node** and the **AV node** in the wall of the **right atrium** of the heart. The modified cardiac muscle fibers in these nodes exhibit spontaneous rhythmic depolarization or impulse conduction, which sends a wave of stimulation throughout the myocardium of the heart. Because the cardiac muscle fibers in the SA node depolarize and repolarize faster than those in the AV node, the SA node sets the pace for the heartbeat and is, therefore, called the **pacemaker**.

Intercalated discs bind all cardiac muscle fibers while stimulatory impulses from the SA node are conducted via **gap junctions** to the atrial musculature, causing rapid spread of stimuli throughout the entire cardiac muscle and their contraction. Impulses from the SA node travel through the heart musculature via **internodal pathways** to stimulate the AV node in the interatrial septum. From the AV node, the impulses spread along specialized conducting cardiac fibers, called the **AV bundle (of His)**, located in the interventricular septum (between ventricles). The AV bundle then divides into right and left bundle branches to stimulate both ventricles to contract. Approximately halfway down the interventricular septum, the AV bundle branches become the **Purkinje fibers**, which branch further to transmit the stimulation throughout the entire ventricular musculature.

The pacemaker activities of the heart are influenced by the axons from the **autonomic nervous system** (**ANS**) and by **hormones**. Axons from both the parasympathetic division and the sympathetic division innervate the heart and form a wide plexus at its base. Although these axons innervate the heart myocardium, they do not affect the initiation of rhythmic activity of the nodes. Instead, they affect the heart rate. Stimulation by the sympathetic nerves accelerates the heart rate, whereas stimulation by the parasympathetic nerves produces the opposite effect and decreases the heart rate.

Purkinje Fibers

Purkinje fibers are thicker and larger than cardiac muscle fibers and contain a greater amount of **glycogen** and fewer contractile filaments. Purkinje fibers are part of the conduction system of the heart. These fibers are located beneath the **endocardium** on either side of the interventricular septum and are recognized as separate tracts. Because Purkinje fibers branch throughout the myocardium, they deliver continuous waves of stimulation from the atrial nodes (SA and AV) to the rest of the heart musculature via the **gap junctions**. This stimulation produces ventricular contractions (systole) and the ejection of blood from both ventricular chambers.

Atrial Natriuretic Hormone

Certain cardiac muscle fibers in the atria exhibit dense granules in their cytoplasm. These granules contain **atrial natriuretic hormone** (**ANH**) that is released in response to atrial distention or stretching. The main function of this factor is to decrease blood pressure by regulating blood volume. The ANH inhibits the release of **renin** by kidney cells and **aldosterone** from the adrenal gland cortex that induce the kidneys to excrete more sodium ions and water (diuresis). As a result, the blood volume and blood pressure are reduced decreasing the distention of the atrial wall and further release of the ANH.

Chapter 10 Summary

Circulatory System

CARDIOVASCULAR SYSTEM

- Consists of heart, major arteries, arterioles, capillaries, venules, and veins
- Two major circuits are systemic circulation and pulmonary circulation
- Systemic circulation takes blood to all systems and back to the heart
- Pulmonary circulation takes blood to the lungs for gaseous exchange and back to the heart

TYPES OF ARTERIES

Elastic Arteries

- Are the largest vessels and include aorta, pulmonary trunk, and their major branches
- Wall primarily composed of elastic connective tissue mixed with smooth muscle fibers
- Exhibit resilience and flexibility; walls greatly expand during systole (heart contraction)
- During diastole (heart relaxation), walls recoil and force blood forward

Muscular Arteries, Arterioles, and Capillaries

- Most numerous vessels with their walls lined with smooth muscle fibers
- Control of blood flow through vasoconstriction or vasodilation of lumina
- Smooth muscles in arterial walls controlled by axons from the ANS
- Arterioles are the small blood vessels with one to five layers of smooth muscle
- Terminal arterioles deliver blood to the smallest blood vessels, the capillaries
- Capillaries are the sites of metabolic exchanges between blood and tissues
- Capillaries connect arterioles with venules

STRUCTURAL PLAN OF ARTERIES

- Wall consists of three layers: inner tunica intima, middle tunica media, and outer tunica adventitia
- Tunica intima consists of endothelium and subendothelial connective tissue
- Tunica media is composed mainly of smooth muscle fibers with some elastic fibers
- In elastic and muscular arteries, smooth muscles produce elastic fibers and some collagen
- Tunica adventitia contains primarily collagen type I and elastic fibers
- Internal elastic lamina (IEL) separates tunica intima from tunica media
- Fenestrations in IEL allow diffusion of nutrients to deeper cells
- External elastic lamina (EEL) separates tunica media from tunica adventitia

STRUCTURAL PLAN OF VEINS

- Capillaries unite to form larger vessels called venules and postcapillary venules
- Thinner walls, larger diameters, and more structural variation than arteries
- Blood under low pressure; valves are present to prevent backflow of blood in extremities
- Blood flow toward heart is due to muscular contractions around veins and valves
- Valves absent in veins of the viscera, the CNS, and the inferior and superior venae cavae
- Wall consists of three layers: tunica intima, tunica media, and tunica adventitia
- Tunica intima consists of endothelium and subendothelial connective tissue
- Tunica media is thin, and smooth muscle intermixes with connective tissue fibers
- Tunica adventitia is the thickest layer, with longitudinal smooth muscle fibers

VASA VASORUM

- Found in the thicker walls of large arteries and veins that do not allow diffusion from lumina
- Small adjacent arterial blood vessels supply tunica media and tunica adventitia
- More extensive in the walls of veins than arteries because of poor oxygen content of veins

TYPES OF CAPILLARIES

- Average diameter is about the size of a RBC (about 8 μm)
- Consist of thin endothelium, basal lamina, and pericytes

- Continuous capillaries are most common; endothelium forms solid lining
- Continuous capillaries found in most organs
- Fenestrated capillaries contain pores or fenestrations in endothelium
- Fenestrated capillaries found in endocrine glands, small intestine, and kidney glomeruli
- Sinusoidal capillaries exhibit wide diameters with wide gaps between endothelial cells
- Basement membrane incomplete or absent in sinusoidal capillaries
- Sinusoidal capillaries found in the liver, spleen, and bone marrow

LYMPHATIC VASCULAR SYSTEM

- Associated with the circulatory system and drains extracellular fluid lymph from tissues
- Lymphatic capillaries start as blind dilations and form the lymph drainage system
- Lymph eventually returned to the circulatory system after filtering lymph in lymph nodes
- Vessels are very thin and show greater permeability than capillaries
- Lymph vessels contain valves, and lymph movement is slow
- Lymph movement is assisted by muscular contractions, arterial pulsations, and intrinsic muscular contraction in vessel walls
- Lymph flows through lymph nodes and is exposed to macrophages
- Lymph contains lymphocytes, fatty acids, and immunoglobulins (antibodies)
- Integral component of immune system of the body

ENDOTHELIUM

- Forms a semipermeable barrier between blood and interstitial tissue
- Pinocytotic vesicles in endothelium allow bidirectional movement of molecules
- Provides smooth surface for blood flow without damage to the platelets
- Lined by glycocalyx and secretes prostacyclin to prevent platelet adhesion and blood clotting
- Produces nitrous oxide, which induces vasodilation
- Produces endothelin proteins that counteract nitrous oxide and cause vasoconstriction

- Converts angiotensin I to angiotensin II, a vasoconstrictor that raises blood pressure
- Inactivates certain compounds, degrades lipoproteins, and produces growth factors
- Contains electron-dense Weibel-Palade bodies that store von Willebrand factor
- Releases von Willebrand factor during damage to increase platelet adhesion and blood clotting

HEART WALL: ENDOCARDIUM, MYOCARDIUM, AND EPICARDIUM

Pacemaker

- Impulse conduction by specialized cardiac cells located in SA and AV nodes
- SA and AV nodes located in the wall of the right atrium
- SA node sets the pace for the heart and is the pacemaker of the heart
- Impulse from SA node conducted via gap junctions to all heart musculature
- AV bundles located on right and left sides of the interventricular septum
- AV bundles become Purkinje fibers
- Pacemaker activities influenced by autonomic nervous system (ANS) and hormones
- Sympathetic axons stimulate heart rate; parasympathetic nerves decrease heart rate

Purkinje Fibers

- Larger than cardiac fibers with more glycogen and lighter staining
- Part of the conduction system of the heart
- Located beneath the endocardium on either side of the interventricular septum
- Branch throughout the myocardium and deliver stimuli via gap junctions to the rest of the heart

Atrial Natriuretic Hormone (ANH)

- Certain atrial cells contain granules with ANH
- Released when atrial wall is stretched
- Decreases blood pressure by inhibiting renin and aldosterone release
- Influences kidneys to lose more sodium and water to decrease blood volume and pressure

Chapter 10 Review Questions

QUESTIONS

In the following multiple-choice questions, choose the letter corresponding to the one best answer.

1. **Which part of the heart conduction system branches and stimulates the contraction of ventricular musculature?**

   A. Sinoatrial node
   B. Purkinje fibers
   C. Internodal pathway
   D. Atrioventricular bundle
   E. Atrioventricular node

2. **Purkinje fibers are recognized histologically by:**

   A. containing more contractile filaments.
   B. their location deep in the heart musculature.
   C. being larger and thicker than the cardiac cells.
   D. having little glycogen in their cytoplasm.
   E. containing granules in their cytoplasm.

3. **What causes the release of atrial natriuretic hormone (ANH)?**

   A. Decreased blood volume in the atrium
   B. Decreased heart rate
   C. Decreased blood pressure
   D. Stretching or distention of the atrium
   E. Stretching or distention of the ventricle

4. **The main function of atrial natriuretic hormone (ANH) is to:**

   A. increase blood flow into the atrium.
   B. increase blood pressure.
   C. reduce atrial distention.
   D. reduce ventricular distention.
   E. decrease pacemaker activity.

5. **The sinoatrial (SA) and atrioventricular (AV) nodes are composed of:**

   A. motor or efferent neurons.
   B. sensory or afferent neurons.
   C. the axon terminals of the autonomic nervous system.
   D. unipolar ganglion cells.
   E. modified cardiac muscle fibers.

ANSWERS

1. **Correct Answer: D.** Atrioventricular bundle. This bundle divides into right and left bundle branches to stimulate both ventricles to contract.

2. **Correct Answer: D.** Having little glycogen in their cytoplasm. Purkinje fibers also have fewer contractile elements.

3. **Correct Answer: D.** Stretching or distention of the atrium. This action causes the release of ANH that results in decreased blood pressure and blood volume, reducing the distention of atrial wall.

4. **Correct Answer: C.** The main function of ANH is to reduce atrial distention.

5. **Correct Answer: E.** The SA and AV nodes are composed of modified cardiac muscle fibers.

ADDITIONAL HISTOLOGIC IMAGES

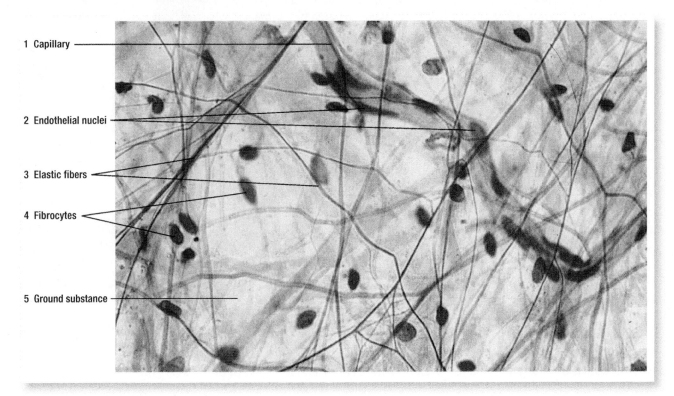

1 Capillary

2 Endothelial nuclei

3 Elastic fibers

4 Fibrocytes

5 Ground substance

FIGURE 10.16 ■ Mesentery spread with a capillary, endothelial nuclei, and the surrounding connective tissue cells and fibers. Stain: hematoxylin and eosin. ×165.

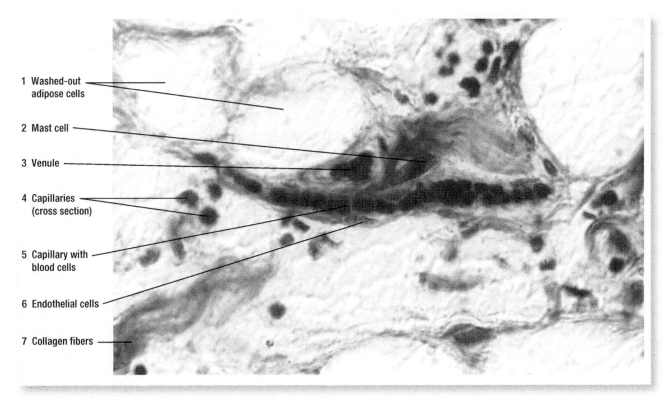

1 Washed-out adipose cells

2 Mast cell

3 Venule

4 Capillaries (cross section)

5 Capillary with blood cells

6 Endothelial cells

7 Collagen fibers

FIGURE 10.17 ■ A section of a mesentery illustrating a capillary with red blood cells, a mast cell, and the surrounding washed-out outlines of adipose cells. Stain: Mallory-Azan. ×205.

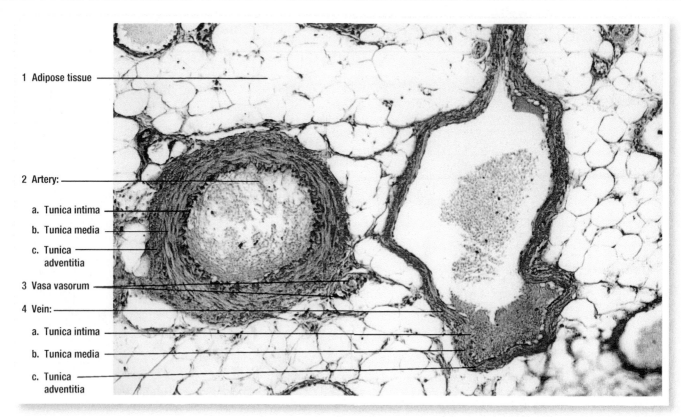

1 Adipose tissue

2 Artery:

   a. Tunica intima

   b. Tunica media

   c. Tunica adventitia

3 Vasa vasorum

4 Vein:

   a. Tunica intima

   b. Tunica media

   c. Tunica adventitia

FIGURE 10.18 ■ Structural comparison between an artery and a vein in the mesentery. Stain: hematoxylin and eosin. ×30.

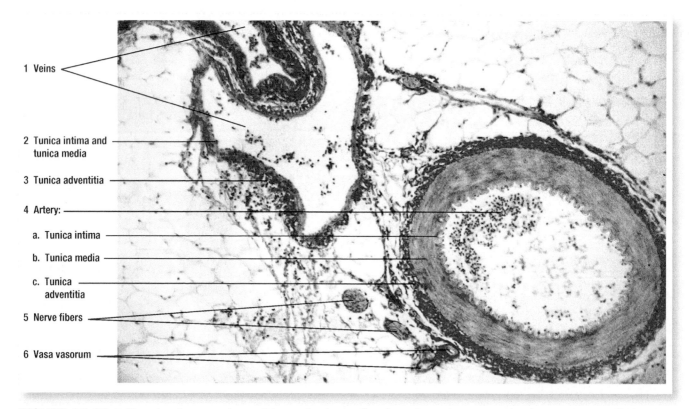

1 Veins

2 Tunica intima and tunica media

3 Tunica adventitia

4 Artery:

   a. Tunica intima

   b. Tunica media

   c. Tunica adventitia

5 Nerve fibers

6 Vasa vasorum

FIGURE 10.19 ■ Structural comparison of layers in the walls of a vein and an artery in the mesentery. Stain: Mallory-Azan. ×50.

1 Loose connective
tissue with
fibrocytes

2 Vein

3 Tunica adventitia

4 Tunica intima

5 Tunica media

6 Valves in vein

7 Nerve fiber

8 Artery

9 Tunica intima

10 Tunica media

11 Tunica adventitia

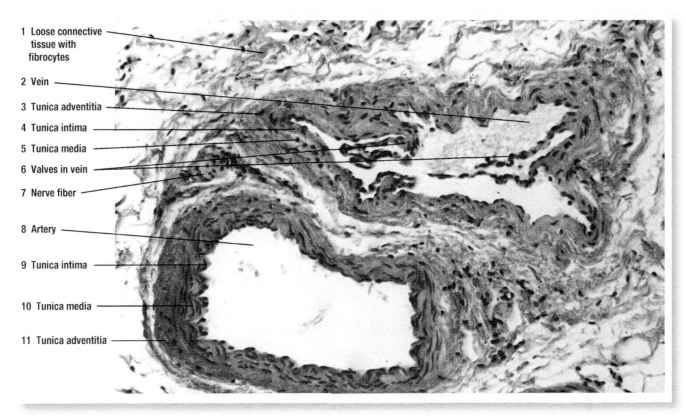

FIGURE 10.20 ■ Comparison of a small artery and a vein with valves surrounded by loose connective tissue with fibrocytes. Stain: hematoxylin and eosin. ×50.

1 Adipose cells

2 Vasa vasorum

3 Artery

4 Endothelial cells

5 Internal elastic
lamina and
tunica intima

6 Tunica media

7 Tunica adventitia

8 Vein

9 Tunica intima

10 Tunica media

11 Tunica adventitia

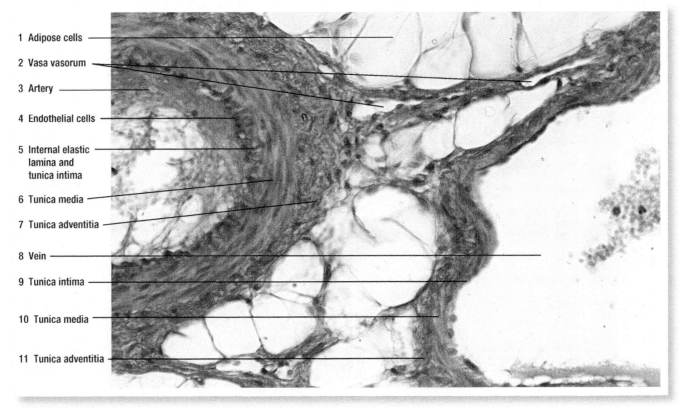

FIGURE 10.21 ■ Higher magnification of an artery and a vein walls with surrounding adipose cells. Stain: hematoxylin and eosin. ×80.

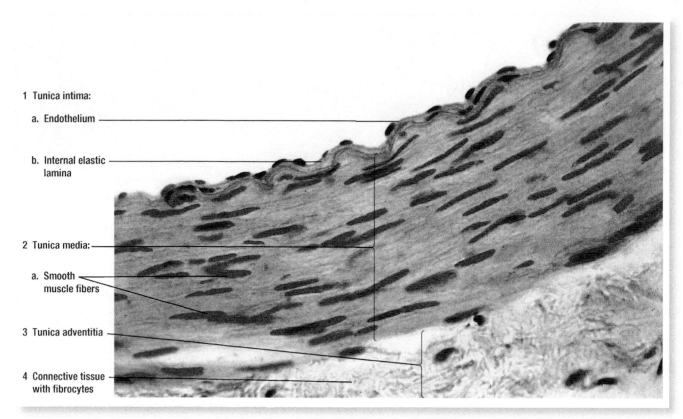

1 Tunica intima:

  a. Endothelium

  b. Internal elastic lamina

2 Tunica media:

  a. Smooth muscle fibers

3 Tunica adventitia

4 Connective tissue with fibrocytes

FIGURE 10.22 ■ Section of an arterial wall illustrating the different layers. Stain: hematoxylin and eosin. ×205.

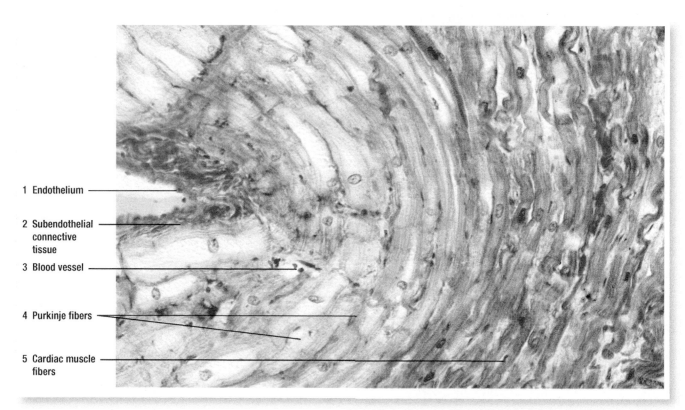

1 Endothelium

2 Subendothelial connective tissue

3 Blood vessel

4 Purkinje fibers

5 Cardiac muscle fibers

FIGURE 10.23 ■ A section of the heart wall near a ventricle illustrating different structures. Stain: Mallory-Azan. ×205.

Immune System

The **immune system** protects the organism against invading pathogens or antigens (bacteria, parasites, and viruses). The immune response occurs as soon as the pathogens enter the organism. As a result, the cells, tissues, and organs of the immune system have wide distribution in the organism so that the immunologic response can quickly counteract the effects of invading foreign substances.

The lymphoid system includes all cells, tissues, and organs that contain aggregates (accumulations) of immune cells called **lymphocytes**. Cells of the immune system, especially lymphocytes, are distributed throughout the body as single cells; as isolated accumulations of cells; as distinct nonencapsulated lymphatic nodules in the loose connective tissue of the **digestive, respiratory**, and **reproductive systems**; or as encapsulated individual lymphoid organs (Fig. 11.1). Lymphoid organs can be divided into two major categories. The **primary lymphoid organs** include the **bone marrow** and the **thymus**. In these organs, the cells of immune system, the **lymphocytes**, are formed, differentiate, and become mature. The **secondary lymphoid organs** include the **lymph nodes, spleen, tonsils**, and the **mucosa-associated lymphoid tissue (MALT)** such as the diffuse lymphoid tissue in the mucosa of the **digestive tract** (gut-associated lymphoid tissue [GALT]), **respiratory tract** (bronchial-associated lymphoid tissue [BALT]), and **Peyer patches**. In the secondary lymphoid organs, most of the lymphocytes encounter foreign antigens, become activated, and produce an immune response to the invading pathogens.

IMMUNE SYSTEM ORGANS: LYMPH NODES, SPLEEN, AND THYMUS

The **lymph nodes** are widely distributed and are primarily found along the paths of lymphatic vessels that are prominent in inguinal and axillary regions. A connective tissue **capsule** surrounds the lymph node and sends its **trabeculae** into its interior. The lymph node exhibits an outer **cortex** and an inner **medulla**. A network of reticular fibers and spherical, nonencapsulated aggregations of lymphocytes called **lymphoid nodules** characterize the cortex, some of which exhibit lighter-staining central areas called **germinal centers**. The medulla consists of **medullary cords** and **medullary sinuses**. Medullary cords are networks of reticular fibers filled with plasma cells, macrophages, and lymphocytes separated by capillary-like channels called medullary sinuses (Fig. 11.2).

The lymph enters the lymph node via **afferent lymphatic vessels** in the capsule on the convex surface. Lymph is then filtered as it flows through the cortex and medullary sinuses to exit the lymph node on the opposite side via the **efferent lymphatic vessels**.

The **spleen** is a large lymphoid organ with a rich blood supply. A connective tissue capsule surrounds the spleen and divides its interior into incomplete compartments called the **splenic pulp**, which consists of white pulp and red pulp. They are so named because of their color when the raw spleen is cut open. **White pulp** consists of dark-staining lymphoid aggregations or **lymphatic nodules** that surround a blood vessel called the **central artery**. This is a misnomer because the central artery is located in an eccentric position in the white pulp. White pulp is located within the blood-rich red pulp. The arterial system ends in **red pulp**, which consists of **splenic cords** and **splenic (blood) sinusoids**. The splenic cords contain networks of reticular fibers with numerous macrophages, lymphocytes, plasma cells, and different blood cells. In contrast, splenic sinuses are interconnected blood channels that drain splenic blood into larger sinuses that leave the spleen via the splenic vein (Fig. 11.3).

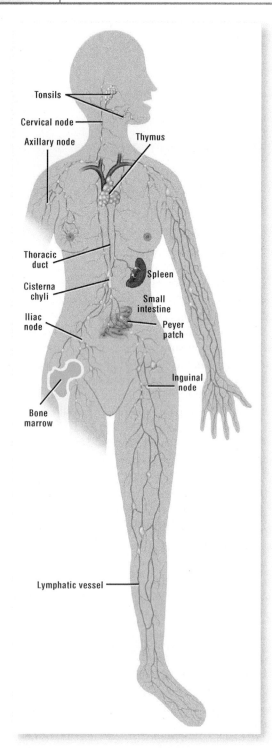

FIGURE 11.1 ■ Location and distribution of the lymphoid organs and lymphatic channels in the body.

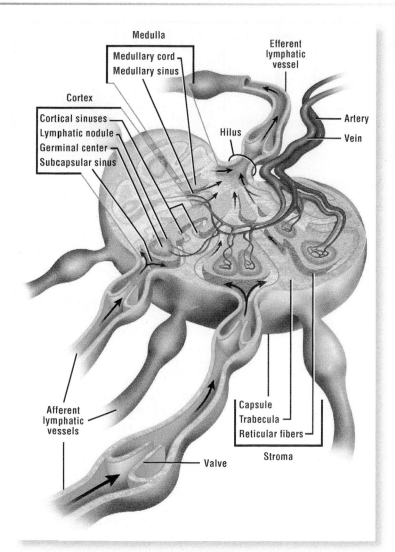

FIGURE 11.2 ■ Internal contents of a lymph node.

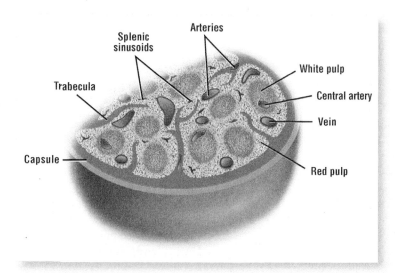

FIGURE 11.3 ■ Internal contents of the spleen.

The **thymus gland** is a soft, lobulated lymphoepithelial organ located in the upper anterior mediastinum and lower part of the neck. The gland is most active during childhood, after which it undergoes slow involution, and, in adults, the organ is filled with adipose tissue. The thymus gland is surrounded by a connective tissue capsule, inferior to the dark-staining **cortex** with a network of interconnecting spaces. These spaces become colonized by **immature lymphocytes** that migrate here from hematopoietic tissues in the developing individual to undergo maturation and differentiation. The epithelial cells of the thymus gland provide structural support for the lymphocyte population. In the lighter-staining **medulla**, the epithelial cells form a coarser framework that contains fewer lymphocytes and whorls of epithelial cells that combine to form **thymic (Hassall) corpuscles**.

IMMUNE SYSTEM CELLS

The cells that carry out immune responses are lymphocytes produced in the primary lymphoid organs and supporting cells. Three major types of lymphocytes are recognized. These are **T lymphocytes (T cells)**, **B lymphocytes (B cells)**, and **natural killer (NK) cells**. Supporting or accessory cells are those that interact with lymphocytes and are antigen-presenting cells (APCs) to lymphocytes for activation and immune response. These include cells from the mononuclear phagocyte system, the tissue **macrophages,** and **dendritic cells** such as **Langerhans** cells in the epidermis of the skin.

All components of the lymphoid system are an essential part of the **immune system**. Different types of lymphocytes are found in blood, lymph, lymphoid tissues, and lymphoid organs. Like all blood cells, lymphocytes originate from precursor **hematopoietic stem cells** in the **bone marrow** and then enter the bloodstream. Morphologically, all lymphocytes appear similar, but, functionally, they are different. Lymphocytes can be distinguished on the basis of where they differentiate, reside, and mature into immunocompetent cells and on the types of surface receptors or markers present on their cell membranes. These criteria allow the lymphocytes to be distinguished into two functionally distinct types, the B lymphocytes (B cells) and subcategories of T lymphocytes (T cells).

T cells originate from lymphocytes that were carried from the bone marrow to the **thymus gland** where they mature, differentiate, and acquire surface receptors and **immunocompetence** before migrating to peripheral lymphoid tissues and organs. The thymus gland produces mature T cells early in life, after which the T cells are distributed throughout the body via the blood and populate lymph nodes, the spleen, and lymphoid aggregates or nodules in connective tissue of the mucosa in the digestive tract (GALT), respiratory tract (BALT), and Peyer patches. Here, the T cells carry out immune responses when stimulated. On encountering an antigen, T cells destroy the antigen either by cytotoxic action or by activating B cells. There are four main subtypes of differentiated T cells: **helper T cells**, **cytotoxic T cells**, **regulatory (suppressor) T cells**, and **memory T cells**.

On encountering an antigen, **helper T cells** assist other lymphocytes by secreting immune chemicals called **cytokines** or **interleukins**. Cytokines are protein hormones that stimulate the proliferation, secretion, differentiation, and maturation of B cells into **plasma cells**, which then produce **antibodies**, or **immunoglobulins**. The immunoglobulins then bind to antigens either to neutralize them or to cause their elimination by macrophage actions. The helper T cells also activate macrophages to become phagocytic and activate cytotoxic T cells.

Cytotoxic T cells recognize antigenically different cells, such as virus-infected cells, foreign cells, or malignant tumor cells, and destroy them. These lymphocytes are activated in the presence of APCs containing antigens that react with their receptors. The cytotoxic T cells then release lysosomes with lytic granules that contain pore-forming protein called **perforin** that creates pores in the membrane of the targeted cell causing **apoptosis**, or cell death.

Regulatory (suppressor) T cells may regulate (moderate or inhibit) specific functions of helper T cells and cytotoxic T cells and, thus, can functionally suppress immune response by influencing the activities of other cells in the immune system.

Memory T cells are the long-living progeny of T cells. They respond rapidly to the same antigens in the body and stimulate the immediate production of cytotoxic T cells. Memory T cells are the counterparts of memory B cells. Memory T cells activate the immune system and directly attack pathogens, whereas B cells produce antibodies that disable or kill the pathogens.

B cells mature and become immunocompetent in bone marrow. After maturation, blood carries B cells to such nonthymic lymphoid organs or tissues as the lymph nodes, spleen, and connective tissue. B cells recognize particular type of antigen due to **antigen receptor complex** on the surface of their cell membrane. Immunocompetent B cells become activated when a specific antigen is encountered that binds to the surface antigen receptor complex of the B cell. The response of B cells to antigens, however, is more intense when APCs, such as **helper T cells**, present the antigens to the B cells. Helper T cells secrete a cytokine (**interleukin 2**) that induces proliferation and differentiation of antigen-activated B cells. The activated B cells enlarge, divide, proliferate, and differentiate into **plasma cells** that secrete **antibodies** specific to the antigen that triggered plasma cell formation. Antibodies react with the antigens and initiate a process that destroys the foreign substance that activated the immune response. The dependence of B cells on helper T cells increases the antibody secretion and produces a strong immune response, such as activation of phagocytes and production of **memory B cells**. Other activated B cells do not become plasma cells but persist in lymphoid organs as memory B cells. These memory cells produce a more rapid and longer-lasting immunologic response should the same antigen reappear.

NK cells develop from the same precursor cells as B and T cells and are the third type of lymphocytes that are genetically programmed to recognize and destroy altered cells. NK cells attack virally infected cells and cancer cells and destroy them in a fashion similar to cytotoxic T cells by releasing perforins and inducing apoptosis (cell death).

In addition to T, B, and NK cells and macrophages, **APCs** are important in immune responses, and they are found in most tissues. These cells phagocytose and process antigens and then present the antigen to T cells, inducing their activation. Most APCs belong to the mononuclear phagocytic system. Included in this group are the connective tissue **macrophages**, **perisinusoidal macrophages** in the liver (Kupffer cells), **Langerhans cells** (also called **dendritic** cells in the skin), and macrophages within the lymphoid organs.

TYPES OF IMMUNE RESPONSES

The mammalian immune system can initiate different types of immune responses to foreign matter. The presence of foreign cells or antigens in the organism stimulates a complex series of immune reactions. The immune responses to invading foreign organisms can be divided into two main types, the innate immune response and the adaptive immune response.

The **innate immune response** is the first line of defense that limits the spread of infection. Its response to antigen invasion involves phagocytic functions that are rapid and involve neutrophils, mast cells, macrophages, dendritic cells, and NK cells. Although the response of the innate immune system is fast, it is **nonspecific** and does not produce memory cells. Stimulation of macrophages and dendritic cells in an innate response produces cytokines (interleukins) that start the inflammatory response.

The **adaptive immune response** targets specific invading foreign organisms and provides **specific**, or adaptive, defenses. This response is slower than the innate immune response, but it produces and retains numerous memory cells that can respond to the second encounter with the particular antigen that is faster, stronger, and longer lasting. Production of long-lived memory cells is the main feature of adaptive immunity. Adoptive immunity also involves two types of specific responses. These are the **humoral immune response** and the **cell-mediated immune response**. These responses produce antibodies that bind to the antigens or stimulate cells that destroy foreign matter. Both the B cells and T cells respond to antigens by different means. **Humoral immunity** is an antibody-mediated immunity because the antibodies are secreted to neutralize pathogens outside the cells. Exposure of **B cells** to an antigen induces proliferation and transformation of some B cells into **plasma cells**. These, in turn, secrete specific **antibodies** into blood and lymph that bind to, inactivate, and destroy the foreign substance or antigens. The activation and proliferation of B cells against antigens require the cooperation of helper T cells that respond to the same antigen and the production of cytokines. The presence of the B cells, plasma cells, and production of antibodies in the blood and lymph is the basis of the humoral immune response.

Cell-mediated immunity involves the activation of phagocytes, **antigen-specific cytotoxic T cells**, and the release of various cytokines in response to antigens. The T cells proliferate and secrete cytokines to stimulate or activate other T cells, B cells, and other cytotoxic T cells. T-cell receptors are bound to the T cells, and the cells themselves bind with antigens. On activation and binding to target cells, cytotoxic T cells destroy foreign cells by inducing **apoptosis**, or programmed cell death, by releasing lytic granules containing perforin. Perforin creates pores in the plasma membrane and kills the cells. T cells may also attack indirectly by activating B cells and increasing their antibody production or stimulating the **macrophages**. T cells provide specific immune protection without secreting antibodies; instead, they have surface receptors for antigens.

thePoint® Supplemental micrographic images are available at **www.thePoint.com/Eroschenko13e** under Lymphoid System.

FIGURE 11.4 | Lymph Node (Panoramic View)

The lymph node consists of lymphocyte aggregations intermixed with dilated lymphatic sinuses that contain lymph and are supported by a framework of fine reticular fibers. A lymph node cut in half shows the outer dark-staining **cortex (4)** and the inner light-staining **medulla (10)**. The lymph node is surrounded by a **pericapsular adipose tissue (1)** with numerous blood vessels (9). A dense connective tissue **capsule (2)** surrounds the lymph node. From the capsule (2), **connective tissue trabeculae (6)** extend into the node, initially between the lymphatic nodules and then throughout the medulla (10). The trabecular connective tissue (6) also exhibits the major **blood vessels (5, 8)**.

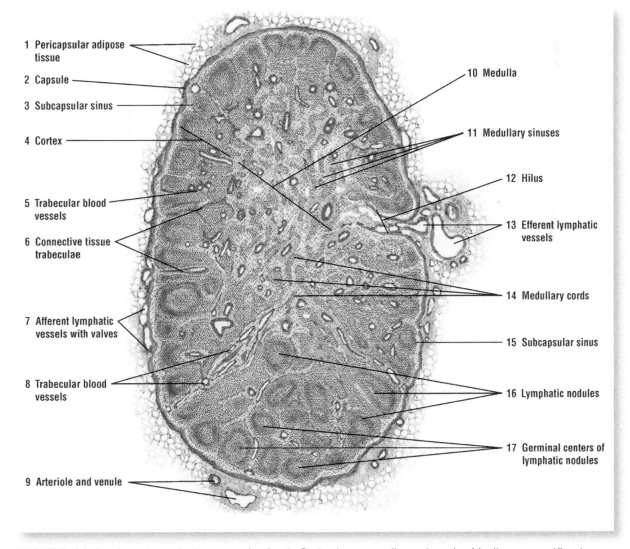

1 Pericapsular adipose tissue

2 Capsule

3 Subcapsular sinus

4 Cortex

5 Trabecular blood vessels

6 Connective tissue trabeculae

7 Afferent lymphatic vessels with valves

8 Trabecular blood vessels

9 Arteriole and venule

10 Medulla

11 Medullary sinuses

12 Hilus

13 Efferent lymphatic vessels

14 Medullary cords

15 Subcapsular sinus

16 Lymphatic nodules

17 Germinal centers of lymphatic nodules

FIGURE 11.4 ■ Lymph node (panoramic view). Stain: hematoxylin and eosin. Medium magnification.

Afferent lymphatic vessels with valves (7) course in the connective tissue capsule (2) of the lymph node and, at intervals, penetrate the capsule to enter a narrow **subcapsular sinus** (3, 15). From here, the sinuses (cortical sinuses) extend along the trabeculae (6) into the **medullary sinuses** (11).

The lymph node cortex (4) contains numerous lymphocyte aggregations called **lymphatic nodules** (16). Some nodules (16) exhibit a lighter-stained area in their center. These are the **germinal centers** (17) of the lymphatic nodules (16) and represent the sites of active lymphocyte proliferation.

In the medulla (10) of the lymph node, the lymphocytes are arranged as irregular cords of lymphatic tissue called **medullary cords** (14) that contain macrophages, plasma cells, and small lymphocytes. The dilated medullary sinuses (11) drain the lymph from the cortical region of the lymph node and course between the medullary cords (14) toward the concavity of the lymph node, the **hilus** (12).

Nerves, blood vessels, and veins that supply and drain the lymph node are located in the **hilus** (12). **Efferent lymphatic vessels** (13) drain the lymph from the medullary sinuses (11) and exit the lymph node in the hilus (12).

FIGURE 11.5 | Lymph Node Capsule, Cortex, and Medulla (Sectional View)

A small section of a cortical region of the lymph node is illustrated at a higher magnification.

A layer of **connective tissue** (1) with a **venule** and an **arteriole** (11) surrounds the lymph node **capsule** (3). In the connective tissue (1) is an afferent **lymphatic vessel** (2) lined with endothelium and exhibiting a **valve** (2). Arising from the inner surface of the capsule (3), the connective tissue **trabeculae** with numerous blood vessels (5, 14, 16) extend through the cortex and medulla. The lymph node cortex is separated from the connective tissue capsule (3) by the **subcapsular (marginal) sinus** (4, 12). The cortex consists of B cell–rich **lymphatic nodules** (13) situated

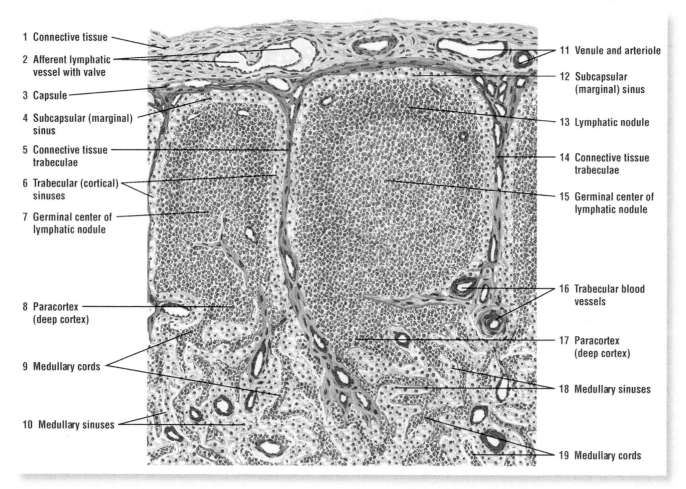

1 Connective tissue
2 Afferent lymphatic vessel with valve
3 Capsule
4 Subcapsular (marginal) sinus
5 Connective tissue trabeculae
6 Trabecular (cortical) sinuses
7 Germinal center of lymphatic nodule
8 Paracortex (deep cortex)
9 Medullary cords
10 Medullary sinuses

11 Venule and arteriole
12 Subcapsular (marginal) sinus
13 Lymphatic nodule
14 Connective tissue trabeculae
15 Germinal center of lymphatic nodule
16 Trabecular blood vessels
17 Paracortex (deep cortex)
18 Medullary sinuses
19 Medullary cords

FIGURE 11.5 ■ Lymph node: capsule, cortex, and medulla (sectional view). Stain: hematoxylin and eosin. Medium magnification.

adjacent to each other but separated by internodular connective tissue trabeculae (5, 14) and **trabecular (cortical) sinuses** (6). In this illustration, two lymphatic nodules (13) are illustrated. Some lymphatic nodules exhibit a central, light-staining **germinal center** (7, 15) surrounded by a denser-staining peripheral portion (13). In the germinal centers (7, 15), the cells are loosely aggregated with the developing lymphocytes showing larger and lighter-staining nuclei with more cytoplasm.

The deeper portion of the lymph node cortex is the **paracortex** (8, 17), a thymus-dependent zone primarily occupied by T cells. This area represents the transition from the lymphatic nodules (7, 13) to the **medullary cords** (9, 19) of the lymph node medulla. The medulla consists of anastomosing cords of lymphatic tissue, the medullary cords (9, 19), interspersed with **medullary sinuses** (10, 18) that drain the lymph from the node into the efferent lymphatic vessels in the hilus (see Fig. 11.2).

Fine reticular connective tissue provides support for the lymph node and forms the core of the lymphatic nodules (13) in the cortex, the medullary cords (9, 19), and all medullary sinuses (10, 18) in the medulla. Because few lymphocytes are seen in the medullary sinuses (10, 18), it is possible to distinguish the reticular framework in the lymphatic nodules (13) and the medullary cords (9, 19). The lymphocytes are so abundant that the fine reticulum is obscured, unless specifically stained, as shown in Figure 11.9. Most of the lymphocytes are small with large, deep-staining nuclei with condensed chromatin and either a small amount of cytoplasm or none at all.

FUNCTIONAL CORRELATIONS 11.1 ■ Lymph Nodes

Lymph nodes are important components of the defense mechanism. They have a strategic location along the paths of **lymphatic vessels** and are most prominent in the **inguinal** and **axillary regions**. Their major functions are **lymph filtration** and the **phagocytosis** of bacteria or foreign substances from the filtered lymph, preventing them from reaching the general circulation. Trapped within the reticular fiber network of each lymph node are fixed or free macrophages that destroy foreign substances. Thus, as lymph is filtered, the nodes localize and prevent the spread of infection into the general circulation and other organs.

Lymph nodes also produce, store, and activate **B cells** and **T cells**. Here the lymphocytes proliferate, and the B cells can transform into plasma cells. As a result, lymph that leaves the lymph nodes via the efferent vessels may contain antibodies that can be distributed to the entire body. In the lymph node, the B cells congregate in the **lymphatic nodules** in the outer cortex, whereas the T cells concentrate below the lymphatic nodules in the deep **cortical** or **paracortical (paracortex) regions**. Lymph nodes are also the sites of **antigenic recognition** and **antigenic activation** of B cells, giving rise to **plasma cells** and **memory B cells**. When B cells are activated by the APCs, these lymphocytes proliferate in the central region of the lymphatic nodule and form lighter-staining germinal centers surrounded by darker-staining lymphocytes. Lymphatic nodules that lack the light-staining germinal centers and only exhibit the dense aggregations of lymphocytes are considered as inactive **primary lymphatic nodules**. After **antigenic stimulation**, primary lymphatic nodules become **secondary**

lymphatic nodules with a lighter-staining **germinal centers** surrounded by dense staining lymphocytes. Germinal centers become the major sites for various B-cell proliferation and differentiation, whereas the T cells undergo the same process in the paracortex of the lymph node beneath and between the lymphatic nodules. Continuous lymphocyte circulation between blood and lymph takes place in the lymph nodes, tonsils, Peyer patches, and spleen. B cells and T cells enter the lymph nodes through the incoming arteries. Lymph formed in the body eventually reaches the blood, and lymphocytes that leave the lymph nodes via the efferent lymph vessels also return to the bloodstream. The arteries supplying lymph nodes branch into capillaries in the cortex and paracortex, which provide an entryway for lymphocytes into the lymph nodes. Most lymphocytes enter the lymph nodes through the postcapillary venules in the paracortex. Here, the postcapillary venules are called **high endothelial venules** because they are lined by tall cuboidal or columnar endothelium and are the sites of entry by **diapedesis** of lymphocytes into the lymph node. B cells and T cells recognize special **adhesion molecules** on the high endothelial cells in these venules and leave the bloodstream to enter the lymph node. This pathway allows the movement of lymphocytes to travel in lymph to other lymph nodes, eventually entering the systemic circulation. Movement of B cells and T cells across the high endothelial venules into lymph nodes is considered homing. These specialized venules are also present in Peyer patches in the small intestine, tonsils, appendix, and cortex of the thymus; high endothelial venules are absent from the spleen.

FIGURE 11.6 | Cortex and Medulla of Lymph Node

This low-power photomicrograph illustrates the lymph node cortex and medulla. A loose connective tissue **capsule** (**4**) with blood vessels and **adipose cells** (**7**) covers the lymph node. Inferior to the capsule (4) is the **subcapsular** (**marginal**) **sinus** (**5**), which overlies the darker-staining and peripheral lymph node **cortex** (**3**). The cortex (3) exhibits numerous **lymphatic nodules** (**1, 6**), some with a lighter-staining **germinal center** (**2**).

The central region of the lymph node is the lighter-staining **medulla** (**9**), characterized by the dark-staining **medullary cords** (**12**) and the light-staining lymphatic channels, the **medullary sinuses** (**11**). The medullary sinuses (11) drain the lymph that enters the lymph node through the afferent lymphatic vessels in the capsule (see Fig. 11.5) and converges toward the hilum of the lymph node (see Fig. 11.2) that contains numerous **arteries** (**8**) and veins. The lymph leaves the lymph node via the **efferent lymphatic vessels** with **valves** (**10**) at the hilum.

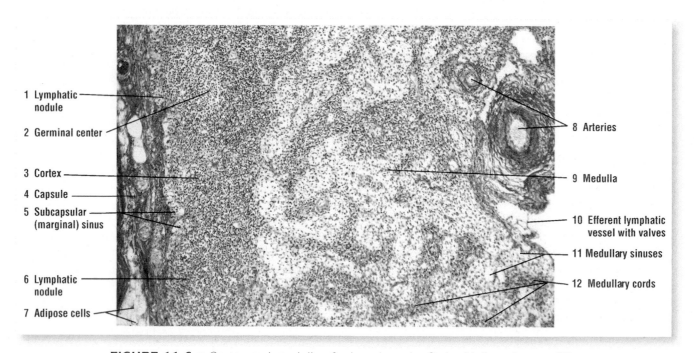

1 Lymphatic nodule
2 Germinal center
3 Cortex
4 Capsule
5 Subcapsular (marginal) sinus
6 Lymphatic nodule
7 Adipose cells

8 Arteries
9 Medulla
10 Efferent lymphatic vessel with valves
11 Medullary sinuses
12 Medullary cords

FIGURE 11.6 ■ Cortex and medulla of a lymph node. Stain: Mallory-Azan. ×25.

FIGURE 11.7 | Lymph Node: Subcortical Sinus and Lymphatic Nodule

This figure illustrates, at a higher magnification and in greater detail, a portion of the lymph node with the connective tissue **capsule** (**3**), **trabecula** (**4**), and **subcapsular sinus** (**1**) that continue on both sides of the trabecula (**4**) as trabecular sinuses (**12**) into the interior of the lymph node.

The reticular connective tissue, the **reticular cells** (**8, 11**), is seen in different regions of the node. Reticular cells (**8, 11**) are visible in the subcapsular sinus (**1**), trabecular sinuses (**12**), and the **germinal center** (**9**) of the **lymphatic nodule** (**14**). Numerous free **macrophages** (**2, 6, 16**) are also seen in the subcapsular sinus (**1**), trabecular sinuses (**12**), and the germinal center (**9**) of the lymphatic nodule (**14**).

A lymphatic nodule with a small section of its **peripheral zone** (**14**) and a germinal center (**9**) with developing lymphocytes are visible. **Endothelial cells** (**5, 13**) line the sinuses (**1, 12**) and form an incomplete cover over the surface of the lymphatic nodules (**14**).

The dense peripheral zone of the lymphatic nodule (**14**) contains an aggregation of **small lymphocytes** (**7**), characterized by dark-staining nuclei, condensed chromatin, and little or no cytoplasm. Small lymphocytes (**7**) are also present in the subcapsular sinus (**1**) and trabecular sinuses (**12**).

The germinal center (**9**) of the lymphatic nodule (**14**) contains **medium-sized lymphocytes** (**10**) characterized by larger, lighter nuclei and more cytoplasm than in the small lymphocytes (**7**). The nuclei of medium-sized lymphocytes (**10**) exhibit variations in the size and density of the chromatin. The largest cells, with less condensed chromatin, are the **lymphoblasts** (**17**) visible in the germinal center (**9**) as large cells with a broad band of cytoplasm and a large vesicular nucleus with one or more nucleoli. **Lymphoblasts** (**15**) produce other lymphoblasts and medium-sized lymphocytes (**10**). With mitotic divisions of lymphoblasts (**15**), the chromatin condenses and the cells decrease in size, producing small lymphocytes (**7**).

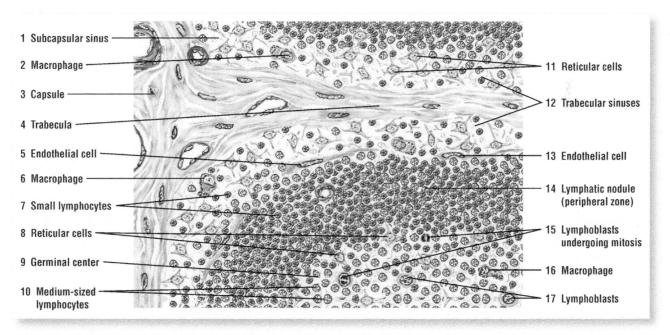

1 Subcapsular sinus
2 Macrophage
3 Capsule
4 Trabecula
5 Endothelial cell
6 Macrophage
7 Small lymphocytes
8 Reticular cells
9 Germinal center
10 Medium-sized lymphocytes

11 Reticular cells
12 Trabecular sinuses
13 Endothelial cell
14 Lymphatic nodule (peripheral zone)
15 Lymphoblasts undergoing mitosis
16 Macrophage
17 Lymphoblasts

FIGURE 11.7 ■ Lymph node: subcortical sinus, trabecular sinus, reticular cells, and lymphatic nodule. Stain: hematoxylin and eosin. High magnification.

FIGURE 11.8 | Lymph Node: High Endothelial Venule in Paracortex (Deep Cortex) of Lymph Node

The paracortex of lymph nodes contains postcapillary venules with an unusual morphology to facilitate the **migration of lymphocytes** from the blood into the lymph node. This image shows a **high endothelial venule** (**2**) lined by tall cuboidal endothelium, instead of the usual squamous endothelium. Several **migrating lymphocytes** (**3**) are seen moving through the venule wall between the high endothelium (**2**) into the **paracortex**. Surrounding the high endothelial venule (**2**) are **lymphocytes** of the paracortex (**5**), a **medullary sinus** (**1**), and a **venule** (**4**) with blood cells.

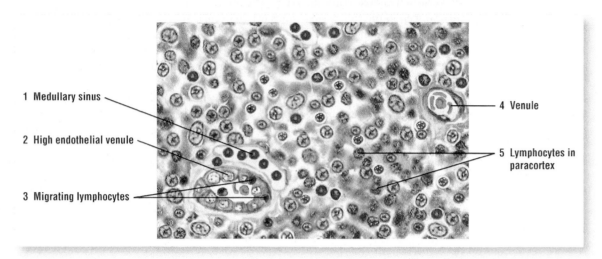

1 Medullary sinus
2 High endothelial venule
3 Migrating lymphocytes
4 Venule
5 Lymphocytes in paracortex

FIGURE 11.8 ■ Lymph node: high endothelial venule in the paracortex (deep cortex) of a lymph node. Stain: hematoxylin and eosin. High magnification.

FIGURE 11.9 | Lymph Node: Subcapsular Sinus, Trabecular Sinus, and Supporting Reticular Fibers

A section of a lymph node, stained with the silver method, illustrates the intricate arrangement of the supporting **reticular fibers** (**6, 9**) of a lymph node. The thicker and denser collagen fibers in the connective tissue **capsule** (**3**) stain pink. Both the capsule and the lymph node are supported by delicate reticular fibers (**6, 9**) that stain black and form a fine meshwork throughout the organ.

The zones illustrated in Figure 11.5 and stained with hematoxylin and eosin are recognizable with the silver stain. A connective tissue **trabecula** (**4**) from the capsule (**3**) penetrates the interior of the lymph node between two **lymphatic nodules** (**8, 12**). Inferior to the capsule (**3**) are **subcapsular (marginal) sinuses** (**1, 7**) that continue on each side of the trabecula (**4**) as **trabecular sinuses** (**2, 5**) into the medulla of the node and eventually to exit through the efferent lymph vessels in the hilum. Also visible are **medullary cords** (**10**) and **medullary sinuses** (**11**).

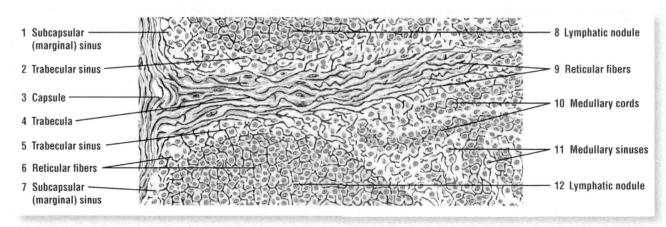

1 Subcapsular (marginal) sinus
2 Trabecular sinus
3 Capsule
4 Trabecula
5 Trabecular sinus
6 Reticular fibers
7 Subcapsular (marginal) sinus
8 Lymphatic nodule
9 Reticular fibers
10 Medullary cords
11 Medullary sinuses
12 Lymphatic nodule

FIGURE 11.9 ■ Lymph node: subcapsular sinus, trabecular sinus, and supporting reticular fibers. Stain: silver stain. Medium magnification.

FIGURE 11.10 | Thymus Gland (Panoramic View)

The thymus gland, located in the upper chest region and anterior to the heart, is a lobulated lymphoid organ enclosed by a connective tissue **capsule** (**1**) from which arise connective tissue **trabeculae** (**2, 10**) that extend into the organ and subdivide the thymus gland into incomplete **lobules** (**8**). Each lobule consists of a dark-staining outer **cortex** (**3, 13**) and a light-staining inner **medulla** (**4, 12**). Because the lobules are incomplete, the medulla shows continuity between the neighboring lobules (**4, 12**). **Blood vessels** (**5, 14**) pass into the thymus gland via the connective tissue capsule (**1**) and the trabeculae (**2, 10**).

The cortex (**3, 13**) of each lobule contains densely packed lymphocytes that do not form lymphatic nodules. In contrast, the medulla (**4, 12**) contains fewer lymphocytes but more epithelial reticular cells. The medulla also contains numerous **thymic (Hassall) corpuscles** (**6, 9**) that characterize the thymus gland.

The histology of the thymus gland varies with age. The thymus gland is highly developed shortly after birth. By puberty, thymus glands begin to involute with gradual regression and degeneration. As a consequence, lymphocyte production declines, and the thymic (Hassall) corpuscles (**6, 9**) become more prominent. In addition, the parenchyma or cellular portion of the gland is gradually replaced by loose **connective tissue** (**10**) and **adipose cells** (**7, 11**). The thymus gland depicted in this illustration exhibits adipose tissue accumulation and signs of involution associated with aging.

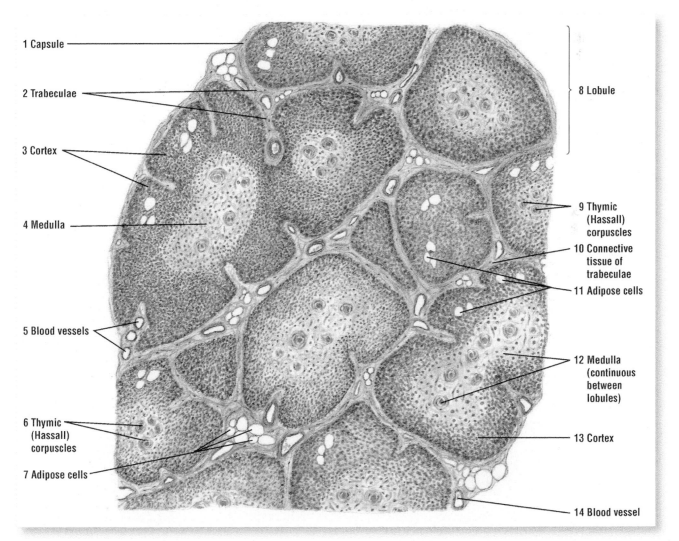

1 Capsule
2 Trabeculae
3 Cortex
4 Medulla
5 Blood vessels
6 Thymic (Hassall) corpuscles
7 Adipose cells
8 Lobule
9 Thymic (Hassall) corpuscles
10 Connective tissue of trabeculae
11 Adipose cells
12 Medulla (continuous between lobules)
13 Cortex
14 Blood vessel

FIGURE 11.10 ■ Thymus gland (panoramic view). Stain: hematoxylin and eosin. Low magnification.

FIGURE 11.11 | Thymus Gland (Sectional View)

A small section of the **cortex** and medulla of a thymus gland lobule is illustrated at a higher magnification. The thymic lymphocytes in the **cortex (1, 5)** form dense aggregations. In contrast, the **medulla (3)** contains only a few lymphocytes but more **epithelial reticular cells (7, 10)**.

The **thymic (Hassall) corpuscles (8, 9)** are oval structures consisting of round or spherical aggregations (whorls) of flattened epithelial cells. The thymic corpuscles also exhibit calcification or **degeneration centers (9)** that stain pink or eosinophilic. **Blood vessels (6)** and **adipose cells (4)** are present in both the thymic lobules and in a connective tissue **trabecula (2)**.

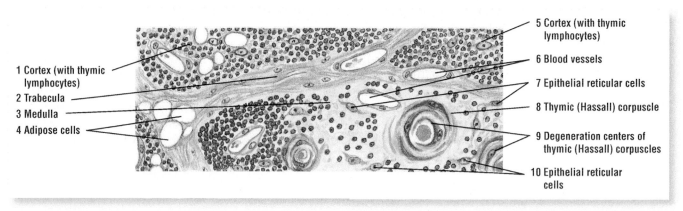

1 Cortex (with thymic lymphocytes)
2 Trabecula
3 Medulla
4 Adipose cells

5 Cortex (with thymic lymphocytes)
6 Blood vessels
7 Epithelial reticular cells
8 Thymic (Hassall) corpuscle
9 Degeneration centers of thymic (Hassall) corpuscles
10 Epithelial reticular cells

FIGURE 11.11 ■ Thymus gland (sectional view). Stain: hematoxylin and eosin. High magnification.

FIGURE 11.12 | Cortex and Medulla of Thymus Gland

A low-magnification photomicrograph shows a portion of the lobule of the thymus gland. A **connective tissue trabecula (1)** subdivides the gland into incomplete lobules. Each lobule consists of the darker-staining **cortex (2)** and the lighter-staining **medulla (3)**. A characteristic **thymic (Hassall) corpuscle (4)** is present in the center of the medulla in one of the lobules.

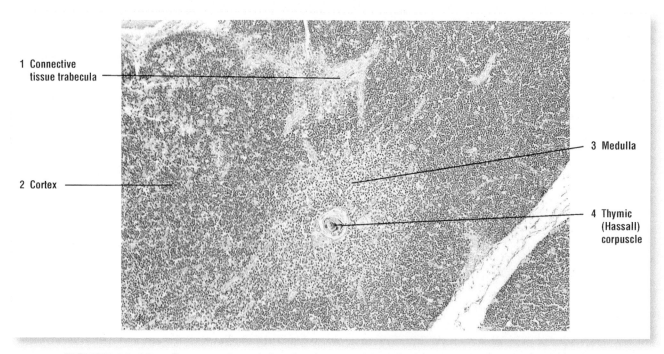

1 Connective tissue trabecula

2 Cortex

3 Medulla

4 Thymic (Hassall) corpuscle

FIGURE 11.12 ■ Cortex and medulla of a thymus gland. Stain: hematoxylin and eosin. ×30.

FUNCTIONAL CORRELATIONS 11.2 ■ Thymus Gland

The primary function of **thymus gland** is to promote the development of cells of the **immune system**, the T cells (lymphocytes, also called **thymocytes**), to recognize and respond to antigens. This gland performs an important role early in childhood in developing the immune system. Undifferentiated **lymphocytes** are carried from the bone marrow via the bloodstream to the thymus gland. In the thymic cortex, the **epithelial reticular cells**, also called **thymic nurse cells**, surround the lymphocytes and promote their differentiation, proliferation, and maturation. Here, the lymphocytes mature into **immunocompetent T cells**, **helper T cells**, and **cytotoxic T cells**, whereby they acquire various surface receptors for the recognition of antigens. Furthermore, the developing lymphocytes are prevented from exposure to blood borne antigens by a physical **blood–thymus barrier**, formed by endothelial cells, epithelial reticular cells, and macrophages. Macrophages outside of the capillaries ensure that substances in the blood vessels do not interact with the developing T cells in the cortex and induce an autoimmune response against the body's own cells or tissues. After maturation, the T cells leave the thymus gland via the bloodstream and populate the **lymph nodes**, **spleen**, and other thymus-dependent **lymphatic tissues** in the organism.

The maturation and selection of T cells within the thymus gland is a complicated process that includes the **positive** and **negative** selection of T cells. Only a small fraction of lymphocytes generated in the thymus gland reach maturity. As maturation progresses in the cortex, the T cells are presented with self- and foreign antigens by APCs. T cells that are unable to recognize self-antigens or that recognize self-antigens die and are eliminated by macrophages (**negative selection**), which is about 95% of the total cells. Those lymphocytes that recognize the foreign antigens (**positive selection**) survive, reach maturity, enter the medulla from the cortex, and are then distributed in the bloodstream to other sites in the body. The macrophages that are close to the perivascular areas and form the blood–thymus barrier are also involved in phagocytosis of apoptotic (dead) lymphocyte that occurred during their differentiation and clonal selection.

In addition to forming the blood–thymus barrier, the epithelial reticular cells secrete hormones necessary for the proliferation, differentiation, and maturation of T cells and the expression of their surface markers. These hormones are **thymulin**, **thymopoietin**, **thymosin**, **thymic humoral factor**, **interleukins**, and **interferon**. The epithelial reticular cells also form distinctive whorls called **thymic (Hassall) corpuscles** in the medulla of the gland, which are characteristic features in identifying the thymus gland. It is believed that thymic corpuscles produce **cytokine thymic stromal lymphopoietin** that induces antigen-presenting cells ([APCs] also known as dendritic cells) to promote development of the regulatory T cells. The thymus gland involutes after puberty and becomes filled with adipose tissue, and the production of T cells decreases. However, because T-lymphocyte progeny has been established, immunity is maintained without new T-cell production. However, if the thymus gland is removed from a newborn, the lymphoid organs will not receive the immunocompetent T cells, and the individual will not acquire the immunologic competence to fight pathogens. Death may occur early in life as a result of complications of an infection and the lack of a functional immune system.

FIGURE 11.13 | Spleen (Panoramic View)

The spleen is surrounded by a dense connective tissue **capsule (1)** from which arise connective tissue **trabeculae (3, 5, 11)** that extend into the spleen's interior. The main trabeculae enter the spleen at the hilus and extend throughout the organ. Located within the trabeculae (3, 5, 11) are **trabecular arteries (5b)** and **trabecular veins (5a)**. Trabeculae that are cut in transverse section (11) appear round or nodular and may contain blood vessels. The spleen is subdivided into white pulp and red pulp, so named because of their appearance in fresh state.

The spleen is characterized by numerous **lymphatic nodules (4, 6)** that constitute the **white pulp (4, 6)**. Included in the white pulp are the **germinal centers (8, 9)** and blood vessels called **central arteries (2, 7, 10)** located in the peripheries of the lymphatic nodules (4, 6). Central arteries (2, 7, 10) are branches of trabecular arteries (5b) that become ensheathed with lymphatic tissue as they leave the connective tissue trabeculae (3, 5, 11). These periarterial lymphatic sheaths (PALS) form the lymphatic nodules (4, 6) of the white pulp (4, 6) of the spleen.

Surrounding the lymphatic nodules (4, 6) and the connective tissue trabeculae (3, 5, 11) is a diffuse cellular meshwork that makes up the bulk of the organ and constitutes the **red** or **splenic pulp (12, 13)**. In fresh preparations, red pulp color is due to its extensive vascular tissue. Present in the red pulp (12, 13) are **pulp arteries (14)**, **venous sinuses (13)**, and **splenic cords (of Billroth) (12)**. The splenic cords (12) appear as diffuse strands of lymphatic tissue between the venous sinuses (13) that form a meshwork of reticular connective tissue.

The spleen does not exhibit a cortex and a medulla, as seen in lymph nodes; however, lymphatic nodules (4, 6) are found throughout the organ. In addition, the spleen contains venous sinuses (13), in contrast to lymphatic sinuses of the lymph nodes. The spleen also does not exhibit subcapsular or trabecular sinuses. The capsule (1) and trabeculae (3, 5, 11) in the spleen are thicker than those in the lymph nodes and with some smooth muscle fibers.

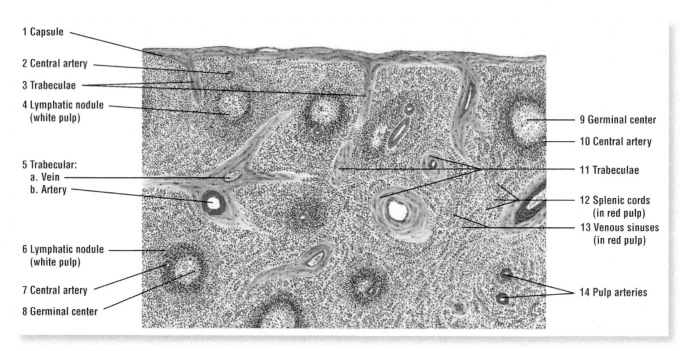

1 Capsule
2 Central artery
3 Trabeculae
4 Lymphatic nodule (white pulp)
5 Trabecular:
   a. Vein
   b. Artery
6 Lymphatic nodule (white pulp)
7 Central artery
8 Germinal center
9 Germinal center
10 Central artery
11 Trabeculae
12 Splenic cords (in red pulp)
13 Venous sinuses (in red pulp)
14 Pulp arteries

FIGURE 11.13 ■ Spleen (panoramic view). Stain: hematoxylin and eosin. Low magnification.

FIGURE 11.14 | Spleen: Red and White Pulp

A higher magnification of a section of the spleen illustrates the red and white pulp and associated connective tissue trabeculae, blood vessels, venous sinuses, and splenic cords.

The large **lymphatic nodule** (3) represents the white pulp of the spleen. Each nodule exhibits a peripheral zone—the periarterial lymphatic sheath—with densely packed small lymphocytes. The **central artery** (4) in the lymphatic nodule (3) has a peripheral, or an eccentric, position; however, because the artery occupies the center of the periarterial lymphatic sheath, it is called the central artery. The cells in the periarterial lymphatic sheath are mainly T cells. A **germinal center** (5) may not always be present. In the more lightly stained germinal center (5) are found B cells, many medium-sized lymphocytes, some small lymphocytes, and lymphoblasts.

The red pulp contains the **splenic cords** (of Billroth) (**1, 8**) and **venous sinuses** (**2, 9**) that course between the cords. The splenic cords (1, 8) are thin aggregations of lymphatic tissue containing small lymphocytes, associated cells, and various blood cells. Venous sinuses (2, 9) are dilated vessels lined with the modified endothelium of elongated cells that appear cuboidal in transverse sections.

Also present in the red pulp are the **pulp arteries** (**10**), branches of the central artery (4) after it leaves the lymphatic nodule (3). Capillaries and pulp veins (venules) are also present.

Connective tissue trabeculae with a **trabecular artery** (**6**) and **trabecular vein** (**7**) are evident.

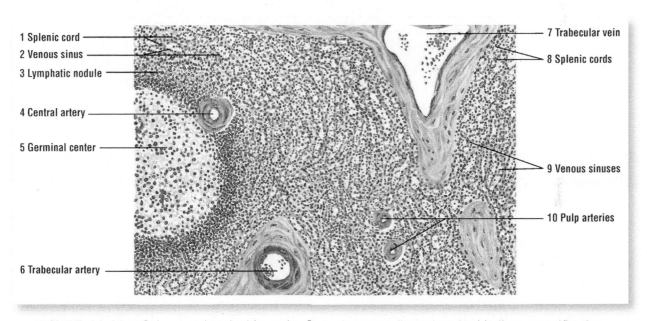

1 Splenic cord
2 Venous sinus
3 Lymphatic nodule
4 Central artery
5 Germinal center
6 Trabecular artery
7 Trabecular vein
8 Splenic cords
9 Venous sinuses
10 Pulp arteries

FIGURE 11.14 ■ Spleen: red and white pulp. Stain: hematoxylin and eosin. Medium magnification.

FIGURE 11.15 | Red and White Pulp of Spleen

A low-magnification photomicrograph illustrates a section of the spleen. A dense irregular **connective tissue capsule** (**1**) covers the organ. From the capsule (**1**), **connective tissue trabeculae** (**3**) with blood vessels extend into the interior of the organ. **White pulp** (**2**) consists of lymphocytes and **lymphatic nodules** (**2a**) with a **germinal center** (**2b**), and a **central artery** (**2c**) is located off-center. Surrounding the white pulp lymphatic nodules (**2**) is the **red pulp** (**4**), primarily composed of **venous sinuses** (**4a**) and **splenic cords** (**4b**).

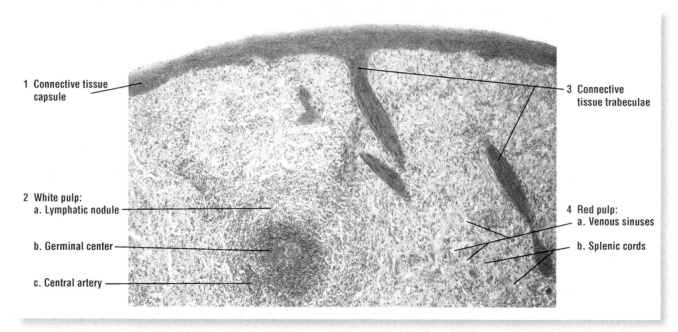

1 Connective tissue capsule

2 White pulp:
a. Lymphatic nodule
b. Germinal center
c. Central artery

3 Connective tissue trabeculae

4 Red pulp:
a. Venous sinuses
b. Splenic cords

FIGURE 11.15 ■ Red and white pulp of the spleen. Stain: Mallory-Azan. ×21.

FUNCTIONAL CORRELATIONS 11.3 ■ Spleen

The **spleen** is the largest lymphoid organ with an extensive blood supply. It filters blood and is the site of immune responses to blood-borne antigens. The two major components of the spleen are the red pulp and white pulp. **Red pulp** consists of a dense network of reticular fibers that contains erythrocytes, lymphocytes, plasma cells, macrophages, and other granulocytes. The main function of the red pulp is to filter the blood. It removes antigens, microorganisms, platelets, and aged or abnormal erythrocytes from the blood. The **white pulp** is the immune component of the spleen and consists of accumulated lymphocytes in the lymphatic nodules that surround the central artery or arteriole. Lymphocytes around the **central arteries** of the white pulp form the **periarteriolar lymphatic sheaths** (**PALS**) and contain primarily **T cells**, **macrophages**, and **antigen-presenting cells** (**APCs**). The lymphatic nodules contain mainly **B cells**. The cells in the spleen detect trapped bacteria and antigens and initiate immune responses against them. As a result, T cells and B cells interact, become activated, proliferate, and perform their immune response.

Macrophages in the spleen also break down the **hemoglobin** of worn-out **erythrocytes**, recycle the iron from hemoglobin, and return it to the **bone marrow**, where it is reused for synthesis of new hemoglobin by developing erythrocytes. The heme from the hemoglobin is further degraded and excreted into **bile** by the liver cells.

During fetal life, the spleen is a **hematopoietic organ**, producing **granulocytes** and **erythrocytes**. This hematopoietic capability, however, ceases after birth. The spleen also serves as an important **reservoir** for blood. Because it has a spongelike microstructure, much blood can be stored in its interior. When needed, the stored blood is returned from the spleen to the general circulation. Although the spleen performs various important functions in the body, it is not an essential organ for life.

FIGURE 11.16 | Palatine Tonsil

The paired palatine tonsils consist of aggregates of lymphatic nodules located in the oral cavity. The palatine tonsils are not surrounded by a connective tissue capsule. As a result, the surface of the palatine tonsil is covered by a **stratified squamous nonkeratinized epithelium** (**1, 6**) that also covers the rest of the oral cavity. Each tonsil is invaginated by deep grooves called **tonsillar crypts** (**3, 9**) that are also lined by stratified squamous nonkeratinized epithelium (1, 6).

Below the epithelium (1, 6) in the connective tissue are **lymphatic nodules** (**2**) distributed along the lengths of the tonsillar crypts (3, 9). The lymphatic nodules (2) frequently merge with each other and usually exhibit lighter-staining **germinal centers** (**7**).

A dense connective tissue underlies the palatine tonsil and forms its **capsule** (**4, 10**). The connective tissue **trabeculae**, some with **blood vessels** (**8**), arise from the capsule (4, 10) and pass toward the surface of the tonsil between the lymphatic nodules (2).

Below the connective tissue capsule (10) are sections of **skeletal muscle** (**5**) fibers.

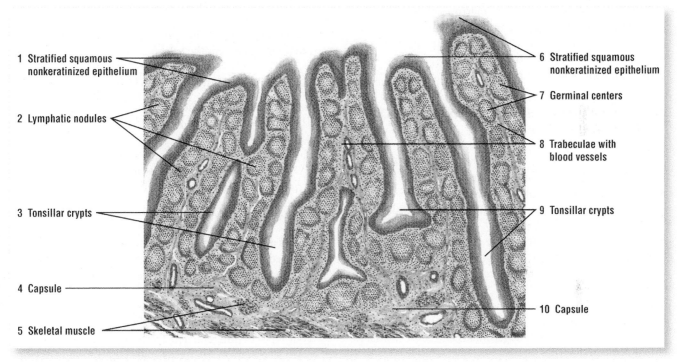

1 Stratified squamous nonkeratinized epithelium

2 Lymphatic nodules

3 Tonsillar crypts

4 Capsule

5 Skeletal muscle

6 Stratified squamous nonkeratinized epithelium

7 Germinal centers

8 Trabeculae with blood vessels

9 Tonsillar crypts

10 Capsule

FIGURE 11.16 ■ Palatine tonsil. Stain: hematoxylin and eosin. Low magnification.

Chapter 11 Summary

IMMUNE SYSTEM

- Protects organism against invading pathogens and has wide distribution
- Contains aggregates of immune cells (lymphocytes) in nodules or lymphoid organs
- Major organs are subdivided into primary and secondary lymphoid organs
- Primary lymph organs are bone marrow and thymus
- Secondary lymph organs are the lymph nodes, tonsils, spleen, and mucosa-associated lymphoid tissue (MALT)
- MALT is in the digestive tract (GALT), respiratory tract (BALT), bone, and Peyer patches

ORGANS OF IMMUNE SYSTEM: LYMPH NODES, THYMUS, AND SPLEEN

Lymph Nodes

- Distributed along the paths of lymphatic vessels
- Most prominent in inguinal and axillary regions
- Major function is lymph filtration and phagocytosis of foreign material from lymph
- Surrounded by connective tissue capsule that sends trabeculae into the interior of the organ
- Exhibit an outer dark-staining cortex and an inner light-staining medulla
- Lymphatic nodules, some with germinal centers, are aggregated in the cortex
- Lymphatic nodules without germinal centers are primary lymphatic nodules
- Lymphatic nodules with antigen stimulation and lighter germinal centers are secondary nodules
- Afferent lymph vessels with valves penetrate the capsule and enter subcapsular sinus
- Major blood vessels present in connective tissue trabeculae
- Medullary cords in the medulla contain plasma cells, macrophages, and lymphocytes
- Medullary sinuses are capillary channels that drain lymph from cortical regions
- Efferent lymphatic vessels drain lymph from the medullary sinuses to exit at the hilus
- Produce and store B and T cells
- B cells accumulate in lymphatic nodules and when activated form germinal centers
- Deeper region of the cortex is the paracortex, occupied by T cells

- T cells concentrate in deep cortical or paracortex regions
- Activate B cells to give rise to plasma cells and memory B cells
- B and T cells enter lymph nodes through postcapillary high endothelial venules
- High endothelium in postcapillary venules contains adhesive molecules as homing receptors for lymphocytes
- Both B and T cells leave bloodstream through high endothelial venules
- High endothelial venules present in numerous other lymphoid organs except the spleen

CELLS OF THE IMMUNE SYSTEM

- Include lymphocytes and different supporting cells
- Three types of lymphocytes are T cells, B cells, and NK cells
- Supporting or accessory cells are antigen-presenting cells (APCs), including macrophages and dendritic cells
- Originate from hemopoietic stem cells in the bone marrow

T Lymphocytes (T Cells)

- T cells arise from lymphocytes that were carried to and matured in the thymus gland
- After maturation, T cells are distributed to all lymph tissues and organs
- On encountering antigens, T cells destroy them by cytotoxic action or by activating B cells
- Four types of differentiated T cells: helper T cells, cytotoxic T cells, memory T cells, and suppressor T cells
- Helper T cells secrete cytokines or interleukins when they encounter antigens
- Cytokines stimulate B cells to differentiate into plasma cells and to secrete antibodies
- Cytotoxic T cells attack and destroy virus-infected, foreign, or malignant cells via perforating protein perforin
- Memory T cells are the long-living progeny of T cells and respond to the same antigens
- Suppressor T cells decrease or inhibit the functions of helper T cells and cytotoxic T cells
- Maturation of T cells is a very complicated process, involving positive and negative selection
- Most T cells recognize self-antigens and die (negative selection)
- T cells that recognize foreign antigens reach maturity and enter the bloodstream (positive selection)

B LYMPHOCYTES (B CELLS)

- B cells remain and mature in the bone marrow, then move to nonthymic lymphoid tissues and organs
- Recognize antigens as a result of antigen receptors on cell membranes and become activated
- Response is more intense when antigen-presenting helper T cells present antigens to B cells
- Cytokines secreted by helper T cells increase the proliferation of activated B cells
- B cells differentiate into plasma cells and secrete antibodies to destroy foreign substances
- Other activated B cells remain as memory B cells for future defense against the same antigens

Natural Killer (NK) Cells and Antigen-Presenting Cells (APCs)

- Develop from the same precursors as B cells and T cells
- NK cells attack virally infected cells and cancer cells as do cytotoxic T cells
- APCs phagocytose and present antigens to T cells for response
- APCs belong to the mononuclear phagocytic system
- APCs include connective tissue macrophages, perisinusoidal macrophages (Kupffer cells) in the liver, Langerhans cells (dendritic) in the skin, and macrophages in the lymphoid organs

TYPES OF IMMUNE RESPONSES

Innate Immune Response

- First line of defense that limits the spread of infection
- Response composed of the rapid response of phagocytic cells and their functions
- Response is nonspecific and does not produce memory cells

Adaptive Immune Response

- Targets specific invading **organisms** and provides specific or adaptive response
- Response is slower than innate response but produces memory cells that can respond to secondary encounters
- Production of long-lived memory cells is main function of adaptive immunity
- Two types of specific responses are humoral and mediated immune responses
- In humoral-mediated response, antigens induce B cells to transform into plasma cells
- Plasma cells, in turn, secrete specific antibodies to destroy antigens
- In cell-mediated response, T cells are activated, release cytokines, stimulate other T and B cells, bind to target cells, and destroy them

SPLEEN

- Largest lymphoid organ with extensive blood supply; filters blood and serves as a blood reservoir
- Surrounded by a connective tissue capsule that divides it into red and white pulp
- White pulp consists of lymphatic nodules with a germinal center around a central artery
- T predominant in periarteriolar lymphatic sheets (PALS) around central arteries
- Red pulp consists of splenic cords and splenic (blood) sinusoids
- Splenic cords contain macrophages, lymphocytes, plasma cells, and different blood cells
- Does not exhibit cortex and medulla but contains lymphatic nodules
- White pulp is the site of immune response to blood-borne antigens
- T cells surround the central arteries, whereas B cells are mainly in the lymphatic nodules
- APCs and macrophages are found in white pulp
- Breaks down hemoglobin from worn-out erythrocytes and recycles iron to bone marrow
- Degrades heme from hemoglobin, which is then excreted in the bile
- During fetal life is an important hematopoietic organ and in adults serves as blood reservoir

THYMUS GLAND

- Lobulated lymphoepithelial organ with dark-staining cortex and light-staining medulla
- Most active in childhood and has an important role early in life in immune system development
- Site where immature lymphocytes from the bone marrow mature into T cells, helper T cells, and cytotoxic T cells
- Thymic nurse cells promote lymphocyte differentiation, proliferation, and maturation
- Blood–thymus barrier prevents developing lymphocytes contacting blood-borne antigens
- Sends mature T cells to populate the lymph nodes, the spleen, and the lymphatic tissues
- Epithelial reticular cells secrete numerous hormones needed for lymphocyte maturation
- Epithelial reticular cells form thymic (Hassall) corpuscles in the medulla
- Maturation of T cells involves positive and negative selection
- Involutes and becomes filled with adipose tissues as the individual ages
- Removal early in life results in loss of immunologic competence

Chapter 11 Review Questions

QUESTIONS

In the following multiple-choice questions, choose the letter corresponding to the one best answer.

1. **The positive selection of lymphocytes in the thymus gland means that:**
   A. lymphocytes that recognize foreign antigens survive and reach maturity.
   B. lymphocytes that recognize self-antigens survive and reach maturity.
   C. lymphocytes unable to recognize self-antigens are eliminated by macrophages.
   D. lymphocytes that recognize foreign antigens die.
   E. lymphocytes are unable to recognize self-antigens.

2. **The main function of red pulp in the spleen is to:**
   A. provide more lymphocytes for the system.
   B. provide residence for B lymphocytes.
   C. increase the presence of antigen-presenting cells.
   D. provide new blood cells during blood loss.
   E. filter blood and remove antigens from it.

3. **The white pulp of the spleen consists mainly of:**
   A. connective tissue and reticular fibers.
   B. white blood cells and red blood cells.
   C. lymphocytes and macrophages around the central artery.
   D. blood sinusoids and blood vessels.
   E. connective tissue trabeculae and fibers.

4. **The immune system organ that exhibits both an afferent and efferent lymph vessel is the:**
   A. lymph node.
   B. spleen.
   C. thymus.
   D. tonsil.
   E. lymphatic nodule.

5. **The spleen is also a hematopoietic organ. When does this function take place?**
   A. During the life of the individual
   B. During severe infection and immune response
   C. Right after birth
   D. During fetal life
   E. Following severe blood loss

ANSWERS

1. **Correct Answer: A.** Lymphocytes that recognize foreign antigens survive and reach maturity. These cells then enter the medulla and are distributed in blood to other lymphatic sites.

2. **Correct Answer: E.** The main function of red pulp in the spleen is to filter blood and remove antigens from it.

3. **Correct Answer: C.** The white pulp of the spleen consists mainly of lymphocytes and macrophages around the central artery. These cells form the periarteriolar lymphatic sheaths (PALS) around the central artery.

4. **Correct Answer: A.** Lymph node. Lymph enters the lymph nodes via afferent lymph vessels and leaves via the efferent lymph vessels in the hilum of the node.

5. **Correct Answer: D.** The spleen is a hematopoietic organ during fetal life.

ADDITIONAL HISTOLOGIC IMAGES

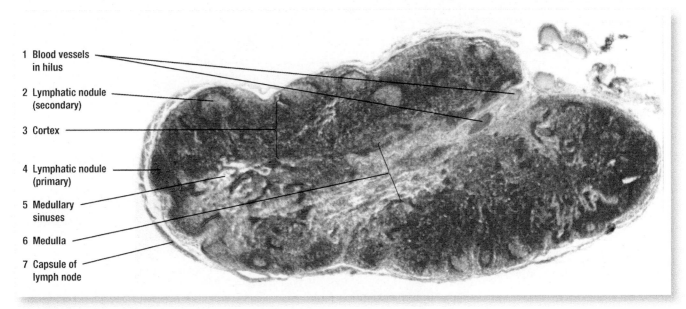

1 Blood vessels in hilus
2 Lymphatic nodule (secondary)
3 Cortex
4 Lymphatic nodule (primary)
5 Medullary sinuses
6 Medulla
7 Capsule of lymph node

FIGURE 11.17 ■ A low-power section of a primate lymph node illustrating its internal components. Stain: hematoxylin and eosin. ×8.

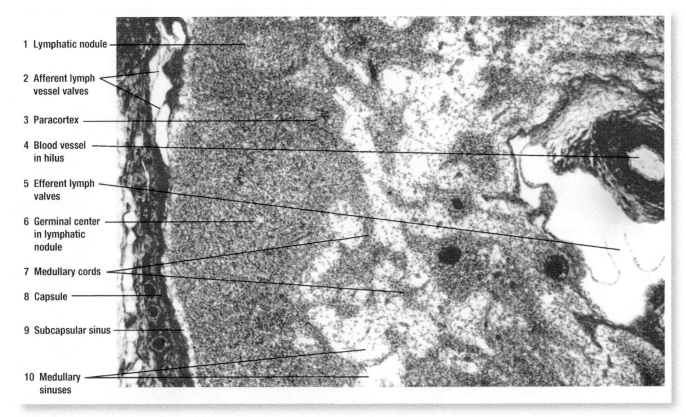

1 Lymphatic nodule
2 Afferent lymph vessel valves
3 Paracortex
4 Blood vessel in hilus
5 Efferent lymph valves
6 Germinal center in lymphatic nodule
7 Medullary cords
8 Capsule
9 Subcapsular sinus
10 Medullary sinuses

FIGURE 11.18 ■ Medium magnification of a section of primate cortex and medulla of a lymph node. Stain: Mallory-Azan. ×50.

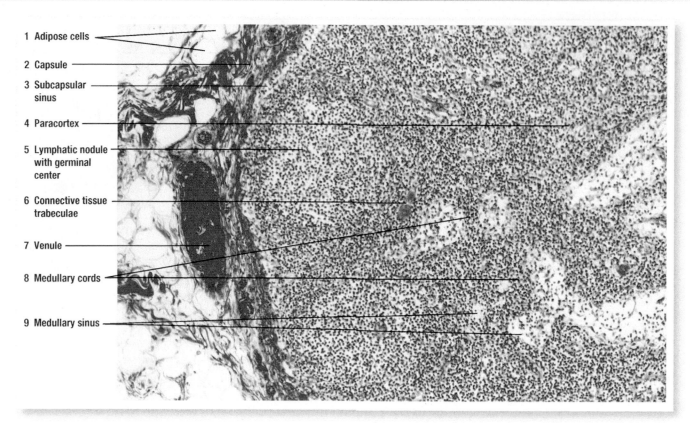

1 Adipose cells

2 Capsule

3 Subcapsular sinus

4 Paracortex

5 Lymphatic nodule with germinal center

6 Connective tissue trabeculae

7 Venule

8 Medullary cords

9 Medullary sinus

FIGURE 11.19 ■ Higher magnification of a primate lymph node illustrating its contents. Stain: Mallory-Azan. ×80.

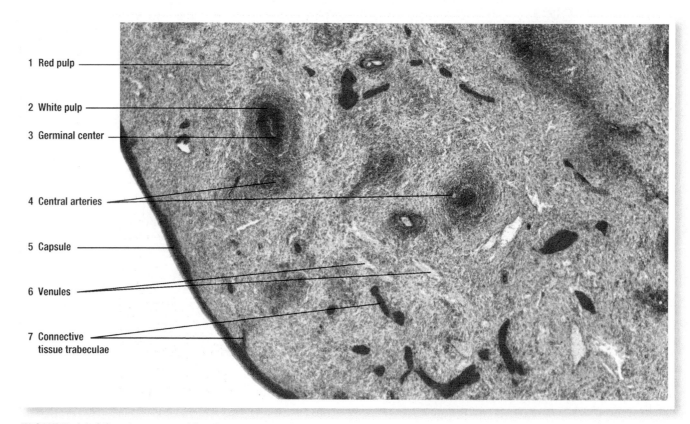

1 Red pulp

2 White pulp

3 Germinal center

4 Central arteries

5 Capsule

6 Venules

7 Connective tissue trabeculae

FIGURE 11.20 ■ Low-magnification section of human spleen illustrating its contents. Stain: Mallory-Azan. ×21.

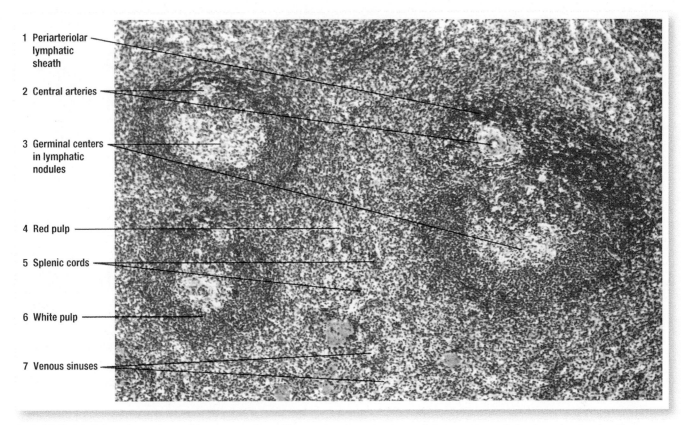

1 Periarteriolar lymphatic sheath

2 Central arteries

3 Germinal centers in lymphatic nodules

4 Red pulp

5 Splenic cords

6 White pulp

7 Venous sinuses

FIGURE 11.21 ■ A section of human spleen illustrating lymphatic nodules, periarteriolar lymphatic sheath (PALS), and the red and white pulp. Stain: hematoxylin and eosin. ×65.

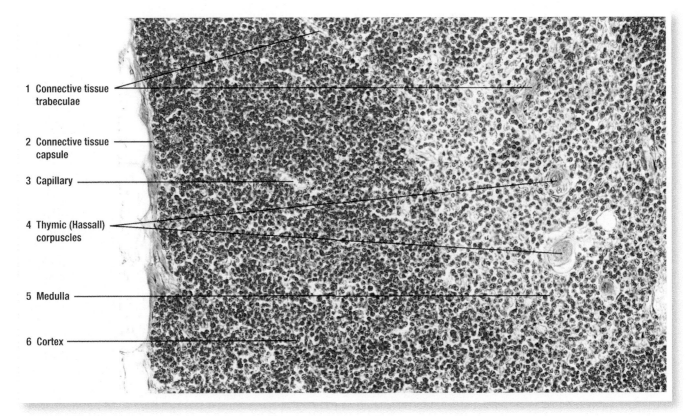

1 Connective tissue trabeculae

2 Connective tissue capsule

3 Capillary

4 Thymic (Hassall) corpuscles

5 Medulla

6 Cortex

FIGURE 11.22 ■ A section of primate thymus gland illustrating the cortex and medulla and their contents. Stain: Mallory-Azan. ×65.

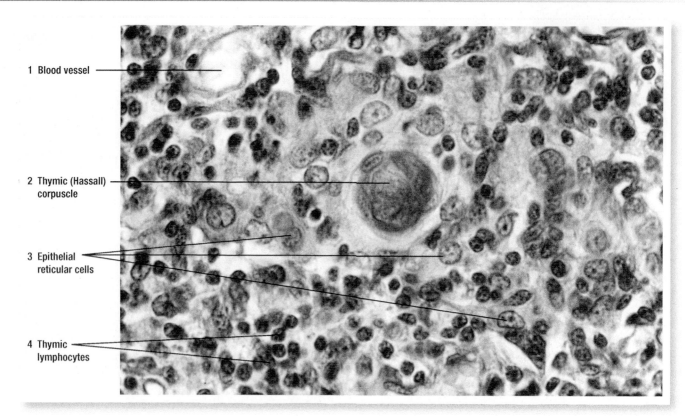

1 Blood vessel

2 Thymic (Hassall) corpuscle

3 Epithelial reticular cells

4 Thymic lymphocytes

FIGURE 11.23 ■ A section of human thymus cortex with the thymic (Hassall) corpuscle and the surrounding cells. Stain: hematoxylin and eosin. ×100.

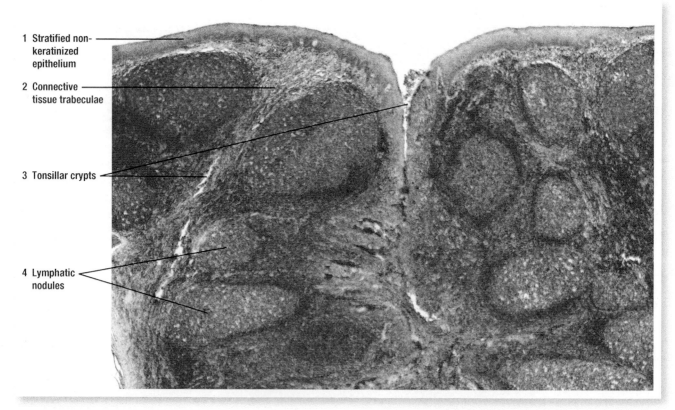

1 Stratified non-keratinized epithelium

2 Connective tissue trabeculae

3 Tonsillar crypts

4 Lymphatic nodules

FIGURE 11.24 ■ Human palatine tonsil illustrating the crypts and the internal structures. Stain: hematoxylin and eosin. ×6.5.

12

Integumentary System

GENERAL OVERVIEW

Skin is the largest organ in the body. Its derivatives and appendages form the **integumentary system**. In humans, skin derivatives include nails, hair, and several types of sweat and sebaceous glands. The surfaces of the body are covered either by thin skin or thick skin. Skin, or **integument**, consists of two distinct regions—the superficial epidermis and a deep dermis. The surface layer of the skin, or the **epidermis**, is nonvascular and is lined by **keratinized stratified squamous epithelium** with distinct cell types and different cell layers. Inferior to the epidermis is the vascular **dermis**, characterized by dense irregular connective tissue, blood vessels, nerves, and various glands. In some areas, numerous hair follicles are visible in the dermis. Beneath the dermis is the **hypodermis**, or a **subcutaneous layer** of connective tissue and adipose tissue that forms the superficial fascia of gross anatomy.

DERMIS: PAPILLARY AND RETICULAR LAYERS

Dermis is the inferior connective tissue layer that binds to the epidermis. A **basement membrane** separates the epidermis from the dermis in which are found such epidermal derivatives as the sweat glands, sebaceous glands, and hair follicles.

The junction of the dermis with the epidermis is irregular. The superficial layer of the dermis forms numerous raised projections called **dermal papillae**, which interdigitate with evaginations of the epidermis, called **epidermal ridges**. This region of the skin is the **papillary layer**. It contains loose irregular connective tissue fibers, capillaries, blood vessels, fibroblasts, macrophages, and other loose connective tissue cells.

The deeper layer of the dermis is the **reticular layer**. This layer is thicker, is characterized by dense irregular connective tissue fibers (mainly type I collagen), and is less cellular than the papillary layer. Also, this layer can withstand more mechanical stresses and supports nerves, blood vessels, hair follicles, and all the sweat glands. There is no distinct boundary between the two dermal layers; the papillary layer blends with the reticular layer. Also, the dermis blends inferiorly with the **hypodermis**, or the **subcutaneous layer**, which contains the superficial fascia and adipose tissue.

The connective tissue of the dermis is highly vascular and contains blood vessels, lymph vessels, and nerves. Certain regions of the skin exhibit **arteriovenous anastomoses** used for temperature regulation. Here, blood passes directly from the arteries into the veins. In addition, the dermis contains such sensory receptors as **Meissner corpuscles** that are located in dermal papillae and **Pacinian corpuscles** deeper in the connective tissue of the dermis.

FUNCTIONAL CORRELATIONS 12.1 ■ Epidermal Cells and Cell Layers

There are four cell types in the epidermis of the skin, with the **keratinocytes** being the most dominant cells. Keratinocytes divide, grow, migrate up, undergo **keratinization**, or **cornification**, and form the protective epidermal and surface layer for the skin. The epidermis is composed of stratified keratinized squamous epithelium. There are other less abundant cell types in the epidermis. These are the melanocytes, Langerhans cells, and Merkel cells, which are interspersed among the keratinocytes in the epidermis. In thick skin, five distinct and recognizable cell layers can be identified.

STRATUM BASALE (GERMINATIVUM)—THE DEEPEST LAYER

The **stratum basale** is the deepest or basal layer in the epidermis. It consists of a single layer of columnar to cuboidal cells that rest on a **basement membrane** separating the dermis from the epidermis. The cells are attached to one another by cell junctions, the **desmosomes**, and to the underlying basement membrane by **hemidesmosomes**. Cells in the stratum basale serve as stem cells for the epidermis; thus, increased mitotic activity is seen in this layer. The cells in this layer continually divide and mature as they migrate up toward the superficial layers. All cells in the stratum basale produce **intermediate keratin filaments** that increase in number as the cells move superficially. These filaments eventually form the components of keratin in the superficial cell layer.

STRATUM SPINOSUM—THE SECOND LAYER

As the keratinocytes divide by mitosis, they move upward in the epidermis and form the second cell layer of keratinocytes, or **stratum spinosum**. This layer consists of four to six rows of cells. Routine histologic preparations with different chemicals cause these cells to shrink. As a result, the developed intercellular spaces between cells appear to form numerous cytoplasmic extensions, or spines, that project from their surfaces. The spines represent the sites where **desmosomes** are anchored to bundles of intermediate keratin filaments, or **tonofilaments**, and to neighboring cells. The synthesis of keratin filaments continues in this layer, which are assembled into bundles of tonofilaments to provide cohesion among

cells and resistance to the abrasion of the epidermis as they terminate at desmosomes.

STRATUM GRANULOSUM—THE THIRD LAYER

Maturing cells that move above the stratum spinosum accumulate dense basophilic **keratohyalin granules** and form the third layer, the **stratum granulosum** that consists of three to five layers of flattened cells. These secretory granules are not surrounded by a membrane and consist of the protein **filaggrin**, which induces the aggregation of keratin tonofilaments into tight bundles. This combination of keratin tonofilaments with protein filaggrin produces **keratin** through the process of keratinization. The keratin formed by this process is the soft keratin of the skin. In addition, the cells of stratum granulosum contain membrane-bound **lamellar granules** (bodies) containing lipid bilayers. These lamellar granules are discharged into the intercellular spaces between the stratum granulosum and the next layer, the stratum corneum (or stratum lucidum if present), as a **lipid** layer to form an impermeable water barrier that seals and waterproofs the epidermis of the skin.

STRATUM LUCIDUM—THE FOURTH LAYER

In thick skin only, the **stratum lucidum** is translucent and barely visible; it lies just superior to the stratum granulosum and inferior to the stratum corneum. The tightly packed cells lack nuclei or organelles and are dead. The flattened cells contain densely packed keratin filaments cross-linked with filaggrin. This layer is not visible in thin skin, although individual cells may be present.

STRATUM CORNEUM—THE FIFTH LAYER

The **stratum corneum** is the fifth and most superficial layer of the skin. All nuclei and organelles have disappeared from the cells of this layer that now consists of flattened, dead cells filled with soft **keratin filaments**. The keratinized, superficial cells from this layer are continually shed, or **desquamated**, and are replaced by new cells arising from the deep stratum basale. During the keratinization process, the hydrolytic enzymes disrupt the nucleus and all cytoplasmic organelles, which disappear as the cells fill with keratin.

OTHER SKIN CELLS

In addition to the **keratinocytes** that form and become the superficial layer of keratinized epithelium, the epidermis also contains three less abundant cell types. These are melanocytes, Langerhans cells, and Merkel cells. Unless the skin is prepared with special stains, these cells are not distinguishable in histologic slides prepared with only hematoxylin and eosin.

Melanocytes are derived from the neural crest cells. They have long, irregular cytoplasmic or dendritic extensions that branch into the epidermis and establish contact with nearby cells. Melanocytes are located between the stratum basale and the stratum spinosum of the epidermis and in hair matrices. Melanocytes synthesize the dark brown pigment **melanin** from the amino acid tyrosine. The formed melanin granules in the melanocytes then migrate to the tips of the cytoplasmic or dendritic extensions, from which they are phagocytized by keratinocytes in the basal cell layers of the epidermis. Melanin imparts a dark color to the skin, and exposure of the skin to sunlight promotes synthesis of melanin. The main function of melanin is to protect the skin from the damaging effects of ultraviolet radiation.

Langerhans cells are monocyte-derived dendritic cells that originate in bone marrow, migrate via the bloodstream, and reside mainly in the stratum spinosum of the skin epidermis. Similar to melanocytes, the dendritic processes of Langerhans cells extend among the cells of stratum spinosum. These dendritic-type cells participate in the body's immune responses. Langerhans cells recognize, phagocytose, and process foreign **antigens** and then present them to T lymphocytes for an immune response. Thus, these cells function as **antigen-presenting cells (APCs)** and are part of the immunologic defense of the skin.

Merkel cells are found in the stratum basale layer of the epidermis and are most abundant in the fingertips. These cells are associated with surrounding keratinocytes and also contact the afferent (sensory) **unmyelinated axons**. As a result, Merkel cells function as **mechanoreceptors** for cutaneous sensation.

MAJOR SKIN FUNCTIONS

The skin comes in direct contact with the external environment and performs numerous protective functions.

Protection

The **keratinized stratified epithelium** of the epidermis protects the body surfaces from mechanical abrasion and forms a physical barrier to pathogens or foreign microorganisms. Because of a **glycolipid layer** between the cells of the stratum granulosum, the epidermis is **impermeable** to water and prevents the loss of fluids through dehydration. Increased synthesis of the pigment melanin by melanocytes further protects the skin against the damaging ultraviolet radiation.

Temperature Regulation

Physical exercise or a warm environment increases **sweating** that reduces the body temperature due to **evaporation** of sweat from the skin. In addition to sweating, temperature regulation also involves increased **dilation** of blood vessels that brings more blood to the superficial layers of the skin where cooling of the blood increases heat loss. Conversely, in cold temperatures, body heat is conserved by **constriction** of superficial blood vessels, decreased blood flow to the skin, and maintaining more heat in the body core.

Sensory Perception

The skin is a large **sensory organ** for the external environment. Numerous encapsulated and free **sensory nerve endings** within the skin respond to stimuli for temperature (heat and cold), touch, pain, and pressure.

Excretion

Through the production of sweat by the **sweat glands**, water, sodium salts, urea, and nitrogenous wastes are excreted through the surface of the skin.

Formation of Vitamin D

The skin is a major source of **vitamin D**. The keratinocytes are not only the primary source of vitamin D for the body but also possess the enzymes to metabolize vitamin D to its active metabolite. Vitamin D is formed from precursor molecules synthesized in the epidermis during exposure of the skin to **ultraviolet rays** from the sun. Vitamin D becomes essential for **calcium absorption** from the intestinal mucosa and for proper mineral metabolism.

thePoint° Supplemental micrographic images are available at **www.thePoint.com/Eroschenko13e** under Skin System.

SECTION 1 Thin Skin

Most surfaces of the body that are not exposed to increased abrasion and wear and tear are covered by **thin skin** (Fig. 12.1). In these regions, the epidermis is thinner, and its cellular composition is simpler than that of thick skin. Present in thin skin are **hair follicles**, **sebaceous glands**, and different types of **sweat glands** (**apocrine** and **eccrine**). Attached to the connective tissue sheath of hair follicles and the connective tissue of the dermis are smooth muscle fibers, called **arrector pili**. Associated with the hair follicles are numerous sebaceous glands. Thus, the terms "thick skin" and "thin skin" refer only to the thickness of the epidermis and do not include the layers below it, which can vary in thickness, depending on the location in the body.

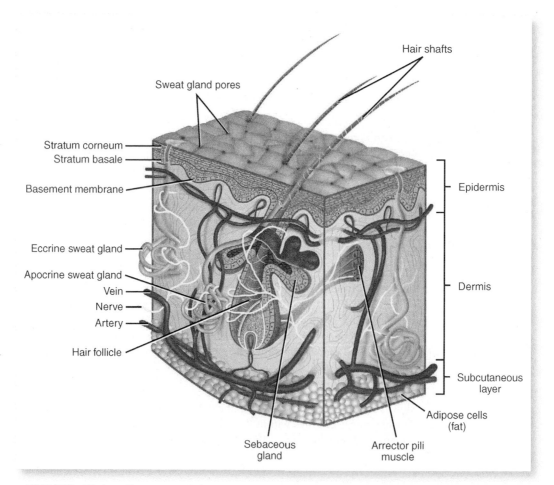

FIGURE 12.1 ■ Contents of the connective tissue dermis of the thin skin of the arm.

FIGURE 12.2 | Thin Skin: Epidermis and Contents of Dermis

This illustration depicts a section of thin skin from body surface, where wear and tear is minimal. To differentiate between the cellular and connective tissue components of the skin, the collagen fibers stain blue, and the cellular components stain red.

The skin consists of two layers: the **epidermis** (**10**) and **dermis** (**14**). The epidermis (10) is the superficial cellular layer with different cell types. The dermis (14), located directly inferior to the epidermis (10), contains connective tissue and cellular components of epidermal origin.

In thin skin, the epidermis (10) exhibits a stratified squamous epithelium and a thin layer of keratinized cells called the **stratum corneum** (**1**), from which the most superficial cells constantly shed or desquamate. Also, the stratum corneum (1) of thin skin is much thinner in contrast to that of thick skin, in which the stratum corneum (1) is much thicker. In this illustration, a few rows of polygonal cells are visible in the epidermis (10). These cells form the **stratum spinosum** (**2**).

The narrow zone of irregular, lighter-staining connective tissue directly below the epidermis (10) is the **papillary layer** (**11**) of the dermis (14) that indents the base of the epidermis to form the **dermal papillae** (**3**). The deeper **reticular layer** (**12**) comprises the bulk of the dermis (14) and consists of dense irregular connective tissue. A portion of the hypodermis (13), the underlying subcutaneous **adipose tissue** (**9**), is also illustrated.

Skin appendages, such as the **sweat gland** (**7**) and **hair follicles** (**8**), develop from the epidermis (10) and are located in the dermis (14). The sweat gland (7) is illustrated in greater detail in Figure 12.4. The expanded terminal portion of the hair follicle (8) observed in the longitudinal section is the **hair bulb** (**8a**) with the base indented by the connective tissue to form a **dermal papilla** (**8b**). Each dermal papilla (8b) contains a capillary network that is vital for sustaining the hair follicle (8). Attached to hair follicles (8) are thin strips of smooth muscle called the **arrector pili muscles** (**5**). Also associated with hair follicles (8) are numerous **sebaceous glands** (**6**).

Found in the reticular layer (12) of the dermis (14) are cross sections of a coiled portion of the sweat gland (7). The elongated portions of the sweat gland (7) that continue to the surface of the skin are the excretory **ducts** of the **sweat glands** (**4, 7a**). The more circular and deeper-lying parts of the sweat gland are the **secretory** (**7b**) portions of the sweat gland (7).

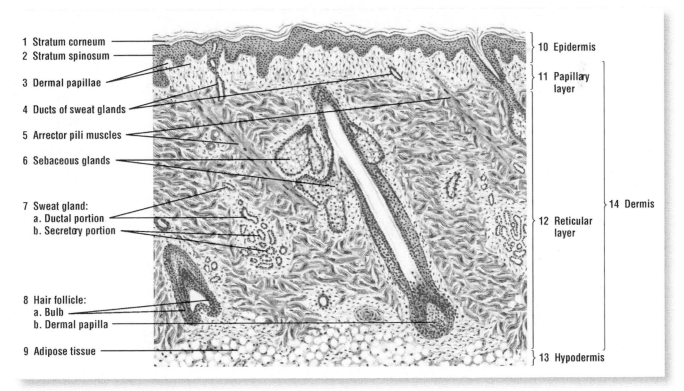

FIGURE 12.2 ■ Thin skin: epidermis and the contents of the dermis. Stain: Masson trichrome (blue stain). Low magnification.

FIGURE 12.3 | Skin: Epidermis, Dermis, and Hypodermis in Scalp

This low-magnification section of the thin skin of the scalp illustrates both the epidermis and dermis and some skin derivatives in the deeper connective tissue layers. The epidermis stains darker than the underlying dermis connective tissue. Visible in the epidermis are the cell layers **stratum corneum** (1), with desquamating superficial cells; the **stratum spinosum** (2); and the basal cell layer, the **stratum basale** (3), with brown **melanin (pigment) granules** (3).

The **connective tissue dermal papillae** (4) indent the underside of the epidermis. A thin connective tissue papillary layer of the dermis is located immediately inferior to the epidermis. The thicker connective tissue **reticular layer** (12) of the dermis extends from just below the epidermis to the **subcutaneous layer** with **adipose tissue** (8). Located inferior to the subcutaneous layer (8) are **skeletal muscle fibers** (9), sectioned in transverse and longitudinal planes.

Hair follicles (13) in the skin of the scalp are numerous, closely packed, and oriented at an angle to the surface. A complete hair follicle in longitudinal section is illustrated with

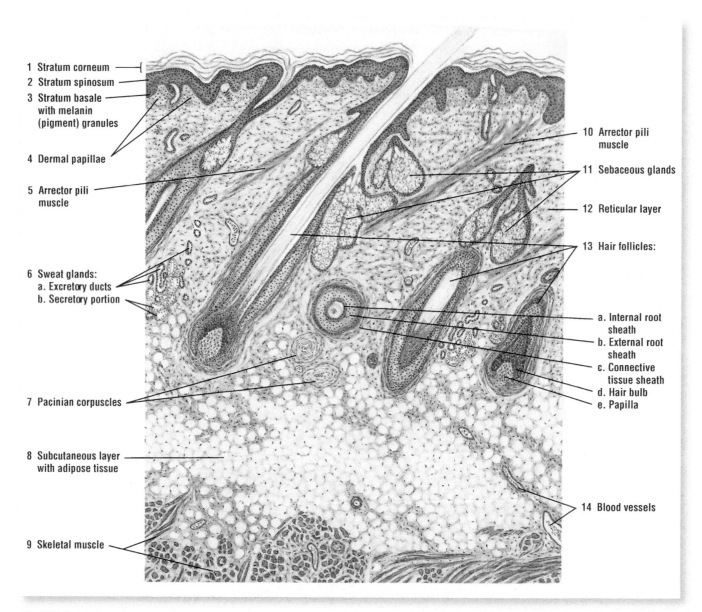

1 Stratum corneum
2 Stratum spinosum
3 Stratum basale with melanin (pigment) granules
4 Dermal papillae
5 Arrector pili muscle
6 Sweat glands:
   a. Excretory ducts
   b. Secretory portion
7 Pacinian corpuscles
8 Subcutaneous layer with adipose tissue
9 Skeletal muscle

10 Arrector pili muscle
11 Sebaceous glands
12 Reticular layer
13 Hair follicles:
   a. Internal root sheath
   b. External root sheath
   c. Connective tissue sheath
   d. Hair bulb
   e. Papilla
14 Blood vessels

FIGURE 12.3 ■ Skin: epidermis, dermis, and hypodermis in the scalp. Stain: hematoxylin and eosin. Low magnification.

parts of other hair follicles (13) sectioned in different planes. A hair follicle (13) that is cut in a transverse plane exhibits the following: the cuticle, **internal root sheath (13a)**, **external root sheath (13b)**, **connective tissue sheath (13c)**, **hair bulb (13d)**, and the connective tissue dermal **papilla (13e)**. The hair passes upward through the follicle (13) to the skin surface. Numerous **sebaceous glands (11)** surround each hair follicle (13). The sebaceous glands (11) are aggregates of clear cells that are connected to a duct that opens into the hair follicle (13) (see Figs. 12.4 and 12.5).

The **arrector pili muscles (5, 10)** are smooth muscles aligned at an oblique angle to the hair follicles (13) and attach to the papillary layer of the dermis and to the connective tissue sheath (13c) of the hair follicle (13). The contraction of arrector pili muscles (5, 10) moves the hair shaft into a more vertical position.

Deep in the dermis or subcutaneous layer (8) are the basal portions of the coiled sweat glands (6). Sections of the **sweat gland (6)** that exhibit lightly stained columnar epithelium are the **secretory portions (6b)** of the gland. These are distinct from the **excretory ducts (6a)** of the sweat glands (6), which are lined by the stratified cuboidal epithelium of smaller, darker-stained cells. Each sweat gland duct (6a) is coiled deep in the dermis but straightens out in the upper dermis and follows a spiral course through the epidermis to the surface of the skin (see Fig. 12.3).

The skin contains many **blood vessels (14)** and sensory receptors. These are the **Pacinian corpuscles (7)** for pressure and vibration located in the subcutaneous tissue (8). The Pacinian corpuscles (7) are illustrated in greater detail and higher magnification in Figure 12.13.

FIGURE 12.4 | Hairy Thin Skin of Scalp: Hair Follicles and Surrounding Structures

This low-power photomicrograph illustrates a section of the thin skin of the scalp. In the **epidermis (1)**, the **stratum corneum (1a)**, **stratum granulosum (1b)**, and **stratum spinosum (1c)** layers are thinner than the same layers in the thick skin. In the dense irregular connective tissue of the **dermis (4)** are **hair follicles (3)** and **sebaceous glands (2, 5)**. An **arrector pili muscle (6)** extends from the deep connective tissue sheath around the hair follicle (3) to the connective tissue of the dermal papillary layer beneath the epidermis.

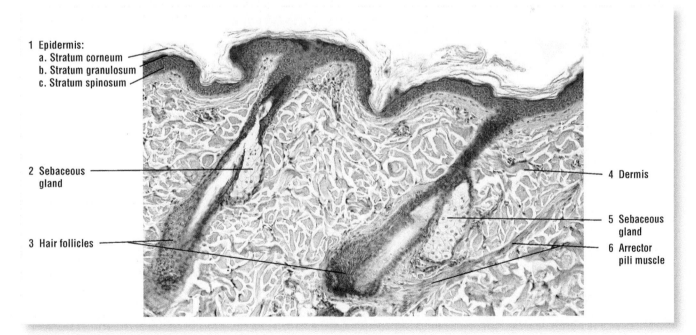

1 Epidermis:
  a. Stratum corneum
  b. Stratum granulosum
  c. Stratum spinosum

2 Sebaceous gland

3 Hair follicles

4 Dermis

5 Sebaceous gland

6 Arrector pili muscle

FIGURE 12.4 ■ Hairy thin skin of the scalp: hair follicles and surrounding structures. Stain: hematoxylin and eosin. ×40.

FIGURE 12.5 | Section of Hair Follicle with Surrounding Structures

This figure illustrates a longitudinal section of a hair follicle with surrounding structures. The different layers of the hair follicle are identified on the *right side*. The hair follicle is surrounded by an outer **connective tissue sheath** (**15**) of the **dermis** (**7**) under which is the **external root sheath** (**14**) composed of several cell layers. These cell layers are continuous with the epithelial layer of the epidermis. The **internal root sheath** (**13**) is composed of a thin, pale epithelial stratum (the Henle layer) and a thin, granular epithelial stratum (the Huxley layer). These two cell layers become indistinguishable as their cells merge in the **hair bulb** (**21**). Internal to the cell layers of the internal root sheath (**13**) are cells that produce the **cuticle** (**12**) and the keratinized **cortex** (**11**) of the hair follicle, which appears as a yellow layer. The **hair root** (**16**) and the **dermal papilla** (**18**) form the hair bulb (**21**) where the external root sheath (**14**) and internal root sheath (**13**) merge into the **hair matrix** (**17**), situated above the dermal papilla (**18**). Cell mitoses and **melanin pigment** (**19**) produced by melanocytes are seen in the matrix cells (**17**). Numerous **capillaries** (**20**) supply the connective tissue of the dermal papilla (**18**).

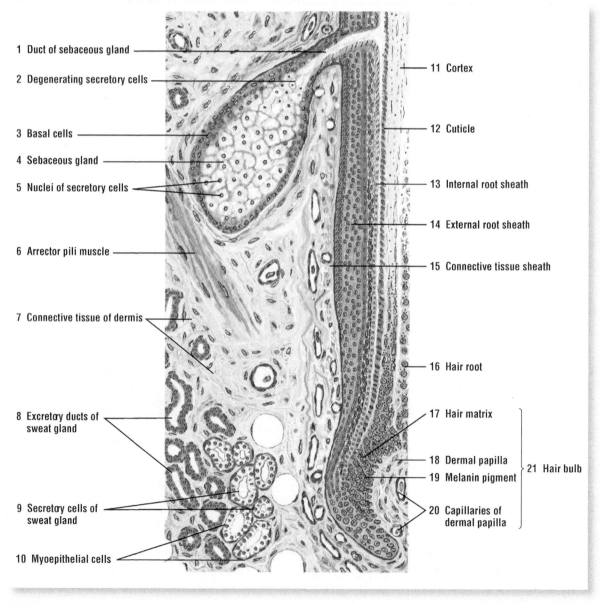

1 Duct of sebaceous gland

2 Degenerating secretory cells

3 Basal cells

4 Sebaceous gland

5 Nuclei of secretory cells

6 Arrector pili muscle

7 Connective tissue of dermis

8 Excretory ducts of sweat gland

9 Secretory cells of sweat gland

10 Myoepithelial cells

11 Cortex

12 Cuticle

13 Internal root sheath

14 External root sheath

15 Connective tissue sheath

16 Hair root

17 Hair matrix

18 Dermal papilla

19 Melanin pigment

20 Capillaries of dermal papilla

21 Hair bulb

FIGURE 12.5 ■ Hair follicle: bulb of the hair follicle, sweat gland, sebaceous gland, and arrector pili muscle. Stain: hematoxylin and eosin. Medium magnification.

In the connective tissue of the dermis (7) and adjacent to the hair follicle are transverse sections of a coiled **sweat gland** (**8, 9**). The **secretory cells** (**9**) of the sweat gland are tall, stain light, and their bases are surrounded by flattened contractile **myoepithelial cells** (**10**). The **excretory ducts** (**8**) of the sweat gland are smaller in diameter, are lined with a stratified cuboidal epithelium, and stain darker than the secretory cells (9).

A **sebaceous gland** (**4**) connected to the hair follicle is sectioned through the middle. This gland (4) is lined with a stratified epithelium that continues with the external root sheath (14) of the hair follicle. The epithelium of the sebaceous gland is modified, and along its base is a row of columnar or cuboidal cells, the **basal cells** (**3**). These cells rest on a basement membrane, surrounded by the connective tissue of the dermis (7). The basal cells (3) of the sebaceous gland (4) divide and fill the acinus of the gland with larger, polyhedral **secretory cells** (**5**) that enlarge, accumulate secretory material, and undergo **degeneration** (**2**). This process produces the oily secretory product of the gland, called sebum. Sebum passes through the short **duct** of the **sebaceous gland** (**1**) into the lumen of the hair follicle.

Each hair follicle is surrounded by numerous sebaceous glands (4) that lie in the connective tissue of the dermis (7) and in the angle between the hair follicle and the smooth muscle strip called the **arrector pili muscle** (**6**). When the arrector pili muscle contracts, the hair stands up, forming a dimple or a goose bump on the skin, at the same time forcing the sebum out of the sebaceous gland (4) into the lumen of the hair follicle and the epidermis.

SECTION 2 Thick Skin

The basic histology of skin is similar in different regions of the body, except in the thickness of the epidermis. **Palms** and **soles** are constantly exposed to increased wear, tear, and abrasion. As a protective measure, the epidermis in these regions is thick, especially the outermost stratified keratinized layer (Fig. 12.6). Because of the increased thickness of the epidermis, the skin on the palms and soles is called **thick skin**. Thick skin also contains numerous **sweat glands**, but it lacks hair follicles, sebaceous glands, and smooth muscle fibers.

thePoint® Supplemental micrographic images are available at **www.thePoint.com/Eroschenko13e** under Skin System.

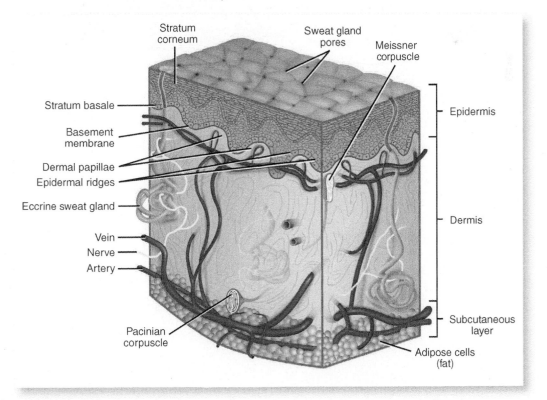

FIGURE 12.6 ■ Contents of the connective tissue dermis of the thick skin of the palm.

FIGURE 12.7 | Thick Skin: Epidermis, Dermis, and Hypodermis of Palm

A low-power photomicrograph illustrates the superficial and deep structures in the thick skin of the palm. The cell layers in the **epidermis** are (6) **stratum corneum** (7), **stratum granulosum** (8), and **stratum basale** (9). Inferior to the epidermis (6) is the dense irregular connective tissue dermis (5). Dermal papillae (11) from the **dermis** (5) indent the base of the epidermis (6). Deep in the dermis (5) and the **hypodermis** (4) are cross sections of the coiled simple tubular **sweat glands** (3) and their **excretory ducts** (10). A layer of **adipose tissue** (1) deep to the dermis (5) is the hypodermis (4) or the superficial fascia. The hypodermis (4) is not part of the integument. Two sensory receptors called the **Pacinian corpuscles** (2) are seen inferior to the adipose tissue (1) of the hypodermis (4).

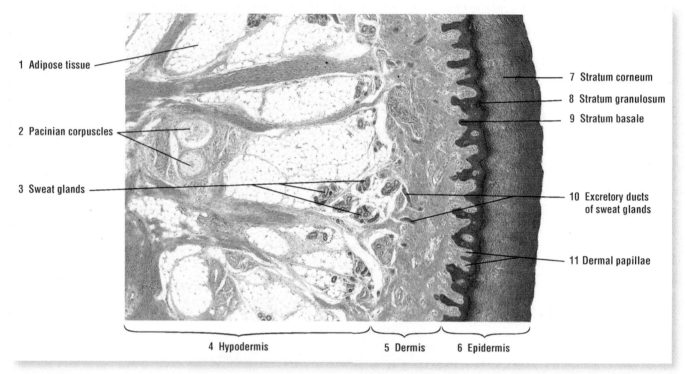

1 Adipose tissue

2 Pacinian corpuscles

3 Sweat glands

7 Stratum corneum

8 Stratum granulosum

9 Stratum basale

10 Excretory ducts of sweat glands

11 Dermal papillae

4 Hypodermis   5 Dermis   6 Epidermis

FIGURE 12.7 ■ Thick skin: epidermis, dermis, and hypodermis of the palm. Stain: hematoxylin and eosin. ×17.

FIGURE 12.8 | Thick Skin of Palm, Superficial Cell Layers, and Melanin Pigment

Thick skin is best illustrated by examining a section from the palm. The epidermis of thick skin exhibits five cell layers and is thicker than thin skin (see Figs. 12.2 to 12.4). The different cell layers of the epidermis are illustrated below in greater detail and at higher magnification.

The outermost layer of thick skin is the **stratum corneum** (**1, 9**), a wide layer of flattened, dead, or keratinized cells that are constantly shed, or **desquamated** (**8**), from the skin surface. Inferior to the stratum corneum (1, 9) is a narrow, lightly stained **stratum lucidum** (**2**) that is difficult to see in most slide preparations. At a higher magnification, the outlines of flattened cells and eleidin droplets in this layer are occasionally seen.

Located below the stratum lucidum (2) is the **stratum granulosum** (**3, 11**), in which the cells are filled with dark-staining **keratohyalin granules** (**3**). Directly under the stratum granulosum (3, 11) is the thick **stratum spinosum** (**4, 12**) composed of several layers of polyhedral cells. These cells are connected to each other by spinous processes or intercellular bridges that represent the desmosomes (macula adherens).

The deepest cell layer in the skin is the columnar or cuboidal **stratum basale** (**5, 13**) that rests on the **basement membrane** (**6, 15**). Mitotic activity and the brown melanin pigment (5, 13) are seen in the deeper layers of the stratum spinosum (4, 12) and stratum basale (5, 13).

The **excretory duct** of a **sweat gland** (**10**) located deep in the dermis penetrates the epidermis, loses its epithelial wall, and spirals through the epidermal cell layers (1 to 5) to the skin surface as small channels with a thin lining.

Dermal papillae (**7**) are prominent in thick skin, where they indent the inferior surface of the epidermis. Some dermal papillae (7) may contain tactile or sensory **Meissner corpuscles** (**14**) and **capillary loops** (**16**).

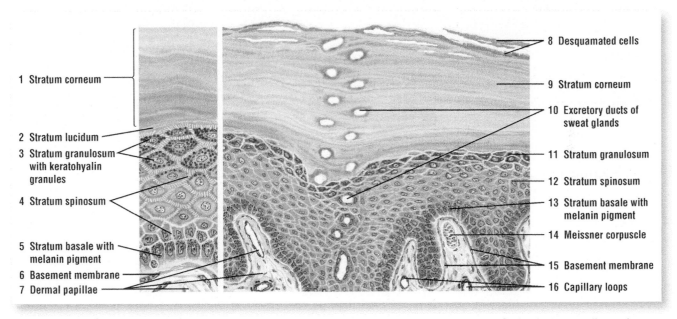

1 Stratum corneum
2 Stratum lucidum
3 Stratum granulosum with keratohyalin granules
4 Stratum spinosum
5 Stratum basale with melanin pigment
6 Basement membrane
7 Dermal papillae

8 Desquamated cells
9 Stratum corneum
10 Excretory ducts of sweat glands
11 Stratum granulosum
12 Stratum spinosum
13 Stratum basale with melanin pigment
14 Meissner corpuscle
15 Basement membrane
16 Capillary loops

FIGURE 12.8 ■ Thick skin of the palm, superficial cell layers, and melanin pigment. Stain: hematoxylin and eosin. Medium magnification.

FIGURE 12.9 | Thick Skin: Epidermis and Superficial Cell Layers

A higher-magnification photomicrograph shows the different cell layers in the **epidermis (1)** of the thick skin of the palm. The outermost and the thickest layer is the **stratum corneum (1a)**. Inferior to the stratum corneum (1a) are two to three layers of cells filled with dark granules. This is the **stratum granulosum (1b)**. Below the stratum granulosum (1b) is the **stratum spinosum (1c)**, a thicker layer of polyhedral cells. The deepest cell layer in the epidermis (1) is the **stratum basale (1d)**. The cells in this layer contain brown **melanin granules (6)**. The stratum basale (1d) is attached to a thin connective tissue **basement membrane (4)** that separates the epidermis (1) from the **dermis (2)**. The connective tissue of the dermis (2) indents the epidermis (1) to form **dermal papillae (5)**. Passing through the dermis (2) and all cell layers of the epidermis (1) is the **excretory duct (3)** of a sweat gland that is located deep in the dermis.

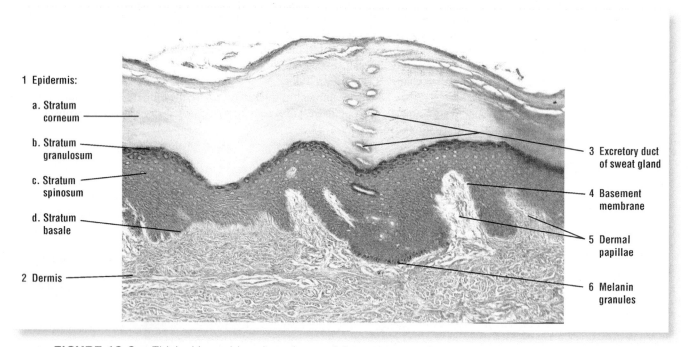

1 Epidermis:

    a. Stratum corneum

    b. Stratum granulosum

    c. Stratum spinosum

    d. Stratum basale

2 Dermis

3 Excretory duct of sweat gland

4 Basement membrane

5 Dermal papillae

6 Melanin granules

FIGURE 12.9 ■ Thick skin: epidermis and superficial cell layers. Stain: hematoxylin and eosin. ×40.

FIGURE 12.10 | Apocrine Sweat Glands: Secretory and Excretory Portions of Sweat Gland

The apocrine glands are large, coiled sweat glands that deliver their secretions into the **hair follicle** (7). This illustration shows cross sections of an apocrine sweat gland and secretory units of an eccrine sweat gland for comparison. The **secretory portion** of the **apocrine sweat gland** (3) consists of wide and dilated lumina. The gland is located deep in the **connective tissue** of the **dermis** (5) or hypodermis with **adipose cells** (4) and numerous **blood vessels** (8). In comparison, the **secretory portion** of an eccrine sweat gland (6) is smaller and with smaller lumina. The cuboidal secretory cells of the apocrine sweat gland (3) are surrounded by **myoepithelial cells** (2) located at the base of the secretory cells. When cut at an oblique angle, the myoepithelial cells (2) loop over the secretory cells to surround them. The **excretory portion** of the **sweat gland** (1) is lined by a double layer of dark-staining or stratified cuboidal cells, which is similar to the excretory duct of the eccrine sweat gland.

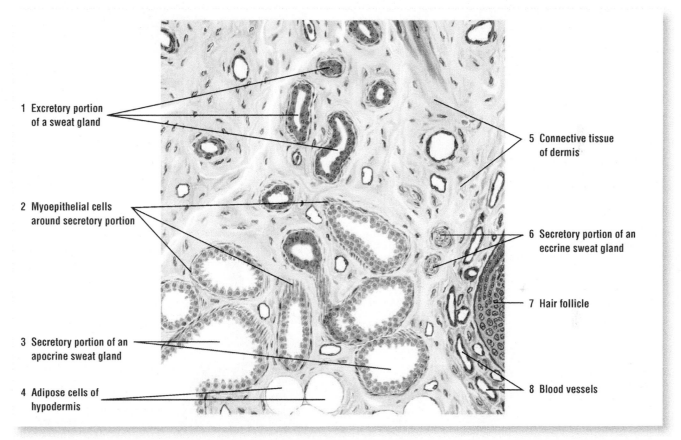

1 Excretory portion of a sweat gland

2 Myoepithelial cells around secretory portion

3 Secretory portion of an apocrine sweat gland

4 Adipose cells of hypodermis

5 Connective tissue of dermis

6 Secretory portion of an eccrine sweat gland

7 Hair follicle

8 Blood vessels

FIGURE 12.10 ■ Apocrine sweat gland: secretory and excretory portions of the sweat gland. Stain: hematoxylin and eosin. Medium magnification.

FIGURE 12.11 | Cross Section and Three-Dimensional Appearance of Eccrine Sweat Gland

The eccrine sweat gland is a simple, coiled tubular gland that extends deep into the dermis or the upper hypodermis. To illustrate this, the sweat gland is shown in both cross-sectional (**left side**) and three-dimensional views (**right side**) as it makes its way through the dermis and **epidermis** (**1, 6**).

Part of the coiled portion of the sweat gland that lies deep in the dermis is the **secretory portion** (**9**). Here, **secretory cells** (**4**) are large, columnar, and stain lightly eosinophilic. Surrounding

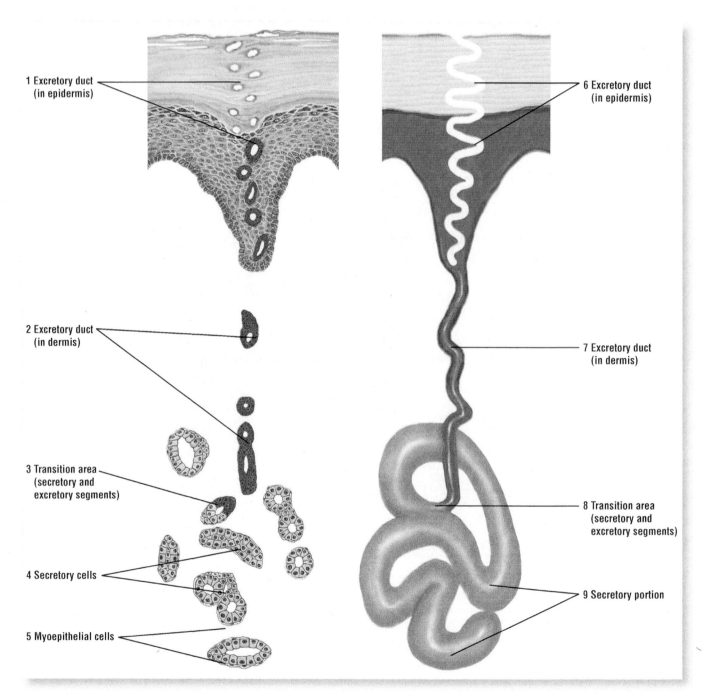

1 Excretory duct
(in epidermis)

2 Excretory duct
(in dermis)

3 Transition area
(secretory and
excretory segments)

4 Secretory cells

5 Myoepithelial cells

6 Excretory duct
(in epidermis)

7 Excretory duct
(in dermis)

8 Transition area
(secretory and
excretory segments)

9 Secretory portion

FIGURE 12.11 ■ Cross section and three-dimensional appearance of an eccrine sweat gland. Stain: hematoxylin and eosin. Low magnification.

the bases of the secretory cells (4) are thin, spindle-shaped **myoepithelial cells** (5) located between the base of the secretory cells (4) and the surrounding basement membrane (not illustrated). Where the light-staining secretory cells (4, 9) change to dark-staining **excretory duct** (2, 7) represents the **transition area** (3, 8) between the secretory and excretory regions of the sweat gland.

The cells of the excretory ducts (2, 7) are smaller than the secretory cells (4). Also, the excretory ducts (2, 7) have smaller diameters and are lined by denser-staining and, stratified cuboidal cells without any myoepithelial cells (2, 7). As the excretory ducts (2, 7) ascend through the connective tissue of the dermis, they straighten out, penetrate the cell layers of the epidermis (1, 6), lose the epithelial wall, and follow a spiral course through the skin cells to the surface.

FUNCTIONAL CORRELATIONS 12.2 ■ Skin Derivatives or Appendages

Nails, **hairs**, and **sweat glands** are derivatives of the skin that develop from the downgrowth of the surface epithelium of the epidermis. During development, these appendages grow into and reside deep within the connective tissue of the **dermis**. Hairs are the hard, cornified, cylindrical structures that arise from **hair follicles** in the skin. One portion of the hair projects through the epithelium of the skin to the exterior; the other portion remains in the dermis. Hair grows from the expanded portion at the base of the hair follicle called the **hair bulb**, which consists of a **matrix** with dividing cells that produce hair growth. Also present around the hair bulb are melanocytes that provide the pigment for the hair. The base of the hair bulb is indented by a **connective tissue papilla**, a vascularized region that brings nutrients to hair follicle and where the hair cells divide, grow, cornify, and form the hairs.

Associated with each hair follicle are one or more **sebaceous glands** that produce an oily secretion called **sebum**. Sebaceous glands also develop from epidermal cells. The secretory product, sebum, forms in sebaceous glands when cells die and is expelled from the glands onto the shaft of the hair follicle. Also, extending from the connective tissue around the hair follicle to the **papillary layer** of the **dermis** are bundles of smooth muscle called **arrector pili**. The sebaceous glands are located between the arrector pili muscle and the hair follicle. Arrector pili muscles are controlled by the **autonomic nervous system** and contract during strong emotions, fear, and cold. Contraction of the arrector pili muscle erects the hair shaft, depresses the skin where it inserts, and produces a small bump on the surface of skin, called a goose bump. In addition, this contraction forces the sebum from sebaceous glands onto the hair follicle and skin. Sebum oils keep the skin smooth, waterproof it, prevent it from drying, and give it some antibacterial protection.

Sweat glands are widely distributed in skin and are of two types: eccrine and apocrine. **Eccrine** sweat glands are simple, coiled tubular glands. Their **secretory portion** is deep in the dermis, from which a coiled, stratified cuboidal **excretory duct** leads to the skin surface. The eccrine sweat glands contain two cell types: **clear cells** without secretory granules and **dark cells** with secretory granules. Secretion from the dark cells is primarily glycoproteins, whereas secretion from clear cells contains water and electrolytes, primarily Na^+ and Cl^+ of sweat. Surrounding the basal region of the secretory portion of each sweat gland are **myoepithelial cells**, whose contraction expels the secretion (sweat) from sweat glands. Eccrine sweat glands are most numerous in the skin of the palms and soles and have an important role in temperature regulation through evaporation of water from sweat. Also, as excretory structures, sweat glands excrete water, sodium salts, ammonia, uric acid, and urea.

Apocrine sweat glands are also found in the dermis and are primarily limited to the axilla, anus, and areolar regions of the breast. These glands also develop from the downgrowth of the epidermis. These sweat glands are also larger than eccrine sweat glands, and their ducts open into the **hair follicle** canal. The secretory portion of the gland is coiled and tubular. However, in contrast to eccrine sweat glands, the lumina of the secretory portion of the gland are wide and dilated, and the secretory cells are low cuboidal. The excretory ducts of the apocrine glands are also stratified cuboidal and are similar to eccrine sweat glands. Similarly, the secretory portions of the apocrine glands are surrounded by contractile **myoepithelial cells**. The apocrine sweat glands become functional at puberty, when the **sex hormones** are produced. The glands produce a **viscous secretion**, which acquires a distinct and unpleasant odor after bacterial decomposition.

FIGURE 12.12 | Glomus in Dermis of Thick Skin

Arteriovenous anastomoses are numerous in the thick skin of the fingers and toes. In some arteriovenous anastomoses, there is a direct connection between the artery and vein. In others, the arterial portion of the anastomosis forms a thick-walled structure called the **glomus** (2). The blood vessel in the glomus (2) is coiled, or convoluted, and, as a result, more than one lumen of the coiled vessel may be seen in a transverse section (2).

The smooth muscle cells in the tunica media of the glomus artery (2) have enlarged and become **epithelioid cells** (6) that become thin again before the artery empties into a venule at the **arteriovenous junction** (5).

All arteriovenous anastomoses have rich innervation and are supplied by blood vessels. A **connective tissue sheath** (7) encloses the glomus (2). The **dermis** (4) around the glomus (2) contains **blood vessels** (8), peripheral **nerves** (1), and excretory **ducts of sweat glands** (3).

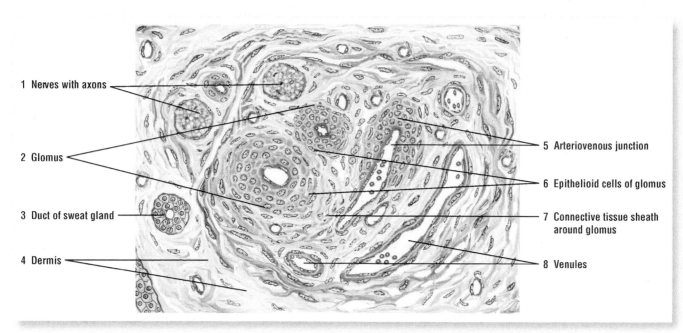

1 Nerves with axons
2 Glomus
3 Duct of sweat gland
4 Dermis
5 Arteriovenous junction
6 Epithelioid cells of glomus
7 Connective tissue sheath around glomus
8 Venules

FIGURE 12.12 ■ Glomus in the dermis of thick skin. Stain: hematoxylin and eosin. High magnification.

FUNCTIONAL CORRELATIONS 12.3 ■ **Arteriovenous Anastomoses and the Glomus**

In numerous tissues, direct communications between arteries and veins called **arteriovenous anastomoses** bypass the capillaries. Their main functions are to regulate blood pressure, blood flow, and temperature and conservation of body heat. A more complex structure for shunts is a **glomus** that consists of a highly coiled arteriovenous shunt surrounded by collagenous connective tissue. The function of the glomus is also to regulate blood flow and conserve body heat. These structures are found in the fingertips, external ear, and other peripheral areas that are exposed to extremely cold temperatures and where arteriovenous shunts are needed.

FIGURE 12.13 | **Pacinian Corpuscles in Dermis of Thick Skin (Transverse and Longitudinal Sections)**

Located deep in the **dermis** (3) of the thick skin are the **Pacinian corpuscles** (2, 9). One Pacinian corpuscle is illustrated in a longitudinal section (2) and the other in transverse section (9).

Each Pacinian corpuscle (2, 9) is ovoid with an elongated central **myelinated axon** (2b, 9b) that is surrounded by **concentric lamellae** (2a, 9a) of compact collagenous fibers that form the **connective tissue capsule** (2c, 9c). Between the connective tissue lamellae (2c, 9c) is a small amount of lymphlike fluid. In a transverse section, the layers of connective tissue lamellae (9a) surrounding the central axon (9b) of the Pacinian corpuscle (9) resemble a sliced onion.

In the dermis (3) around the Pacinian corpuscles (2, 9) are **adipose cells** (5), blood vessel **venule** (10), peripheral **nerves** (4, 6), and cross sections of an **excretory duct** (1) and the **secretory portion** of the **sweat gland** (8). The contractile **myoepithelial cells** (7) surround the secretory portion of the sweat gland (8).

The Pacinian corpuscles (2, 9) are important sensory receptors for pressure, vibration, and touch.

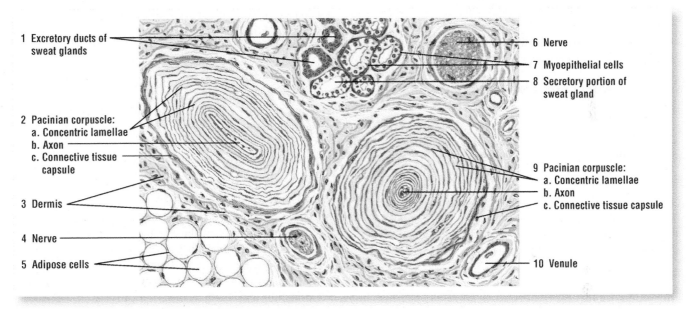

1 Excretory ducts of sweat glands

2 Pacinian corpuscle:
  a. Concentric lamellae
  b. Axon
  c. Connective tissue capsule

3 Dermis

4 Nerve

5 Adipose cells

6 Nerve

7 Myoepithelial cells

8 Secretory portion of sweat gland

9 Pacinian corpuscle:
  a. Concentric lamellae
  b. Axon
  c. Connective tissue capsule

10 Venule

FIGURE 12.13 ■ Pacinian corpuscles in the dermis of thick skin (transverse and longitudinal sections). Stain: hematoxylin and eosin. High magnification.

Chapter 12 Summary

Integumentary System

GENERAL OVERVIEW

- Skin is the largest organ; skin and its derivatives form the integumentary system
- Consists of the superficial epidermis and deeper dermis
- Nonvascular epidermis is covered by keratinized stratified squamous epithelium
- Vascular dermis contains irregular connective tissue, blood vessels, nerves, and glands
- Beneath the dermis is the hypodermis, or subcutaneous, layer of connective tissue or fascia

DERMIS: PAPILLARY AND RETICULAR LAYERS

Papillary Layer

- Basement membrane separates the dermis from the epidermis
- Is the superficial layer in the dermis and contains loose irregular connective tissue
- Dermal papillae and epidermal ridges form evaginations and interdigitations
- Connective tissue filled with fibers, cells, and blood vessels
- Sensory receptors (Meissner corpuscles) are present in the dermal papillae

Reticular Layer

- Is the deeper and thicker layer in the dermis, filled with dense irregular connective tissue
- Few cells are present, and collagen is type I
- No distinct boundary between the papillary and reticular layers
- Blends inferiorly with the hypodermis or subcutaneous layer (hypodermis) of superficial fascia
- Contains arteriovenous anastomoses and sensory receptors Pacinian corpuscles
- Concentric lamellae of collagen fibers surround myelinated axons in Pacinian corpuscles

EPIDERMAL CELL LAYERS

Stratum Basale (Germinativum): First Layer

- Deepest or basal single layer of cells that rests on the basement membrane

- Cells attached by desmosomes and by hemidesmosomes to the basement membrane
- Cells serve as stem cells for the epidermis and show increased mitotic activity
- Cells mature and migrate upward in the epidermis and produce intermediate keratin filaments

Stratum Spinosum: Second Layer

- Is the layer above the stratum basale that consists of four to six rows of cells
- During histologic preparation, cells shrink and intercellular spaces appear as spines
- Cells continue to synthesize keratin filaments that become assembled into tonofilaments
- Spines represent sites of desmosome attachments to keratin tonofilaments

Stratum Granulosum: Third Layer

- Cells above the stratum spinosum and consists of three to five cell layers of flattened cells
- Cells filled with dense keratohyalin granules and membrane-bound lamellar granules
- Keratohyalin granules consist of the protein filaggrin that cross-links with keratin filaments
- Combination of keratin tonofilaments with keratohyalin granules produces soft keratin
- Lamellar granules discharge lipid material between cells and waterproof the skin

Stratum Lucidum: Fourth Layer

- Lies superior to the stratum granulosum, found in thick skin only; translucent and barely visible
- Hydrolytic enzymes disrupt cell contents and pack them with keratin filaments

Stratum Corneum: Fifth Layer

- Most superficial layer and consists of flat, dead cells filled with soft keratin
- Keratinized cells continually shed or desquamated from the surface and replaced by new cells
- During keratinization, hydrolytic enzymes eliminate the nucleus and organelles

OTHER SKIN CELLS

Melanocytes

- Arise from neural crest cells and are located between the stratum basale and stratum spinosum
- Long irregular cytoplasmic or dendritic extensions branch into the epidermis
- Synthesize from amino acid tyrosine a dark brown pigment: melanin
- Melanin in cytoplasmic extensions phagocytized by keratinocytes in basal cell layers
- Melanin darkens skin color and protects it from ultraviolet radiation

Langerhans Cells

- Dendritic-type cells originate from the bone marrow and migrate via the blood to the skin
- Reside primarily in the stratum spinosum and are part of the immune system of the skin
- Are antigen-presenting cells of the skin and are part of immune system of the skin

Merkel Cells

- Present in the basal layer of the epidermis and most abundant in fingertips
- Associated with keratinocytes and afferent axons and function as sensory mechanoreceptors

EPIDERMIS: THICK VERSUS THIN SKIN

- Palms and soles, because of wear and tear, are covered by thick skin
- Thick skin contains sweat glands but lacks hair, sebaceous glands, and smooth muscle
- Thin skin contains sebaceous glands, hair, sweat glands, and arrector pili smooth muscle
- Keratinocytes are the predominant cell type in the epidermis
- Less numerous epidermal cells are the melanocytes, Langerhans cells, and Merkel cells

MAJOR SKIN FUNCTIONS

- Protection through the keratinized epidermis from abrasion and the entrance of pathogens
- Impermeable to water, owing to lipid layer in the epidermis
- Body temperature regulation as a result of sweating and changes in vessel diameters
- Sensory perception of touch, pain, pressure, and temperature changes because of nerve endings
- Excretions through sweat of water, sodium salts, urea, and nitrogenous waste
- Formation of vitamin D from precursor molecules produced in the epidermis when exposed to the sun

SKIN DERIVATIVES

Hairs

- Develop from the surface epithelium of the epidermis and reside deep in the dermis
- Are hard cylindrical structures that arise from hair follicles
- Surrounded by external and internal root sheaths
- Grow from the expanded hair bulb of the hair follicle
- Hair bulb indented by connective tissue (dermal) papilla that is highly vascularized
- Hair matrix situated above the papilla contains mitotic cells and melanocytes

Sebaceous Glands

- Numerous sebaceous glands associated with each hair follicle
- Cells in sebaceous glands grow, accumulate secretions, die, and become oily secretion sebum
- Smooth muscles arrector pili attach to the papillary layer of the dermis and to the sheath of the hair follicle
- Contraction of the arrector pili muscle stands hair up and forces sebum into the lumen of the hair follicle

Sweat Glands

- Widely distributed in the skin and are of two types: eccrine and apocrine
- Assist in temperature regulation and excretion of water, salts, and some nitrogenous waste

Eccrine Sweat Glands

- Are simple coiled glands located deep in the dermis in the skin of palms and soles
- Consist of clear and dark secretory cells and excretory duct
- Clear cells secrete watery product, whereas dark cells secrete mainly mucus
- Contractile myoepithelial cells surround only the secretory cells
- Excretory duct is thin, dark staining, and lined by stratified cuboidal cells
- Excretory duct ascends, straightens, and penetrates the epidermis to reach the surface of the skin

Apocrine Sweat Glands

- Found coiled in the deep dermis of the axilla, anus, and areolar regions of the breast
- Ducts of glands open into hair follicles
- Lumina are wide and dilated, with low cuboidal epithelium
- Contractile myoepithelial cells surround the secretory portion of the glands
- Become functional at puberty when sex hormones are present
- Secretion has an unpleasant odor after bacterial decomposition

Chapter 12 Review Questions

QUESTIONS

In the following multiple choice questions, choose the letter corresponding to the one best answer.

1. **Skin derivatives, such as hair and sweat glands, originate from the:**
   - A. dermis.
   - B. hypodermis.
   - C. neural crest.
   - D. connective tissue.
   - E. epithelium of the epidermis.

2. **Sweat gland secretions are expelled from the secretory portions of the gland by:**
   - A. the contraction of arrector pili muscles.
   - B. the contraction of smooth muscles around the gland.
   - C. the contraction of myoepithelial cells.
   - D. pressure from the secretory cells.
   - E. the influence of hormones.

3. **Secretions from the sebaceous gland are expelled by:**
   - A. the contraction of arrector pili muscles.
   - B. the contraction of smooth muscles around the gland.
   - C. the contraction of myoepithelial cells.
   - D. pressure from the secretory cells.
   - E. the influence of hormones.

4. **Langerhans cells originate in the:**
   - A. thymus gland.
   - B. lymph nodes.
   - C. dermis of the skin.
   - D. bone marrow.
   - E. epidermis of the skin.

5. **Meissner corpuscles are found:**
   - A. in the epidermis.
   - B. around the hair follicles.
   - C. in the stratum granulosum.
   - D. in the hypodermis.
   - E. in the dermal papillae.

ANSWERS

1. **Correct Answer: E.** Epithelium of the epidermis. Epithelial cells from the epidermis grow downward into the dermis where they form the skin derivatives.

2. **Correct Answer: C.** The contraction of myoepithelial cells. Myoepithelial cells surround the secretory portions of the glands like a basket. When they contract, the secretion is expelled from the gland.

3. **Correct Answer: A.** The contraction of arrector pili muscles. These smooth muscle fibers are attached to the connective tissue of the hair follicle and the dermis. Sebaceous glands are located between the arrector pili muscle and the hair follicle. When arrector muscle fibers contract, the sebaceous gland secretion is expelled.

4. **Correct Answer: D.** Bone marrow. From here, the cells are carried to the epidermis of the skin, where they reside and perform immune functions.

5. **Correct Answer: E.** In the dermal papilla. Dermis indents the epidermis, and Meissner corpuscles are found in some of these indentations.

ADDITIONAL HISTOLOGIC IMAGES

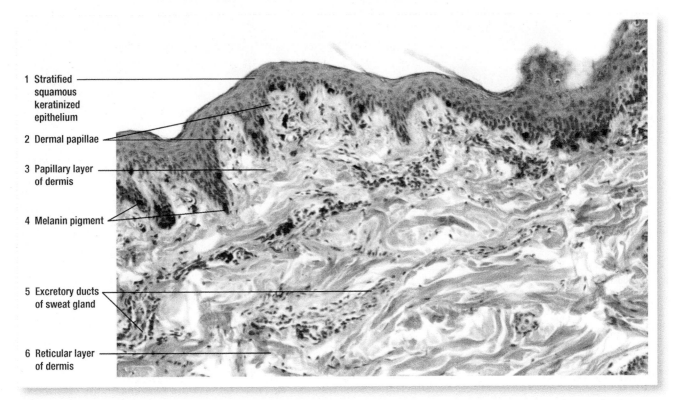

1 Stratified squamous keratinized epithelium

2 Dermal papillae

3 Papillary layer of dermis

4 Melanin pigment

5 Excretory ducts of sweat gland

6 Reticular layer of dermis

FIGURE 12.14 ■ Hairy thin skin of the human scalp illustrating hair follicles and surrounding tissues in the dermis. Stain: hematoxylin and eosin. ×40.

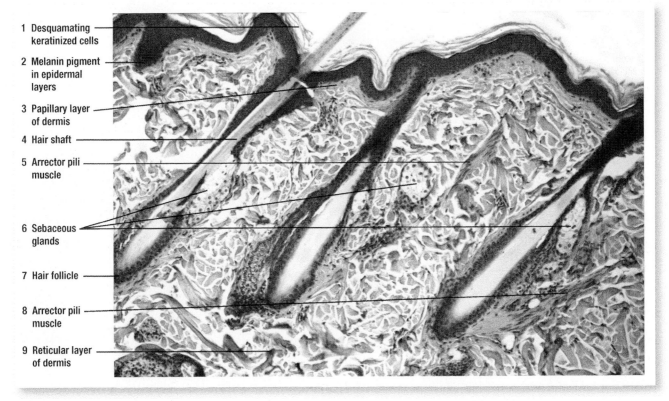

1 Desquamating keratinized cells

2 Melanin pigment in epidermal layers

3 Papillary layer of dermis

4 Hair shaft

5 Arrector pili muscle

6 Sebaceous glands

7 Hair follicle

8 Arrector pili muscle

9 Reticular layer of dermis

FIGURE 12.15 ■ A section of primate thin skin illustrating the contents of the epidermis and dermis. Stain: hematoxylin and eosin. ×40.

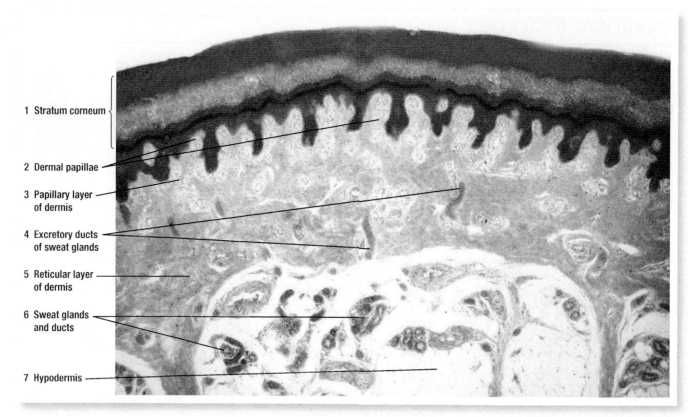

1 Stratum corneum

2 Dermal papillae

3 Papillary layer
  of dermis

4 Excretory ducts
  of sweat glands

5 Reticular layer
  of dermis

6 Sweat glands
  and ducts

7 Hypodermis

FIGURE 12.16 ■ A section of human thick skin (palm) illustrating the epidermis, dermis, and their contents. Stain: hematoxylin and eosin. ×25.

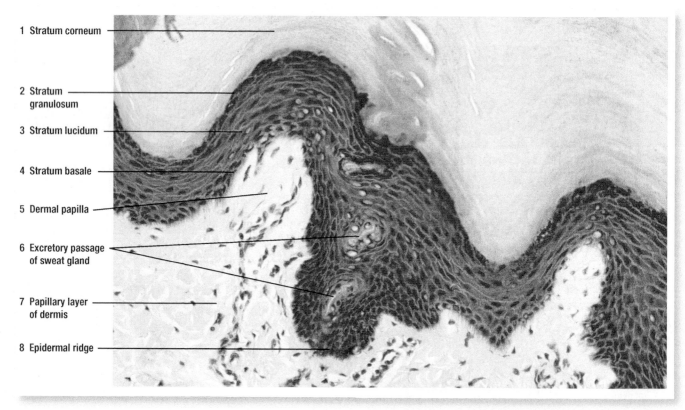

1 Stratum corneum

2 Stratum
  granulosum

3 Stratum lucidum

4 Stratum basale

5 Dermal papilla

6 Excretory passage
  of sweat gland

7 Papillary layer
  of dermis

8 Epidermal ridge

FIGURE 12.17 ■ A section of human thick skin illustrating the layers of epidermis. Stain: hematoxylin and eosin. ×40.

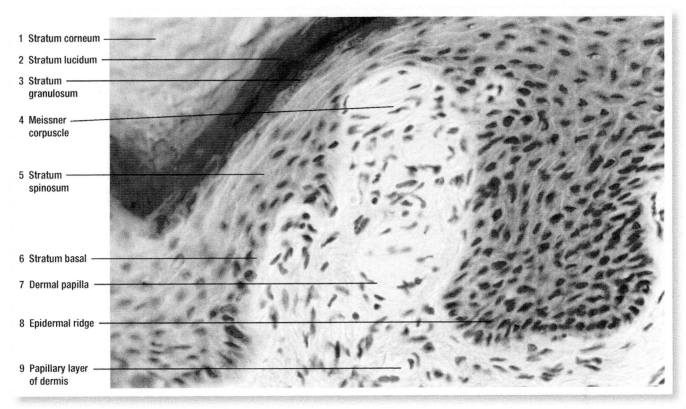

1 Stratum corneum
2 Stratum lucidum
3 Stratum granulosum
4 Meissner corpuscle
5 Stratum spinosum
6 Stratum basal
7 Dermal papilla
8 Epidermal ridge
9 Papillary layer of dermis

FIGURE 12.18 ■ High-magnification section of human thick skin illustrating the epidermal layers, a Meissner corpuscle, and the underlying dermis. Stain: hematoxylin and eosin. ×205.

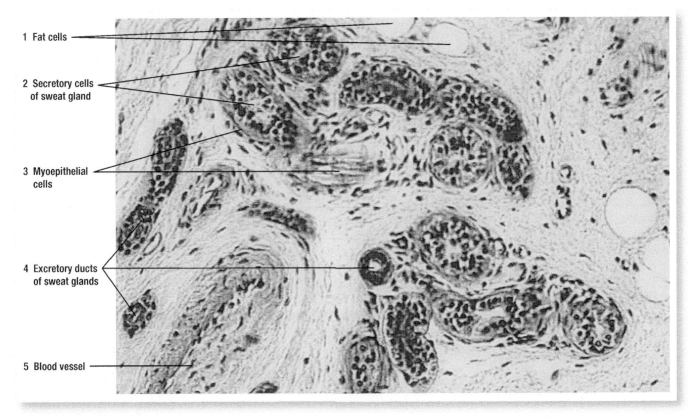

1 Fat cells
2 Secretory cells of sweat gland
3 Myoepithelial cells
4 Excretory ducts of sweat glands
5 Blood vessel

FIGURE 12.19 ■ A section of human dermis with excretory ducts and the secretory cells of the sweat glands surrounded by myoepithelial cells. Stain: hematoxylin and eosin. ×100.

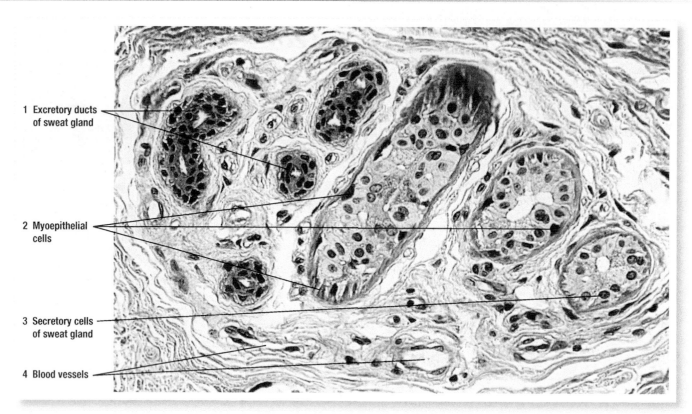

1 Excretory ducts
  of sweat gland

2 Myoepithelial
  cells

3 Secretory cells
  of sweat gland

4 Blood vessels

FIGURE 12.20 ■ Higher magnification of a human sweat gland with excretory ducts, secretory cells, and myoepithelial cells. Stain: Mallory-Azan. ×130.

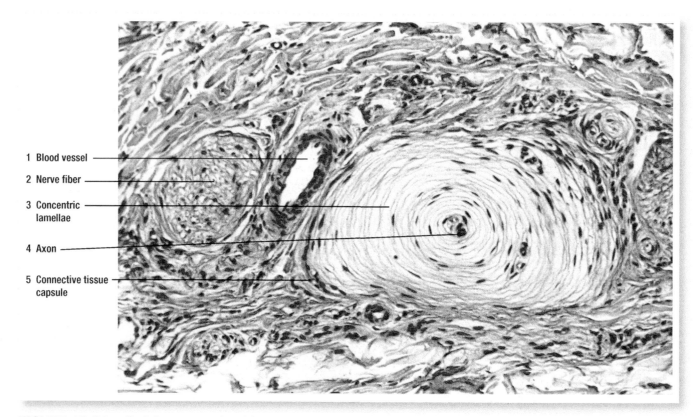

1 Blood vessel

2 Nerve fiber

3 Concentric
  lamellae

4 Axon

5 Connective tissue
  capsule

FIGURE 12.21 ■ Pacinian corpuscle with surrounding structures in the dermis of a male primate organ. Stain: hematoxylin and eosin. ×80.

Digestive System Part I: Oral Cavity and Major Salivary Glands

The digestive system consists of a long **hollow tube**, or tract, that starts at the oral cavity and terminates at the anus. The system consists of the **oral cavity, esophagus, stomach, small intestine, large intestine, rectum**, and **anal canal**. Associated with the digestive tract are the **salivary glands, liver**, and **pancreas** that are located outside the digestive tract. Their secretory products are delivered to the digestive tract through excretory ducts that penetrate the digestive tract wall and deliver their secretory products into the digestive tube.

SECTION 1 Oral Cavity

In the oral cavity, ingested food is masticated (chewed) by teeth (Fig. 13.1) and lubricated by saliva for swallowing. Because food is broken down in the oral cavity, this region is lined with a protective, nonkeratinized, **stratified squamous epithelium**, which also lines the inner or labial surface of the lips.

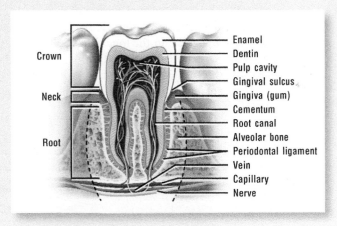

Crown

Neck

Root

Enamel
Dentin
Pulp cavity
Gingival sulcus
Gingiva (gum)
Cementum
Root canal
Alveolar bone
Periodontal ligament
Vein
Capillary
Nerve

FIGURE 13.1 ■ Sagittal section of a tooth.

LIPS

The oral cavity is formed, in part, by the lips and cheeks. The lips are lined with a very thin skin covered by a stratified squamous keratinized epithelium. Blood vessels are close to the lip surface, imparting a red color to the lips. The outer surface of the lip contains hair follicles, sebaceous glands, and sweat glands. The lips also contain skeletal muscle called **orbicularis oris**. Inside the free margin of the lip, the outer lining changes to a thicker stratified squamous nonkeratinized oral epithelium. Beneath the oral epithelium are found mucus-secreting **labial glands**.

TONGUE

The **tongue** is a muscular organ located in the oral cavity (Fig. 13.2). The core of the tongue consists of **connective tissue** and interlacing bundles of **skeletal muscle fibers**. The distribution and random orientation of individual skeletal muscle fibers in the tongue allows for its increased movement during chewing, swallowing, and speaking. The dorsal surface of the tongue is divided into an anterior two-thirds and a posterior one-third section by a V-shaped depression called the **sulcus terminalis**.

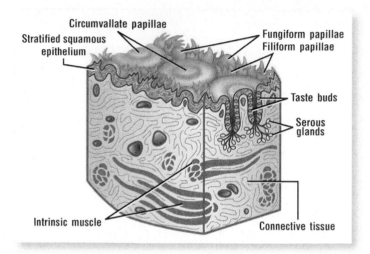

FIGURE 13.2 ■ A section of posterior tongue showing the circumvallate papillae, the location of the taste buds, and the associated serous glands.

Papillae

The epithelium on the dorsal surface of the tongue exhibits numerous elevations or projections called **papillae** (Fig. 13.3). These are indented by the underlying connective tissue called **lamina propria**. All papillae on the tongue are covered by **stratified squamous epithelium** that shows partial or incomplete **keratinization**. In contrast, the epithelium on the ventral surface of the tongue is smooth and nonkeratinized.

There are four types of papillae on the dorsal surface of the tongue: filiform, fungiform, circumvallate, and foliate (not shown).

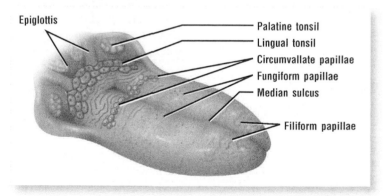

FIGURE 13.3 ■ Dorsal surface of the tongue, showing the location of different papillae and tonsils.

Filiform Papillae

The most numerous and smallest papillae on the surface of the tongue are the narrow, conical, or pointed, **filiform papillae**. They cover the entire anterior dorsal surface of the tongue and are keratinized. Filiform papillae of the tongue do not contain taste buds.

Fungiform Papillae

The less numerous but larger, broader, and taller than the filiform papillae are the **fungiform papillae**. These papillae exhibit a mushroom-like shape, project above the filiform papillae, and are prevalent in the anterior region and tip of the tongue. Fungiform papillae are scattered among the filiform papillae of the tongue surface.

Circumvallate Papillae

Circumvallate papillae are larger than the fungiform or filiform papillae. About 8 to 12 circumvallate papillae are located in the posterior region of the tongue in humans. These papillae are characterized by deep moats or **furrows** that encircle them. Numerous excretory ducts from underlying **serous (von Ebner) glands** located in the connective tissue of the tongue empty their serous secretions into the base of these furrows. Numerous taste buds are located in the stratified epithelium on the lateral sides of each papilla.

Foliate Papillae

Foliate papillae are well developed in some animals but are rudimentary or poorly developed in humans.

Taste Buds

Located in the confines of the stratified epithelium of the foliate and fungiform papillae, and on the lateral sides of the circumvallate papillae, are barrel-shaped **taste buds** (Fig. 13.4). In addition to the tongue, taste buds are found in the epithelium of the soft palate, pharynx, and epiglottis. The epithelial surface of each taste bud contains an opening called the **taste pore**. Each taste bud occupies the full thickness of the epithelium and contains three main cell types.

Located within each taste bud are elongated **gustatory (neuroepithelial or taste) cells** that extend from the base of the taste bud to the taste pore. The apices of each taste cell exhibit numerous **microvilli** that protrude through the taste pore. The bases of these taste cells form **synapses** with small afferent axons. Also present in the taste buds are elongated, supporting **sustentacular cells** that are less numerous and not sensory. At the base of each taste bud are the **basal cells** that are undifferentiated and serve as **stem cells** for the other two cell types.

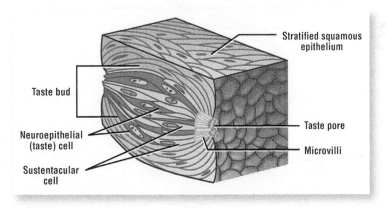

FIGURE 13.4 ■ A section of the tongue epithelium showing the taste bud and its cells spanning the entire width of the stratified squamous epithelium.

Lymphoid Aggregations: Tonsils (Palatine, Pharyngeal, and Lingual)

The tonsils are aggregates of diffuse lymphoid tissue and lymphoid nodules that are located in the oral pharynx. The **palatine tonsils** are located on the lateral walls of the oral part of the pharynx. These tonsils are lined with stratified squamous nonkeratinized epithelium and exhibit numerous **crypts**. A connective tissue capsule separates the tonsils from the adjacent tissue. The **pharyngeal tonsil** is a single structure situated in the superior and posterior portions of the pharynx. It is covered by pseudostratified ciliated epithelium. The **lingual tonsils** are located on the dorsal surface of the posterior third of the tongue and are visible as numerous small bulges composed of massed lymphoid aggregations. The lingual tonsils are lined with a stratified squamous nonkeratinized epithelium. Each tonsil is invaginated by the covering epithelium to form crypts, around which are found lymphatic nodules with germinal centers.

thePoint° Supplemental micrographic images are available at **www.thePoint.com/Eroschenko13e** under Digestive System Part I: Oral Cavity.

FIGURE 13.5 | Lip (Longitudinal Section)

Thin skin lines the external surface of the lip. The **epidermis** (**11**) exhibits stratified squamous keratinized epithelium with **desquamating surface cells** (**10**). Beneath the epidermis (**11**) is the **dermis** (**14**) with **sebaceous glands** (**2, 12**) associated with **hair follicles** (**4, 15**) and the simple tubular **sweat glands** (**16**) deeper in the dermis (**14**). The **arrector pili muscles** (**3, 13**) attach to the hair follicles (**4, 15**). Also visible in the periphery are blood vessels, an **artery** (**6a**), and a **venule** (**6b**). The core of the lip contains striated muscles, the **orbicularis oris** (**5, 17**).

The **transition zone** (**1**) between the skin epidermis (**11**) and the oral epithelium is a mucocutaneous junction. The internal or oral surface of the lip is lined with a moist, stratified, squamous nonkeratinized **oral epithelium** (**8**) that is thicker than the epithelium of the epidermis (**11**). The surface cells of the oral epithelium (**8**), without cornification, are sloughed off (desquamated) into the fluids of the **mouth** (**10**). Deeper connective tissue contains tubuloacinar and mucus-secreting **labial glands** (**9, 18**). The secretions from these glands moisten the oral mucosa. The small excretory ducts of the labial glands (**9, 18**) open into the oral cavity.

The connective tissue of the lip also contains numerous **adipose cells** (**7**), blood vessels (**6**), and numerous capillaries. Because the blood vessels (**6**) are close to the surface, the color of the blood shows through the overlying thin epithelium, giving the lips a characteristic red color.

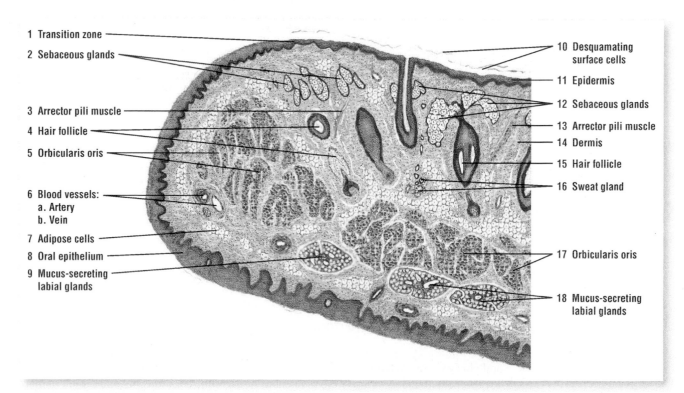

1 Transition zone
2 Sebaceous glands
3 Arrector pili muscle
4 Hair follicle
5 Orbicularis oris
6 Blood vessels:
  a. Artery
  b. Vein
7 Adipose cells
8 Oral epithelium
9 Mucus-secreting labial glands

10 Desquamating surface cells
11 Epidermis
12 Sebaceous glands
13 Arrector pili muscle
14 Dermis
15 Hair follicle
16 Sweat gland
17 Orbicularis oris
18 Mucus-secreting labial glands

FIGURE 13.5 ■ Lip (longitudinal section). Stain: hematoxylin and eosin. Low magnification.

FIGURE 13.6 | Anterior Region of Tongue: Apex (Longitudinal Section)

This illustration shows a longitudinal section of the anterior portion of the tongue. The oral cavity is lined with a protective **mucosa (5)** that consists of an outer epithelial layer (**epithelium**) **(5a)** and an underlying connective tissue layer, the **lamina propria (5b).**

The dorsal surface of the tongue is rough due to numerous mucosal projections called **papillae (1, 2, 6).** In contrast, the mucosa **(5)** of the ventral surface of the tongue is smooth. The slender, cone-shaped **filiform papillae (2, 6)** are the most numerous and cover the entire dorsal surface of the tongue. The tips of the filiform papillae **(2, 6)** show keratinization.

Less numerous are the **fungiform papillae (1)** with a broad, round surface of noncornified epithelium and a prominent core of **lamina propria (5b).**

The core of the tongue consists of crisscrossing bundles of **skeletal muscle (3, 7).** As a result, the skeletal muscles of the tongue are typically seen in longitudinal, transverse, or oblique planes of section. In the **connective tissue (9)** around the muscle bundles are **arteries (4a, 8a), veins (4b, 8b),** and **nerve fibers (11).**

In the lower half of the tongue and surrounded by skeletal muscle fibers **(3, 7)** is a section of the **anterior lingual gland (10).** This gland is of a mixed type and contains both **mucous acini (10b)** and **serous acini (10c),** as well as mixed acini. The **interlobular ducts (10a)** from the anterior lingual gland **(10)** pass into the larger **excretory duct** of the **lingual gland (12)** that opens into the oral cavity on the ventral surface of the tongue.

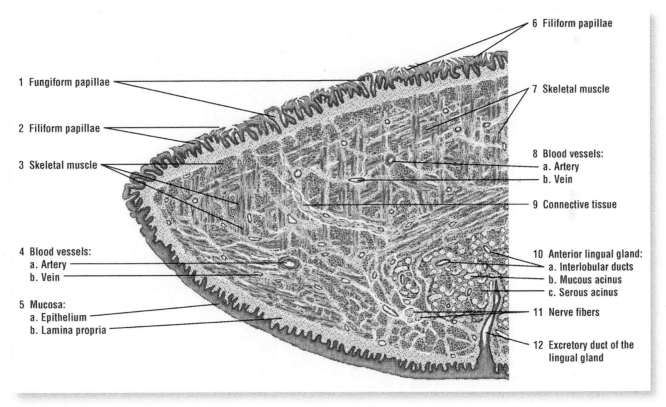

FIGURE 13.6 ■ Anterior region of the tongue: apex (longitudinal section). Stain: hematoxylin and eosin. Low magnification.

FIGURE 13.7 | Tongue: Circumvallate Papilla (Cross Section)

A cross section of a circumvallate papilla of the tongue is illustrated. The **lingual epithelium** (2) that covers the circumvallate papilla is **stratified squamous epithelium** (1). The underlying connective tissue, the **lamina propria** (3), exhibits numerous **secondary papillae** (7) that project into the overlying epithelium (1, 2) of the papilla. A deep trench, or **furrow** (5, 10), surrounds the base of each circumvallate papilla.

The oval **taste buds** (4, 9) are located in the epithelium of the lateral surfaces of the circumvallate papilla and in the epithelium on the outer wall of the furrow (5, 10). (Fig. 13.9 illustrates the taste buds in greater detail with higher magnification.)

Located deep in the lamina propria (3) and core of the tongue are numerous, **tubuloacinar serous (von Ebner) glands** (6, 11), whose **excretory ducts** (6a, 11a) open at the base of the circular furrows (5, 10). The secretory product from the **serous acini** (6b, 11b) produces solvents for taste-inducing substances.

Most of the core of the tongue consists of interlacing bundles of **skeletal muscles** (12). Examples of skeletal muscle fibers sectioned in **longitudinal** (12a) and **transverse** (12b) **planes** are abundant. This interlacing arrangement of skeletal muscles (12) gives the tongue the necessary mobility for phonating and chewing and swallowing of food. The lamina propria (3) surrounding the serous glands (6, 11) and muscles (12) also contains an abundance of **blood vessels** (8).

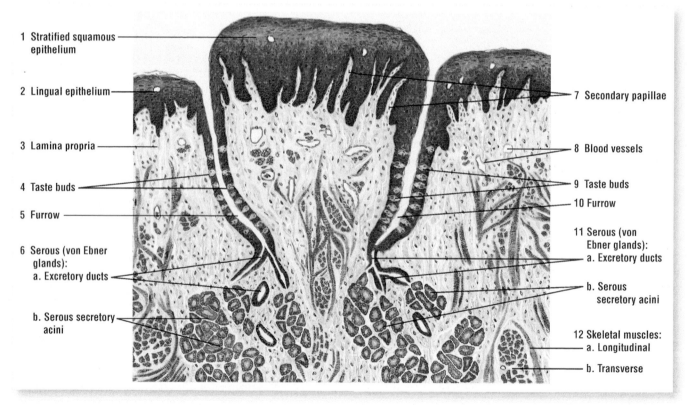

1 Stratified squamous epithelium

2 Lingual epithelium

3 Lamina propria

4 Taste buds

5 Furrow

6 Serous (von Ebner glands):
   a. Excretory ducts

   b. Serous secretory acini

7 Secondary papillae

8 Blood vessels

9 Taste buds

10 Furrow

11 Serous (von Ebner glands):
   a. Excretory ducts

   b. Serous secretory acini

12 Skeletal muscles:
   a. Longitudinal

   b. Transverse

FIGURE 13.7 ■ Tongue: circumvallate papilla (cross section). Stain: hematoxylin and eosin. Medium magnification.

FIGURE 13.8 | **Tongue: Filiform and Fungiform Papillae**

This low-power photomicrograph shows the dorsal surface of the tongue with a large **fungiform papilla** (**2**). The surface of this papilla (2) is covered by **stratified squamous epithelium** (**3**) that is not cornified or keratinized. The fungiform papilla (2) also exhibits numerous **taste buds** (**4**) located in the epithelium on the apical surface of the papilla, in contrast to the circumvallate papillae, in which the taste buds are located in the peripheral epithelium (see Fig. 13.7).

The underlying **lamina propria** (**5**) projects into the surface epithelium of the fungiform papilla (2) to form numerous indentations. Surrounding the fungiform papilla (2) are the slender **filiform papillae** (**1**), whose conical tips are covered by stratified squamous epithelium that exhibits partial keratinization.

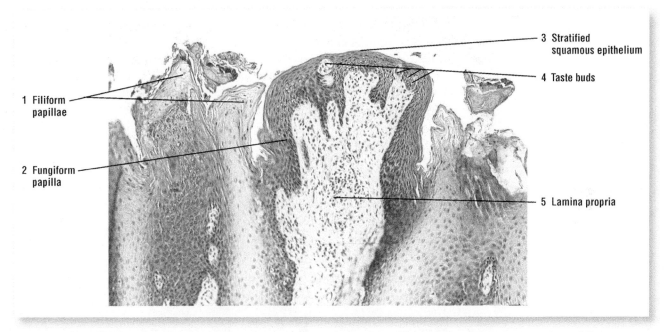

1 Filiform papillae

2 Fungiform papilla

3 Stratified squamous epithelium

4 Taste buds

5 Lamina propria

FIGURE 13.8 ■ Tongue: filiform and fungiform papillae. Stain: hematoxylin and eosin. ×25.

FUNCTIONAL CORRELATIONS 13.1 ■ Tongue and Taste Buds

The main functions of the tongue during food processing are to perceive **taste** and to assist with mastication (chewing) and swallowing of the food mass, called a **bolus**. In the oral cavity, taste sensations are detected by receptor taste cells in the **taste buds** of the **fungiform** and **circumvallate papillae** of the tongue. In addition to the tongue, taste buds are also found in the mucous membrane of the **soft palate**, **pharynx**, and **epiglottis**.

Substances to be tasted are first dissolved in the **saliva** in the oral cavity and then contact the taste cells by entering the taste pores. In addition to saliva, taste buds located in the epithelium of circumvallate papillae are continuously washed by secretions produced by the underlying **serous (von Ebner) glands**. This secretion enters the **furrow** at the base of the papillae to dissolve different substances, which enter the **taste pores** in taste buds. The receptor taste cells are stimulated by direct contact with the molecules of dissolved substances, which in turn stimulate the afferent nerve fibers with which the taste cells synapse and conduct the information to the brain for taste interpretation and detection. Fully tasting food requires olfaction in addition to taste bud activation.

There are four basic taste sensations: **sour**, **salt**, **bitter**, and **sweet**. A fifth type of taste, called **umami** (savory), is sensed by receptors for glutamate, found in salt form as monosodium glutamate. All remaining taste sensations are various combinations of the basic four tastes. It is now believed that the sensitivity to all tastes is equally distributed across the entire tongue. However, it is also believed that some areas of the tongue may be more sensitive to a certain specific type of taste than to others.

FIGURE 13.9 | Tongue: Taste Buds

The taste **buds** (**5, 12**) at the bottom of a **furrow** (**14**) of the circumvallate papilla are illustrated in greater detail. The taste buds (5, 12) are embedded within and extend the full thickness of the stratified **lingual epithelium** (**1**). The taste buds (5, 12) are distinguished from the surrounding stratified epithelium (1) by their oval shapes and elongated cells (modified columnar) that are arranged perpendicular to the epithelium (1).

Three different types of cells can be identified in the taste buds (5, 12). The supporting, or **sustentacular cells** (**3, 8**), are elongated and exhibit a darker cytoplasm and a slender, dark nucleus. The **taste cells**, or **gustatory cells** (**7, 11**), exhibit a lighter cytoplasm and a more oval, lighter nucleus. The **basal cells** (**13**) are located at the periphery of the taste bud (5, 12) near the basement membrane. The basal cells (13) give rise to both the sustentacular cells (3, 8) and the gustatory cells (7, 11).

Each taste bud (5, 12) exhibits a small opening onto the epithelial surface called the **taste pore** (**9**). The apical surfaces of both the sustentacular cells (3, 8) and the gustatory cells (7, 11) exhibit long **microvilli (taste hairs)** (**4**) that extend into and protrude through the taste pore (9) into the furrow (14) around the circumvallate papilla.

The underlying **lamina propria** (**2**) adjacent to the epithelium and the taste buds (5, 12) consists of a loose connective tissue with numerous **blood vessels** (**6, 10**) and nerve fibers.

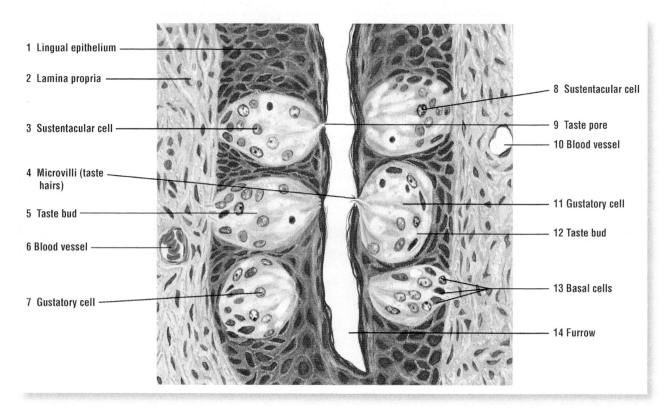

1 Lingual epithelium
2 Lamina propria
3 Sustentacular cell
4 Microvilli (taste hairs)
5 Taste bud
6 Blood vessel
7 Gustatory cell
8 Sustentacular cell
9 Taste pore
10 Blood vessel
11 Gustatory cell
12 Taste bud
13 Basal cells
14 Furrow

FIGURE 13.9 ■ Tongue: taste buds. Stain: hematoxylin and eosin. High magnification.

FIGURE 13.10 | **Posterior Tongue: Behind Circumvallate Papilla and Near Lingual Tonsil (Longitudinal Section)**

The anterior two thirds of the tongue are separated from the posterior third of the tongue by a depression or a sulcus terminalis. The posterior region is located behind the circumvallate papillae and near the lingual tonsils. The dorsal surface of the posterior region exhibits large **mucosal ridges** (1) and elevations or **folds** (7) that resemble the large fungiform papillae of the anterior tongue. A **stratified squamous epithelium** (6) without keratinization covers the mucosal ridges (1) and the folds (7). The filiform and fungiform papillae of the anterior region of the tongue are absent from the posterior tongue. Lymphatic nodules of the lingual tonsils can be seen in these folds (7).

The lamina **propria** (7) of the mucosa is wider but similar to the anterior two thirds of the tongue. Under the stratified squamous epithelium (6) are aggregations of diffuse **lymphatic tissue** (2) and **adipose tissue** (4), **nerve fibers** (3) (in longitudinal section), blood vessels, an **artery** (8), and a **vein** (9).

Deep in the connective tissue of the lamina propria (7) and between the interlacing **skeletal muscle fibers** (5) are mucous acini of the **posterior lingual glands** (11) whose **excretory ducts** (10) open onto the dorsal surface of the tongue, between bases of the mucosal ridges and folds (1, 7).

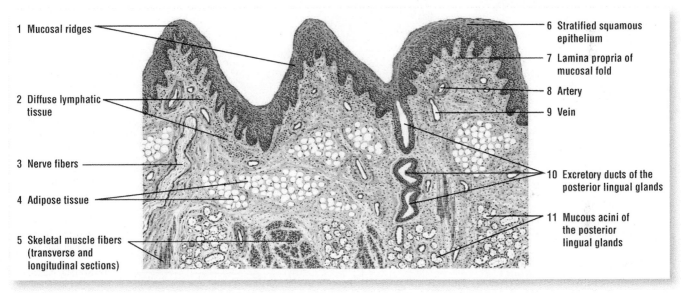

1 Mucosal ridges

2 Diffuse lymphatic tissue

3 Nerve fibers

4 Adipose tissue

5 Skeletal muscle fibers (transverse and longitudinal sections)

6 Stratified squamous epithelium

7 Lamina propria of mucosal fold

8 Artery

9 Vein

10 Excretory ducts of the posterior lingual glands

11 Mucous acini of the posterior lingual glands

FIGURE 13.10 ■ Posterior tongue: behind circumvallate papillae and near lingual tonsil (longitudinal section). Stain: hematoxylin and eosin. Low magnification.

FIGURE 13.11 | Lingual Tonsils (Transverse Section)

Lingual tonsils are aggregations of small, individual tonsils, each with its **tonsillar crypt (2, 8)** that are situated on the dorsal surface of the posterior region or the root of the tongue. A nonkeratinized **stratified squamous epithelium (1)** lines the tonsils and their crypts (2, 8). The tonsillar crypts (2, 8) form deep invaginations and may extend into the **lamina propria (5)**.

Lymphatic **nodules (3, 9)**, some with **germinal centers (3, 9)**, are located in the lamina propria (5) below the stratified squamous surface epithelium (1). Dense **lymphatic infiltration (4, 10)** surrounds the individual lymphatic nodules (3, 9). Also in the lamina propria (5) are fat cells of the **adipose tissue (7)** and the secretory **mucous acini** of the **posterior lingual glands (11)**. Small excretory ducts from the lingual glands (11) form larger **excretory ducts (6)** that often open into the tonsillar crypts (2, 8). Others open directly on the lingual surface. Interspersed among the connective tissue of the lamina propria (5), the adipose tissue (7), and the secretory mucous acini of the posterior lingual glands (11) are **skeletal muscle fibers (12)** of the tongue.

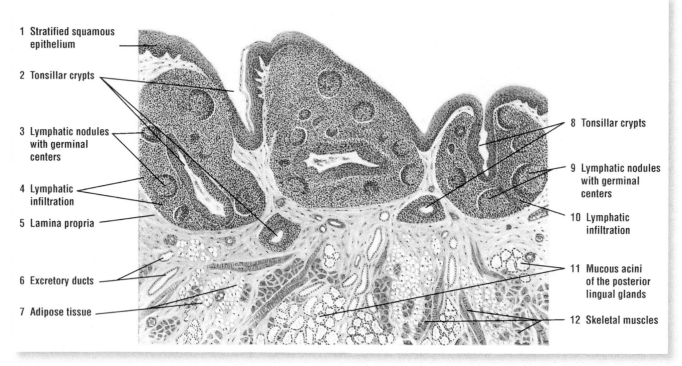

1 Stratified squamous epithelium

2 Tonsillar crypts

3 Lymphatic nodules with germinal centers

4 Lymphatic infiltration

5 Lamina propria

6 Excretory ducts

7 Adipose tissue

8 Tonsillar crypts

9 Lymphatic nodules with germinal centers

10 Lymphatic infiltration

11 Mucous acini of the posterior lingual glands

12 Skeletal muscles

FIGURE 13.11 ■ Lingual tonsils (transverse section). Stain: hematoxylin and eosin. Low magnification.

FIGURE 13.12 | Dried Tooth (Longitudinal Section)

This illustration shows a longitudinal section of a dried, nondecalcified, and unstained tooth. The mineralized parts of a tooth are the enamel, dentin, and cementum. **Dentin** (**3**) is covered by **enamel** (**1**) in the region that projects above the gum. Enamel is not present at the root of the tooth, and dentin is covered by **cementum** (**6**). Cementum (6) contains lacunae with the cementum-producing cells called cementocytes and their connecting canaliculi. Dentin (3) surrounds both the **pulp cavity** (**5**) and its extension into the root of the tooth as the **root canal** (**11**). In life, the pulp cavity and root canal are filled with fine connective tissue, fibroblasts, histiocytes, and dentin-forming cells, the odontoblasts. Blood capillaries and nerves enter the pulp cavity (5) through an **apical foramen** (**13**) at the tip of each root.

Dentin (3) exhibits wavy, parallel dentinal tubules. The earlier, or primary, dentin is located at the periphery of the tooth. The latter, or secondary, dentin lies along the pulp cavity, where it is formed throughout life by odontoblasts. In the crown of a dried tooth at the **dentinoenamel junction** (**2**) are numerous irregular, air-filled spaces that appear black in the section. In life, these **interglobular spaces** (**4**, **10**) are filled with incompletely calcified dentin (interglobular dentin). Similar areas, but smaller and spaced closer together, are present in the root, close to the dentinal–cementum junction, where they form the **granular layer (of Tomes)** (**12**).

The dentin in the crown of the tooth is covered with a thicker layer of enamel (1), composed of enamel rods or prisms held together by an interprismatic cementing substance. The **lines of Retzius** (**7**) represent the variations in the rate of enamel deposition. Light rays passing through a dried section of the tooth are refracted by twists that occur in the enamel rods as they course toward the surface; these are the light **lines of Schreger** (**8**). Poor calcification of enamel rods during enamel formation can produce **enamel tufts** (**9**) that extend from the dentinoenamel junction into the enamel (see Fig. 13.13).

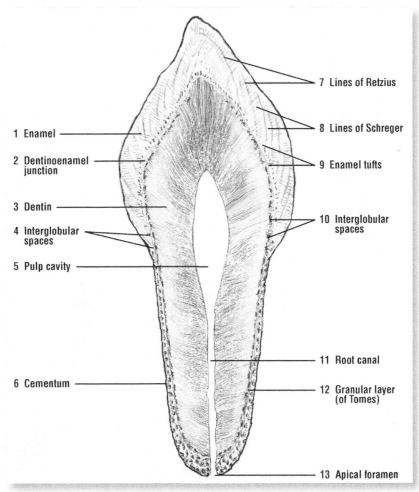

FIGURE 13.12 ■ Dried tooth (longitudinal section). Ground and unstained. Low magnification.

FIGURE 13.13 | Dried Tooth: Dentinoenamel Junction

A section of the **dentin matrix** (4) and **enamel** (5) at the **dentinoenamel junction** (1) is illustrated at a higher magnification. The enamel is produced by cells called ameloblasts as successive segments that form elongated **enamel rods** or **prisms** (7). The **enamel tufts** (6), which are the poorly calcified, twisted enamel rods or prisms, extend from the dentinoenamel junction (1) into the enamel (5). The dentin matrix (4) is produced by cells called odontoblasts. The odontoblastic processes of the odontoblasts occupy tunnel-like spaces in the dentin, forming the clearly visible **dentin tubules** (3) and black, air-filled **interglobular spaces** (2).

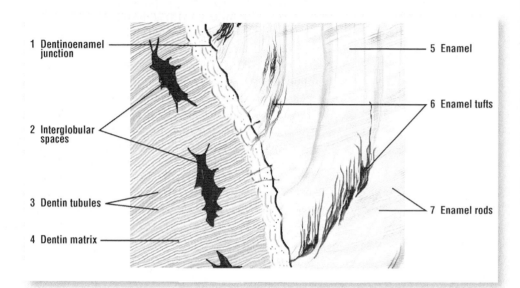

FIGURE 13.13 ■ Dried tooth: dentinoenamel junction. Ground and unstained. Medium magnification.

FIGURE 13.14 | Dried Tooth: Cementum and Dentin Junction

The junction between the **dentin matrix** (5) and **cementum** (2) is illustrated at a higher magnification. At the junction of the cementum (2) with the dentin matrix (5) is a layer of small interglobular spaces, the **granular layer of Tomes** (7). Internal to this layer in the dentin matrix (5) are the large, irregular **interglobular spaces** (4, 8) commonly seen in the crown of the tooth, but may also be seen in the root of the tooth.

Cementum (2) is a thin layer of bony material secreted by cells cementoblasts (mature forms, cementocytes) with **lacunae** (1) that house the cementocytes and exhibit **canaliculi** (3) for the cytoplasmic processes of cementocytes.

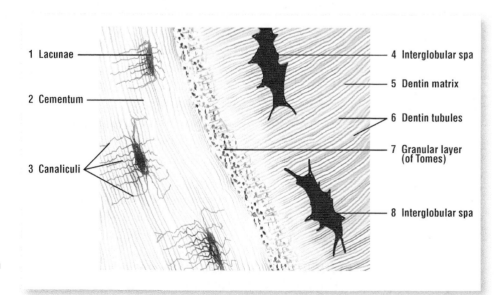

FIGURE 13.14 ■ Dried tooth: cementum and dentin junction. Ground and unstained. Medium magnification.

FIGURE 13.15 | **Developing Tooth (Longitudinal Section)**

A developing tooth is shown embedded in a socket, the **dental alveolus (23)** in the jaw **bone (9)**. The stratified squamous nonkeratinized **oral epithelium (1, 11)** covers the developing tooth and the underlying connective tissue **lamina propria (2, 12)**. A downgrowth from the oral epithelium (1, 11) invades the lamina propria (2, 12) and the primitive connective tissue as the **dental lamina (3)**. The primitive **connective tissue (8, 17)** surrounds the developing tooth and forms a **dental sac (8, 17)** around the tooth.

The dental lamina (3) from the oral epithelium (1, 11) proliferates and gives rise to a cap-shaped enamel organ that consists of the **external enamel epithelium (4)**, the extracellular **stellate reticulum (5, 14)**, and the enamel-forming **ameloblasts** of the **inner enamel epithelium (6)**. The ameloblasts of the inner enamel epithelium (6) secrete the hard **enamel (7, 13)** around the **dentin (16)**. The enamel (7, 13) appears as a narrow band of dark, red-staining material.

At the concave or the opposite end of the enamel organ, the **dental papilla (21)** originates from the primitive connective tissue **mesenchyme (21)** and forms the dental pulp or core of the developing tooth. **Blood vessels (20)** and nerves innervate the dental papilla (21) from below. The mesenchymal cells in the dental papilla (21) differentiate into **odontoblasts (15, 19)** and form the outer margin of the dental papilla (21). The odontoblasts (15) secrete an uncalcified dentin called **predentin (18)** that calcifies and forms a layer of pink-staining dentin (16) adjacent to the dark-staining enamel (7, 13).

At the base of the tooth, the external enamel epithelium (4) and the ameloblasts of the inner enamel epithelium (6) grow downward and form the bilayered **epithelial root sheath (of Hertwig) (10, 22)** that induces the adjacent mesenchyme (21) cells to differentiate into odontoblasts (15, 19) and to form dentin (16).

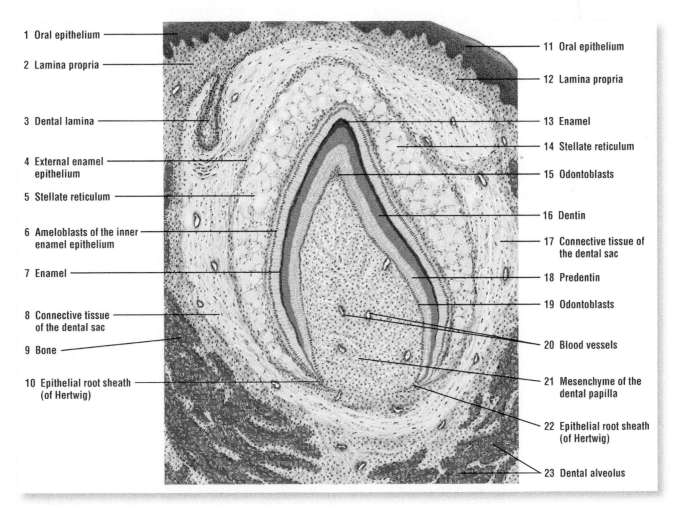

1 Oral epithelium
2 Lamina propria
3 Dental lamina
4 External enamel epithelium
5 Stellate reticulum
6 Ameloblasts of the inner enamel epithelium
7 Enamel
8 Connective tissue of the dental sac
9 Bone
10 Epithelial root sheath (of Hertwig)

11 Oral epithelium
12 Lamina propria
13 Enamel
14 Stellate reticulum
15 Odontoblasts
16 Dentin
17 Connective tissue of the dental sac
18 Predentin
19 Odontoblasts
20 Blood vessels
21 Mesenchyme of the dental papilla
22 Epithelial root sheath (of Hertwig)
23 Dental alveolus

FIGURE 13.15 ■ Developing tooth (longitudinal section). Stain: hematoxylin and eosin. Low magnification.

FIGURE 13.16 | Developing Tooth: Dentinoenamel Junction in Detail

A section of the dentinoenamel junction from a developing tooth is illustrated at high magnification. On the left side is an area of **stellate reticulum** (**1**) of the enamel adjacent to the columnar **ameloblasts** (**2**) that secrete the **enamel** (**3**). During enamel (3) formation, the apical extensions of ameloblasts are transformed into terminal processes (of Tomes). The mature enamel (3) consists of calcified, elongated enamel rods (4) or prisms that are barely visible in the dark-stained enamel (3). The **enamel rods** (**4**) extend through the thickness of the enamel (3).

The right side shows the nuclei of **mesenchymal cells** in the **dental papilla** (**5**). The **odontoblasts** (**6**) are located adjacent to the dental papilla (5) and secrete the uncalcified organic matrix of **predentin** (**8**) that calcifies into **dentin** (**9**). The odontoblasts (6) exhibit slender **processes (of Tomes)** (**7**) that penetrate both the predentin (8) and the dentin (9).

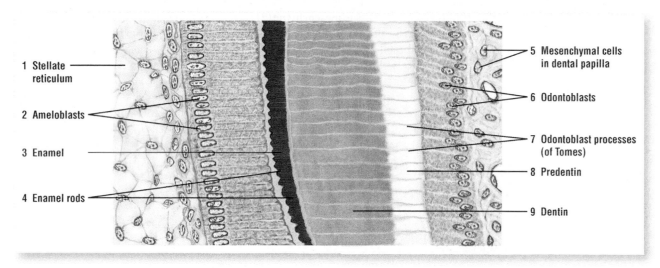

1 Stellate reticulum
2 Ameloblasts
3 Enamel
4 Enamel rods

5 Mesenchymal cells in dental papilla
6 Odontoblasts
7 Odontoblast processes (of Tomes)
8 Predentin
9 Dentin

FIGURE 13.16 ■ Developing tooth: dentinoenamel junction in detail. Stain: hematoxylin and eosin. High magnification.

SECTION 2 Major Salivary Glands

There are three major **salivary glands** for the oral cavity: parotid, submandibular, and sublingual. Salivary glands are located outside the oral cavity and convey their secretions into the mouth via **excretory ducts**. The paired **parotid glands** are the largest of the salivary glands, located anterior and inferior to the external ear. The smaller and also paired **submandibular (submaxillary) glands** are located inferior to the mandible in the floor of the mouth. The smallest salivary glands are the **sublingual glands**; these are aggregates of smaller glands located inferior to the tongue.

Salivary glands are surrounded by dense connective tissue capsules from which septa subdivide the secretory areas into lobes and lobules. Each salivary gland is composed of cellular **secretory units** called **acini** (singular, acinus) and **excretory ducts** with variable histologic features, depending on their location in the gland. The secretory units are small, saclike dilations located at the beginning of the first segment of the excretory duct system called the **intercalated ducts**.

CELLS OF SALIVARY GLAND ACINI

Secretory cells of salivary glands are of two types: serous or mucous. The acini exhibit either serous cells that produce protein-rich watery secretions or mucous cells that secrete mucus or a mixture of acini cells that produce both types of secretions (Fig. 13.17).

Serous cells in the acini are pyramidal in shape. Their spherical nuclei are displaced basally due to accumulation of secretory granules in the upper or apical regions of the cytoplasm.

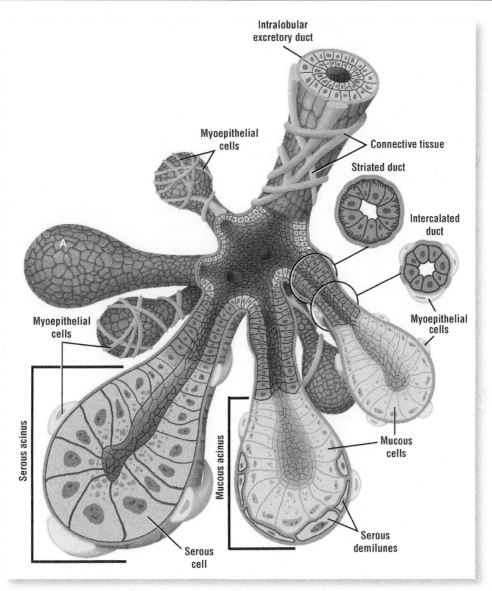

FIGURE 13.17 ■ Salivary glands. The different types of acini (serous, mucous, and mixed, with serous demilunes), different duct types (intercalated, striated, and interlobular), and myoepithelial cells of a salivary gland are illustrated.

Mucous cells are similar in shape to serous cells, except their cytoplasm is completely filled with light-staining, secretory product **mucus** that flattens the nucleus and displaces it to the base of the cytoplasm.

In some salivary glands, both mucous and serous cells are in the same secretory acinus. In these mixed acini, where mucous cells predominate, serous cells form a crescent, or moon-shaped, cap over the mucous cells. In routine histologic preparations, these serous crescent-like structures are called **serous demilunes**. With new rapid freezing techniques, however, it is believed that these demilunes may be artifacts of fixation. The secretions from serous cells in the demilunes enter the lumen of the acinus through tiny intercellular canaliculi between mucous cells.

Contractile **myoepithelial cells** are flattened cells that surround both the serous and mucous acini and the initial portion of the duct system, the intercalated ducts. They are sometimes called "basket cells" because they surround the acini with their cytoplasmic branches like a basket. Myoepithelial cells are located between the cell membrane of the secretory cells in acini and the surrounding basement membrane.

SALIVARY GLAND DUCTS

Connective tissue fibers subdivide the salivary glands into numerous **lobules**, which contain the secretory units and their excretory ducts.

Intercalated Ducts

Serous and mucous, as well as mixed seromucous acini, empty their secretions into the initial and smallest **intercalated ducts** with tiny lumina lined with a low cuboidal epithelium. Contractile myoepithelial cells surround the acini and portions of intercalated ducts.

Striated Ducts

Several intercalated ducts merge to form the larger **striated ducts**. These ducts are lined with a columnar epithelium and, with proper staining, exhibit tiny basal striations that correspond to the basal infoldings of the cell membrane and the cellular interdigitations. Located in the basal infoldings are numerous and elongated mitochondria.

Serous glands have well-developed intercalated ducts and striated ducts in contrast to mucous glands that exhibit poorly developed intercalated ducts and striated ducts.

Excretory Intralobular Ducts

Striated ducts join to form larger **intralobular ducts** of gradually increasing size, surrounded by increasing layers of connective tissue.

Interlobular and Interlobar Ducts

Intralobular ducts join to form the larger **interlobular ducts** and **interlobar ducts**. The terminal portion of these large ducts conveys saliva from salivary glands to the oral cavity and constitutes the main ducts of each salivary gland. As the interlobular and interlobar excretory ducts increase in size, the lining epithelium may be lined with either stratified low cuboidal or stratified columnar cells (see Fig. 13.17).

thePoint®   Supplemental micrographic images are available at **www.thePoint.com/Eroschenko13e** under Digestive System Part I: Oral Cavity.

FIGURE 13.18 | Parotid Salivary Gland

The parotid salivary gland is a large serous gland classified as a compound tubuloacinar gland. This illustration depicts a section of the parotid gland at a lower magnification, with details of specific structures represented at a higher magnification in separate boxes below.

The parotid gland is surrounded by a capsule from which arise numerous **interlobular connective tissue septa** (6) that subdivide the gland into lobes and lobules. Located in the connective tissue septa (6) are **arteriole** (9), **venule** (1), and **interlobular excretory ducts** (2, 13, IV).

Each salivary gland lobule contains pyramid-shaped secretory cells arranged around a lumen forming the **serous acini** (5, 8, I). The spherical nuclei of the serous cells (I) are located at the base of the slightly basophilic cytoplasm. In certain sections, the lumen in serous acini (5, 8, I) is not always visible. At a higher magnification, small **secretory granules** (I) are visible in the apices of these cells (5, 8, I). The number of secretory granules in serous cells varies with the functional activity of the gland. All serous acini (5, 8, I) are surrounded by thin, contractile **myoepithelial cells** (7, I) located between the basement membrane and the serous cells (5, 8, I). Because of their small size, in some sections, only the myoepithelial cells nuclei are visible (7, I). Some parotid gland lobules may contain **adipose cells** (3) that appear as clear oval structures surrounded by darker-staining serous acini (5, 8, I).

The secretory serous acini (5, 8, I) empty their product into the narrow **intercalated ducts** (10, 12, II). These ducts have small lumina, are lined with a simple squamous or a low cuboidal epithelium, and are often surrounded by myoepithelial cells (see Fig. 13.19). The secretory product from the intercalated ducts (10, 12, II) drains into larger **striated ducts** (11, III) with larger lumina that are lined with simple columnar cells that exhibit basal striations (11, III). The striations in the striated ducts (11, III) are formed by deep infoldings of the basal cell membrane.

The striated ducts (11, III), in turn, empty their product into the **intralobular excretory ducts** (**4**) located within the lobules of the gland. These ducts join larger interlobular excretory ducts (2, 13, IV) in the connective tissue septa (6) around the salivary gland lobules. The lumina of interlobular excretory ducts (2, 13, IV) become progressively wider and the epithelium can increase from columnar to pseudostratified or even stratified columnar in large excretory (lobar) ducts that drain the parotid gland lobes.

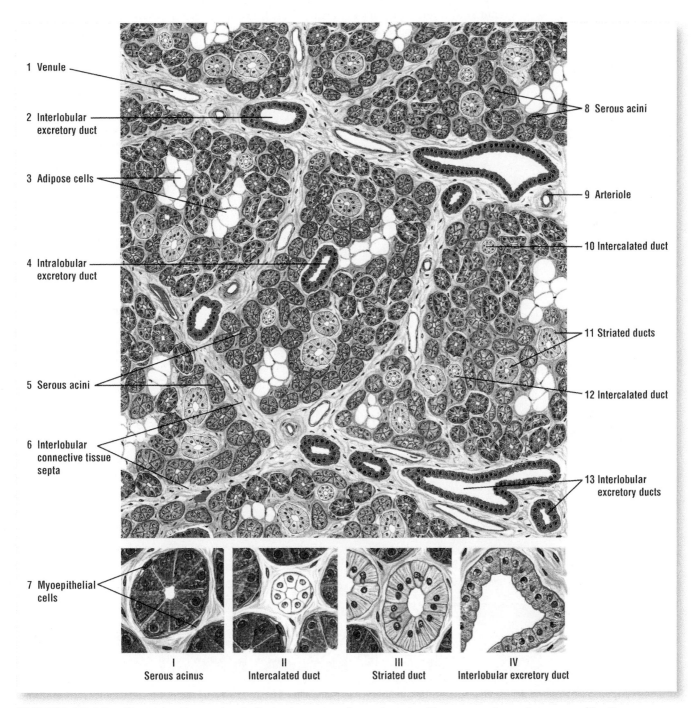

1 Venule

2 Interlobular excretory duct

3 Adipose cells

4 Intralobular excretory duct

5 Serous acini

6 Interlobular connective tissue septa

7 Myoepithelial cells

8 Serous acini

9 Arteriole

10 Intercalated duct

11 Striated ducts

12 Intercalated duct

13 Interlobular excretory ducts

| I | II | III | IV |
| Serous acinus | Intercalated duct | Striated duct | Interlobular excretory duct |

FIGURE 13.18 ■ Parotid salivary gland. Stain: hematoxylin and eosin. *Upper panel:* medium magnification. *Lower panel:* high magnification.

FIGURE 13.19 | Submandibular Salivary Gland

The submandibular salivary gland is a mixed compound tubuloacinar gland with both serous and mucous acini, with serous acini predominating. The presence of serous and mucous acini distinguishes the submandibular gland from the parotid gland, which is a purely serous gland.

This illustration depicts several lobules of the submandibular gland in which **mucous acini** (**5, 11, 13, II**) are intermixed with **serous acini** (**6, I**). The detailed features of different acini and ducts of the gland are illustrated at a higher magnification in separate boxes below.

The serous acini (6, I) are similar to those in the parotid gland (Fig. 13.18). They are characterized by smaller, darker-stained pyramidal cells, spherical basal nuclei, and apical secretory granules. In contrast, the mucous acini (5, 11, 13, II) are larger, have larger lumina, and exhibit variable sizes and shapes. The mucous cells (5, 11, 13, II) are columnar with pale or almost colorless cytoplasm after staining with flattened nuclei pressed against the base of the cell membrane.

In mixed seromucous acini, the mucous acini are normally surrounded or capped by one or more serous cells, forming a crescent-shaped **serous demilune** (**7, 10**). The thin, contractile

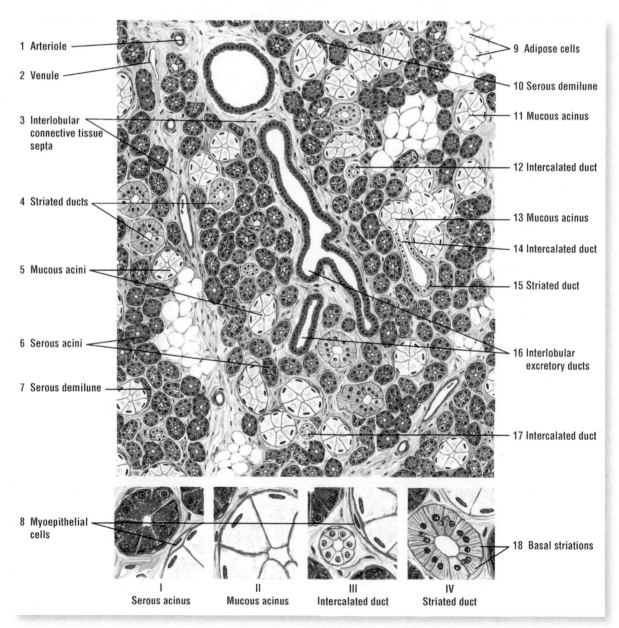

1 Arteriole
2 Venule
3 Interlobular connective tissue septa
4 Striated ducts
5 Mucous acini
6 Serous acini
7 Serous demilune
8 Myoepithelial cells

9 Adipose cells
10 Serous demilune
11 Mucous acinus
12 Intercalated duct
13 Mucous acinus
14 Intercalated duct
15 Striated duct
16 Interlobular excretory ducts
17 Intercalated duct
18 Basal striations

I	II	III	IV
Serous acinus	Mucous acinus	Intercalated duct	Striated duct

FIGURE 13.19 ■ Submandibular salivary gland. Stain: hematoxylin and eosin. *Upper panel:* medium magnification. *Lower panel:* high magnification.

myoepithelial cells (8) surround the serous (I) and mucous (II) acini and the **intercalated ducts (III)**.

The duct system of the submandibular gland is similar to that of the parotid gland. The small intralobular **intercalated ducts (12, 14, 17, III)** have small lumina and are shorter, whereas the **striated ducts (4, 15, IV)** with distinct **basal striations (18)** in the cells are longer than in the parotid gland. This figure illustrates a mucous acinus (13) opening into an intercalated duct (14) that joins a larger striated duct (15). Interlobular excretory ducts (16) are located in the **interlobular connective tissue septa (3)** with nerves, an **arteriole (1)**, a **venule (2)**, and **adipose cells (9)**.

FIGURE 13.20 | Sublingual Salivary Gland

The sublingual salivary gland is also a compound, mixed tubuloacinar gland that resembles the submandibular gland because it contains both **serous (11)** and the conspicuous **mucous acini (9, I, II)**. Most of the acini, however, are mucous (9, I, II) and are capped with **serous**

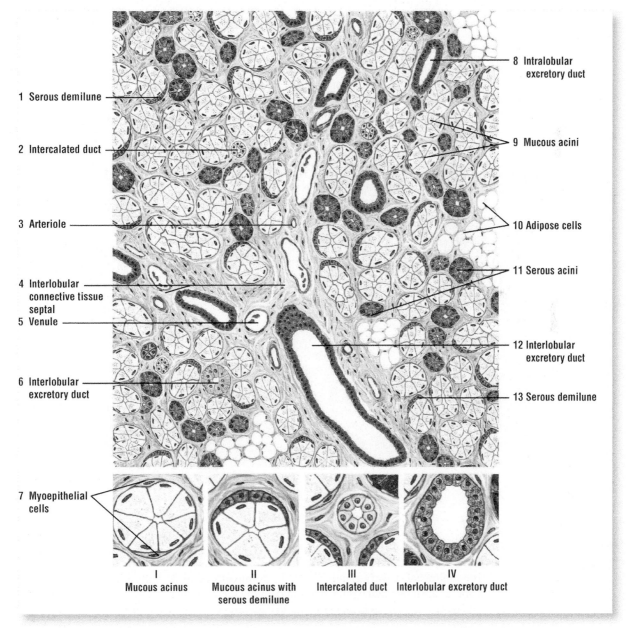

1 Serous demilune

2 Intercalated duct

3 Arteriole

4 Interlobular connective tissue septal

5 Venule

6 Interlobular excretory duct

7 Myoepithelial cells

8 Intralobular excretory duct

9 Mucous acini

10 Adipose cells

11 Serous acini

12 Interlobular excretory duct

13 Serous demilune

I	II	III	IV
Mucous acinus	Mucous acinus with serous demilune	Intercalated duct	Interlobular excretory duct

FIGURE 13.20 ■ Sublingual salivary gland. Stain: hematoxylin and eosin. *Upper panel:* medium magnification. *Lower panel:* high magnification.

demilunes (**1, 13, II**). Purely serous acini (**11**) are less numerous in the sublingual gland; however, the seromucous composition of each gland varies. In this illustration, serous acini (**11**) appear frequently, whereas in other sections of the sublingual gland, serous acini (**11**) may be absent. At a higher magnification, the **myoepithelial cells** (**7, I**) surround individual serous and mucous acini (**I**).

In comparison with other salivary glands, the duct system of the sublingual gland is different. The **intercalated ducts** (**2, III**) are short or absent and not readily observed. In contrast, the nonstriated **intralobular excretory ducts** (**6, 8, IV**) are more prevalent. These excretory ducts (**6, 8, IV**) are equivalent to the striated ducts of the submandibular and parotid glands but lack the membrane infolding and basal striations.

The **interlobular connective tissue septa** (**4**) are more abundant in the sublingual glands than in the parotid and submandibular glands. An **arteriole** (**3**), a **venule** (**5**), nerve fibers, and **interlobular excretory ducts** (**12**) are seen in the septa. The epithelial lining of the interlobular excretory ducts (**12**) varies from low columnar in the smaller ducts to pseudostratified or stratified columnar in the larger ducts. In addition, the oval **adipose cells** (**10**) are seen scattered in the connective tissue.

FIGURE 13.21 | Serous Salivary Gland: Parotid Gland

This photomicrograph illustrates a section of the parotid salivary gland. In humans, the parotid gland is entirely composed of serous acini (**1**) and excretory ducts. In this illustration, the **serous acini** (**1**) are filled with tiny secretory granules. A small **intercalated duct** (**2**) with its cuboidal epithelium is surrounded by the serous acini (**1**). Also on the right side is a larger, lighter-stained excretory duct, the **striated duct** (**3**).

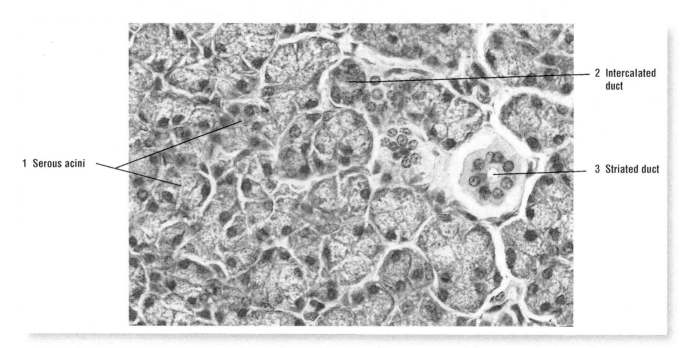

1 Serous acini
2 Intercalated duct
3 Striated duct

FIGURE 13.21 ■ Serous salivary gland: parotid gland. Stain: hematoxylin and eosin. ×165.

FIGURE 13.22 | Mixed Salivary Gland: Sublingual Gland

The sublingual salivary gland exhibits both **mucous acini** (**2**) and **serous acini** (**3**). The mucous acini (**2**) are larger and lighter staining than the serous acini (**3**), and their cytoplasm is filled with **mucus** (**1**). The serous acini (**3**) are darker staining with tiny secretory granules in the apical cytoplasm. The serous acini (**3**) around the mucous acini (**2**) form crescent-shaped structures called **serous demilunes** (**4**). A tiny excretory **intercalated duct** (**5**), lined with a cuboidal epithelium, and a larger **striated duct** (**6**) with columnar epithelium, are also visible in the gland.

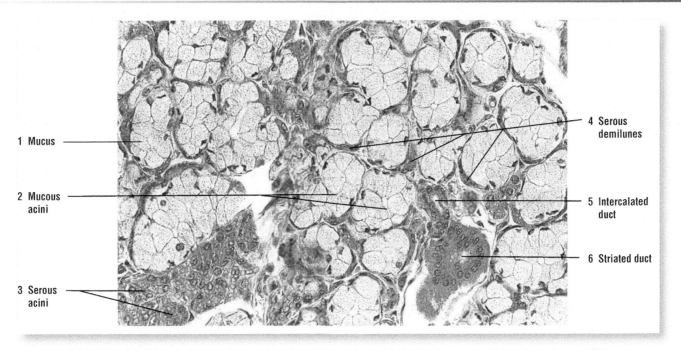

1 Mucus

2 Mucous acini

3 Serous acini

4 Serous demilunes

5 Intercalated duct

6 Striated duct

FIGURE 13.22 ■ Mixed salivary gland: sublingual gland. Stain: hematoxylin and eosin. ×165.

FUNCTIONAL CORRELATIONS 13.2 ■ Salivary Glands, Saliva, and Salivary Ducts

Salivary glands produce about 1 L/day of a watery secretion called **saliva**, which enters the oral cavity via large excretory ducts. **Myoepithelial cells** surround the secretory acini and the initial portions of intercalated ducts, and as a result of nervous stimulation, the contractions of myoepithelial expel the secretory products into the oral cavity.

Saliva is a mixture of secretions produced by cells in different salivary glands. Although the major composition of saliva is **water**, it also contains ions, proteins, mucus, enzymes, and antibodies (immunoglobulins). The sight, smell, thought, taste, or actual presence of food in the mouth causes an **autonomic stimulation** of the salivary glands that increases production of saliva and its release into the oral cavity.

Saliva performs numerous functions. It moistens the chewed food and provides solvents that allow it to be tasted. Saliva lubricates the bolus of chewed food for easier swallowing and in its passage through the esophagus to the stomach. Saliva also contains numerous **electrolytes** (calcium, potassium, sodium, chloride, bicarbonate ions, and others). A digestive enzyme, **salivary amylase**, mainly produced by the **serous acini**, initiates the breakdown of starch into smaller carbohydrates during the time that food is in the oral cavity. Once the bolus enters the stomach, it is acidified by gastric juices. This action decreases amylase activity and carbohydrate digestion.

Saliva also controls **bacterial flora** in the oral cavity and protects it against oral pathogens. The bacterial enzyme, **lysozyme**, secreted by serous cells hydrolyzes cell walls of bacteria and inhibits their growth in the oral cavity. In addition, saliva contains salivary **antibodies** primarily immunoglobulin A, produced by the **plasma cells** located in the connective tissue of salivary glands. Salivary acinar cells secrete a protein component that binds to and transports the immunoglobulins from plasma cells in the connective tissue into saliva. The antibodies then form complexes with antigens and assist in immunologic defense against oral bacteria.

As saliva flows through the duct system of salivary glands, the salivary ducts modify its ionic content by selective transport, resorption, or secretions of ions. The **striated ducts** actively reabsorb **sodium** and chloride ions from saliva, whereas **potassium** and bicarbonate ions, the buffering ions produced in the striated ducts, are added to the salivary secretions, forming a hypotonic saliva. The numerous infoldings of the basal cell membrane or striations in the striated ducts contain elongated mitochondria that provide the necessary energy for fluid and electrolyte transports across the cell membranes.

The striated ducts of each lobule drain into interlobular or excretory ducts that eventually form the main duct for each gland, which ultimately empties its contents into the oral cavity.

Chapter 13 Summary

Digestive System Part I: Oral Cavity and Salivary Glands

OVERVIEW

- Hollow tube consisting of oral cavity, esophagus, stomach, small intestine, large intestine, rectum, and anal canal
- Salivary glands, liver, and pancreas are accessory organs located outside the tube
- Secretory products from all accessory organs delivered to the tube via excretory ducts

ORAL CAVITY

- Lined with stratified squamous epithelium for protection
- Food masticated here, and saliva lubricates food for swallowing

Lips

- Lined with thin skin covered by stratified squamous keratinized epithelium
- Blood vessels close to the surface impart red color
- Contain hairs, sebaceous and sweat glands, and mucus-secreting labial glands
- Core contains skeletal muscle orbicularis oris

Tongue

- Consists of connective tissue and interlacing skeleton muscle fibers
- Dorsal surface divided into anterior two thirds and posterior third by sulcus terminalis
- Dorsal surface covered by elevations called filiform, fungiform, and circumvallate papillae
- Filiform papillae are most numerous, smallest, and keratinized; lack taste buds
- Fungiform papillae are less numerous, larger, mushroom-like, and contain taste buds
- Circumvallate papillae are largest, are in the back of the tongue, and are encircled by furrows
- Numerous taste buds located on the lateral sides of each papilla
- Underlying serous glands empty serous secretions into the base of furrows
- Foliate papillae are rudimentary in humans
- Posterior lingual glands in the connective tissue open onto dorsal surface of tongue

Taste Buds

- Located in foliate, fungiform, and circumvallate papillae; pharynx; palate; and epiglottis
- Exhibit tastes pores and occupy thickness of epithelium; microvilli protrude through taste pore
- Neuroepithelial cells synapse with afferent axons and are the receptors for taste
- Also contain supportive sustentacular cells, whereas basal cells can serve as stem cells
- Substances that are tasted are first dissolved in saliva and then enter taste pore
- Serous glands wash peripheral taste buds in the furrows of circumvallate papillae
- Five basic taste sensations are sour, salt, bitter, sweet, and umami
- Sensitivity to all tastes distributes across entire tongue
- Some areas of tongue may be more sensitive to certain tastes

Lymphoid Aggregations: Tonsils

- Diffuse lymphoid tissue and nodules in the oral pharynx
- Palatine and lingual tonsils covered by stratified squamous epithelium and show crypts
- Pharyngeal tonsil is single and covered by pseudostratified ciliated epithelium
- Some lymphatic nodules contain germinal centers

Teeth

- Developing teeth found in dental alveolus in the jawbone
- Downward growth from oral epithelium forms dental lamina and gives rise to ameloblasts
- Mesenchyme gives rise to dental papilla and odontoblasts
- Odontoblasts secrete dentin, whereas ameloblasts produce enamel of tooth

MAJOR SALIVARY GLANDS

- Parotid, submandibular, and sublingual are major salivary glands that produce saliva
- Composed of secretory acini and excretory ducts that bring saliva into oral cavity
- Cells are serous or mucous; serous cells form serous demilunes around mucous acini
- Contractile myoepithelial cells surround serous and mucous acini and part of intercalated ducts

- Serous, mucous, and mixed secretory acini empty secretions into intercalated ducts
- Intercalated ducts merge into larger striated ducts with basal membrane infoldings
- Striated ducts form larger interlobular ducts that empty into interlobar excretory ducts
- Glands produce about 1 L of saliva per day, which is mostly water
- Saliva formed after autonomic stimulation

- Saliva contains electrolytes and carbohydrate-digesting enzyme salivary amylase
- Saliva contains antibodies produced by plasma cells and lysozyme to control oral bacteria
- Saliva is modified by transport of ions as it passes intercalated ducts and striated ducts
- Striated ducts absorb sodium and chloride from saliva, whereas potassium and bicarbonate ions are added to produce hypotonic saliva

Chapter 13 Review Questions

QUESTIONS

In the following multiple choice questions, choose the letter corresponding to the one best answer.

1. **Intercalated ducts in salivary glands modify the saliva that passes through them by:**

   A. secreting bicarbonate ions and absorbing chloride.
   B. absorbing sodium and adding potassium and bicarbonate ions.
   C. secreting bicarbonate and potassium ions.
   D. adding water and enzymes.
   E. absorbing bicarbonate and chloride ions.

2. **Striated ducts in salivary glands modify the saliva that passes through them by:**

   A. secreting bicarbonate ions and absorbing chloride.
   B. absorbing sodium and adding potassium and bicarbonate ions.
   C. secreting bicarbonate and potassium ions.
   D. adding water and enzymes.
   E. absorbing bicarbonate and chloride ions.

3. **What is the main function of salivary amylase?**

   A. Breaking down starch in the oral cavity
   B. Moistening and lubricating the bolus
   C. Increasing the production of antibodies in the saliva
   D. Controlling bacterial flora in the oral cavity
   E. Stimulating increased production of saliva

4. **What is the main function of myoepithelial cells?**

   A. To add more electrolytes to saliva
   B. To increase enzyme content in the oral cavity
   C. To constrict intercalated and striated ducts
   D. To contract secretory acini to expel secretions
   E. To lubricate the food bolus in the oral cavity

5. **The immunoglobulins found in the saliva are produced by:**

   A. serous acini in salivary glands.
   B. mucous acini in salivary glands.
   C. striated ducts.
   D. plasma cells in the salivary acini and striated ducts.
   E. plasma cells in the connective tissue around salivary glands.

ANSWERS

1. **Correct Answer: A.** Secreting bicarbonate ions and absorbing chloride. The exchanges of these ions form a hypotonic saliva for the oral cavity.

2. **Correct Answer: B.** Absorbing sodium and adding potassium and bicarbonate ions. This action buffers and produces a hypotonic saliva.

3. **Correct Answer: A.** Breaking down starch in the oral cavity. Although starch is in the oral cavity, amylase breaks it down before it is swallowed.

4. **Correct Answer: D.** To contract secretory acini to expel secretions. The contractile myoepithelial cells surround the secretory acini and, by contracting, cause expulsion of the secretory products into the excretory ducts.

5. **Correct Answer: E.** Plasma cells in the connective tissue around salivary glands. The proteins secreted by acinar cells bind to and transport immunoglobulins from plasma cells into saliva.

ADDITIONAL HISTOLOGIC IMAGES

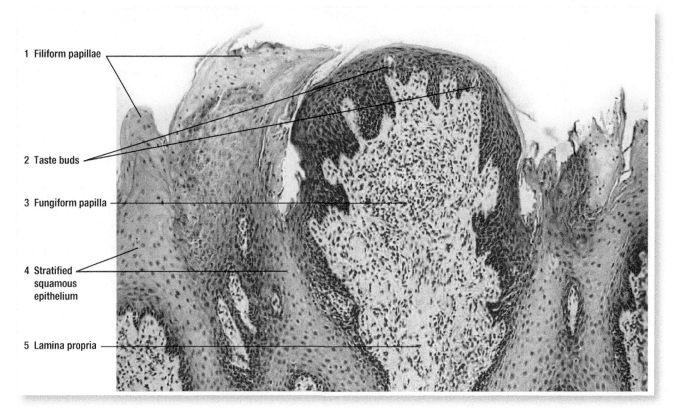

1 Filiform papillae
2 Taste buds
3 Fungiform papilla
4 Stratified squamous epithelium
5 Lamina propria

FIGURE 13.23 ■ Dorsal surface of the human tongue illustrating the filiform and fungiform papillae with taste buds. Stain: hematoxylin and eosin. ×25.

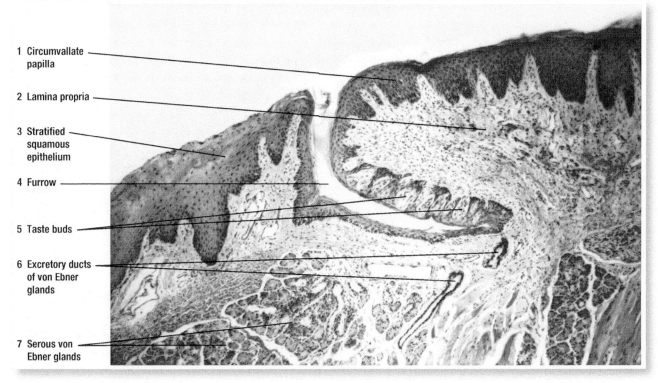

1 Circumvallate papilla
2 Lamina propria
3 Stratified squamous epithelium
4 Furrow
5 Taste buds
6 Excretory ducts of von Ebner glands
7 Serous von Ebner glands

FIGURE 13.24 ■ Dorsal surface of the human tongue illustrating the circumvallate papilla with surrounding structures. Stain: hematoxylin and eosin. ×25.

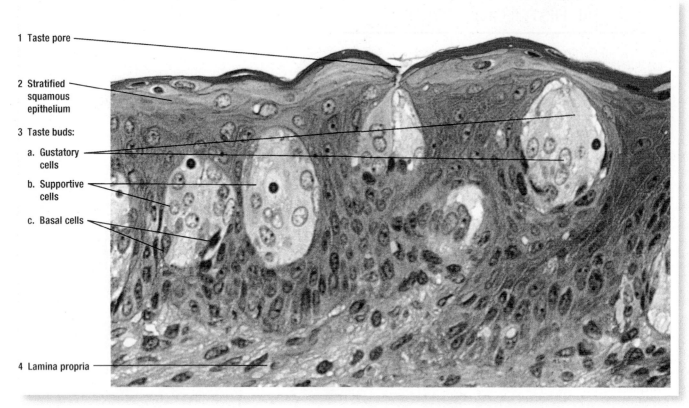

1 Taste pore

2 Stratified squamous epithelium

3 Taste buds:

  a. Gustatory cells

  b. Supportive cells

  c. Basal cells

4 Lamina propria

FIGURE 13.25 ■ Plastic section of the fungiform papilla on a primate tongue illustrating taste buds. Stain: hematoxylin and eosin. ×130.

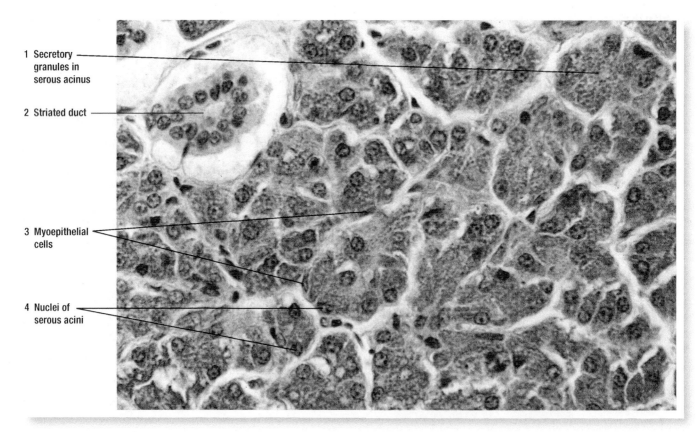

1 Secretory granules in serous acinus

2 Striated duct

3 Myoepithelial cells

4 Nuclei of serous acini

FIGURE 13.26 ■ Section of a primate serous parotid salivary gland illustrating a striated duct and serous acini. Stain: hematoxylin and eosin. ×165.

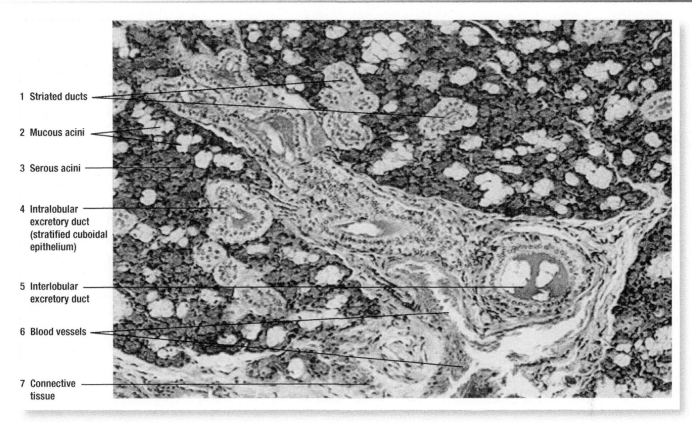

1 Striated ducts

2 Mucous acini

3 Serous acini

4 Intralobular
excretory duct
(stratified cuboidal
epithelium)

5 Interlobular
excretory duct

6 Blood vessels

7 Connective
tissue

FIGURE 13.27 ■ Seromucous (submandibular) primate gland illustrating serous and mucous acini and different excretory ducts. Stain: hematoxylin and eosin. ×60.

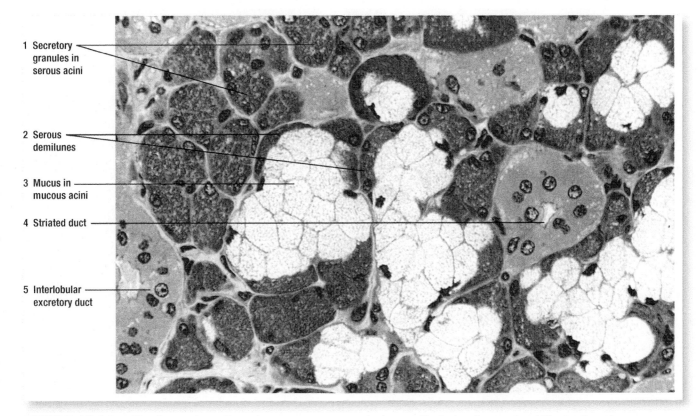

1 Secretory
granules in
serous acini

2 Serous
demilunes

3 Mucus in
mucous acini

4 Striated duct

5 Interlobular
excretory duct

FIGURE 13.28 ■ Plastic section of a primate seromucous (submandibular) salivary gland illustrating the serous and mucous acini. Stain: hematoxylin and eosin. ×160.

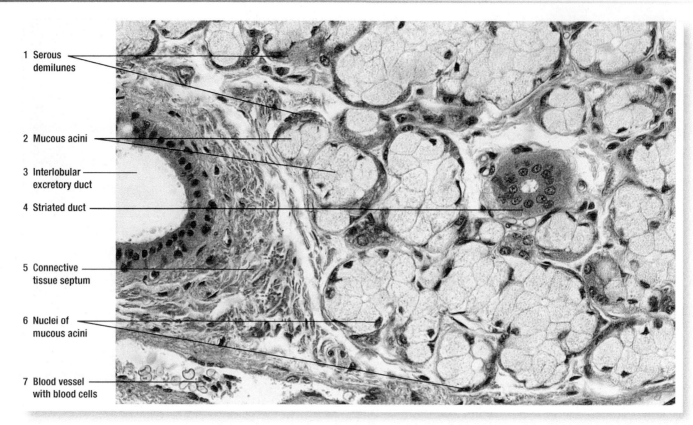

1 Serous demilunes

2 Mucous acini

3 Interlobular excretory duct

4 Striated duct

5 Connective tissue septum

6 Nuclei of mucous acini

7 Blood vessel with blood cells

FIGURE 13.29 ■ A section of primate seromucous (sublingual) gland with mucous acini, serous demilunes, and excretory ducts. Stain: hematoxylin and eosin. ×130.

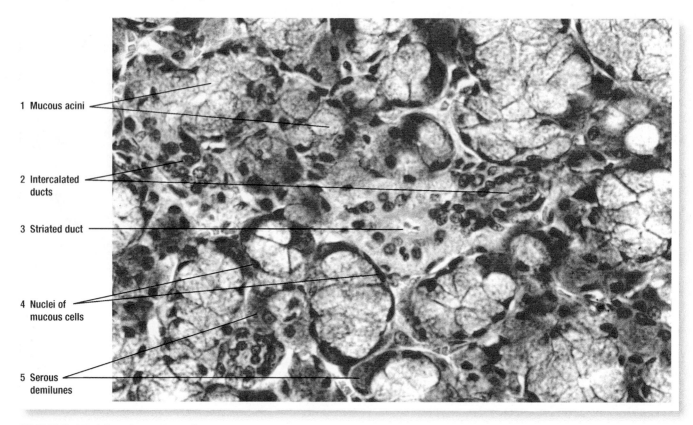

1 Mucous acini

2 Intercalated ducts

3 Striated duct

4 Nuclei of mucous cells

5 Serous demilunes

FIGURE 13.30 ■ A section of primate seromucous (sublingual) gland illustrating the mucous acini, serous demilunes, and excretory ducts. Stain: hematoxylin and eosin. ×165.

Digestive System Part II: Esophagus and Stomach

GENERAL PLAN OF DIGESTIVE SYSTEM—AN OVERVIEW

The digestive (gastrointestinal) tract is a long hollow tube extending from the esophagus to the rectum. It includes the esophagus, stomach, small intestine (duodenum, jejunum, and ileum), large intestine (colon), and rectum. The wall of the digestive tube shows four distinct layers that represent the basic histologic organization of the entire tract. These layers are the mucosa, submucosa, muscularis externa, and serosa (or adventitia). Because the digestive tract performs different functions during the digestive processes, the morphology of these layers exhibits variations. These are primarily evident in the epithelium and indicate the specific functions for each section of the tract.

Mucosa

The **mucosa** is the innermost layer of the digestive tube that consists of a lining **epithelium** and glands that extend into the underlying layer of loose connective tissue called the **lamina propria**. A thin inner circular and an outer longitudinal layer of smooth muscle, called the **muscularis mucosae**, form the outer boundary of the mucosa.

Submucosa

The **submucosa** is located inferior to the mucosa. It consists of dense irregular connective tissue with numerous blood and lymph vessels and a **submucosal (Meissner) nerve plexus** that contains postganglionic parasympathetic neurons. The neurons and axons of the submucosal nerve plexus control the motility of the mucosa and secretory activities of mucosal glands. In the initial portion of the small intestine, the duodenum, the submucosa contains numerous branched mucous glands.

Muscularis Externa

The **muscularis externa** is a thick, smooth muscle layer located inferior to submucosa. Except for the large intestine, this contains an inner layer of circular smooth muscle and an outer layer of longitudinal smooth muscle. Situated between the two smooth muscle layers are connective tissue and another nerve plexus called the **myenteric (Auerbach) nerve plexus**. This plexus also contains postganglionic parasympathetic neurons and controls the motility of smooth muscles in the muscularis externa.

Serosa

The serosa is the outermost layer of the abdominal portion of the esophagus, stomach, and small intestine and is continuous with the mesentery and the lining of the abdominal cavity. The serosa is a serous membrane of simple squamous epithelium called **mesothelium** and a thin underlying loose connective tissue that surrounds the visceral organs. If mesothelium covers the visceral organs, the organs are **intraperitoneal** and the outermost layer is called serosa. Serosa also covers ascending and descending colon only on the anterior and lateral surfaces. The posterior surfaces of the colon are bound to the posterior abdominal body wall and are not covered by the mesothelium or suspended by a mesentery.

Adventitia

When the digestive tube is not covered by mesothelium, it lies outside the peritoneal cavity and is called **retroperitoneal**. Here, the outermost layer of the organ adheres to the body wall and consists only of a connective tissue called **adventitia**.

The characteristic features of each layer of the digestive tube and their functions are discussed in detail with illustration of the different parts of the digestive tract.

SECTION 1 Esophagus

The **esophagus** is a tube about 10 in long extending from the **pharynx** to the **stomach**. It is located posterior to the trachea in the mediastinum of the **thoracic cavity**. After descending the thoracic cavity, the esophagus penetrates the muscular **diaphragm** with a short section present in the abdominal cavity before terminating at the stomach. In the thoracic cavity, the esophagus is surrounded by the connective tissue **adventitia** (Fig. 14.1). In the abdominal cavity, a simple squamous mesothelium covers the outermost wall of the short segment of the esophagus, forming the **serosa**.

The esophageal lumen is lined with a moist, **nonkeratinized stratified squamous epithelium**. An empty esophagus exhibits numerous but temporary **longitudinal folds** of mucosa in its lumen that are due to the contractions of the esophageal muscles. The wall of the esophagus contains two types of glands that secrete mucus; however, they are located in different parts of the organ. In the lamina propria of the proximal and distal parts of the esophagus near the stomach are the **esophageal cardiac glands** because they resemble the mucous glands located in the cardiac region of the stomach. In the submucosa are the **esophageal glands proper** that are scattered along the entire length of the esophagus. The mucus from these glands lubricates the lumen of the esophagus, protects the mucosa, and facilitates smooth passage of food material (bolus) through the esophagus to the stomach.

The outer wall of the esophagus, the **muscularis externa**, contains both skeletal and smooth muscles fibers. In the upper third of the esophagus, both layers of the muscularis externa contain striated **skeletal muscle fibers**. In the middle third of the esophagus, the muscularis externa

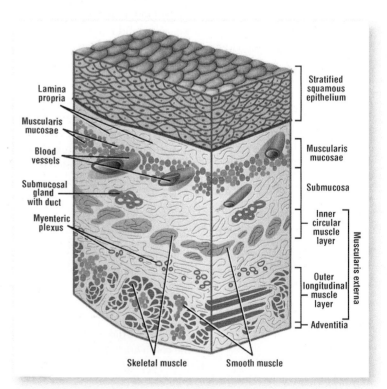

FIGURE 14.1 ■ Four layers (mucosa, submucosa, muscularis externa, and adventitia) in the wall of the esophagus and their characteristic contents.

Lamina propria

Muscularis mucosae

Blood vessels

Submucosal gland with duct

Myenteric plexus

Stratified squamous epithelium

Muscularis mucosae

Submucosa

Inner circular muscle layer

Outer longitudinal muscle layer

Adventitia

Muscularis externa

Skeletal muscle

Smooth muscle

contains a mixture of both **skeletal** and **smooth muscle** fibers, whereas in the lower third of the esophagus, both layers are **smooth muscle fibers** (see Fig. 14.1).

thePoint° Supplemental micrographic images are available at **www.thePoint.com/Eroschenko13e** under Digestive System Part II: Esophagus and Stomach.

FIGURE 14.2 | **Wall of Upper Esophagus (Transverse Section)**

The esophagus is a long, hollow tube whose wall consists of the mucosa, submucosa, muscularis externa, and adventitia. In this illustration, the upper portion of the esophagus has been sectioned in a transverse plane.

The **mucosa (1)** of the esophagus consists an inner lining of nonkeratinized **stratified squamous epithelium (1a)**; an underlying thin layer of fine connective tissue, the **lamina propria (1b)**; and a layer of longitudinal smooth muscle fibers, the muscularis mucosae (1c), shown in transverse plane. The **connective tissue papillae (9)** of the lamina propria (1b) indent the

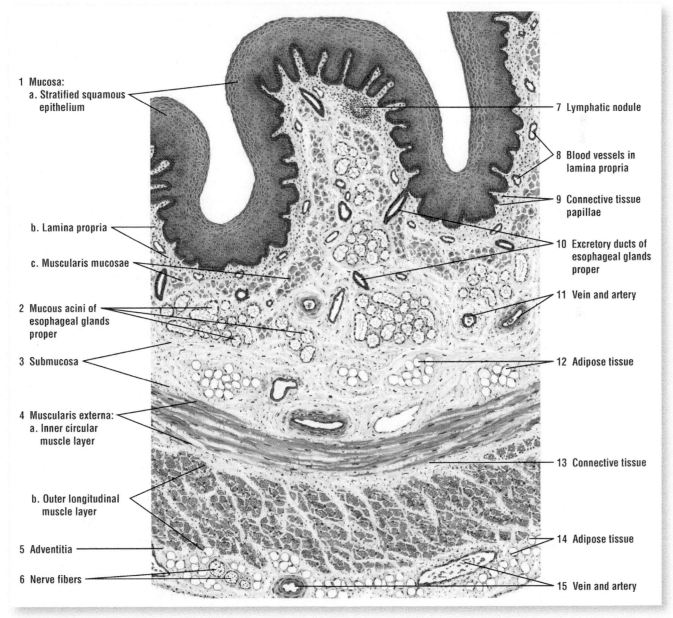

1 Mucosa:
  a. Stratified squamous
    epithelium

7 Lymphatic nodule

8 Blood vessels in
  lamina propria

9 Connective tissue
  papillae

b. Lamina propria

c. Muscularis mucosae

10 Excretory ducts of
   esophageal glands
   proper

11 Vein and artery

2 Mucous acini of
  esophageal glands
  proper

3 Submucosa

12 Adipose tissue

4 Muscularis externa:
  a. Inner circular
    muscle layer

13 Connective tissue

b. Outer longitudinal
  muscle layer

14 Adipose tissue

5 Adventitia

6 Nerve fibers

15 Vein and artery

FIGURE 14.2 ■ Wall of the upper esophagus (transverse section). Stain: hematoxylin and eosin. Low magnification.

epithelium (1a). Found in the lamina propria (1b) are small **blood vessels** (8), diffuse lymphatic tissue, and a small **lymphatic nodule** (7).

The **submucosa** (3) is a wide layer of moderately dense irregular connective tissue with some **adipose tissue** (12). The **mucous acini** of **esophageal glands proper** (2) are in the submucosa (3) at intervals throughout the length of the esophagus. The **excretory ducts** (10) of these glands (2) pass through the muscularis mucosae (1c) and the lamina propria (1b) to open into the esophageal lumen. The dark-staining ductal epithelium of the glands merges with the stratified squamous surface epithelium (1a) of the esophagus (see Fig. 14.3). Numerous **blood vessels** (11) are found in the submucosa (3).

Located inferior to the submucosa (3) is the **muscularis externa** (4), composed of two muscle layers, an **inner circular muscle layer** (4a) and the outer **longitudinal muscle layer** (4b), whose muscle fibers are shown here sectioned in a transverse plane. A thin layer of **connective tissue** (13) lies between the inner circular muscle layer (4a) and the outer longitudinal muscle layer (4b).

In humans, the muscularis externa (4) in the upper third of the esophagus consists of striated skeletal muscles. In the middle third of the esophagus, the inner circular layer (4a) and the outer longitudinal layer (4b) exhibit a mixture of both smooth muscle and skeletal muscle fibers. In the lower third of the esophagus, only smooth muscle is present.

The **adventitia** (5) consists of a loose connective tissue layer that blends with the adventitia of the trachea and the surrounding structures. **Adipose tissue** (14), large blood vessels, an **artery** and a **vein** (15), and **nerve fibers** (6) are numerous in the connective tissue of the adventitia (5).

FIGURE 14.3 | Upper Esophagus (Transverse Section)

The next two histologic sections illustrate the difference between the upper and the lower esophageal wall.

The mucosa of the upper esophagus (as in Fig. 14.2) consists of a stratified squamous nonkeratinized **epithelium** (1), a connective tissue **lamina propria** (2), and smooth muscle **muscularis mucosae** (3) (transverse plane). A **lymphatic nodule** (4) is visible in the lamina propria (2). In the **submucosa** (7) are adipose cells and **mucous acini of esophageal glands proper** (6) and their **excretory ducts** (5). The muscularis externa consists of an **inner circular layer** (10) and an **outer longitudinal layer** (14) of skeletal muscles, separated by **connective tissue** (11). The outermost layer is the connective tissue **adventitia** (8) with adipose tissue, **nerves** (13), a **vein** (9), and an **artery** (12).

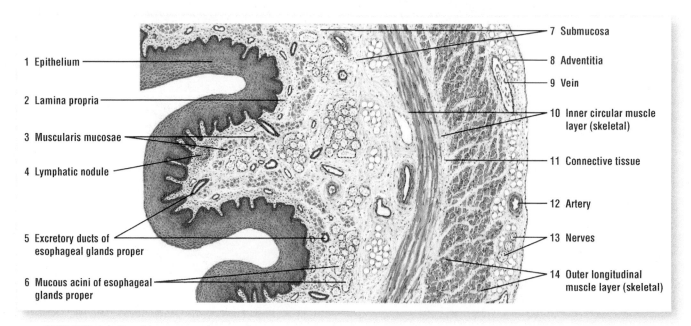

1 Epithelium
2 Lamina propria
3 Muscularis mucosae
4 Lymphatic nodule
5 Excretory ducts of esophageal glands proper
6 Mucous acini of esophageal glands proper
7 Submucosa
8 Adventitia
9 Vein
10 Inner circular muscle layer (skeletal)
11 Connective tissue
12 Artery
13 Nerves
14 Outer longitudinal muscle layer (skeletal)

FIGURE 14.3 ■ Upper esophagus (transverse section). Stain: hematoxylin and eosin. Low magnification.

FIGURE 14.4 | Lower Esophagus (Transverse Section)

This illustration shows the terminal portion of the esophagus near the stomach.

As in the upper esophagus, the **mucosa** (**1**) of the lower esophagus consists of stratified squamous nonkeratinized **epithelium** (**1a**), the connective tissue **lamina propria** (**1b**), and a smooth muscle layer **muscularis mucosae** (**1c**) (transverse section). Also visible are the **connective tissue papillae** (**2**) that indent the epithelium (**1a**) and a **lymphatic nodule** (**3**).

The **submucosa** (**6**) contains mucous acini of the **esophageal glands proper** (**5**), their **excretory ducts** (**4**), and **adipose tissue** (**7**). In some regions of the esophagus, these glands may be absent.

The major differences between the upper and lower esophagus are seen in the next two layers. The **muscularis externa** (**10**) in the lower esophagus consists of smooth muscle layers, an **inner circular muscle layer** (**10a**) and an **outer longitudinal muscle layer** (**10b**). The outermost layer of the lower esophagus is the **serosa** (**8**) or visceral peritoneum. Serosa (**8**) consists of a connective tissue layer lined with a simple squamous layer mesothelium. In contrast, the connective tissue adventitia surrounds the esophagus in the thoracic region.

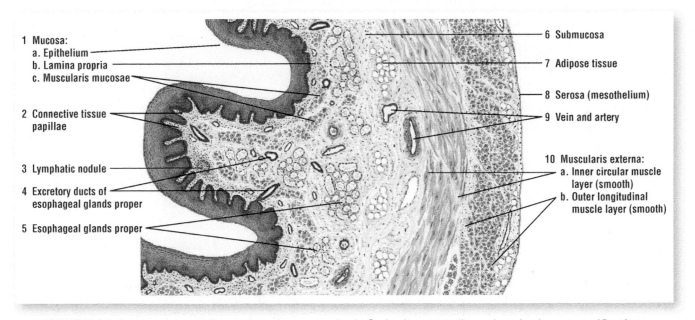

1 Mucosa:
a. Epithelium
b. Lamina propria
c. Muscularis mucosae

2 Connective tissue papillae

3 Lymphatic nodule

4 Excretory ducts of esophageal glands proper

5 Esophageal glands proper

6 Submucosa

7 Adipose tissue

8 Serosa (mesothelium)

9 Vein and artery

10 Muscularis externa:
a. Inner circular muscle layer (smooth)
b. Outer longitudinal muscle layer (smooth)

FIGURE 14.4 ■ Lower esophagus (transverse section). Stain: hematoxylin and eosin. Low magnification.

FIGURE 14.5 | Upper Esophagus: Mucosa and Submucosa (Longitudinal Section)

This higher-magnification illustration of the upper esophagus has been sectioned longitudinally to show a different perspective. The smooth muscle fibers of the muscularis mucosae (9) exhibit a longitudinal orientation, and the fibers of the inner circular muscle layer are cut in a transverse section.

The esophagus is lined with a stratified squamous **epithelium** (7). The connective tissue **lamina propria** (8) contains numerous blood vessels, aggregates of lymphocytes, and a small **lymphatic nodule** (2). **Connective tissue papillae** (1) from the lamina propria (8) indent the surface epithelium (7). The **muscularis mucosae** (9) is illustrated as bundles of smooth muscle fibers sectioned in a longitudinal plane.

The underlying **submucosa** (3, 10) contains **mucous acini of esophageal glands proper** (4). Small **excretory ducts** (11) from these glands (4), lined with a simple epithelium, join the larger excretory ducts with stratified epithelium. One of the excretory ducts joins the stratified squamous epithelium (7) of the esophageal lumen. In the submucosa (3, 10) are **blood vessels** (12), **nerves** (5), and **adipose cells** (6).

The **inner circular muscle layer** (13 in the muscularis externa) consists of skeletal muscle that is illustrated in a transverse plane at the bottom of the figure.

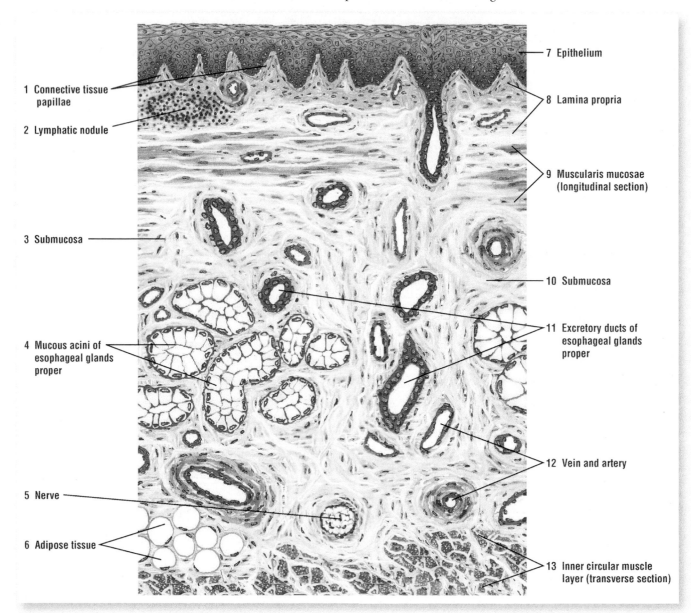

1 Connective tissue papillae
2 Lymphatic nodule
3 Submucosa
4 Mucous acini of esophageal glands proper
5 Nerve
6 Adipose tissue

7 Epithelium
8 Lamina propria
9 Muscularis mucosae (longitudinal section)
10 Submucosa
11 Excretory ducts of esophageal glands proper
12 Vein and artery
13 Inner circular muscle layer (transverse section)

FIGURE 14.5 ■ Upper esophagus: mucosa and submucosa (longitudinal view). Stain: hematoxylin and eosin. Medium magnification.

FIGURE 14.6 | **Lower Esophagus Wall (Transverse Section)**

This low-magnification photomicrograph illustrates the lower portion of the esophagus. The mucosa consists of a thick but nonkeratinized **stratified squamous epithelium** (**1**), a connective tissue **lamina propria** (**2**), and a thin strip of smooth **muscle muscularis mucosae** (**3**). Below the muscularis mucosae are the esophageal glands in the submucosa, and closer to the stomach are the esophageal cardiac glands in the lamina propria.

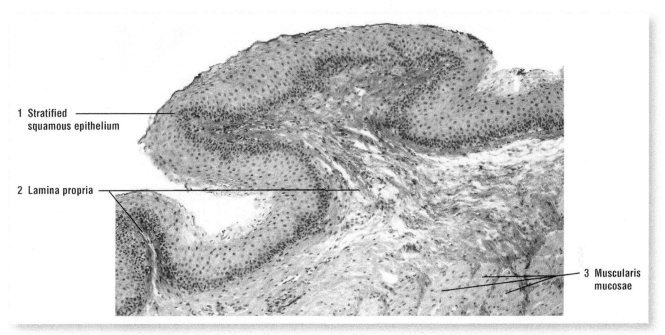

FIGURE 14.6 ■ Lower esophageal wall (transverse section). Stain: Mallory-Azan. ×30.

FUNCTIONAL CORRELATIONS 14.1 ■ Esophagus

The major function of the esophagus is to convey liquids or chewed food (bolus) from the oral cavity to the stomach. For this function, the lumen of the esophagus is lined with a protective nonkeratinized stratified squamous epithelium. Aiding in this function are esophageal glands in lamina propria. The esophageal cardiac glands are in the lamina propria of the upper and lower regions of the esophagus and exhibit morphology similar to those found in the cardia of the stomach, where the esophagus terminates.

Esophageal glands proper are located in the submucosa. Both types of glands produce mucus to lubricate the esophageal lumen and protect it during the passage of ingested solid material. The swallowed material is moved from one end of the esophagus to the other by strong muscular contractions called peristalsis. At the lower end of the esophagus, a muscular gastroesophageal sphincter constricts the lumen and prevents the regurgitation of swallowed material into the esophagus.

FIGURE 14.7 | Esophageal–Stomach Junction

At its terminal end, the esophagus joins the stomach and forms the esophageal–stomach junction. The nonkeratinized **stratified squamous epithelium** (**1**) of the esophagus abruptly changes to simple columnar, mucus-secreting **gastric epithelium** (**10**) of the cardiac region of the **stomach**.

At the esophageal–stomach junction, the **esophageal glands proper** (**7**) may be seen in the **submucosa** (**8**) with their **excretory ducts** (**4, 6**) coursing through the **muscularis mucosae** (**5**) and the **lamina propria** (**2**) of the esophagus into its lumen. In the lamina propria (**2**) of the esophagus near the stomach junction are the **esophageal cardiac glands** (**3**). Both the esophageal glands proper (**7**) and the cardiac glands (**3**) secrete mucus.

The lamina propria of the esophagus (**2**) continues into the lamina propria of the stomach (**12**), where it is filled with **glands** (**16, 17**) and diffuse lymphatic tissue. The lamina propria of the stomach (**12**) is penetrated by shallow **gastric pits** (**11**) into which empty the gastric glands (**16, 17**).

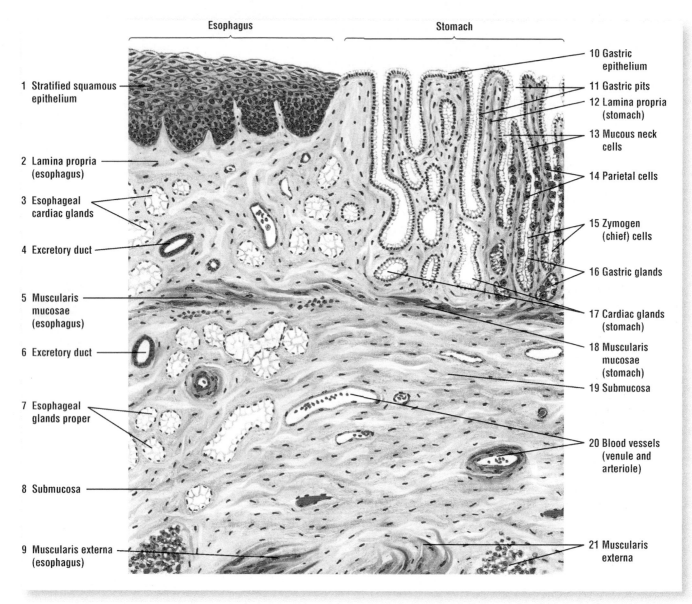

FIGURE 14.7 ■ Esophageal–stomach junction. Stain: hematoxylin and eosin. Low magnification.

The simple tubular **cardiac glands** (**17**) are limited to the transition region, the cardia of the stomach, and are lined with pale-staining, mucus-secreting columnar cells. Below the cardiac region of the stomach are the simple tubular **gastric glands** (**16**), some showing basal branching.

In contrast to the cardiac glands (**17**), the gastric glands (**16**) contain four cell types: the pale-staining **mucous neck cells** (**13**); large, eosinophilic **parietal cells** (**14**); basophilic chief or **zymogenic cells** (**15**); and several endocrine cells (not illustrated), collectively called the entero-endocrine cells.

The **muscularis mucosae** of the esophagus (**5**) also continue with the muscularis mucosae of the **stomach** (**18**). In the esophagus, the muscularis mucosae (**5**) are usually a single layer of longitudinal smooth muscle fibers, whereas in the stomach, a second layer of the inner circular layer of smooth muscle is added.

The **submucosa** (**8, 19**) and the **muscularis externa** (**9, 21**) of the esophagus are continuous with those of the stomach. **Blood vessels** (**20**) are found in the submucosa (**8, 19**) from which smaller blood vessels are distributed to other regions of the stomach.

FIGURE 14.8 | **Esophageal–Stomach Junction (Transverse Section)**

This low-magnification photomicrograph illustrates the esophagus–stomach junction that is characterized by an abrupt transition from the thick **stratified squamous epithelium** (**1**) of the esophagus to the simple **columnar epithelium** (**4**) of the stomach. Inferior to the epithelium (**1**) is the **lamina propria** (**2**), below which is the smooth muscle **muscularis mucosae** (**3**). The lamina propria (**2**) indents the undersurface of the esophageal epithelium to form the connective tissue papillae. The surface of the stomach exhibits numerous **gastric pits** (**5**), which open from below the **gastric glands** (**6**). The **lamina propria** (**7**) of the stomach, in contrast esophagus, is seen as thin strips of connective tissue between the tightly packed gastric glands (**6**).

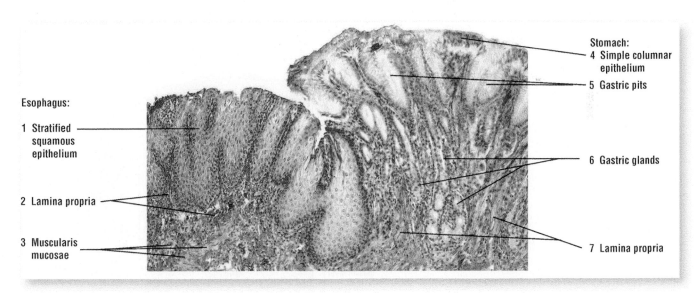

FIGURE 14.8 ■ Esophageal–stomach junction (transverse section). Stain: Mallory-Azan. ×30.

SECTION 2 Stomach

The stomach is an expanded hollow organ situated between the esophagus and the small intestine. At the abrupt transition esophageal–stomach junction, the **simple columnar epithelium** of the stomach is lined by cells that produce a large quantity of mucus. The mucus adheres to the surface epithelium and protects the stomach lining from the corrosive gastric juices of the gastric glands.

The stomach **cardia** is where the esophagus terminates. The upper dome-shaped portion is the **fundus**, below which is located the **body** or **corpus** of the stomach. The funnel-shaped, lower terminal region of the stomach is the **pylorus**. The fundus and the body compose about two thirds of the stomach, have identical histology, and form the major portions of the stomach. As a result, the stomach has three distinct histologic regions: cardiac, fundus/body, and pylorus. Also, all stomach regions exhibit **rugae**, the longitudinal folds of the mucosa and submucosa that are temporary, but disappear when the stomach is distended with fluid or solid material.

The luminal surface of the stomach is pitted with numerous tiny openings called **gastric pits** (Fig. 14.9). These pits are formed by the luminal epithelium that invaginates the underlying **lamina propria** of the **mucosa**. The **gastric glands** are located below the surface (luminal) epithelium and open directly into the gastric pits that deliver their secretions into the stomach lumen. The gastric glands descend through the lamina propria to the **muscularis mucosae**. The stomach mucosa consists of different cell types and deep gastric glands that produce most of the gastric secretions or juices for digestion.

Below the mucosa is the dense connective tissue **submucosa** with large blood vessels and nerves. The thick **muscularis externa** exhibits three muscle layers instead of the two that are normally seen in the esophagus and the small intestine. The outer layer of the stomach is covered by the **serosa**, or visceral peritoneum (see Fig. 14.9).

thePoint® Supplemental micrographic images are available at **www.thePoint.com/Eroschenko13e** under Digestive System Part II: Esophagus and Stomach.

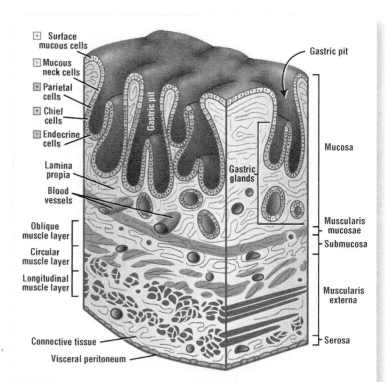

FIGURE 14.9 ■ Four layers (mucosa, submucosa, muscularis externa, and serosa) in the wall of the stomach and their characteristic contents.

FIGURE 14.10 | Stomach: Fundus and Body Region (Transverse Section)

The three histologic regions of the stomach are the cardia, the fundus and body, and the pylorus. The fundus and body constitute the most extensive region in the stomach. The stomach wall exhibits four general regions: **mucosa** (**1, 2, 3**), **submucosa** (**4**), **muscularis externa** (**5, 6, 7**), and **serosa** (**8**).

The **mucosa** consists of the **surface epithelium** (**1**), lamina propria (**2**), and **muscularis mucosae** (**3**). The surface of the stomach is lined with a **simple columnar epithelium** (**1, 11**) that extends into and lines the **gastric pits** (**10**), which are tubular infoldings of the surface epithelium (**11**). In the fundus, the gastric pits (**10**) are not deep and extend into the mucosa about one fourth of its thickness. Beneath the epithelium is the **lamina propria** (**2, 12**) that fills the spaces between the gastric glands. A thin, smooth muscle **muscularis mucosae** (**3, 15**), consisting of an inner circular and an outer longitudinal layer, forms the outer boundary of the mucosa. Thin strands of

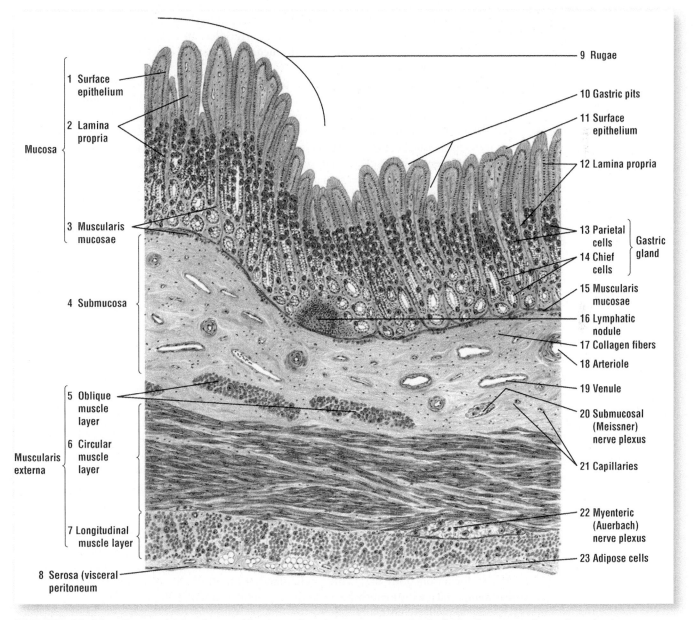

FIGURE 14.10 ■ Stomach: fundus and body region (transverse section). Stain: hematoxylin and eosin. Low magnification.

smooth muscle from the muscularis mucosae (3, 15) extend into lamina propria (2, 12) between the **gastric glands (13**, **14)** toward the surface epithelium (1, 11), which are illustrated at a higher magnification in Figure 14.11, label 8.

The gastric glands (13, 14) are packed in the lamina propria (2, 12), occupy the entire mucosa (1, 2, 3), and open into the bottom of the gastric pits (10). The surface epithelium of the gastric mucosa, from the cardiac to the pyloric region, consists of the same cell type. However, the cells in the gastric glands distinguish the regional differences of the stomach. Two distinct cell types can be identified in the gastric glands. The acidophilic **parietal cells (13)** are located in the upper portions of the glands, whereas the basophilic **chief (zymogenic) (14)** cells occupy the lower regions. The subglandular regions of the lamina propria (2, 12) may contain either lymphatic tissue or small **lymphatic nodules (16)**.

The mucosa of the empty stomach exhibits temporary folds called **rugae (9)** that form during the contractions of the muscularis mucosae (3, 15). As the stomach fills, the rugae disappear and form a smooth mucosa.

The **submucosa (4)** lies inferior to muscularis mucosae (3, 15). In an empty stomach, submucosa (4) can extend into the rugae (9). The submucosa (4) contains dense irregular connective tissue and more **collagen fibers (17)** than the lamina propria (2, 12). In addition, the submucosa (4) contains lymph vessels, **capillaries (21)**, large **arterioles (18)**, and **venules (19)**. Isolated clusters of parasympathetic ganglia of the **submucosal (Meissner) nerve plexus (20)** can be seen deeper in the submucosa.

The **muscularis externa (5, 6, 7)** consists of three layers of smooth muscle, each oriented in a different plane: an inner **oblique (5)**, a middle **circular (6)**, and an outer **longitudinal (7)** layer. The oblique layer is not complete and is not always seen in sections of the stomach wall. In this illustration, the circular layer has been sectioned longitudinally and the longitudinal layer transversely. Located between the circular and longitudinal smooth muscle layers is a **myenteric (Auerbach) nerve plexus (22)** of parasympathetic ganglia and nerve fibers.

The **serosa (8)** consists of a thin outer layer of connective tissue that overlies the muscularis externa (5, 6, 7) and is covered by a simple squamous mesothelium of the **visceral peritoneum (8)**. The serosa can contain **adipose cells (23)**.

FIGURE 14.11 | Stomach: Mucosa of Fundus and Body (Transverse Section)

The mucosa and submucosa of the fundic region are illustrated at a higher magnification. The simple columnar **surface epithelium (1**, **13)** extends into the **gastric pits (11)** into which open the tubular **gastric glands (5)**. The **lamina propria (6)** fills the spaces between the packed gastric glands (5) and extends from the surface epithelium (1) to the **muscularis mucosae (9)**.

The lamina propria (6) and collagen fibers are better seen in the **mucosal ridges (2)**. Scattered throughout the lamina propria (6) are the fibroblast nuclei, lymphoid **lymphatic nodule (17)**, lymphocytes, and other loose connective tissue cells.

The gastric glands (5) extend the length of the mucosa and in deeper regions the gastric glands may branch. As a result, the gastric glands appear as transverse and oblique sections. Each gastric gland consists of three regions. At the junction of the gastric pit with the gastric gland is the **isthmus (14)**, lined with surface epithelial cells (1, 13) and **parietal cells (4)**. Lower in the gland is the **neck (15)**, containing mainly **mucous neck cells (3)** and some parietal cells (4). The base or **fundus (16)** is the deep portion of the gland, composed predominantly of **chief (zymogenic) cells (7)** and a few parietal cells (4). The fundic glands also contain undifferentiated cells and enteroendocrine cells (not illustrated) that secrete different hormones to regulate the digestive system.

Three types of cells can be identified in the fundic gastric glands. The mucous neck cells (3) are located just below the gastric pits (11) and are interspersed between the parietal cells (4) in the neck region of the glands. The parietal cells (4) stain uniformly acidophilic (pink), which distinguishes them from other cells in the fundic glands. In contrast, the chief cells (zymogenic) (7) are basophilic and are distinguishable from the acidophilic parietal cells (4).

The muscularis mucosae (9) in the stomach are composed of two thin strips of smooth muscle: the **inner circular layer (9a)** and **outer longitudinal layer (9b)**. In this illustration, the inner circular layer (9a) is sectioned longitudinally, and the outer layer (9b) is sectioned transversely. Extending upward from the muscularis mucosae (9) to the surface epithelium (1, 13) are strands of **smooth muscle (8, 12)**.

Inferior to the muscularis mucosa (9) is the **submucosa (10)** with denser connective tissue, **collagen fibers (18)**, the nuclei of **fibroblasts (19)**, **arterioles (20)**, **venules (21)**, lymphatics, and capillaries in addition to adipose cells.

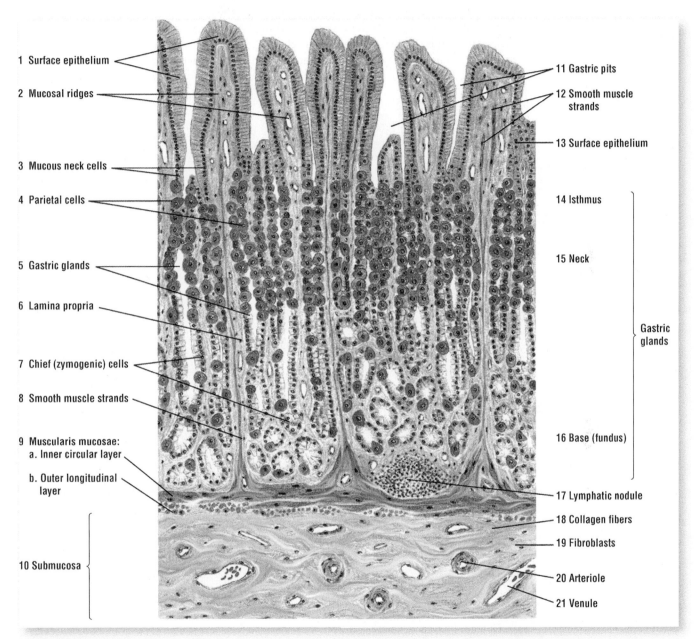

1 Surface epithelium
2 Mucosal ridges
3 Mucous neck cells
4 Parietal cells
5 Gastric glands
6 Lamina propria
7 Chief (zymogenic) cells
8 Smooth muscle strands
9 Muscularis mucosae:
   a. Inner circular layer
   b. Outer longitudinal layer
10 Submucosa

11 Gastric pits
12 Smooth muscle strands
13 Surface epithelium
14 Isthmus
15 Neck
16 Base (fundus)
17 Lymphatic nodule
18 Collagen fibers
19 Fibroblasts
20 Arteriole
21 Venule

Gastric glands

FIGURE 14.11 ■ Stomach: mucosa of the fundus and body (transverse section). Stain: hematoxylin and eosin. Medium magnification.

FIGURE 14.12 | Stomach: Fundus and Body Region (Plastic Section)

This low-magnification photomicrograph illustrates the mucosa of the stomach wall. The fundus and body regions of the stomach have identical histology. The stomach surface is lined with a mucus-secreting, **simple columnar epithelium** (1) that extends down into the **gastric pits** (2). In the fundus and body, the gastric pits (2) are shallow. Draining into the gastric pits (2) are the **gastric glands** (5) with different cell types that are packed, and their lumina are not clearly visible. The large, pale-staining cells in the gastric glands (5) are the acid-secreting **parietal cells** (3), which are more numerous in the upper regions of the gastric glands (5). The darker-staining cells are the **chief (zymogenic) cells** (6), and they are mostly confined to the basal regions of the gastric glands (5). Between the gastric glands (5) are strips of the **lamina propria** (7). A thin **muscularis mucosae** (8) separate the mucosa from the **submucosa** (4).

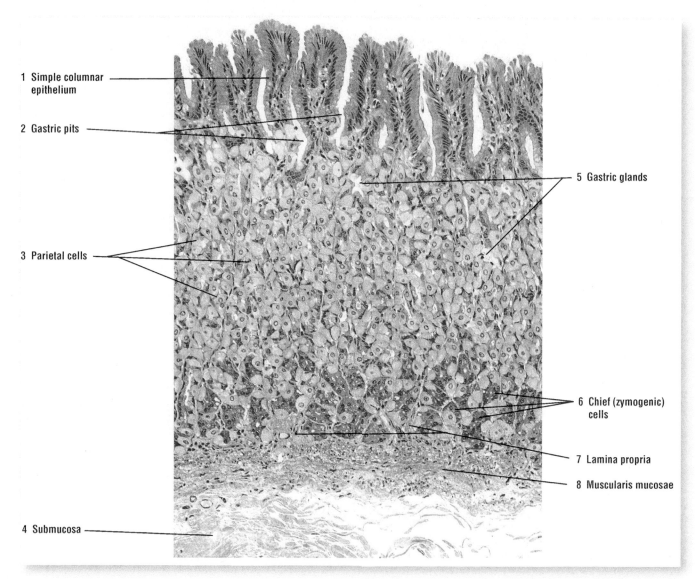

1 Simple columnar epithelium

2 Gastric pits

3 Parietal cells

5 Gastric glands

6 Chief (zymogenic) cells

7 Lamina propria

8 Muscularis mucosae

4 Submucosa

FIGURE 14.12 ■ Stomach: fundus and body region (plastic section). Stain: hematoxylin and eosin. ×50.

FUNCTIONAL CORRELATIONS 14.2 ■ Gastric Pits and Cells of Gastric Glands in the Stomach

The **cardia** and **pylorus** are located at opposite ends of the stomach. The cardia surrounds the entrance of the esophagus into the stomach. At the esophageal–stomach junction are the **cardiac glands**. The pylorus is the most inferior, funnel-shaped region of the stomach that terminates at the border of the small intestine called the duodenum. In the cardiac, the **gastric pits** are shallow, whereas in the pylorus, the gastric pits are deep. However, the histology of gastric glands in both regions is similar, and the cells are predominantly **mucus secreting**.

In contrast, the gastric glands in the fundus and body exhibit different histology and contain three major cell types. Located in gastric glands near the gastric pits are the **mucous neck cells**. The large polygonal cells with eosinophilic cytoplasm are the **parietal cells** that are primarily located in the upper half of the gastric glands, squeezed between gland cells. Located predominantly in the lower region of the gastric glands are basophilic staining cuboidal **chief (zymogenic) cells**.

In addition to cells in gastric glands, the mucosa of the digestive tract also contains **enteroendocrine** or gastrointestinal endocrine cells that are part of the diffuse neuroendocrine system. These cells are distributed in different digestive organs and are located among and between exocrine cells. Unless digestive organs are prepared with special stains, the diffuse neuroendocrine cells are difficult to see in normal histologic sections.

In addition, there are undifferentiated stem cells in the neck regions of the gastric glands that continuously renew the cells in the gastric mucosa. These stem cells move upward to replace lost or worn-out surface cells or downward to replace the cells deep in the glands.

FIGURE 14.13 | Stomach: Superficial Region of Gastric (Fundic) Mucosa

Higher magnification of the superficial region of the stomach shows the cells that constitute the mucosa of the fundus and body.

The columnar **surface epithelium (1)** exhibits basal oval nuclei and a lightly stained cytoplasm owing to the presence of mucigen droplets. The epithelium (1) is separated from the **lamina propria (3, 7, 8)** by a thin **basement membrane (2)** that extends downward into the gastric pits (4). The lamina propria (3, 7, 8) is vascular and contains **blood vessels (9)**. The **gastric glands (5)** lie in the lamina propria (3, 7, 8) below the **gastric pits (4)**. The neck region of the gastric glands (5) is lined with **mucous neck cells (10)** that have round, basal nuclei. The constricted necks of the gastric glands (5) open into the bottom of the gastric pits (4).

The **parietal cells (6, 11)** are large cells with a pyramidal shape, round nuclei, and acidophilic cytoplasm interspersed among the mucous neck cells (10). They are the most conspicuous cells in the gastric mucosa and are found predominantly in the upper third to upper half of the gastric glands (5). The free surfaces of parietal cells (6, 11) open into the lumen of the gastric glands (5). Some parietal cells (6, 11) may be binucleate (two nuclei).

Deeper in the lower half of the gastric glands (5) are the basophilic **chief (zymogenic) cells (12)**, which also border on the lumen of the gland. Some parietal cells (6, 11) are also seen here.

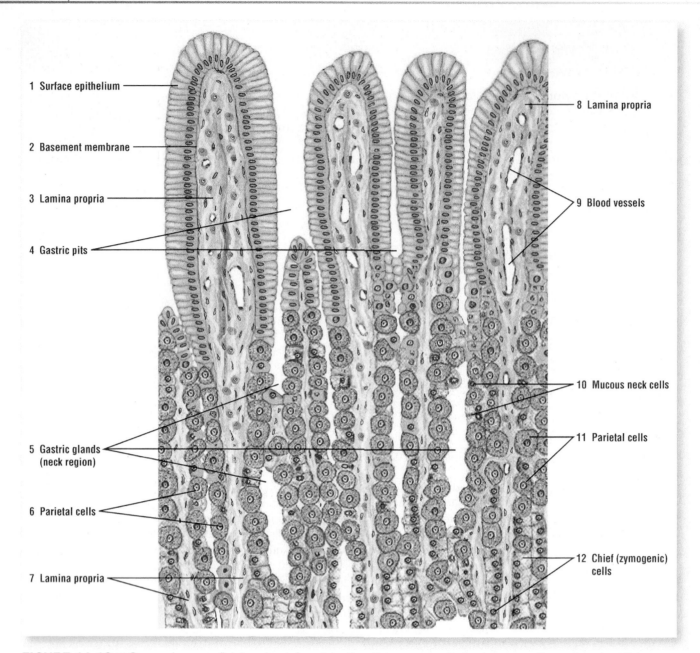

1 Surface epithelium

2 Basement membrane

3 Lamina propria

4 Gastric pits

5 Gastric glands
(neck region)

6 Parietal cells

7 Lamina propria

8 Lamina propria

9 Blood vessels

10 Mucous neck cells

11 Parietal cells

12 Chief (zymogenic)
cells

FIGURE 14.13 ■ Stomach: superficial region of gastric (fundic) mucosa. Stain: hematoxylin and eosin. High magnification.

FIGURE 14.14 | **Stomach: Basal Region of Gastric (Fundic) Mucosa**

The **gastric glands** (**1**, **9**) in the body and fundus of the stomach show **basal branching** (**9**). In the upper regions of the gastric glands, the **chief** or **zymogenic cells** (**6**, **10**) border the lumen of gastric glands (1, 9). In the basal regions, the **parietal cells** (**2**) are wedged against the basement membrane and are not always in direct contact with the lumen.

The **lamina propria** (**3**, **7**) surrounds the gastric glands (1). A small **lymphatic nodule** (**4**) is located in the lamina propria (3) adjacent to the gastric glands (1, 9). The two layers of the **muscularis mucosae** (**5**), the inner circular layer and the outer longitudinal layer, are seen below the gastric glands (1, 9). **Strands of smooth muscle** (**8**) extend upward from the muscularis mucosae (5) into the lamina propria (3, 7) between the gastric glands (1, 9).

Adjacent to the muscularis mucosae (5) is the **submucosa** (**11**).

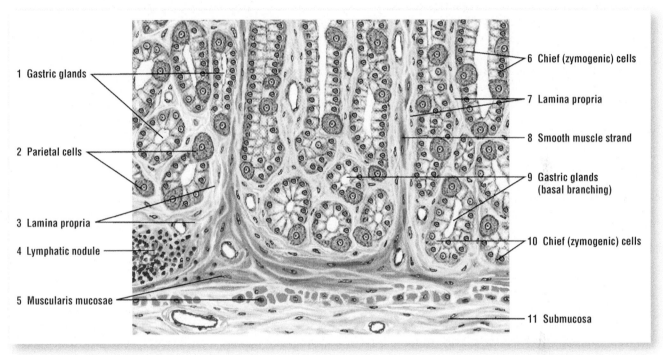

1 Gastric glands
2 Parietal cells
3 Lamina propria
4 Lymphatic nodule
5 Muscularis mucosae

6 Chief (zymogenic) cells
7 Lamina propria
8 Smooth muscle strand
9 Gastric glands (basal branching)
10 Chief (zymogenic) cells
11 Submucosa

FIGURE 14.14 ■ Stomach: basal region of gastric (fundic) mucosa. Stain: hematoxylin and eosin. High magnification.

FUNCTIONAL CORRELATIONS 14.3 ■ Stomach

The stomach **receives**, **stores**, **mixes**, **digests**, and **absorbs** some of the ingested products. In addition, the stomach cells secrete different hormones that regulate digestive functions. Some functions are designed specifically to reduce the mass of ingested food material, or **bolus**, to a semiliquid mass called **chyme**. The reduction of bolus is performed by strong, muscular peristaltic contractions of the stomach wall when food enters the stomach. With the pylorus closed, the muscular contractions churn and mix the stomach contents with **gastric juices** produced by the **gastric glands**. **Neurons** and **axons** located in the **submucosal nerve plexus** and **myenteric nerve plexus** of the stomach wall regulate the peristaltic activity. In addition, the stomach also performs some absorption; however, this is limited to absorption of water, alcohol, salts, and certain drugs.

GASTRIC GLAND CELLS IN CARDIA, BODY, AND FUNDUS OF STOMACH

Cardiac glands are limited to the narrow cardiac region of the stomach that surrounds the esophageal opening. They are primarily mucous cells. The mucus produced by these glands and the cardiac glands of the esophagus neutralize the gastric reflux and protect the esophageal lining.

Chemical reduction or digestion of food in the stomach is the main function of gastric secretions produced by different cells in the gastric glands, especially by cells in the fundus and body of the stomach. The main components of the gastric secretions are **pepsin**, **hydrochloric acid**, **mucus**, **gastric intrinsic factor**, **water**, **lysozyme**, and different **electrolytes**.

The surface or luminal epithelial cells of the stomach and the mucous neck cells of the gastric pits secrete thick layers of **mucus**. This secretion covers, lubricates, and protects the stomach surface from the corrosion by acidic gastric juices secreted by the gastric glands and the ingested material.

The major component of gastric juice is the **hydrochloric acid** (HCL) produced by **parietal cells** of the gastric glands. In humans, parietal cells also produce **gastric intrinsic factor**, a glycoprotein that is necessary for the absorption of **vitamin B$_{12}$** from the terminal portion of the small intestine. Vitamin B$_{12}$ is necessary for **erythrocyte** (red blood cell) production (**erythropoiesis**) in the red bone marrow. Deficiency of this vitamin leads to the development of **pernicious anemia**, a disorder of erythrocyte formation.

Chief (**zymogenic**) **cells** are filled with granules that contain the proenzyme **pepsinogen**, an inactive precursor of **pepsin**. Release of pepsinogen during gastric secretion into the acidic environment of the stomach converts the inactive pepsinogen into the highly active, proteolytic enzyme pepsin. This enzyme digests large protein molecules into smaller peptides, converting almost all of the proteins into smaller molecules. Pepsin is responsible for converting the solid food material into fluid chyme. The chief cells also produce **gastric lipase** for digesting lipids.

The secretory activities of the chief and parietal cells are controlled by the autonomic nervous system and the hormone **gastrin**, secreted by the enteroendocrine cells of the pyloric region of the stomach.

Enteroendocrine cells secrete various **polypeptides** and **proteins** with hormonal activity that influences digestive tract functions. They are called enteroendocrine cells because they produce gastric hormones and are located in the digestive organs. The enteroendocrine cells are also called **APUD** (**amine precursor uptake and decarboxylation**) **cells** because they can take up the precursors of amines and decarboxylate them. These cells are not confined to the gastrointestinal tract, but are also found in the respiratory organs and other organs of the body where they are also known by different names. However, because not all enteroendocrine cells accumulate amine precursors, the APUD designation has now been replaced by the term **diffuse neuroendocrine system** (**DNES**). Additional details, description, and illustration of known enteroendocrine cells are found in Chapter 15.

FIGURE 14.15 | Pyloric Region of Stomach

In the mucosa of the pyloric region of the stomach, the **gastric pits** (3, 8) are deeper than those in the body or fundus regions. The gastric pits (3, 8) extend into the mucosa to about one half or more of its thickness. The surface of the stomach is lined with a simple **columnar mucous epithelium** (1) that also extends into and lines all the gastric pits (3, 8).

The **pyloric glands** (5, 9) open into the bottom of the gastric pits (3, 8), and they are either branched or coiled tubular glands containing mucous secretions, illustrated in both transverse (5)

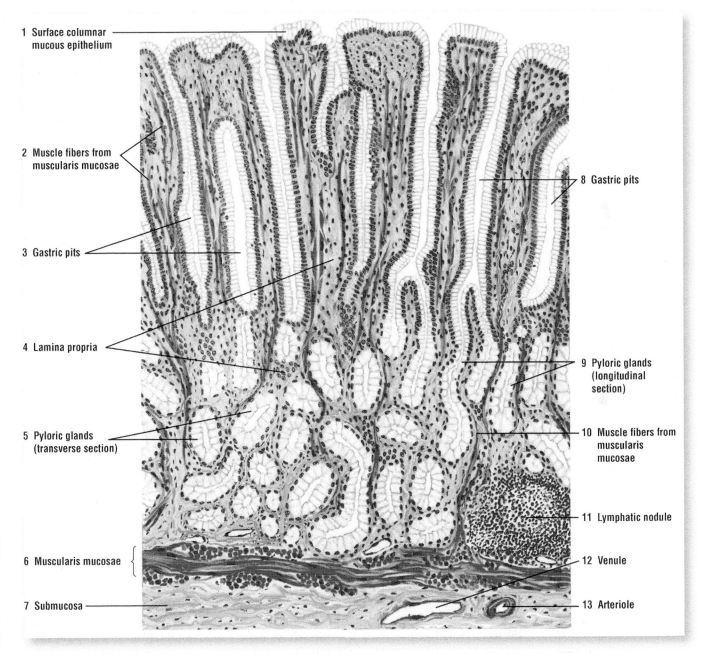

1 Surface columnar mucous epithelium

2 Muscle fibers from muscularis mucosae

3 Gastric pits

4 Lamina propria

5 Pyloric glands (transverse section)

6 Muscularis mucosae

7 Submucosa

8 Gastric pits

9 Pyloric glands (longitudinal section)

10 Muscle fibers from muscularis mucosae

11 Lymphatic nodule

12 Venule

13 Arteriole

FIGURE 14.15 ■ Pyloric region of the stomach. Stain: hematoxylin and eosin. Medium magnification.

and longitudinal (9) sections. Similar to the cardiac region of the stomach, one cell type is found in the epithelium of these glands. The tall columnar cell stains lightly because of its mucigen (mucus) with flattened or oval nuclei that are located at the base. Enteroendocrine cells are also present in this region and can be demonstrated with a special stain.

The remaining structures in the pyloric region of the stomach are similar to those of other regions. The **lamina propria** (4) contains lymphatic tissue and an occasional lymphatic nodule (11). Located below the **lymphatic nodule** (11) is the smooth muscle **muscularis mucosae** (6). Individual **smooth muscle fibers** (2, 10) from the circular layer of the **muscularis mucosae** (6) pass upward between the pyloric glands (5, 9) into the lamina propria (4) and the upper region of the mucosa. Located below the muscularis mucosae (6) is the **submucosa** (7), which contains blood vessels—an **arteriole** (13) and a **venule** (12).

FUNCTIONAL CORRELATIONS 14.4 ■ **Cells in Pyloric Gastric Glands**

Pyloric glands contain the same cell types as those present in cardiac glands in the cardiac region of the stomach. Mucus-secreting cells predominate and the secrete mucus that covers and protects the pyloric mucosa. Other cells in the pyloric gastric glands produce the enzyme **lysozyme** that destroys bacteria in the stomach, and enteroendocrine **gastrin-secreting cells** (**G cells**) secrete gastrin hormone, whose main function is to stimulate HCL production by the parietal cells.

FIGURE 14.16 | Pyloric–Duodenal Junction (Longitudinal Section)

The **pylorus** (1) of the stomach is separated from the **duodenum** (11) of the small intestine by a thick smooth muscle layer called the **pyloric sphincter** (8) formed by the thickened circular layer of the muscularis externa of the **stomach** (9).

At the junction with the duodenum (11), the **mucosal ridges** (4) of the stomach around **gastric pits** (3) become broader, irregular, and more variable in shape. Coiled tubular **pyloric (mucous) glands** (6) in the **lamina propria** (5) open at the bottom of the gastric pits (3). **Lymphatic nodules** (16) are seen between the stomach (1) and the duodenum (11).

The mucus-secreting **stomach epithelium** (2) changes to the **intestinal epithelium** (12) in the duodenum. The intestinal epithelium (12) consists of goblet cells and columnar cells with apical brush borders (microvilli) that are present throughout the length of the small intestine. The duodenum (11) contains **villi** (13), a specialized form of surface modification. Between individual villi are **intervillous spaces** (14) of the intestinal lumen.

Short, simple tubular **intestinal glands** (**crypts of Lieberkühn**) (15) are present in the lamina propria of the duodenum. These glands consist of goblet cells and cells with striated borders (microvilli) of the surface epithelium.

Duodenal glands (Brunner glands) (18) occupy most of the **submucosa** (19) in the upper duodenum (11) and are the characteristic features of this part of the duodenum. The ducts of the duodenal glands (18) penetrate the **muscularis mucosae** (17) and enter the base of the intestinal glands (15), disrupting the muscularis mucosae (17). Except for the esophageal (submucosal) glands proper, the duodenal glands (18) are the only submucosal glands in the digestive tract. In the **muscularis externa of both the stomach** (9) and the **duodenum** (20) are neurons and axons of the **myenteric nerve plexuses** (10, 21).

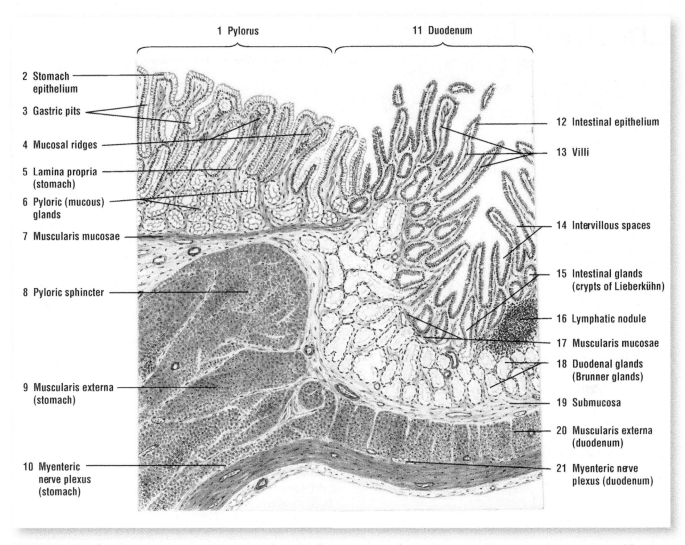

1 Pylorus   11 Duodenum

2 Stomach epithelium

3 Gastric pits

4 Mucosal ridges

5 Lamina propria (stomach)

6 Pyloric (mucous) glands

7 Muscularis mucosae

8 Pyloric sphincter

9 Muscularis externa (stomach)

10 Myenteric nerve plexus (stomach)

12 Intestinal epithelium

13 Villi

14 Intervillous spaces

15 Intestinal glands (crypts of Lieberkühn)

16 Lymphatic nodule

17 Muscularis mucosae

18 Duodenal glands (Brunner glands)

19 Submucosa

20 Muscularis externa (duodenum)

21 Myenteric nerve plexus (duodenum)

FIGURE 14.16 ■ Pyloric–duodenal junction (longitudinal section). Stain: hematoxylin and eosin. Low magnification.

Chapter 14 Summary

Digestive System Part II: Esophagus and Stomach

GENERAL PLAN OF DIGESTIVE SYSTEM: AN OVERVIEW

- Hollow tube extending from the oral cavity to rectum
- Wall exhibits basic organization of the entire tube
- Morphology of the wall and epithelium varies due to different functions

Mucosa

- Is the innermost layer of digestive tract and consists of the epithelium and glands
- Loose connective tissue around glands is the lamina propria
- Smooth muscle layer muscularis mucosae forms the outer layer of mucosae
- Muscularis mucosae has an inner circular and an outer longitudinal smooth muscle layer

Submucosa

- Located inferior to mucosa
- Consists of dense irregular connective tissue with blood vessels, nerves, and lymphatics
- Contains submucosal nerve plexus that controls muscularis mucosae

Muscularis Externa

- Thick, smooth muscle layer inferior to or below submucosa
- Normally contains an inner circular and an outer longitudinal smooth muscle layer
- Myenteric nerve plexus located between inner and outer smooth muscle layers
- Myenteric nerve plexus controls motility of smooth muscles in muscularis externa

Serosa

- Most superficial layer of abdominal portions of the digestive tract
- Thin layer of connective tissue and mesothelium that cover the visceral organs
- Covers abdominal esophagus, stomach, small intestine, and anterior wall of the colon

Adventitia

- Consists only of connective tissue layer without mesothelium lining
- Covers thoracic part of the esophagus and posterior wall of the ascending and descending colon

ESOPHAGUS

- Soft tube that extends from the pharynx to stomach, posterior to the trachea
- Penetrates the diaphragm, and a short portion is in the abdominal cavity before entering stomach
- In the thoracic cavity, outside layer is connective tissue or adventitia
- Lumen lined with moist, nonkeratinized stratified squamous epithelium
- Mucous esophageal glands are in both the lamina propria and the submucosa for lubrication
- In the upper third, muscularis externa contains skeletal muscle
- In the middle, both smooth and skeletal muscles are found in muscularis externa
- In the lower third, muscularis externa contains smooth muscle only
- Muscularis mucosae and submucosa continue with those of stomach layers

STOMACH

- Transition from the esophagus to the stomach is abrupt; stratified squamous to simple columnar epithelium
- Consists of cardiac, fundic and body, and pyloric regions
- When contracted or empty, temporary rugae are seen in the wall
- Fundus and body form the major region and are histologically identical
- Receives, stores, mixes, digests, and absorbs some food products to form liquid chyme
- Converts bolus of ingested food into semiliquid mass called chyme
- Surface is pitted by gastric pits, which are connected to gastric glands in the lamina propria
- Surface is lined with mucus-secreting, simple columnar epithelium for protection
- Gastric glands produce gastric juices rich in hydrochloric acid and protein-digesting enzymes
- Muscularis externa shows internal oblique, middle circular, and outer longitudinal muscle layers

- Submucosal and myenteric nerve plexuses regulate peristaltic activity
- Serosa or visceral peritoneum covers the outer layer of the stomach

Gastric Pits and Cells of Gastric Glands

- In the cardia, gastric pits are shallow; in the pylorus, gastric pits are deep; both produce mucus
- In the body and fundus, parietal cells are large, acidophilic, and are in the upper gland region
- Deeper regions of the gastric glands contain chief or zymogen cells
- In cardiac and pylorus, epithelium and simple tubular gastric glands produce mucus

- Glands in the pylorus also produce mucus and bacteria-destroying enzyme lysozyme
- Pylorus gland G cells also secrete gastrin that stimulates parietal cells to produce HCL
- Parietal cells in the fundus and body produce hydrochloric acid and gastric intrinsic factor
- Gastric intrinsic factor is essential for absorption of vitamin B12 and for erythropoiesis
- Chief cells produce pepsinogen that is converted to pepsin in acidic environment
- Enteroendocrine cells secrete a variety of polypeptides and proteins for digestive functions
- Mucus-secreting stomach cells change to intestinal epithelium in the duodenum

Chapter 14 Review Questions

In the following multiple choice questions, choose the letter corresponding to the one best answer.

1. What induces pepsinogen to convert into pepsin?

A. Mucus secretion by luminal cells

B. Gastric intrinsic factor release

C. Acidic environment containing hydrochloric acid

D. Gastrin secretion

E. Bicarbonate or neutral content of chyme

2. What role does the gastric intrinsic factor play in the digestive process?

A. It increases digestive tract motility and digestion of its contents.

B. It neutralizes pepsinogen and pepsin.

C. It stimulates the production of hydrochloric acid.

D. It is necessary for absorption of vitamin B12 from the small intestine.

E. It activates the enteroendocrine cells to produce hormones.

3. Zymogenic or chief cells of the gastric glands produce:

A. gastric intrinsic factor.

B. pepsinogen.

C. pepsin.

D. hydrochloric acid.

E. gastrin.

4. What role do the surface epithelium cells perform during the digestive process?

A. They add secretions to the gastric juices produced by the gastric glands.

B. They secrete mucus for the stomach lining to protect it against corrosive gastric juices.

C. They secrete additional hydrochloric acid to the gastric juices.

D. They produce pepsinogen.

E. They produce gastric hormones to assist digestive processes.

5. What is found in the lamina propria of the stomach?

A. Connective tissue and gastric glands

B. Different nerve plexuses

C. Longitudinal and all three circular smooth muscle layers

D. Adventitia

E. Large blood vessels and nerves

ANSWERS

1. Correct Answer: C. Acidic environment containing hydrochloric acid. Once pepsinogen reaches the acidity of the stomach, it is converted to the proteolytic enzyme pepsin.

2. Correct Answer: D. It is necessary for absorption of vitamin B12 from the small intestine. This factor is produced by the parietal cells and plays an important role in erythropoiesis in the bone marrow.

3. Correct Answer: B. Pepsinogen. This is an inactive precursor of pepsin that is formed after pepsinogen reaches the acidic environment of the stomach.

4. Correct Answer: B. They secrete mucus for the stomach lining to protect it against corrosive gastric juices. The surface cells produce large amounts of mucus that cover the luminal surface of the stomach.

5. Correct Answer: A. Connective tissue and gastric glands. The connective tissue is squeezed by the gastric glands into strips between the glands.

ADDITIONAL HISTOLOGIC IMAGES

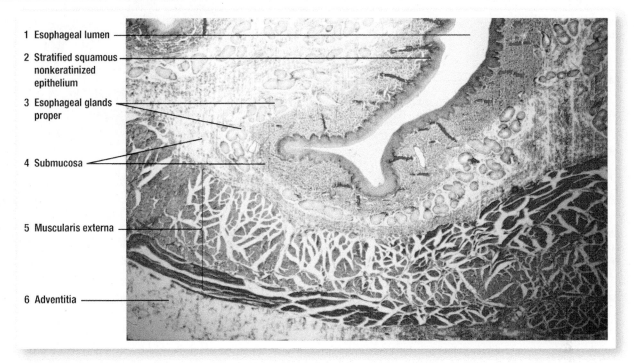

1 Esophageal lumen
2 Stratified squamous nonkeratinized epithelium
3 Esophageal glands proper
4 Submucosa
5 Muscularis externa
6 Adventitia

FIGURE 14.17 ■ A transverse section of a primate esophagus illustrating the contents of its wall. Esophageal glands proper are in the submucosa. Stain: hematoxylin and eosin. ×10.

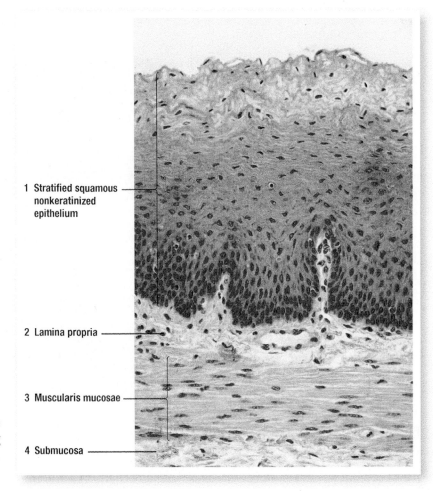

1 Stratified squamous nonkeratinized epithelium
2 Lamina propria
3 Muscularis mucosae
4 Submucosa

FIGURE 14.18 ■ A higher magnification of a human esophageal wall illustrating epithelium and the lamina propria. Stain: hematoxylin and eosin. ×64.

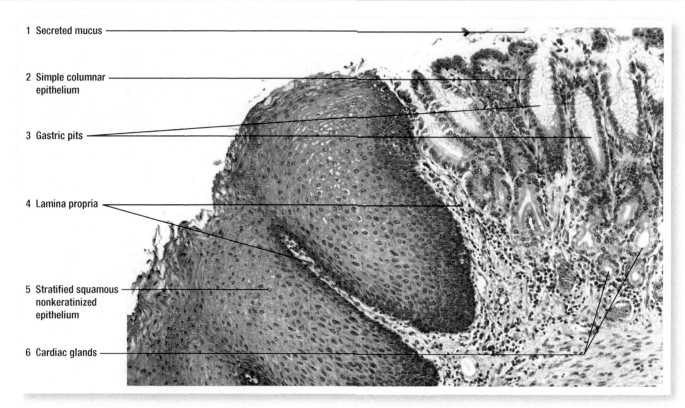

1 Secreted mucus

2 Simple columnar epithelium

3 Gastric pits

4 Lamina propria

5 Stratified squamous nonkeratinized epithelium

6 Cardiac glands

FIGURE 14.19 ■ Esophageal–stomach junction in a human illustrating the abrupt epithelial change at the junction. Stain: hematoxylin and eosin. ×50.

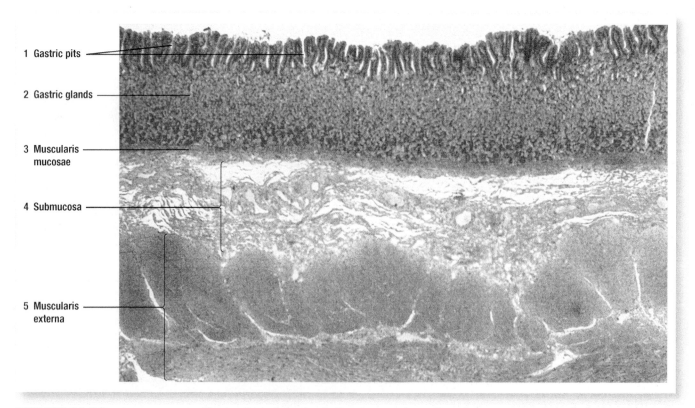

1 Gastric pits

2 Gastric glands

3 Muscularis mucosae

4 Submucosa

5 Muscularis externa

FIGURE 14.20 ■ Lower-power illustration of the body/fundus section of a primate stomach wall. Stain: hematoxylin and eosin. ×6.5.

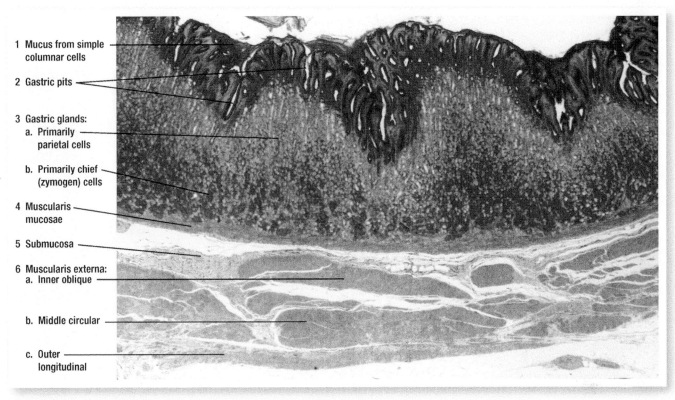

1 Mucus from simple columnar cells

2 Gastric pits

3 Gastric glands:
   a. Primarily parietal cells

   b. Primarily chief (zymogen) cells

4 Muscularis mucosae

5 Submucosa

6 Muscularis externa:
   a. Inner oblique

   b. Middle circular

   c. Outer longitudinal

FIGURE 14.21 ■ Lower-power illustration of the body/fundus section of a human stomach wall. Stain: periodic acid–Schiff. ×8.0.

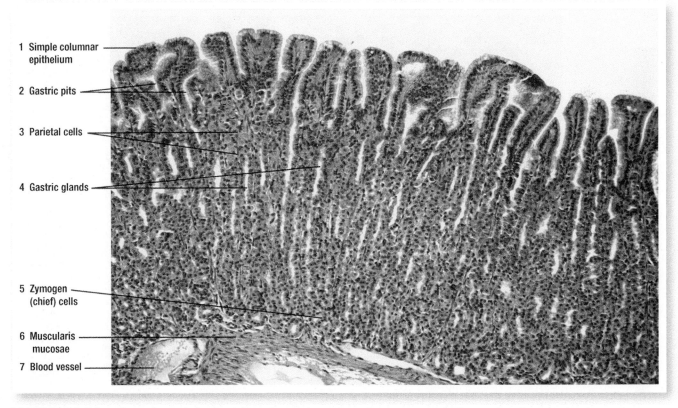

1 Simple columnar epithelium

2 Gastric pits

3 Parietal cells

4 Gastric glands

5 Zymogen (chief) cells

6 Muscularis mucosae

7 Blood vessel

FIGURE 14.22 ■ A section of the body/fundus region of a primate stomach illustrating the gastric pits and gastric glands with different cells. Stain: hematoxylin and eosin. ×25.

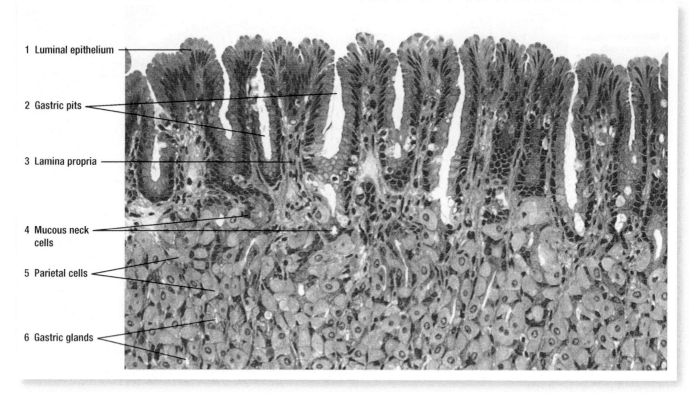

1 Luminal epithelium

2 Gastric pits

3 Lamina propria

4 Mucous neck cells

5 Parietal cells

6 Gastric glands

FIGURE 14.23 ■ A thin plastic section of the luminal surface area of the body/fundus region of a primate stomach. Stain: hematoxylin and eosin. ×65.

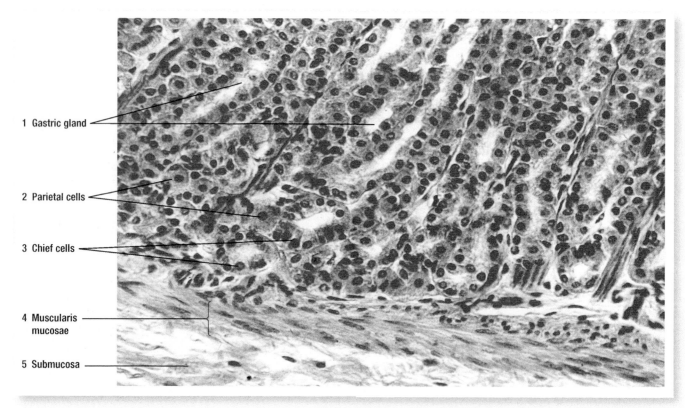

1 Gastric gland

2 Parietal cells

3 Chief cells

4 Muscularis mucosae

5 Submucosa

FIGURE 14.24 ■ A section of the body/fundus region of a primate stomach illustrating bases of the gastric glands. Stain: hematoxylin and eosin. ×65.

Digestive System Part III: Small Intestine and Large Intestine

SECTION 1 Small Intestine

SMALL INTESTINE

The **small intestine** is a convoluted tube about 5 to 7 m long; it is the longest section of the digestive tract. It extends from the junction with the stomach to the **large intestine**, or **colon**. The small intestine is divided into three parts: the **duodenum**, **jejunum**, and **ileum**. The microscopic differences among these three segments are minor; however, these minor differences allow for identification of different segments.

The main function of the small intestine is the digestion of gastric contents and absorption of nutrients into blood capillaries and lymphatic lacteals.

Surface Modifications of Small Intestine for Absorption

The mucosa of the small intestine exhibits structural modifications that increase the cellular surface areas for the absorption of nutrients and fluids. These modifications include three structures: plicae circulares, villi, and microvilli.

In contrast to the rugae of the stomach, the **plicae circulares** are permanent spiral folds or elevations of the mucosa (with a submucosal core) that extend into the intestinal lumen. These structures are most prominent in the proximal portion of the small intestine, the jejunum, where most absorption takes place; they decrease in prominence toward the ileum.

Villi are also permanent finger-like projections of lamina propria of the mucosa that extend into the intestinal lumen. They are covered by **simple columnar epithelium** and are also more prominent in the proximal portion of the small intestine with the height decreasing toward the ileum. The connective tissue core of each villus contains a lymphatic capillary called a **lacteal**, blood capillaries, and individual strands of smooth muscles (Fig. 15.1).

Each villus contains blood vessels, lymphatic capillaries, nerves, smooth muscle, and loose irregular connective tissue, in addition to the **lamina propria** plasma cells, tissue eosinophils, macrophages, and mast cells.

Smooth muscle fibers from the muscularis mucosae extend into the core of individual villi to induce movements. This action increases the contacts of the villi with the digested food products in the intestinal lumen.

Microvilli are cytoplasmic extensions that cover the apices of the intestinal absorptive cells. They are visible under a light microscope as a **brush border** (also called striated border). With transmission electron microscopy, they appear as regular and dense finger-like extensions of the absorptive cell cytoplasm. The microvilli are coated by a glycoprotein coat (glycocalyx), which contains **brush border enzymes**. The microvilli increase the absorptive luminal surface area many fold.

Glands, Cells, and Lymphatic Cells and Nodules in Small Intestine

Intestinal Glands

Located throughout the small intestine are the **intestinal glands** (**crypts of Lieberkühn**). These glands open into the intestinal lumen at the base of the villi. The simple columnar epithelium that

353

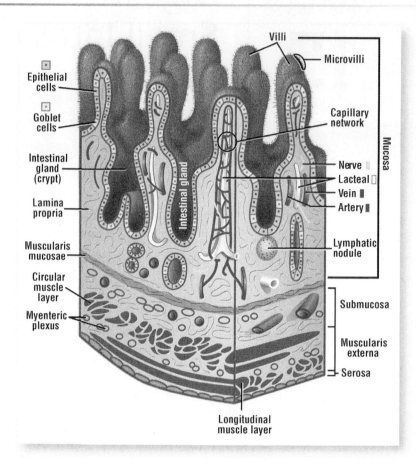

FIGURE 15.1 ■ Different cell types and layers in the wall of the small intestine.

lines the villi is continuous with that of the intestinal glands that contain regenerative stem cells, absorptive cells, goblet cells, Paneth cells, and enteroendocrine cells.

Intestinal Cells

- **Absorptive cells** are the most common cells in the intestinal epithelium. These cells are tall and columnar with a prominent brush border of **microvilli**. A thick **glycocalyx** coat covers and protects the microvilli from the corrosive digestive chemicals.
- **Goblet cells** are interspersed among the columnar absorptive cells of the epithelium. They increase in number toward the distal region of the small intestine (ileum).
- **Enteroendocrine** or diffuse neuroendocrine system (DNES) cells are scattered throughout the epithelium of the villi and intestinal glands.
- **Duodenal (Brunner) glands** are primarily found in the **submucosa** of the initial portion of the duodenum and characterize this region of the small intestine. These are branched, tubuloacinar glands with light-staining **mucous cells**. The ducts of duodenal glands penetrate the muscularis mucosae and discharge their secretory products at the base of intestinal glands located between the villi.
- **Undifferentiated** or **stem cells** are located at the base of intestinal glands, and they exhibit increased mitotic activity. These stem cells replace all worn-out columnar absorptive cells, goblet cells, and intestinal gland cells in the small intestine.
- **Paneth cells** are located at the base of intestinal glands, characterized by deep-staining eosinophilic granules in their cytoplasm.

Lymphatic Nodules and Lymphocytic Cells

Peyer patches are aggregations of closely packed, permanent **lymphatic nodules** that are found primarily in the wall of the terminal portion of the small intestine, the ileum. These nodules occupy a large portion of the lamina propria and submucosa of the ileum. The dispersed lymphocytes and the Peyer patches constitute the **gut-associated lymphoid tissue** (GALT) that serves as an immunologic barrier throughout the gastrointestinal tract.

M cells are specialized epithelial cells that cover the Peyer patches and large lymphatic nodules; they are not found anywhere else in the intestine. Instead of microvilli, these cells exhibit numerous apical microfolds, hence the name "M cells." M cells phagocytose luminal antigens and transport them to the lymphocytes and antigen-presenting dendritic cells located in the lamina propria resulting in adaptive immune responses that produce specific antibodies that are then transported to the intestinal lumen to eliminate harmful pathogens from its surface.

Regional Differences in Small Intestine

The **duodenum** is the shortest segment of the small intestine. Here, the villi are broad, tall, and numerous, with fewer goblet cells in the epithelium. Branched **duodenal (Brunner) glands** with mucus-secreting cells in the submucosa characterize this region. The glands, however, diminish in number toward the end of the duodenum.

The **jejunum** is longer than the duodenum and contains the largest surface area for the absorption of the digested material. Here, the villi are tall and lined with simple columnar epithelium composed of absorptive cells and some mucus-secreting goblet cells. There are also more goblet cells in the epithelium of the jejunum than in the duodenum. The jejunum does not contain any duodenal (Brunner) glands or lymphatic nodule aggregations (Peyer patches).

The **ileum** contains villi that are narrow and short with the epithelium containing more goblet cells than the duodenum or the jejunum. In addition to increased numbers of lymphocytes in the lamina propria, the aggregated lymphatic nodules (Peyer patches) are large and most numerous in the distal ileum. Lymphatic nodules aggregate in the lamina propria and submucosa to form the prominent Peyer patches.

thePoint®   Supplemental micrographic images are available at **www.thePoint.com/Eroschenko13e** under Digestive System Part III: Small Intestine and Large Intestine.

FIGURE 15.2 | **Small Intestine: Duodenum (Longitudinal Section)**

The wall of the duodenum consists of four layers: the mucosa with the **lining epithelium** (7a), the **lamina propria** (7b), and the **muscularis mucosae** (9, 12); the underlying connective tissue **submucosa** with the mucous **duodenal (Brunner) glands** (3, 13); the two smooth muscle layers

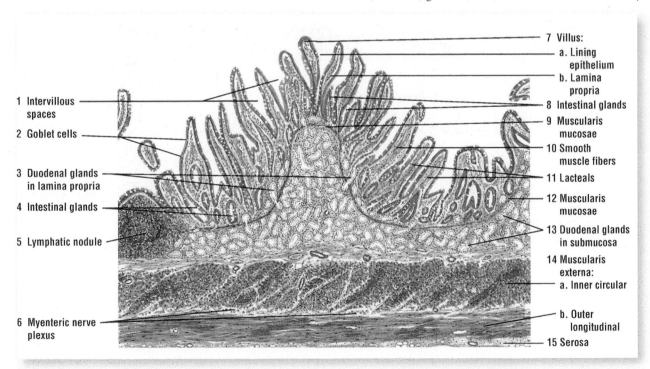

1 Intervillous spaces
2 Goblet cells
3 Duodenal glands in lamina propria
4 Intestinal glands
5 Lymphatic nodule
6 Myenteric nerve plexus

7 Villus:
a. Lining epithelium
b. Lamina propria
8 Intestinal glands
9 Muscularis mucosae
10 Smooth muscle fibers
11 Lacteals
12 Muscularis mucosae
13 Duodenal glands in submucosa
14 Muscularis externa:
a. Inner circular
b. Outer longitudinal
15 Serosa

FIGURE 15.2 ■ Small intestine: duodenum (longitudinal section). Stain: hematoxylin and eosin. Low magnification.

of the **muscularis externa** (**14**); and the visceral peritoneum **serosa** (**15**). These layers are continuous with those of the stomach, small intestine, and large intestine (colon).

The small intestine is characterized by finger-like extensions, **villi** (**7**) (singular, villus); a lining epithelium (**7a**) of columnar cells lined with the microvilli that form the brush borders; light-staining **goblet cells** (**2**); and short, tubular **intestinal glands** (**crypts of Lieberkühn**) (**4, 8**) in the lamina propria (**7b**). Although the duodenal glands (**3, 13**) in the submucosa (**13**) characterize the duodenum, such glands are absent from the rest of the small intestine (jejunum and ileum) and the large intestine.

The villi (**7**) are mucosal surface modifications. Between the villi (**7**) are the **intervillous spaces** (**1**). The lining epithelium (**7a**) covers each villus and the intestinal glands (**4, 8**). Each villus (**7**) contains a core of lamina propria (**7b**), strands of **smooth muscle fibers** (**10**) that extend upward into the villi from the muscularis mucosae (**9, 12**), and a central lymphatic vessel called a **lacteal** (**11**) (see Fig. 15.8 for details).

The intestinal glands (**4, 8**) are located in the lamina propria (**7b**) and open into the intervillous spaces (**1**). In sections of the duodenum, the submucosal duodenal glands (**13**) extend into the lamina propria (**3**). The lamina propria (**7b**) also contains fine connective tissue fibers with reticular cells, diffuse lymphatic tissue, and **lymphatic nodules** (**5**).

The submucosa (**13**) in the duodenum is almost completely filled with branched, tubular duodenal glands (**13**). These glands (**13**) penetrate the muscularis mucosae (**9, 12**) when they project into the lamina propria (**3**). The secretions from the duodenal glands (**3**) enter at the bottom of the intestinal glands (**3, 4, 8**).

In a cross section of the duodenum, the muscularis externa (**14**) consists of an **inner circular layer** (**14a**) and an **outer longitudinal layer** (**14b**) of smooth muscle. However, in this figure, the duodenum has been cut in a longitudinal plane, and the direction of fibers in these two smooth muscle layers is reversed. Parasympathetic ganglion cells of the **myenteric (Auerbach) nerve plexus** (**6**), found in the small and large intestines, are in the connective tissue between the two muscle layers of the muscularis externa (**14**). Similar but smaller plexuses of ganglion cells are also found in the submucosa (not illustrated) in the small and large intestines.

The **serosa** (**visceral peritoneum**) (**15**) contains the connective tissue cells, blood vessels, and adipose cells. The serosa forms the outermost layer of the first part of the duodenum.

FUNCTIONAL CORRELATIONS 15.1 ■ Duodenum

A characteristic feature of the duodenum is the branched tubuloacinar **duodenal (Brunner) glands** in the submucosa whose excretory ducts penetrate the muscularis mucosae at the base of intestinal glands. Duodenal glands release their product into the intestinal lumen in response to the entrance of **acidic chyme** from the stomach and parasympathetic stimulation by the vagus nerve.

The main function of the duodenal glands is to protect the duodenal mucosa from the corrosive gastric acidity. Thus, alkaline **mucus** and **bicarbonate secretions** from the duodenal glands buffer or neutralize the acidic chyme. This action provides a more favorable environment for digestive enzymes that are released into the duodenum from the pancreas.

Enteroendocrine cells located in the secretory acini of duodenal (Brunner) glands also produce a polypeptide hormone called **urogastrone** that inhibits or decreases hydrochloric acid secretion by the parietal cells in the stomach.

FIGURE 15.3 | Small Intestine: Duodenum (Transverse Section)

This low-magnification photomicrograph illustrates a transverse section of the duodenum. The luminal surface exhibits **villi** (2) that are covered by **simple columnar epithelium** (1) with a brush border. The core of each villus (2) contains the **lamina propria** (4, 6) with connective tissue cells, lymphatic cells, plasma cells, macrophages, smooth muscle cells, and others. In addition, the lamina propria (4, 6) contains blood vessels and the dilated, blind-ending lymphatic channels, the **lacteals** (3). Between the villi (2) are the **intestinal glands** (7) that extend to the **muscularis mucosae** (8). Inferior to the muscularis mucosae (8) is the **submucosa** (9). In the duodenum, the submucosa (9) is filled with light-staining, mucus-secreting **duodenal glands** (5), whose ducts pierce the muscularis mucosae (8) to deliver their secretory product at the base of the intestinal glands (7). Surrounding the submucosa (9) and the duodenal glands (5) is the **muscularis externa** (10).

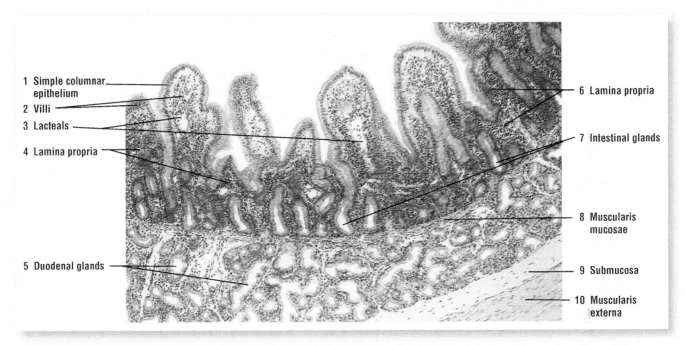

1 Simple columnar epithelium
2 Villi
3 Lacteals
4 Lamina propria
5 Duodenal glands

6 Lamina propria
7 Intestinal glands
8 Muscularis mucosae
9 Submucosa
10 Muscularis externa

FIGURE 15.3 ■ Small intestine: duodenum (transverse section). Stain: hematoxylin and eosin. ×25.

FIGURE 15.4 | Small Intestine: Jejunum (Transverse Section)

The histology of the lower duodenum, jejunum, and ileum is similar to that of the upper duodenum (see Fig. 15.2) except for the duodenal (Brunner) glands; these are limited to the submucosa in the upper part of the duodenum.

This figure illustrates the permanent fold of the **plicae circulares** (**10**) that extends into the jejunal lumen. The core of plicae circulares (10) is formed by **submucosa** (**3, 15**) with numerous **arteries** and **veins** (**13**). The finger-like **villi** (**12**) cover the plica (10). Between the villi (12) are the **intervillous spaces** (**11**), and at the bottom of the villi (12) are the **intestinal glands** (**14**) in the **lamina propria** (**5**). The intestinal glands (crypts of Lieberkühn) (4) open into the intervillous spaces (11).

Each villus (12) exhibits a columnar **lining epithelium** (**1**) with brush border and goblet cells. Below the epithelium (1) in the lamina propria (5) is a **lymphatic nodule** (**6**) with a germinal center. Individual strands of smooth muscle fibers from the **muscularis mucosae** (**2**) extend in the lamina propria of the villi (12). Each villus also contains a central **lacteal** (**4**) and capillaries (see Fig. 15.8).

The small intestine is surrounded by the **muscularis externa** that contains an **inner circular** (**7**) **layer** and an **outer longitudinal smooth muscle** (**8**) layer. Parasympathetic ganglion cells of the **myenteric plexus** (**16**) are present in the connective tissue between the muscle layers of the muscularis externa (7, 8). A similar submucosal plexus is also present in the submucosa, but it is not illustrated in this figure.

A visceral peritoneum, or **serosa** (**17**), surrounds the small intestine under which are connective tissue fibers, blood vessels, and **adipose cells** (**9**).

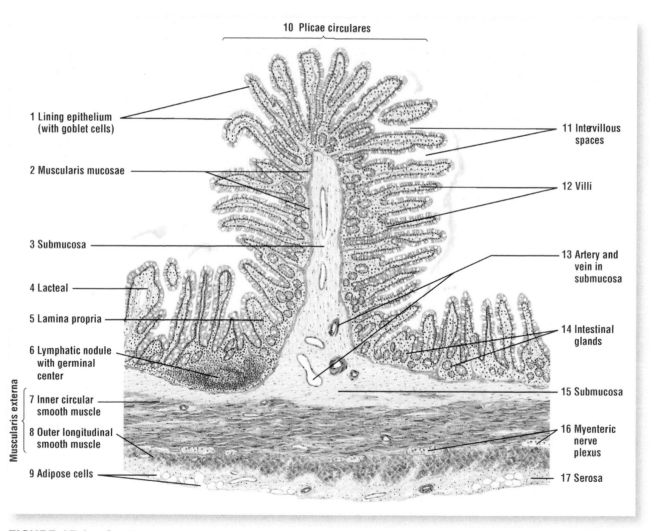

FIGURE 15.4 ■ Small intestine: jejunum (transverse section). Stain: hematoxylin and eosin. Low magnification.

FIGURE 15.5 | Intestinal Glands with Paneth Cells and Enteroendocrine Cells

Extending from the intervillous spaces of the intestinal lumen through the **lamina propria** (**6**) to the smooth muscle **muscularis mucosae** (**5**) are the **intestinal glands** (**1, 8**). This high-magnification illustration shows the bases of the intestinal glands (1, 8) sectioned in longitudinal (1) and cross sections (8). Located in their bases (1, 8) are different cells. The most obvious are the pyramid-shaped cells filled with large, acidophilic granules that displace the nucleus toward the base of the cell. These are the **Paneth cells** (**4, 10**) and are found in the intestinal glands throughout the length of the small intestine. As in the villi, there are also numerous **goblet cells** (**2**) in the intestinal glands (1, 8).

In addition to the goblet cells (2), there are numerous **mitotic cells** (**7**) that serve as stem cells for regeneration of cells that are lost from the intestinal glands (1, 8). Also present are the **enteroendocrine cells** (**3, 9**) that are interspersed among the intestinal gland cells, goblet cells (2), and Paneth cells (4, 10). Enteroendocrine cells (3, 9) contain secretory granules in the basal cytoplasm and are close to the lamina propria (6) and the blood vessels. These cells are part of the **diffuse neuroendocrine system** (**DNES**) and are found in the epithelia of different systems, such as the gastrointestinal tract (the stomach and the small and large intestines), the respiratory tract, pancreas, and thyroid glands.

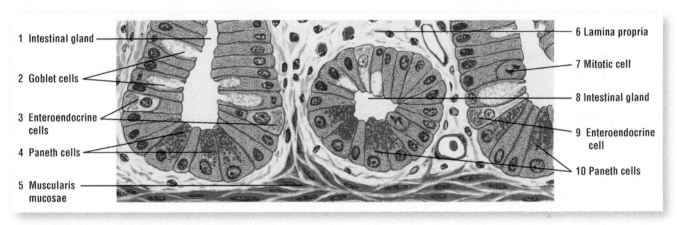

1 Intestinal gland
2 Goblet cells
3 Enteroendocrine cells
4 Paneth cells
5 Muscularis mucosae
6 Lamina propria
7 Mitotic cell
8 Intestinal gland
9 Enteroendocrine cell
10 Paneth cells

FIGURE 15.5 ■ Intestinal glands with Paneth cells and enteroendocrine cells. Stain: hematoxylin and eosin. High magnification.

FIGURE 15.6 | Small Intestine: Jejunum with Paneth Cells

This low-magnification photomicrograph illustrates the mucosa of the jejunum. The **villi** (**1**) are lined with a **simple columnar epithelium** (**2**) with a brush border interspersed with the mucus-filled **goblet cells** (**3**). Located in the **lamina propria** (**6**) of each villus are lymphatic cells, macrophages, smooth muscle cells, **blood vessels** (**7**), and lymphatic lacteals (not visible). Between the villi are the **intestinal glands** (**8**) with red-staining or eosinophilic secretory granules of **Paneth cells** (**9**). The intestinal glands (**8**) end near the **muscularis mucosae** (**4**), inferior to which is the **submucosa** (**5**).

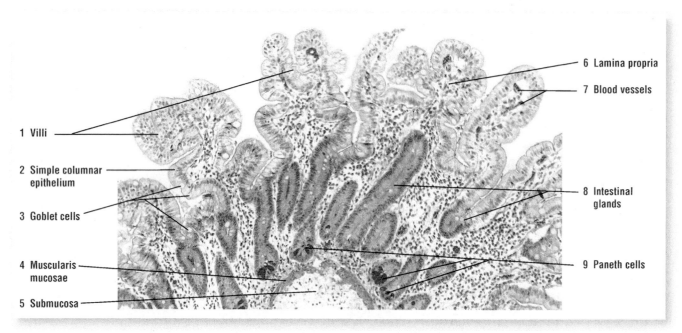

FIGURE 15.6 ■ Small intestine: jejunum with Paneth cells. Stain: Mallory-Azan. ×40.

FUNCTIONAL CORRELATIONS 15.2 ■ Paneth Cells and Enteroendocrine Cells in Small Intestine

Paneth cells, located in the bases of intestinal glands perform **defensive functions** in the digestive tract. Paneth cells produce **lysozyme**, an antibacterial enzyme that digests the bacterial cell walls and membranes of microorganisms. These cells also release the hydrophobic peptide **defensin** in response to microbial presence. Thus, Paneth cells function in controlling the microbial flora in the small intestine and regulating the microenvironment of the intestinal crypts.

Enteroendocrine cells located in the epithelium of the small intestine secrete numerous **regulatory hormones** for the digestive system, including gastric inhibitory peptide, secretin, and cholecystokinin (pan-

creozymin). To release these hormones into the capillaries, the secretory granules in these cells are located in the base of the cells and are adjacent to the lamina propria and the capillaries.

Gastric inhibitory peptide inhibits parietal cell production of hydrochloric acid. Entrance of acidic chyme into the duodenum also causes a release of the hormone **secretin**, which influences the exocrine cells of the pancreas to secrete a bicarbonate-rich fluid that neutralizes the luminal acidity and promotes the action of digestive enzymes in the small intestine. **Cholecystokinin** increases the secretion of pancreatic enzymes into the small intestine and induces gallbladder contractions to expel the stored bile.

FIGURE 15.7 | Small Intestine: Ileum with Lymphatic Nodules (Peyer Patches) (Transverse Section)

In the lamina propria and submucosa of the ileum is a highly developed gut-associated lymphoid tissue (GALT). A characteristic feature of the ileum wall is the aggregations of numerous **lymphatic nodules** (**5, 12**) called **Peyer patches** (**5, 12**) that coalesce with boundaries between them becoming indistinct. Most of these lymphatic nodules (5, 12) exhibit **germinal centers** (**5**).

The lymphatic nodules (5, 12) originate in the diffuse lymphatic tissue of the **lamina propria** (**10**). Villi are absent in the area of the intestinal lumen where the nodules (5, 12) expand to reach the surface of the mucosa and spread out in the **submucosa** (**6**).

Also illustrated are the surface epithelium (1) that covers the villi (2, 8), intestinal glands (4, 11), lacteals in the villi (3, 9), the inner circular layer (14a) and the outer longitudinal layer (14b) of the muscularis externa (14), and the serosa (7).

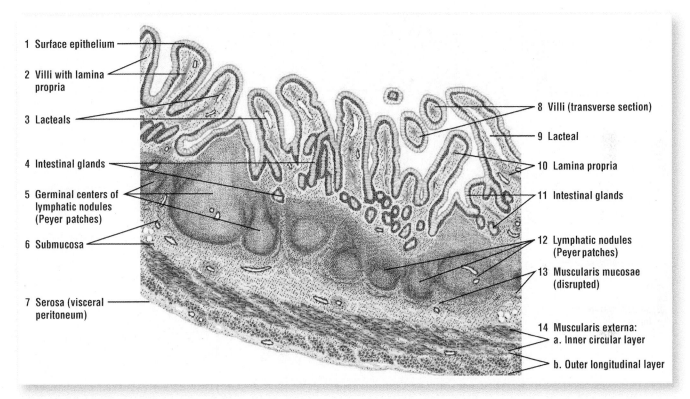

1 Surface epithelium

2 Villi with lamina propria

3 Lacteals

4 Intestinal glands

5 Germinal centers of lymphatic nodules (Peyer patches)

6 Submucosa

7 Serosa (visceral peritoneum)

8 Villi (transverse section)

9 Lacteal

10 Lamina propria

11 Intestinal glands

12 Lymphatic nodules (Peyer patches)

13 Muscularis mucosae (disrupted)

14 Muscularis externa:
a. Inner circular layer
b. Outer longitudinal layer

FIGURE 15.7 ■ Small intestine: ileum with lymphatic nodules (Peyer patches) (transverse section). Stain: hematoxylin and eosin. Low magnification.

FIGURE 15.8 | Small Intestine: Villi (Longitudinal and Transverse Section)

Several **villi** (**1**) are sectioned in the longitudinal and transverse plane and illustrated at a higher magnification. The simple columnar **surface epithelium** (**2**) that covers the villi (**1**) contains mucus-secreting **goblet cells** (**7**) and absorptive cells with **brush borders** (**microvilli**) (**3**). To show mucus, the section was stained for carbohydrates with the goblet cells (**7**) staining magenta-red.

A thin **basement membrane** (**8**) is visible between the surface epithelium (**2**) and the **lamina propria** (**4**) that contains connective tissue cells, collagen fibers, blood cells, and **smooth muscle fibers** (**5**). Also present in each villus (but not always seen in sections) is a **central lacteal** (**6**), a lymphatic vessel lined with endothelium. Arterioles, venules, and **capillaries** (**9**) are also visible in the villi.

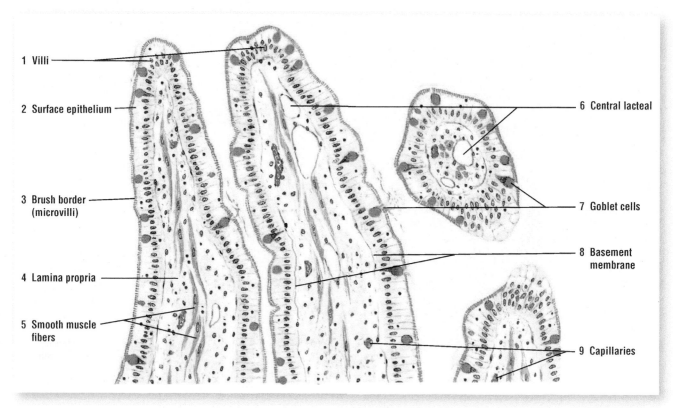

1 Villi

2 Surface epithelium

3 Brush border (microvilli)

4 Lamina propria

5 Smooth muscle fibers

6 Central lacteal

7 Goblet cells

8 Basement membrane

9 Capillaries

FIGURE 15.8 ■ Small intestine: villi (longitudinal and transverse section). Stain: periodic acid–Schiff. Medium magnification.

FIGURE 15.9 | Ultrastructure of Microvilli in Absorptive Cell in Small Intestine

Microvilli are tiny surface projections that appear as a pink-staining brush border on absorptive cells in the intestine, especially when the slides are stained for carbohydrates and examined with a light microscope. With a transmission electron microscope, the brush border is seen as dense finger-like **microvilli** (**1, 5**) that project from the apical plasma membrane of absorptive cells. Although microvilli (1, 5) are seen in different cell types, they are most prevalent lining the villi of the small intestine.

The core of the microvilli (1, 5) consists of vertical actin microfilaments that are attached to the cytoplasm by actin microfilaments called the **terminal web** (**2, 6**). Also seen are numerous **cytoplasmic vesicles** (**4**), **secretory granules** (**3**), and numerous **mitochondria** (**7**), sectioned in different planes.

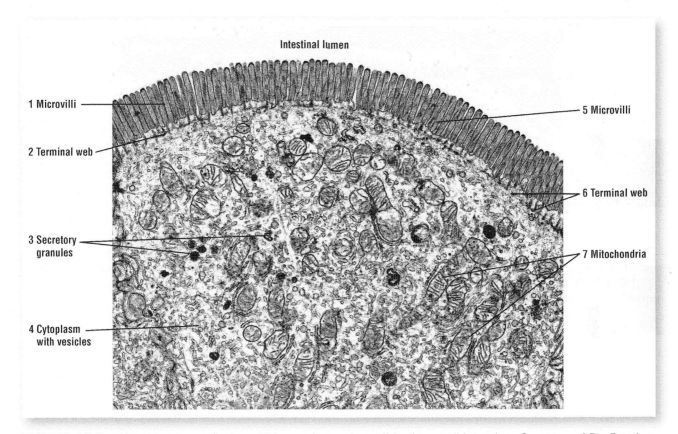

FIGURE 15.9 ■ Ultrastructure of microvilli in an absorptive cell in the small intestine. Courtesy of Dr. Rex A. Hess, Professor Emeritus, Comparative Biosciences, College of Veterinary Medicine, University of Illinois, Urbana, Illinois. ×6,150.

FUNCTIONAL CORRELATIONS 15.3 ■ Peyer Patches in Ileum

The lamina propria and submucosa in the ileum contain numerous aggregates of large lymphatic nodules called **Peyer patches**. Overlying these lymphatic patches are specialized epithelial cells called the **M cells** whose cell membranes show microfolds that contain both macrophages and lymphocytes. The lymphatic nodules of Peyer patches contain numerous **B lymphocytes**, some **T lymphocytes**, **macrophages**, and **plasma cells**. M cells continually sample the **antigens** of the intestinal lumen, ingest the antigens, and present them to the underlying lymphocytes and macrophages in the lamina propria. The antigens that reach the underlying lymphocytes and macrophages then initiate the proper immunologic responses to these foreign molecules. Peyer patches and lymphatic aggregates represent the **gut-associated lymphatic tissue (GALT)**.

SMALL INTESTINE: FUNCTIONAL OVERVIEW

The small intestine performs numerous digestive functions, including (1) continuation and completion of **digestion** (initiated in the oral cavity and the stomach) of food products (chyme) by chemicals and enzymes produced in the liver and pancreas and by cells in its own mucosa, (2) selective **absorption** of nutrients into the blood and lymph capillaries, (3) **transportation** of chyme and digestive waste material to the large intestine, and (4) release of different **hormones** into the bloodstream to regulate the secretory functions and motility of digestive organs.

The epithelial **goblet cells** secrete **mucus** that lubricates, coats, and protects the intestinal surface from the corrosive actions of digestive chemicals and enzymes. The outer **glycocalyx** coat on absorptive cells not only protects the intestinal surface from digestion but also contains **brush border enzymes** required for the final breakdown of ingested food products before absorption. Enzymes such as disaccharidases, peptidases, sucrase, lipase, lactase, and others are produced by absorptive epithelial cells and are an integral part of the membrane proteins of the glycocalyx. Thus, the brush borders not only increase the absorptive surfaces in the intestinal lumen but also become an area where enzymes perform the final digestive processes of carbohydrates and proteins. Absorption of nutrients in the small intestine occurs via diffusion, facilitated diffusion, osmosis, and active transport. Intestinal cells absorb amino acids, glucose, and fatty acids—the end products of protein, carbohydrate, and fat digestion, respectively. Amino acids, water, various ions, and glucose enter the blood capillaries in the lamina propria of each villus, from which they pass to the liver via the portal vein. Most of the long-chain fatty acids and monoglycerides, however, do not enter the capillaries but instead enter the tiny, blind-ending lymphatic vessels (lacteals) also located in the lamina propria of each villus. Smooth muscle fibers in the villi move and contract the villi. This action forces the contents from the lacteals into larger lymph vessels in the submucosa.

SECTION 2   Large Intestine (Colon)

The large intestine is situated between the anus and the terminal end of the ileum. It is shorter and less convoluted than the small intestine. The large intestine consists of the cecum; ascending, transverse, descending, and sigmoid colon; as well as the rectum and anus.

Chyme enters the large intestine from the ileum through the ileocecal valve. Unabsorbed and undigested food residues from the small intestine enter the large intestine following strong peristaltic actions of smooth muscles in the muscularis externa (Fig. 15.10). The residues entering the large intestine are in a semifluid state; however, by terminal portion of the large intestine, these residues become semisolid **feces**.

the**Point**®   Supplemental micrographic images are available at **www.thePoint.com/Eroschenko13e** under Digestive System Part III: Small Intestine and Large Intestine.

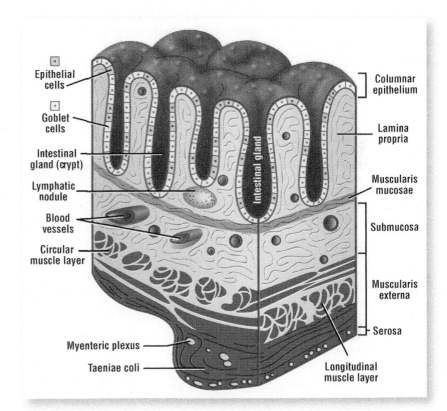

FIGURE 15.10 ■ Different cells and layers in the wall of the large intestine.

FIGURE 15.11 | Large Intestine: Colon and Mesentery (Panoramic View, Transverse Section)

The wall of the colon has the same basic layers as the small intestine. The **mucosa (4–7)** consists of simple columnar **epithelium (4)**, **intestinal glands (5)**, **lamina propria (6)**, and **muscularis mucosae (7)**. The **submucosa (8)** contains connective tissue cells and fibers, various blood vessels, and nerves. Two smooth muscle layers make up the **muscularis externa (13)**. The **serosa (visceral peritoneum and mesentery) (3, 17)** covers the transverse colon and the sigmoid colon.

The colon does not have villi or plicae circulares, and the luminal surface of the mucosa is smooth. In an undistended colon, the mucosa (4–7) and the submucosa (8) exhibit **temporary folds (12)**. In the lamina propria (6) and the submucosa (8) are **lymphatic nodules (9, 11)**.

The smooth muscle layers in the muscularis externa (13) of the colon are different from those of the small intestine. The **inner circular muscle layer (16)** is continuous and surrounds the colon wall, whereas the outer muscle layer is condensed into three broad, longitudinal bands called **taeniae coli (1, 10)**. A very thin **outer longitudinal muscle layer (15)**, which is often discontinuous, is found between the taeniae coli (1, 10). The parasympathetic ganglion cells of the **myenteric (Auerbach) nerve plexus (2, 14)** are found between the two smooth muscle layers of the muscularis externa (13).

The transverse and sigmoid colon are attached to the body wall by a **mesentery (18)**. As a result, the serosa (3, 17) is the outermost layer.

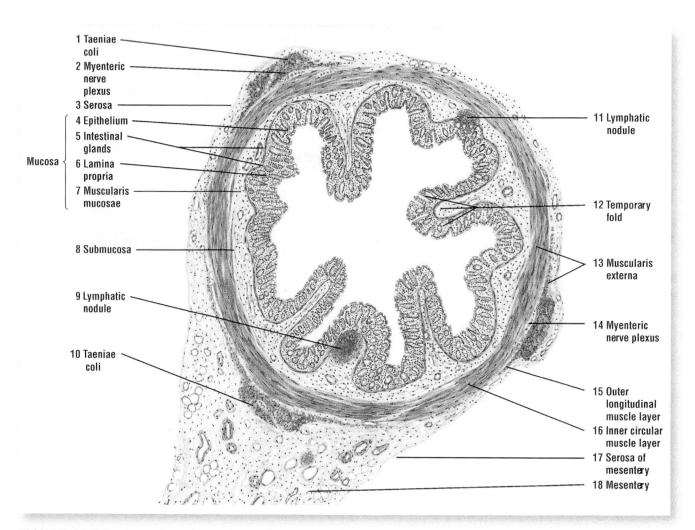

FIGURE 15.11 ■ Large intestine: colon and mesentery (panoramic view, transverse section). Stain: hematoxylin and eosin. Low magnification.

FIGURE 15.12 | **Large Intestine: Colon Wall (Transverse Section)**

This low-magnification photomicrograph illustrates a portion of the colon wall. The simple columnar epithelium contains the **absorptive columnar cells** (1) and the mucus-filled **goblet cells** (2, 6), which increase in number toward the terminal end of the colon. The **intestinal glands** (4) are deep and straight and extend through the **lamina propria** (3) to the **muscularis mucosae** (8). The lamina propria (3) and the **submucosa** (9) are filled with aggregations of lymphatic cells and **lymphatic nodules** (5, 7).

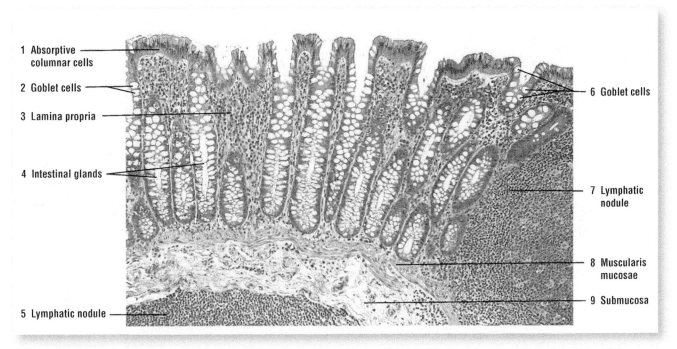

1 Absorptive columnar cells
2 Goblet cells
3 Lamina propria
4 Intestinal glands
5 Lymphatic nodule
6 Goblet cells
7 Lymphatic nodule
8 Muscularis mucosae
9 Submucosa

FIGURE 15.12 ■ Large intestine: colon wall (transverse section). Stain: hematoxylin and eosin. ×30.

FIGURE 15.13 | Large Intestine: Colon Wall (Transverse Section)

The wall of an undistended colon exhibits **temporary folds** (8) that consist of both the **mucosa** (**10–12**) and **submucosa** (**13**) layers. The four layers of the colon wall that are continuous with those of the small intestine are the mucosa (10–12), submucosa (13), **muscularis externa** (**14**), and **serosa** (**5**).

Villi are not present in the colon. The connective tissue **lamina propria** (**11**) contains long **intestinal glands** (**1, 9**) (crypts of Lieberkühn) that continue through the lamina propria (11) to the **muscularis mucosae** (**2, 12**).

The lining **epithelium** (**10**) in the colon is simple columnar and characterized by **goblet cells** (**10**) that also line the intestinal glands (1, 9). In the illustration are intestinal glands (1, 9) that are sectioned both longitudinally and in cross sections (9).

As in the small intestine, the lamina propria (11) contains diffuse lymphatic tissues. A distinct **lymphatic nodule** (**3**) is visible deep in the connective tissue of the lamina propria (11). Some of the larger lymphatic nodules may extend through the muscularis mucosae (2, 12) into the connective tissue of the submucosa (13).

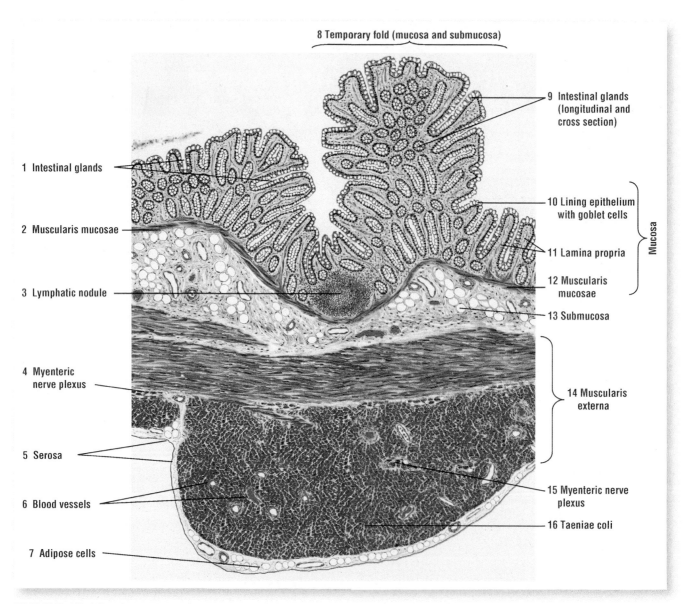

FIGURE 15.13 ■ Large intestine: colon wall (transverse section). Stain: hematoxylin and eosin. Medium magnification.

In contrast to the small intestine, the muscularis externa (14) of the colon is atypical. The longitudinal layer (14) is arranged into strips or bands of smooth muscle called the **taeniae coli (16)** and supplied by **blood vessels (6)**. The parasympathetic ganglia of the **myenteric nerve plexus (4, 15)** are located between the muscle layers of the muscularis externa (14).

The outermost layer, serosa (5), covers the connective tissue and **adipose (fat) cells** (7). However, the serosa (5) covers only the transverse and sigmoid colon. The ascending and descending colon are retroperitoneal, attached to the body wall, and their posterior surfaces lined with the connective tissue adventitia.

FUNCTIONAL CORRELATIONS 15.4 ■ Large Intestine

The principal functions of the large intestine are to absorb **water** and **minerals (electrolytes)** from the remaining indigestible material that was transported from the ileum of the small intestine and to compact it into feces for elimination. The epithelium of the large intestine contains **absorptive cells** similar to those in the small intestine and numerous mucus-secreting **goblet cells** that lubricate the lumen to facilitate passage of the feces. No digestive enzymes are produced by the cells of the large intestine.

HISTOLOGIC DIFFERENCES BETWEEN SMALL AND LARGE INTESTINES (COLON)

The large intestine lacks both plicae circulares and villi that characterize the small intestine. Intestinal glands that are present in the large intestine are similar to those of the small intestine. However, they are deeper (longer) and lack the Paneth cells in their bases. Similar to small intestine, the epithelium of the large intestine also contains enteroendocrine cells.

The **goblet cells** are more numerous in the large intestine epithelium than in the small intestine. Moreover, the number of goblet cells increases from the cecum toward the sigmoid colon of the large intestine. The lamina propria of the large intestine also contains many solitary lymphatic nodules, lymphocyte accumulations, plasma cells, and macrophages. The increased presence of GALT is due to the increased population of bacteria in the colon.

In contrast to the small intestine, the muscularis externa of the large intestine and the cecum exhibit a complete inner circular smooth muscle layer, whereas the outer longitudinal muscle layer is arranged into three longitudinal muscle strips called **taeniae coli**. The contraction, or tonus, in the taeniae coli forms sacculations or compartments in the large intestine, called **haustra** (see Fig. 15.10).

FIGURE 15.14 | Appendix (Panoramic View, Transverse Section)

This figure illustrates a cross section of the vermiform appendix at a low magnification. Its morphology is similar to that of the colon, except for certain modifications.

The **lining epithelium** (1) of the appendix contains goblet cells, the **lamina propria** (3), **intestinal glands** (5) (crypts of Lieberkühn), and a **muscularis mucosae** (2). The intestinal glands (5) are less well developed, shorter, and spaced farther apart than in the colon. **Diffuse lymphatic tissue** (6) in the lamina propria (3) is abundant and often in the **submucosa** (8).

Lymphatic nodules (4, 9) with germinal centers are highly characteristic of the appendix. These nodules originate in the lamina propria (3) and may extend to the submucosa (8).

The submucosa (8) has numerous blood vessels (11). The muscularis externa (7) consists of the inner circular layer (7a) and the outer longitudinal layer (7b). The parasympathetic ganglia (12) of the myenteric plexus (12) are located between the inner (7a) and outer (7b) smooth muscle layers of the muscularis externa.

The outermost layer of the appendix is the **serosa** (10) under which are seen **adipose cells** (13).

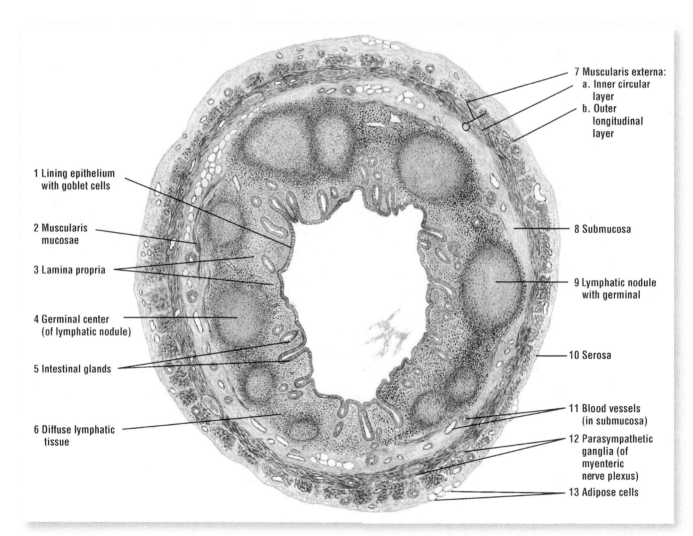

7 Muscularis externa:
 a. Inner circular layer
 b. Outer longitudinal layer

1 Lining epithelium with goblet cells

2 Muscularis mucosae

3 Lamina propria

4 Germinal center (of lymphatic nodule)

5 Intestinal glands

6 Diffuse lymphatic tissue

8 Submucosa

9 Lymphatic nodule with germinal

10 Serosa

11 Blood vessels (in submucosa)

12 Parasympathetic ganglia (of myenteric nerve plexus)

13 Adipose cells

FIGURE 15.14 ■ Appendix (panoramic view, transverse section). Stain: hematoxylin and eosin. Low magnification.

FIGURE 15.15 | Rectum (Panoramic View, Transverse Section)

The histology of the upper rectum is similar to that of the colon.

The surface **epithelium** (**1**) of the **lumen** (**5**) is lined with simple columnar cells with brush borders and goblet cells. The **intestinal glands** (**4**), **adipose cells** (**12**), and **lymphatic nodules** (**10**) in the **lamina propria** (**2**) are similar to the colon. The intestinal glands are longer, closer together, and filled with goblet cells. Beneath the lamina propria (**2**) is the **muscularis mucosae** (**11**).

The longitudinal **folds** (**3**) with a core of **submucosa** (**8**) in the upper rectum and colon are temporary. Permanent longitudinal folds (rectal columns) are found in the lower rectum and the anal canal.

Taeniae coli of the colon continue into the rectum, where the **muscularis externa** (**13**) acquires the **inner circular** (**13a**) and **outer longitudinal** (**13b**) **smooth muscle layers**. Between these two smooth muscle layers are the **parasympathetic ganglia** of the **myenteric (Auerbach) plexus** (**14**).

Adventitia (**9**) covers a portion of the rectum, and serosa covers the remainder. Numerous **blood vessels** (**6, 7, 15**) are in both the submucosa (**8**) and the adventitia (**9**).

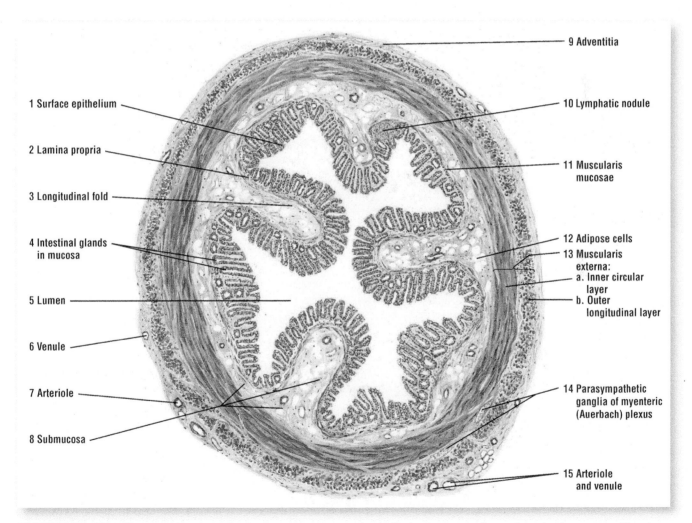

FIGURE 15.15 ■ Rectum (panoramic view, transverse section). Stain: hematoxylin and eosin. Low magnification.

FIGURE 15.16 | Anorectal Junction (Longitudinal Section)

The portion of the anal canal above the **anorectal junction** (**7**) represents the lowermost part of the rectum. The part of the anal canal below the anorectal junction (**7**) shows the transition from the **simple columnar epithelium** (**1**) to the **stratified squamous epithelium** (**8**) of the skin. The change from the rectal mucosa to the anal mucosa occurs at the anorectal junction (**7**).

The rectal mucosa is similar to colon. The **intestinal glands** (**3**) are shorter and spaced farther apart with the **lamina propria** (**2**) more prominent, diffuse lymphatic tissue more abundant, and **lymphatic nodules** (**11**) more numerous.

The **muscularis mucosae** (**4**) and the intestinal glands (**3**) terminate at the anorectal junction (**7**). The lamina propria (**2**) of the rectum is replaced by the dense irregular connective tissue of the **anal canal** (**9**). The **submucosa** (**5**) merges with the connective tissue of the anal canal, a highly vascular region. The **internal hemorrhoidal plexus** (**10**) of veins lies in the mucosa of the anal canal. Blood vessels from this region continue into the submucosa (**5**) of the rectum.

The circular smooth muscle layer of the **muscularis externa** (**6**) increases in thickness in the upper region of the anal canal and forms the **internal anal sphincter** (**6**). Lower in the anal canal, the internal anal sphincter (**6**) is replaced by skeletal muscles of the **external anal sphincter** (**12**). External to the external anal sphincter (**12**) is the skeletal **levator ani muscle** (**13**).

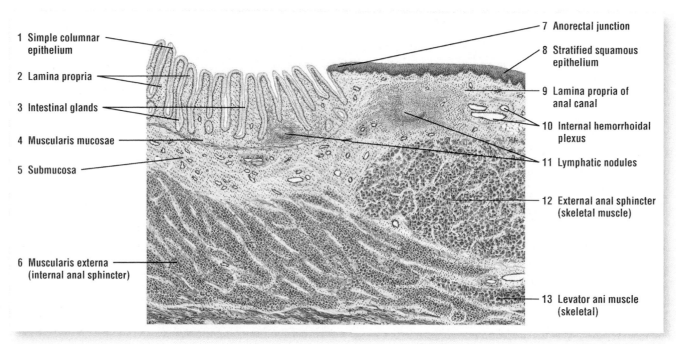

1 Simple columnar epithelium
2 Lamina propria
3 Intestinal glands
4 Muscularis mucosae
5 Submucosa
6 Muscularis externa (internal anal sphincter)

7 Anorectal junction
8 Stratified squamous epithelium
9 Lamina propria of anal canal
10 Internal hemorrhoidal plexus
11 Lymphatic nodules
12 External anal sphincter (skeletal muscle)
13 Levator ani muscle (skeletal)

FIGURE 15.16 ■ Anorectal junction (longitudinal section). Stain: hematoxylin and eosin. Low magnification.

Chapter 15 Summary

Digestive System Part III: Small Intestine and Large Intestine

SMALL INTESTINE

- Long, convoluted tube divided into duodenum, jejunum, and ileum
- Duodenum is the shortest segment with broad, tall, and numerous villi
- Digests gastric contents and absorbs nutrients into blood capillaries and lymphatic lacteals
- Transports chyme and waste products to large intestine
- Releases numerous hormones to regulate secretory functions and motility of digestive organs
- Amino acids, water, ions, glucose, and other substances are absorbed and transported in blood capillaries
- Long-chain fatty acids and monoglycerides are transported by lymphatic lacteals
- Contains numerous permanent surface modifications that increase cellular contact for absorption
- Plicae circulares are spiral folds with submucosa core that extend into intestinal lumen
- Villi are finger-like projections of lamina propria that extend into the intestinal lumen
- Microvilli are cytoplasmic extensions of absorptive cells that extend into the intestinal lumen
- Microvilli are coated with brush border enzymes that perform the final digestion of food products before absorption
- Villi contain a core of connective tissue with capillaries, lacteal, and smooth muscle strands
- Lamina propria is filled with lymphocytes, plasma cells, macrophages, eosinophils, and mast cells
- Smooth muscle strands in lamina propria of villi induce their movement and contractions

Cells of the Small Intestine

- Absorptive cells with microvilli covered by glycocalyx are most common in intestinal epithelium
- Goblet cells, interspersed between absorptive cells, increase in number toward distal region
- Enteroendocrine cells are scattered throughout the epithelium and intestinal glands
- Enteroendocrine cells are part of the diffuse neuroendocrine system (DNES)
- Secretory granules of enteroendocrine cells located at the base of cells and close to capillaries
- Enteroendocrine cells secrete numerous regulatory hormones for the digestive system
- Undifferentiated cells in the base of intestinal glands replace worn-out luminal cells
- Paneth cells with pink eosinophilic granules in cytoplasm are located in the intestinal glands
- Paneth cells have defensive functions by producing the antibacterial enzyme lysozyme and the hydrophobic peptide defensin
- M cells are specialized cells that cover the lymphatic Peyer patches and are part of the immune defense system

Glands of the Small Intestine

- Intestinal glands located between villi throughout the small intestine
- Intestinal glands open into the intestinal lumen at the base of the villi
- Duodenal glands in the submucosa of duodenum are characteristic of this region
- Duodenal glands penetrate muscularis mucosae to discharge mucus and bicarbonate secretions
- Bicarbonate secretions enter base of intestinal glands and protect duodenum from acidic chyme
- Polypeptide urogastrone from enteroendocrine cells from the duodenal glands inhibits hydrochloric acid secretions

Lymphatic Accumulations in the Small Intestine

- Peyer patches are numerous aggregations of permanent lymphatic nodules
- Peyer patches found primarily in the lamina propria and submucosa of the terminal part of the ileum
- Overlying Peyer patches are specialized M cells, which are not found anywhere else in the intestine
- Peyer patches and the lymphatic aggregations are part of gut-associated lymphatic tissue (GALT)
- M cells show deep invaginations or microfolds that contain macrophages and lymphocytes
- M cells sample intestinal antigens and present them to underlying lymphocytes for immunologic responses

LARGE INTESTINE

- Situated between anus and the terminal end of ileum
- Shorter and less convoluted than small intestine
- Consists of cecum and ascending, transverse, descending, and sigmoid sections
- Semifluid chyme enters through ileocecal valve
- At terminal end, semifluid residues become hardened or semisolid feces
- Main function is the absorption of water and electrolytes
- Epithelium consists of simple columnar epithelium with increased number of goblet cells

- Goblet cells produce mucus for lubricating the canal to facilitate passage of feces
- No enzymes or chemicals produced, but enteroendocrine cells are present in the epithelium
- No plicae circulares, villi, or Paneth cells; intestinal glands are deeper
- Increased numbers of solitary lymphatic nodules with cells are present in lamina propria
- Muscularis externa contains inner circular layer with outer layer arranged in three strips, the taeniae coli
- Contractions of taeniae coli form sacculations or haustra

Chapter 15 Review Questions

QUESTIONS

In the following multiple choice questions, choose the letter corresponding to the one best answer.

1. The lacteals of the small intestine are located in the:

   A. submucosa.
   B. lamina propria of the villi.
   C. duodenal glands.
   D. intestinal glands.
   E. absorptive cells.

2. The main function of the large intestine is to:

   A. continue enzymatic digestion of undigested material.
   B. produce enzymes for further digestion.
   C. neutralize undigested material with mucus secretion.
   D. absorb water and electrolytes from undigested material.
   E. finish absorbing nutrients that were started in the small intestine.

3. The large intestine is characterized by the following:

   A. Well-developed plicae circulares
   B. Numerous submucosal glands
   C. Deep intestinal glands and predominance of goblet cells
   D. Numerous Paneth cells in intestinal glands
   E. Numerous villi

4. What characterizes the muscularis externa of the large intestine?

   A. Three longitudinal muscle strips called taeniae coli
   B. Lack of inner circular smooth muscle layer
   C. Three layers of smooth muscles
   D. Skeletal muscle layer
   E. Presence of both smooth and skeletal muscle fibers

5. To increase contact with digested material, individual villi show movement. This is due to:

   A. contraction of the inner layer of muscularis externa.
   B. contraction of the outer layer of muscularis externa.
   C. peristalsis in the wall of the digestive tract.
   D. contraction of the actin filaments in the individual cells of the villi.
   E. smooth muscle fiber contraction from the muscularis mucosae that extend into villi.

ANSWERS

1. **Correct answer: B.** Lamina propria of the villi. Each villus contains tiny, blind-ending channels, lacteals, that transport the fatty acids out of the lacteals into larger lymph vessels.

2. **Correct answer: D.** Absorb water and electrolytes from undigested material. This action hardens the ingested material. There are no other digestive functions in the colon.

3. **Correct answer: C.** Deep intestinal glands and predominance of goblet cells. The goblet cells provide the necessary lubricant for moving the hardened fecal material through the tube.

4. **Correct answer: A.** Three longitudinal muscle strips called taeniae coli. The prominent outer longitudinal muscle layer is condensed into three prominent strips, the taeniae coli.

5. **Correct answer: E.** Smooth muscle fiber contraction from the muscularis mucosae that extend into villi. The movement of the villi and their contractions increases their contact with digested material and moves the fatty acids from the lacteals of the villi into larger lymph vessels.

ADDITIONAL HISTOLOGIC IMAGES

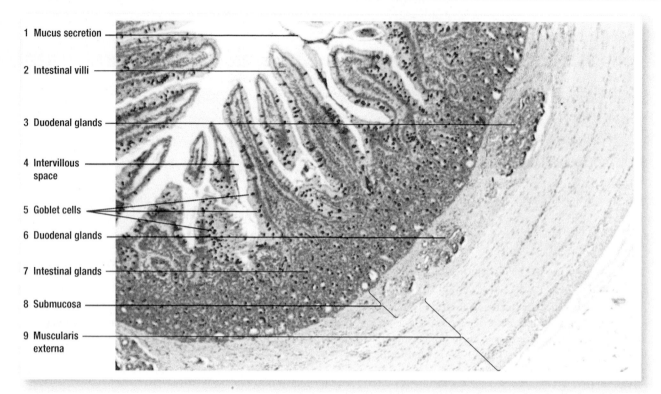

1 Mucus secretion
2 Intestinal villi
3 Duodenal glands
4 Intervillous space
5 Goblet cells
6 Duodenal glands
7 Intestinal glands
8 Submucosa
9 Muscularis externa

FIGURE 15.17 ■ A cross section of feline duodenum illustrating its characteristic features. Cells with mucus secretions stain magenta-red. Stain: iron hematoxylin and Alcian blue. ×25.

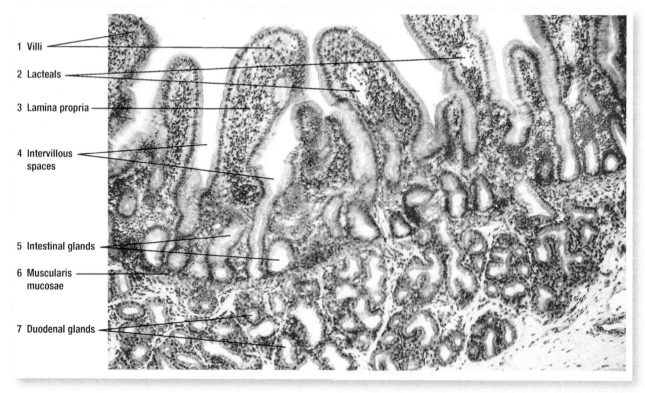

1 Villi
2 Lacteals
3 Lamina propria
4 Intervillous spaces
5 Intestinal glands
6 Muscularis mucosae
7 Duodenal glands

FIGURE 15.18 ■ Higher magnification of a primate duodenum with intestinal and the characteristic duodenal glands. Stain: hematoxylin and eosin. ×130.

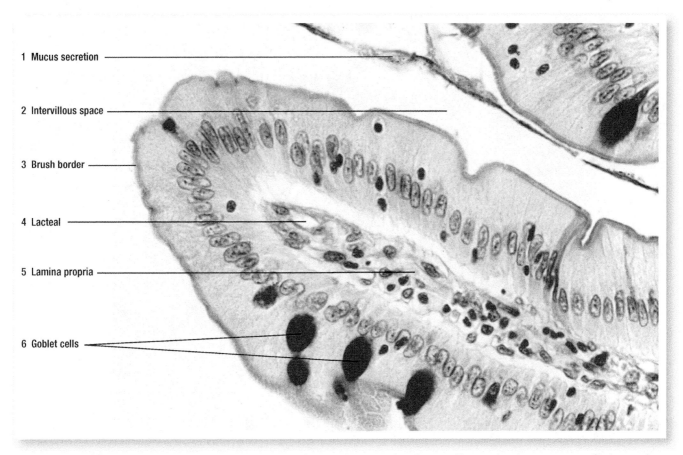

1 Mucus secretion

2 Intervillous space

3 Brush border

4 Lacteal

5 Lamina propria

6 Goblet cells

FIGURE 15.19 ■ High magnification of the villus from a human duodenum illustrating its contents. Stain: periodic acid–Schiff. ×130.

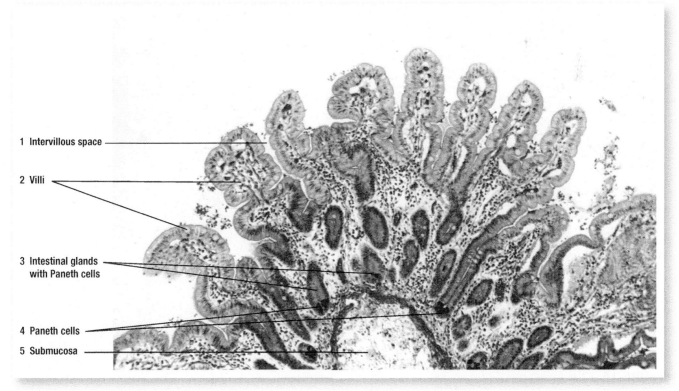

1 Intervillous space

2 Villi

3 Intestinal glands with Paneth cells

4 Paneth cells

5 Submucosa

FIGURE 15.20 ■ A section of human jejunum illustrating the mucosa with Paneth cells in the intestinal glands. Stain: Mallory-Azan. ×30.

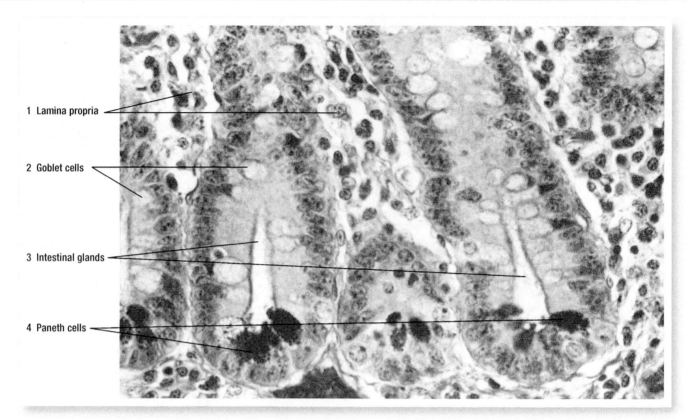

1 Lamina propria

2 Goblet cells

3 Intestinal glands

4 Paneth cells

FIGURE 15.21 ■ A section of feline jejunum illustrating the bases of the intestinal glands with Paneth cells. Stain: periodic acid–Schiff. ×165.

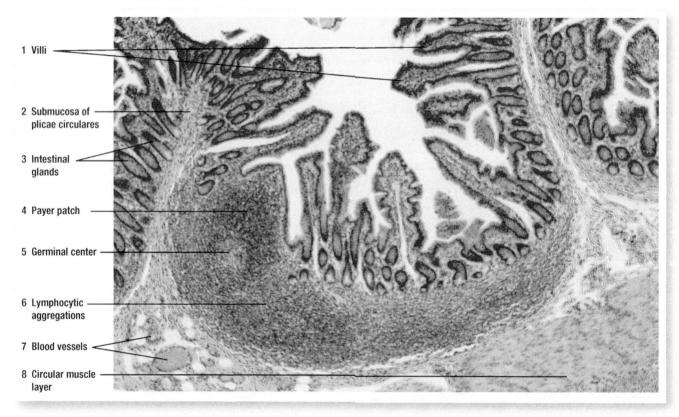

1 Villi

2 Submucosa of plicae circulares

3 Intestinal glands

4 Payer patch

5 Germinal center

6 Lymphocytic aggregations

7 Blood vessels

8 Circular muscle layer

FIGURE 15.22 ■ A section of human ileum illustrating a Peyer patch and the submucosal lymphocytic aggregation. Stain: hematoxylin and eosin. ×25.

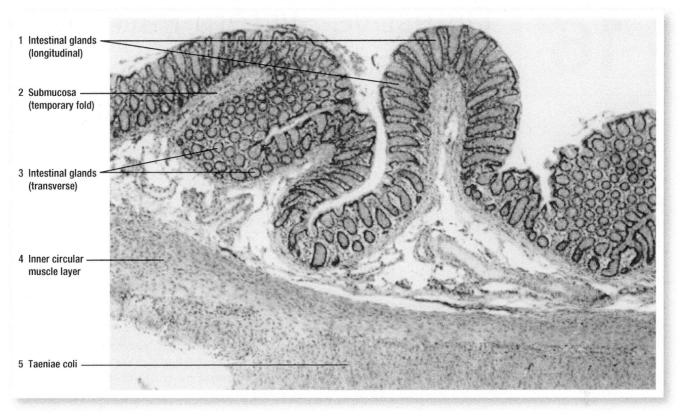

1 Intestinal glands
(longitudinal)

2 Submucosa
(temporary fold)

3 Intestinal glands
(transverse)

4 Inner circular
muscle layer

5 Taeniae coli

FIGURE 15.23 ■ A section of human colon with temporary folds, intestinal glands, and a section of taeniae coli. Stain: hematoxylin and eosin. ×15.

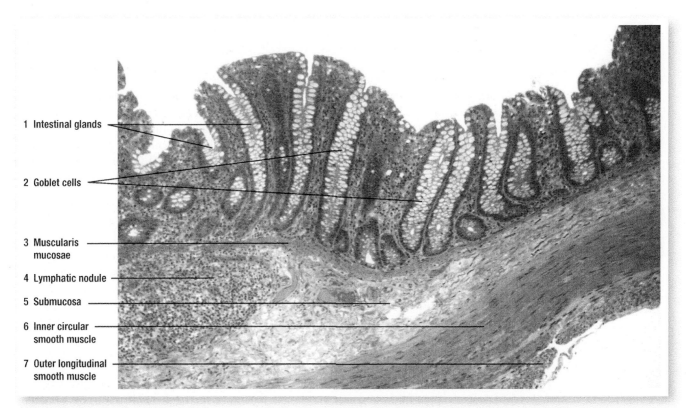

1 Intestinal glands

2 Goblet cells

3 Muscularis
mucosae

4 Lymphatic nodule

5 Submucosa

6 Inner circular
smooth muscle

7 Outer longitudinal
smooth muscle

FIGURE 15.24 ■ A plastic section of primate colon illustrating the contents of its wall. Stain: hematoxylin and eosin. ×60.

16 Digestive System Part IV: Accessory Digestive Organs (Liver, Pancreas, and Gallbladder)

The accessory organs of the digestive system are located outside of the digestive tube. Excretory glands from the salivary glands open into the oral cavity. The **liver**, **pancreas**, and **gallbladder** located in the abdominal cavity deliver their secretory products to the duodenum via excretory ducts. The **common bile duct** from the liver and the **main pancreatic duct** from the pancreas join in the duodenal loop to form a single duct common for both organs that penetrates the duodenal wall and enters its lumen. The gallbladder joins the common bile duct via the cystic duct. Thus, **bile** from the gallbladder and **enzymes** from the pancreas enter the duodenum via a common duct.

SECTION 1 Liver

The liver is one of the largest digestive organs and is located in a very strategic position. All absorbed nutrients and liquids from the intestines enter the liver through the **hepatic portal vein**, except the complex lipid products, which enter and are transported in the **lymph vessels**. The absorbed products percolate through the liver capillaries called **sinusoids** (Fig. 16.1). Nutrient-rich blood in the hepatic portal vein is brought to the liver before it enters the general circulation. Because venous blood from the digestive organs in the hepatic portal vein is poor in oxygen, a **hepatic artery** from the aorta supplies liver cells with oxygenated blood, forming a **dual blood supply** to the liver.

In histologic sections, liver exhibits repeating hexagonal units called liver (**hepatic**) **lobules**. In the center of each lobule is the **central vein**, from which radiate plates of liver cells, called **hepatocytes**, and the blood vessels, sinusoids, toward the periphery. In the periphery, the surrounding connective tissue contains **portal canals**, also called **portal areas** or **portal triads**, where branches of the **hepatic artery**, **hepatic portal vein**, **bile duct**, and **lymph vessels** can be seen. In human liver, three to six portal areas can be seen per hepatic lobule. Venous and arterial blood from the vessels in the peripheral portal area mix in the liver sinusoids as it flows toward the central vein. From here, blood enters the general circulation through the hepatic veins that leave the liver and enter the inferior vena cava.

The hepatic sinusoids are tortuous, dilated blood channels lined with a discontinuous layer of **fenestrated endothelial cells** with discontinuous basal lamina. The hepatic sinusoids are separated from the underlying hepatocytes by a subendothelial **perisinusoidal spaces** (**spaces of Disse**). Located in these spaces are the microvilli of hepatocytes and strands of connective

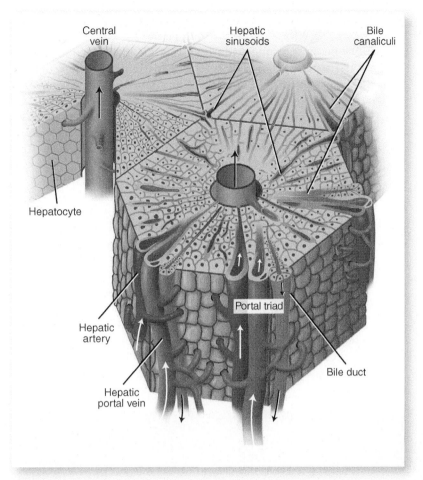

FIGURE 16.1 ■ A section from the liver is illustrated, with emphasis on the details of the liver lobule.

tissue fibers. The microvilli increase the surface area for exchange of metabolites in the flowing blood and the hepatocytes. As a result, ingested material in the sinusoidal blood contacts hepatocytes through the discontinuous endothelial wall, allowing for efficient exchange of materials between hepatocytes and blood. The hepatic sinusoids also contain macrophages called **Kupffer cells**, derived from monocytes, that form part of the endothelium. These cells are large, and their processes may extend across or span the entire lumen of the sinusoid. Other cells in the subendothelial perisinusoidal spaces are the **hepatic stellate cells**, also called the **Ito cells**. These cells are primary fat-storing cells that also accumulate and store much of the body's vitamin A. In addition, under certain pathological conditions, Ito cells differentiate into **myofibroblasts** and produce extracellular connective tissue matrix within the perisinusoidal spaces that results in **liver fibrosis**.

Hepatocytes secrete bile into **bile canaliculi** located between individual hepatocytes. The canaliculi converge at the periphery of liver lobules and empty into short **canals of Hering** that merge in the portal area with the **bile ductules**. These ductules are lined by cuboidal or columnar cells called **cholangiocytes**. From the portal areas, the bile ductules drain into larger right and left hepatic ducts that carry bile out of the liver. Within the liver lobules, bile flows in bile canaliculi toward the bile ductules in the peripheral portal areas, whereas blood in the sinusoids flows in the opposite direction toward the central veins of the liver lobules.

the**Point**®   Supplemental micrographic images are available at **www.thePoint.com/Eroschenko13e** under Digestive System Part IV: Liver, Pancreas, and Gallbladder.

FIGURE 16.2 | Pig Liver (Panoramic View, Transverse Section)

In the pig liver, connective tissue from the hilus extends between the liver lobes as **interlobular septa** (**5, 9**) and defines the **hepatic (liver) lobules** (**7**). A section of pig's liver was stained with Mallory-Azan stain to illustrate the connective tissue septa (**5, 9**) that stain dark blue.

A complete hepatic lobule (on the left) and parts of adjacent hepatic lobules (**7**) are illustrated. The blue-staining interlobular septa (**5, 9**) contain interlobular branches of the **portal vein** (**4, 11**), **bile duct** (**2, 12**), and **hepatic artery** (**3, 13**), which are collectively considered as **portal areas**, portal canals, or portal triads. At the periphery of each lobule are several portal areas within the interlobular septa (**5, 9**) that also contain small lymphatic vessels and nerves, which are usually small and only occasionally seen.

In the center of each hepatic lobule (**7**) is the **central vein** (**1, 8**). Radiating from each central vein (**1, 8**) toward the lobule periphery are **plates of hepatic cells** (**6**). Located between the hepatic plates (**6**) are blood channels, **hepatic sinusoids** (**10**). Arterial and venous blood mixes in the hepatic sinusoids (10) and flows toward the central vein (**1, 8**) of each lobule (**7**).

Bile, produced by hepatocytes, flows through the tiny bile canaliculi between the hepatocytes into the interlobular **bile ducts** (**2, 12**) (see Fig. 16.6).

The interlobular vessels and bile ducts (2 to 4, 11 to 13) are highly branched, and, in a cross section of the liver lobule, more than one section of these structures are seen within a portal area.

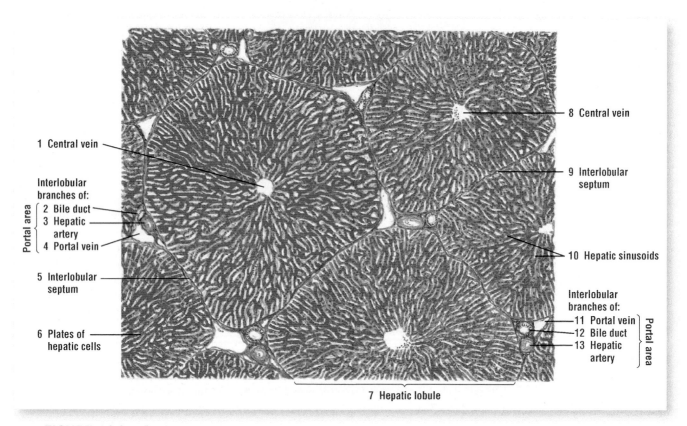

FIGURE 16.2 ■ Pig liver (panoramic view, transverse section). Stain: Mallory-Azan. Low magnification.

FIGURE 16.3 | Primate Liver (Panoramic View, Transverse Section)

In the primate or human liver, the connective tissue septa between individual **hepatic lobules** (8) are not as conspicuous as in the pig, and the liver sinusoids are continuous between lobules. Despite these differences, **portal areas** with interlobular branches of the **portal veins** (**2, 11**), **hepatic arteries** (**3, 13**), and **bile ducts** (**1, 12**) are visible around the lobule (8) peripheries in the **interlobular septa** (**4, 10**).

In the center of each hepatic lobule (8) is the **central vein** (**6, 9**). The **hepatic sinusoids** (5) appear between the **plates of hepatic cells** (7) that radiate from the central veins (6, 9) toward the periphery of the hepatic lobule (8). As illustrated in Figure 16.1, branches of the interlobular vessels and bile ducts are seen within the portal areas of a hepatic lobule (8).

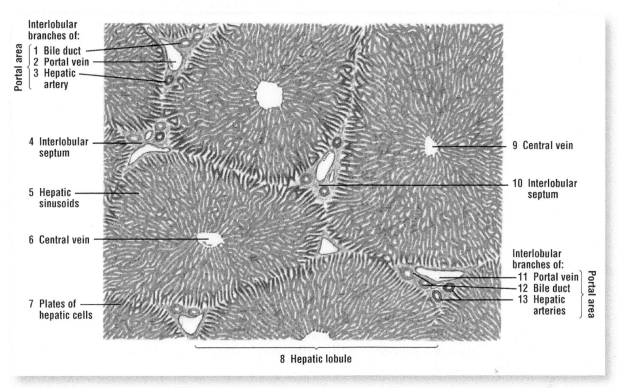

Portal area
Interlobular branches of:
1 Bile duct
2 Portal vein
3 Hepatic artery

4 Interlobular septum

5 Hepatic sinusoids

6 Central vein

7 Plates of hepatic cells

9 Central vein

10 Interlobular septum

Interlobular branches of:
11 Portal vein
12 Bile duct
13 Hepatic arteries
Portal area

8 Hepatic lobule

FIGURE 16.3 ■ Primate liver (panoramic view, transverse section). Stain: hematoxylin and eosin. Low magnification.

FUNCTIONAL CORRELATIONS 16.1 ■ Liver

The liver hepatocytes perform more functions than any other cell in the body. In addition, the liver cells exhibit both endocrine and exocrine roles by secreting substances into a duct and into the blood sinusoids, respectively. In addition, the liver performs vital functions early in life, functioning as the site of **hematopoiesis** or blood cell production in the fetus.

EXOCRINE FUNCTIONS

One major **exocrine function** of hepatocytes is to synthesize and release about 500 to 1,200 mL of **bile** per day. The bile enters the **bile canaliculi** and flows through the liver via a system of small ductules and larger ducts that carry the bile from the liver to the **gallbladder** where it is stored and concentrated

by removal of water. Release of bile from the liver and gallbladder is regulated by regulatory hormones. Bile flow is increased when a hormone **cholecystokinin** is released by the mucosal enteroendocrine cells (DNES) of the duodenum by the presence of fats or fatty meal in the duodenum. Cholecystokinin causes intermittent contraction of smooth muscles in the gallbladder wall and relaxation of the sphincter (of Oddi), expelling the bile into the duodenum.

Bile salts in the bile emulsify partially digested fats into smaller molecules for more efficient completion of digestion by **pancreatic lipases** produced by the pancreas. The digested fats are absorbed in the small intestine, and the long fatty acid chains enter the blind-ending lymphatic **lacteals** in the lamina

(continued)

FUNCTIONAL CORRELATIONS 16.1 ■ Liver (*Continued*)

propria of individual villi. From the lacteals, fats are carried into larger lymphatic ducts that eventually drain into the major veins and systemic circulation.

Hepatocytes also excrete **bilirubin**, a toxic chemical formed after degradation of worn-out erythrocytes by liver macrophages **Kupffer cells**. Bilirubin is taken up by hepatocytes from the blood and added to and excreted into bile.

ENDOCRINE FUNCTIONS

Hepatocytes are also **endocrine cells**, releasing substances directly into the bloodstream. The arrangement of hepatocytes in a liver lobule allows hepatocytes direct contact with the contents of the blood to take up and metabolize carbohydrates, proteins, and fats and store them in their cytoplasm. Hepatocytes then release many of the metabolized products back into the bloodstream, as the blood flows through the sinusoids and contacts hepatocytes. The hepatocytes also synthesize most of the circulating plasma proteins, including albumins, lipoproteins,

glycoproteins, and the blood-clotting factors prothrombin and fibrinogen. The liver cells also store essential nutrients, fats, various vitamins, minerals, and carbohydrates as glycogen. When needed, the stored glycogen in the liver is converted back into glucose and released into the bloodstream.

PHAGOCYTIC FUNCTIONS

Hepatocytes detoxify the blood of drugs and toxic substances as it percolates through the sinusoids. Kupffer cells that line the sinusoids are fixed liver phagocytes that originated from blood monocytes. These large, branching cells span the sinusoids and are filled with lysosomes. They filter and phagocytose the particulate material, bacteria, cellular debris, and worn-out or damaged erythrocytes that flow through the sinusoids.

In addition, antibodies (immunoglobulins) produced by plasma cells in the intestinal lamina propria are taken up from blood by hepatocytes and transported into bile canaliculi and bile. From here, antibodies enter the intestinal lumen to control its bacterial flora.

FIGURE 16.4 | **Bovine Liver: Liver Lobule (Transverse Section)**

This lower-magnification photomicrograph of a bovine liver illustrates hepatic (liver) lobules. The portal area of the lobule contains the branches of the **portal vein** (**5**), the **hepatic artery** (**6**), and, normally, a bile duct, which is not seen in this micrograph. From the **central vein** (**1**) radiate the **plates of hepatic cells** (**2**) toward the lobule periphery. Located between the plates of hepatic cells (**2**) are the blood **sinusoids** (**3**) that convey blood from the portal vein (**5**) and hepatic artery (**6**) to the central vein (**1**). Both the central vein (**1**) and the sinusoids (**3**) are lined with a discontinuous and fenestrated type of **endothelium** (**4**).

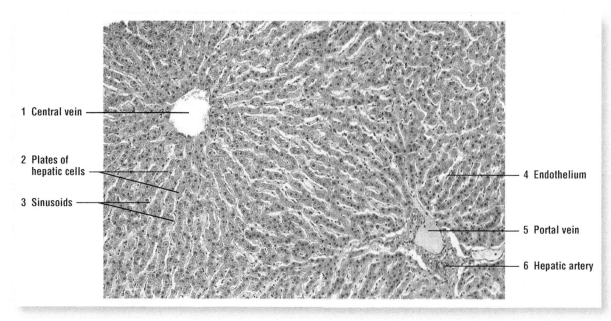

FIGURE 16.4 ■ Bovine liver: liver lobule (transverse section). Stain: hematoxylin and eosin. ×30.

FIGURE 16.5 | Hepatic (Liver) Lobule (Sectional View, Transverse Section)

A section of the hepatic lobule between the **central vein (9)** and connective tissue **interlobular septum (1, 6)** of the portal area is illustrated in greater detail. In the interlobular septum (1, 6) are seen **portal vein (4), hepatic arteries (3), bile ducts (5),** and a **lymphatic vessel (2).** Multiple cross sections of hepatic arteries (3) and bile ducts (5) are attributable to their branching in the septum or their passage into and out of the septum.

Branches of the portal vein (4) and hepatic artery (3) penetrate the interlobular septum (1, 6) and form the **sinusoids (8, 10)** that are situated between **plates of hepatic cells (7).** Discontinuous **endothelial cells (10)** line the sinusoids (8, 10) and the central vein (9). **Blood cells** (erythrocytes and leukocytes) in **sinusoids (8)** drain toward the central vein (9) of each lobule. Also present in the sinusoids (10) are fixed macrophages, the Kupffer cells (see Fig. 16.7).

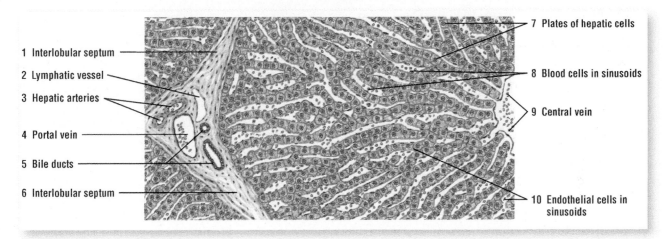

1 Interlobular septum
2 Lymphatic vessel
3 Hepatic arteries
4 Portal vein
5 Bile ducts
6 Interlobular septum

7 Plates of hepatic cells
8 Blood cells in sinusoids
9 Central vein
10 Endothelial cells in sinusoids

FIGURE 16.5 ■ Hepatic (liver) lobule (sectional view, transverse section). Stain: hematoxylin and eosin. High magnification.

FIGURE 16.6 | Bile Canaliculi in Liver Lobule (Osmic Acid Preparation)

Preparation of a liver section with osmic acid and staining with hematoxylin and eosin reveals the **bile canaliculi (3, 5),** the tiny channels between individual hepatocytes in the **hepatic plates (4).** The canaliculi (3, 5) follow an irregular course between the hepatic plates (4) and branch freely within the hepatic plates (4).

The **sinusoids (6)** are lined with discontinuous **endothelial cells (1)** and drain toward and open into the **central vein (2).**

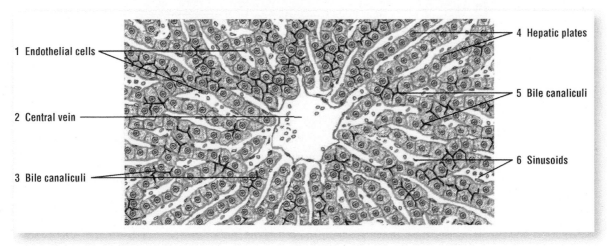

1 Endothelial cells
2 Central vein
3 Bile canaliculi

4 Hepatic plates
5 Bile canaliculi
6 Sinusoids

FIGURE 16.6 ■ Bile canaliculi in a liver lobule (osmic acid preparation). Stain: hematoxylin and eosin. High magnification.

FIGURE 16.7 | Kupffer Cells in Liver Lobule (India Ink Preparation)

The majority of cells that line the liver **sinusoids** (5) are **endothelial cells** (2) with an attenuated cytoplasm and a small nucleus. To demonstrate the phagocytic cells in the liver sinusoids (5), an animal was intravenously injected with India ink. The phagocytic **Kupffer cells** (3, 7) ingest the carbon particles from the ink, filling their cytoplasm with black deposits and becoming prominent in the sinusoids (5) between the **hepatic plates** (6). Kupffer cells (3, 7) are large cells with several processes and an irregular or stellate outline that protrudes into the sinusoids (5). The nuclei of Kupffer cells (3, 7) are obscured by the ingested carbon particles.

Visible on the periphery of the lobule is a section of the **interlobular septum** (1) and a part of the **bile duct** (4) lined with cuboidal cells.

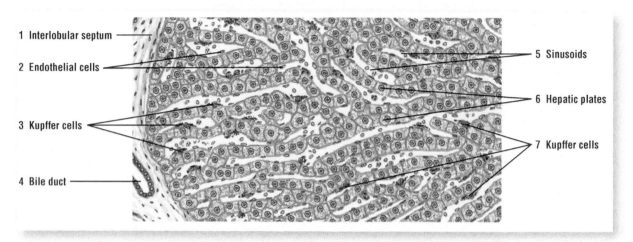

FIGURE 16.7 ■ Kupffer cells in a liver lobule (India ink preparation). Stain: hematoxylin and eosin. High magnification.

FIGURE 16.8 | Glycogen Granules in Liver Cells (Hepatocytes)

The cytoplasm of hepatocytes varies in appearance depending on nutritional status. After a meal, liver **hepatocytes** (1) store glycogen in their cytoplasm. With the periodic acid–Schiff stain, the **glycogen granules** (2, 4) in the hepatocyte (1) cytoplasm stain bright red and exhibit an irregular distribution within the cytoplasm.

Also visible in this illustration are hepatic **sinusoids** (3) and flattened **endothelial cells** (5) in their lumina.

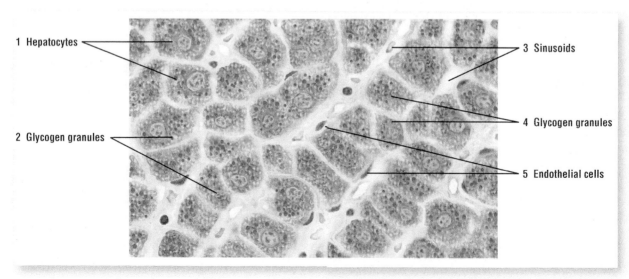

FIGURE 16.8 ■ Glycogen granules in liver cells (hepatocytes). Stain: periodic acid–Schiff with blue counterstain for nuclei. Oil immersion.

FIGURE 16.9 | **Reticular Fibers in Liver Lobule**

Fine reticular **fibers** (**6**, **8**) provide the supporting connective tissue of the liver. In this illustration, the reticular fibers stain black, and the liver cells stain pale pink or violet. The reticular fibers (6, 8) line the **sinusoids** (**8**), support the endothelial cells, and form a denser network of reticular fibers in the wall of the **central vein** (**7**). The reticular fibers (6, 8) also merge with the **collagen fibers** in the **interlobular septum** (**1**), where they surround the **portal vein** (**2**) and the **bile duct** (**3**).

Also visible in the reticular network are the pink-staining **nuclei of hepatocytes** (**4**) and the **hepatic plates** (**5**) that radiate from the central vein (7) toward the interlobular septum (1).

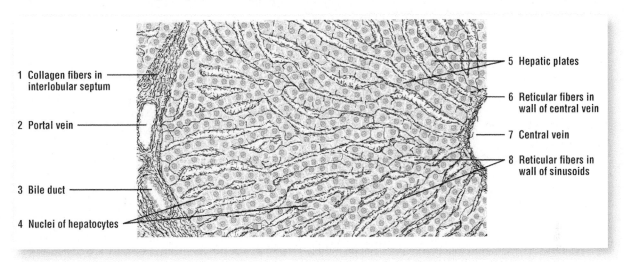

1 Collagen fibers in interlobular septum

2 Portal vein

3 Bile duct

4 Nuclei of hepatocytes

5 Hepatic plates

6 Reticular fibers in wall of central vein

7 Central vein

8 Reticular fibers in wall of sinusoids

FIGURE 16.9 ■ Reticular fibers in a liver lobule. Stain: reticulin method. Medium magnification.

FIGURE 16.10 | **Liver Sinusoids, Space of Disse, Hepatocytes, and Endothelial Cells in Liver Lobule**

This high-magnification micrograph shows details of the cells and structures in a liver lobule. The **sinusoids** (**1**, **7**) are lined with discontinuous **endothelial cells** (**6**, **8**). The narrow separations between the endothelial cells (6, 8) and **hepatocytes** (**9**) show the **space of Disse** (**3**, **5**). Also visible in the sinusoids (1, 7) are the larger phagocytic **Kupffer cells** (**4**, **10**) that can span the sinusoid (1, 7). Located between the hepatocytes (9) are tiny channels that in the cross section appear as dots; these are the **bile canaliculi** (**2**).

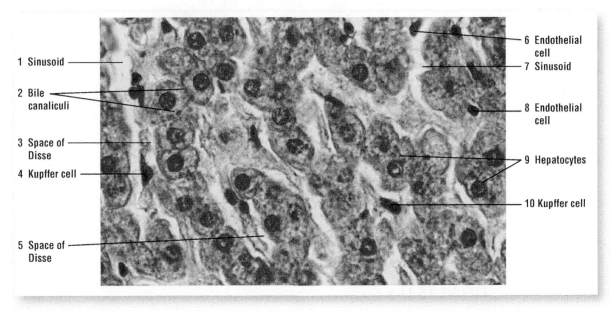

1 Sinusoid

2 Bile canaliculi

3 Space of Disse

4 Kupffer cell

5 Space of Disse

6 Endothelial cell

7 Sinusoid

8 Endothelial cell

9 Hepatocytes

10 Kupffer cell

FIGURE 16.10 ■ Liver sinusoids, space of Disse, hepatocytes, and endothelial cells in a liver lobule. Stain: hematoxylin and eosin. ×205.

SECTION 2 Pancreas

EXOCRINE PANCREAS

The pancreas is a soft, elongated organ located posterior to the stomach. The **head** of the pancreas lies in the duodenal loop, and the **tail** extends across the abdominal cavity to the spleen. Most of the pancreas is an **exocrine gland**. The exocrine secretory units or acini contain pyramid-shaped **acinar cells**, whose apices are filled with secretory granules. These granules contain the precursors of several pancreatic **digestive enzymes** that are secreted into the intestinal lumen via the excretory duct in an **inactive form**.

The secretory acini of the pancreas are subdivided into **lobules** and bound together by loose connective tissue. The **excretory ducts** in the exocrine pancreas start from within the center of individual acini as pale-staining **centroacinar cells** and continue with the lining cells of the short **intercalated ducts** that are located outside of the acini (Fig. 16.11). Intercalated ducts from different acini merge to form **intralobular ducts** in the connective tissue, which, in turn, join to form larger **interlobular ducts** that empty into the **main pancreatic duct**. Excretory ducts of the pancreas do not exhibit striations in their cells, and there are no striated ducts or myoepithelial cells.

ENDOCRINE PANCREAS

The endocrine units of the pancreas are scattered among the exocrine acini as isolated, pale-staining, and highly vascularized units called **pancreatic islets (of Langerhans)**. Each islet is surrounded by fine fibers of the reticular connective tissue. With special immunocytochemical staining, three cell types are identified in each pancreatic islet: **alpha**, **beta**, and **delta**. Other cells in the pancreatic islets, including the **pancreatic polypeptide** (**PP**) cells, are considered as minor cells. Each group of these cells secretes a single hormone.

Alpha cells constitute about 20% of the islets and are located around the islet periphery. The most numerous beta cells constitute about 70% of the islet cells and are concentrated in

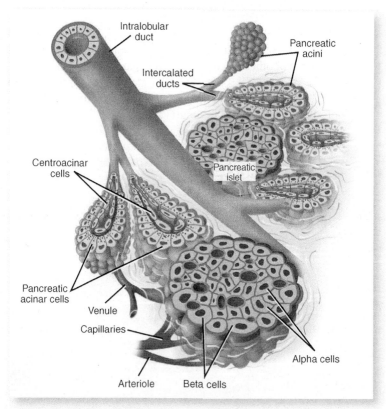

FIGURE 16.11 ■ A section from the pancreas is illustrated, with emphasis on the details of the duct system of the exocrine pancreas.

the center of the islet. The remaining cell types are few in number and are located throughout the islets.

thePoint®   Supplemental micrographic images are available at **www.thePoint.com/Eroschenko13e** under Digestive System Part IV: Liver, Pancreas, and Gallbladder.

FIGURE 16.12 | Exocrine and Endocrine Pancreas (Sectional View)

The pancreas is a mixed organ; it contains both endocrine and exocrine components. The exocrine component forms the majority of the pancreas and consists of packed secretory **serous acini** and **zymogenic cells (5)** arranged in small lobules. The lobules are surrounded by thin intralobular and **interlobular connective tissue septa (1)** with **blood vessels (2, 10)**, **interlobular ducts (6)**, nerves, and, occasionally, a sensory receptor **pacinian corpuscle (8)**. Between serous acini **(5)** are the isolated **cells of pancreatic islets** (of Langerhans) **(3, 11)**. These islets **(3, 11)** represent the endocrine portion of pancreas and are the characteristic features of the organ.

Each pancreatic acinus **(5)** consists of pyramid-shaped, protein-secreting **zymogenic** cells **(5)** surrounding a small central lumen. The initial parts of each excretory duct of the acinus **(5)** are visible as pale-staining **centroacinar cells (7, 9)** located in the middle of the acinus. The secretory products leave the acini via **intercalated (intralobular) ducts (4)** that are lined with a low cuboidal epithelium. The centroacinar cells **(7, 9)** are continuous with the epithelium of the intercalated ducts **(4)**.

The intercalated ducts **(4)**, in turn, drain into interlobular ducts **(6)** in the interlobular connective tissue septa **(4)**. The interlobular ducts **(6)** are lined with a simple cuboidal epithelium that becomes taller and stratified as the ducts increase in size.

Pancreatic islets **(3, 11)** are demarcated from the surrounding exocrine acini **(5)** tissue by a thin layer of reticular fibers. The islets **(3, 11)** are larger than the acini and are clusters of epithelial cells permeated by fenestrated **capillaries (11)**. The cells of a pancreatic islet **(3, 7)** are illustrated at a higher magnification in Figures 16.13 and 16.14.

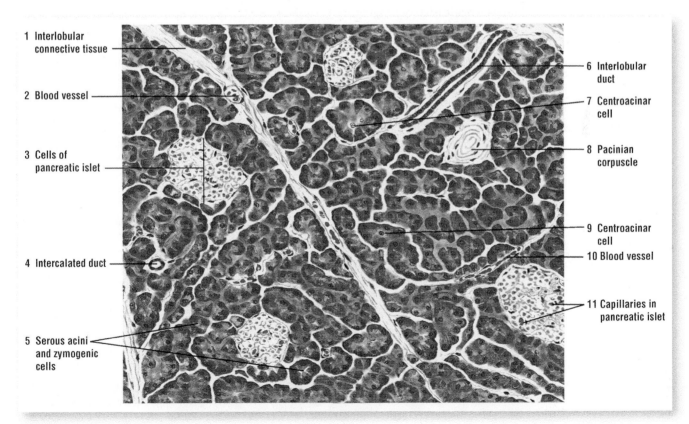

1 Interlobular connective tissue
2 Blood vessel
3 Cells of pancreatic islet
4 Intercalated duct
5 Serous acini and zymogenic cells

6 Interlobular duct
7 Centroacinar cell
8 Pacinian corpuscle
9 Centroacinar cell
10 Blood vessel
11 Capillaries in pancreatic islet

FIGURE 16.12 ■ Exocrine and endocrine pancreas (sectional view). Stain: hematoxylin and eosin. Low magnification.

FUNCTIONAL CORRELATIONS 16.2 ■ Exocrine Pancreas

The exocrine and endocrine functions of the pancreas are performed by separate cells. The pancreas produces digestive enzymes that exit the gland through a major excretory duct, whereas the hormones produced by the pancreatic islets are transported from the pancreas via blood vessels.

Both hormones and vagal stimulation regulate pancreatic exocrine secretions. Two intestinal hormones, **secretin** and **cholecystokinin (CCK)**, secreted by the **enteroendocrine (DNES) cells** in the duodenal mucosa into the bloodstream, are the principal hormones that regulate exocrine pancreatic secretions.

The presence of acidic chyme in the small intestine (duodenum) stimulates the release of the hormone **secretin**, which, in turn, induces the exocrine pancreatic cells to produce increased amounts of a watery fluid rich in **sodium bicarbonate ions**. This fluid is primarily produced by **centroacinar cells** in the pancreatic acini and cells in the **intercalated ducts**. The bicarbonate fluid neutralizes the acidic

chyme, stops the action of the proteolytic enzyme pepsin secreted by gastric glands in the stomach, and creates a neutral environment in the duodenum for the digestive pancreatic enzymes.

The presence of fats and proteins in the small intestine induces CCK release that stimulates the pancreatic acinar cells to secrete digestive enzymes. These are **pancreatic amylase** for carbohydrate digestion, **pancreatic lipase** for lipid digestion, **deoxyribonuclease** and **ribonuclease** for digestion of nucleic acids, and the **proteolytic enzymes trypsinogen**, **chymotrypsinogen**, and **procarboxypeptidase**.

Pancreatic enzymes are produced in the acinar cells, released in an **inactive form** after hormonal stimulation, and are indirectly activated only in the lumen of the duodenum by the hormone **enterokinase** secreted by the intestinal mucosa. Enterokinase, in turn, converts trypsinogen to trypsin, and trypsin then converts all inactive pancreatic enzymes into active digestive enzymes in the chyme.

FIGURE 16.13 │ Pancreatic Islet

A **pancreatic islet** (of Langerhans) (**2**) is illustrated at a higher magnification. The endocrine cells of the islet (**2**) are arranged in cords and clumps, between which are found fine connective tissue fibers and an extensive **capillary** (**3**) network. A thin **connective tissue capsule** (**5**) separates the endocrine pancreatic islet from the surrounding exocrine serous acini (**4, 6**). Some of the serous **acini** (**4, 6**) exhibit a centrally located **centroacinar cells** (**4, 6**), which form the initial part of the

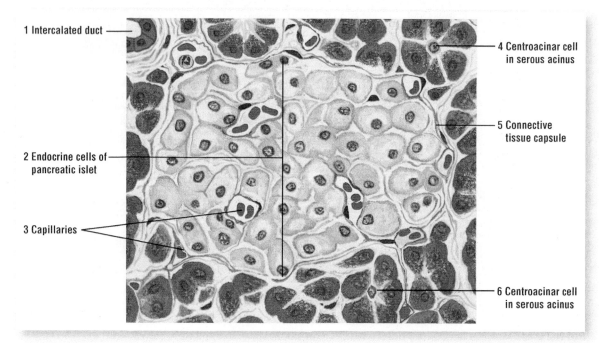

1 Intercalated duct

4 Centroacinar cell in serous acinus

5 Connective tissue capsule

2 Endocrine cells of pancreatic islet

3 Capillaries

6 Centroacinar cell in serous acinus

FIGURE 16.13 ■ Pancreatic islet. Stain: hematoxylin and eosin. High magnification.

duct system that leads to the excretory intercalated duct. In contrast to secretory acini in other glands, there are no myoepithelial cells surrounding the secretory acini.

In routine histologic preparations, the cells that secrete different hormones from the pancreatic islet (2) cannot be identified. However, with different staining, the hormone-secreting cells can be identified and is illustrated in Figures 16.14 and 16.16.

FIGURE 16.14 | Pancreatic Islet (Special Preparation)

This pancreas has been prepared with a stain to distinguish the glucagon-secreting **alpha** (A) **cells** (**1**) from the insulin-secreting **beta** (B) **cells** (**3**). The cytoplasm of alpha cells (1) stains pink, whereas the cytoplasm of beta cells (3) stains blue. The alpha cells (1) are situated more peripherally in the islet, and the beta cells (3) more centrally. Also, the predominant beta cells (3) constitute about 70% of the islet. Delta (D) cells (not illustrated) are also present in the islets. These cells are least abundant in the islets, have a variable cell shape, and may occur anywhere in the pancreatic islet.

Capillaries (**2**) around the endocrine cells demonstrate the rich vascularity of the pancreatic islets. The thin **connective tissue capsule** (**4**) separates the islet cells from the **serous acini** (**6**). **Centroacinar cells** (**5**) are visible in some of the acini.

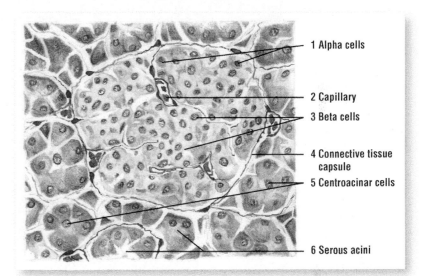

1 Alpha cells

2 Capillary

3 Beta cells

4 Connective tissue capsule

5 Centroacinar cells

6 Serous acini

FIGURE 16.14 ■ Pancreatic islet (special preparation). Stain: Gomori chrome alum hematoxylin and phloxine. High magnification.

FUNCTIONAL CORRELATIONS 16.3 ■ Endocrine Pancreas

The endocrine components of the pancreas are the **pancreatic islets (of Langerhans)** that secrete two major hormones that regulate blood glucose levels and glucose metabolism.

Alpha cells produce the hormone **glucagon** that is released in response to low blood glucose levels. Glucagon elevates blood glucose levels by accelerating the conversion of glycogen, amino acids, and fatty acids in the liver cells into glucose for release into the bloodstream.

Beta cells produce the hormone **insulin**, whose release is stimulated by elevated blood glucose levels after a meal. Insulin lowers blood glucose levels by accelerating transmembrane transport of glucose into hepatocytes, muscle cells, and adipose cells.

Insulin also accelerates the conversion of glucose into glycogen in hepatocytes. The effects of insulin on blood glucose levels are exactly opposite to that of glucagon.

Delta cells secrete the hormone **somatostatin**. This hormone decreases and inhibits secretory activities of both alpha (glucagon-secreting) and beta (insulin-secreting) cells through local action within the pancreatic islets. It also inhibits the production of bicarbonate and enzymes by the exocrine cells of the pancreas.

Pancreatic polypeptide (PP) cells produce the hormone **pancreatic polypeptide**. This hormone inhibits the production of bile and intestinal motility, inhibits pancreatic enzymes and bicarbonate secretions, and stimulates the gastric chief (zymogen) cells.

FIGURE 16.15 | Pancreas: Endocrine (Pancreatic Islet) and Exocrine Regions

This high-magnification photomicrograph of the pancreas illustrates both exocrine and endocrine components. In the center is the light-staining endocrine **pancreatic islet** (3). A thin **connective tissue capsule** (2) separates the pancreatic islet (3) from the exocrine **secretory acini** (5). The pancreatic islet (3) contains rich vascularization (6). The exocrine secretory acini (5) consist of pyramid-shaped cells arranged around small lumina whose centers contain one or more light-staining **centroacinar cells** (4).

The smallest excretory duct in the pancreas is the **intercalated duct** (1) lined with a simple cuboidal epithelium.

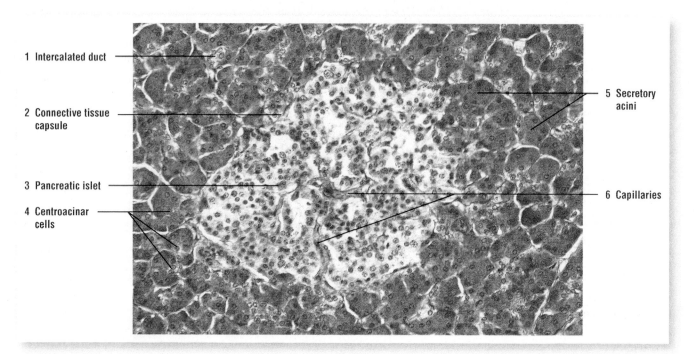

1 Intercalated duct

2 Connective tissue capsule

3 Pancreatic islet

4 Centroacinar cells

5 Secretory acini

6 Capillaries

FIGURE 16.15 ■ Pancreas: endocrine (pancreatic islet) and exocrine regions. Stain: periodic acid–Schiff and hematoxylin. ×80.

FIGURE 16.16 | Immunohistochemical Preparation of Mammalian Pancreatic Islet

With immunohistochemical preparation, different cell types are visible in the pancreatic islet. This high-magnification image shows precise distribution of the two major cell types in the pancreatic islet. The **glucagon-producing cells** (**A cells**) are stained bright red and are located peripherally in the islet. The **insulin-producing cells** (**B cells**) are stained bright **green** and are located on the inside of the islet surrounded by the peripheral A cells.

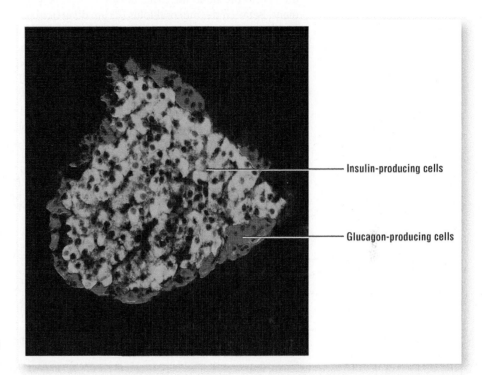

Insulin-producing cells

Glucagon-producing cells

FIGURE 16.16 ■
Immunohistochemical preparation of a mammalian pancreatic islet. Courtesy of Dr. Ernest Adeghate, Professor and Chairman, Department of Anatomy, Faculty of Medicine and Health Sciences, UAE University, Al Ain, United Arab Emirates. ×200.

SECTION 3 Gallbladder

The gallbladder is a small, hollow organ attached to the inferior surface of the liver. Bile is produced by liver hepatocytes that leaves the liver and flows to, is stored, and is concentrated in the gallbladder. Upon hormonal stimulation, bile leaves the gallbladder via the cystic duct and enters the duodenum via the **common bile duct** through the **major duodenal papilla**, a finger-like protrusion of the duodenal wall into the lumen.

The gallbladder is not a gland. Its main function is to store and concentrate bile by absorbing its water. Bile is released into the digestive tract as a result of hormonal stimulation after a meal that contains fatty foods. When the gallbladder is empty, the mucosa exhibits deep **folds**.

thePoint° Supplemental micrographic images are available at **www.thePoint.com/Eroschenko13e** under Digestive System Part IV: Liver, Pancreas, and Gallbladder.

FIGURE 16.17 | Wall of Gallbladder

The gallbladder is a muscular sac. Its wall consists of the mucosa, the muscularis externa, and the adventitia or serosa. The gallbladder wall does not contain a muscularis mucosae or submucosa.

The mucosa consists of a **simple columnar epithelium** (**1**) with underlying **lamina propria** (**2**) with loose connective tissue, some diffuse lymphatic tissue, and blood vessels—**venule and arteriole** (**9**). In the nondistended state, the gallbladder wall shows temporary **mucosal folds** (**7**) that disappear when the gallbladder becomes distended with bile. The mucosal folds (**7**) resemble the villi in the small intestine; however, they vary in size and shape, with an irregular arrangement. Between the mucosal folds (**7**) are **diverticula** or **crypts** (**3, 8**) that form deep indentations in the mucosa. In cross section, the diverticula, or crypts (**3, 8**), in the lamina propria (**2**) resemble tubular glands. However, there are no glands in the gallbladder, except in the neck region.

External to the lamina propria (**2**) is the muscularis with bundles of randomly oriented **smooth muscle fibers** (**10**) without distinct layers and interlacing **elastic fibers** (**4**).

Surrounding smooth muscle fibers (**10**) is a thick layer of dense **connective tissue** (**6**) with blood vessels—**artery** and **vein** (**11**)—lymphatics, and **nerves** (**5**).

Serosa (**12**) covers the entire unattached gallbladder surface. Where the gallbladder is attached to the liver surface, this connective tissue layer is the adventitia.

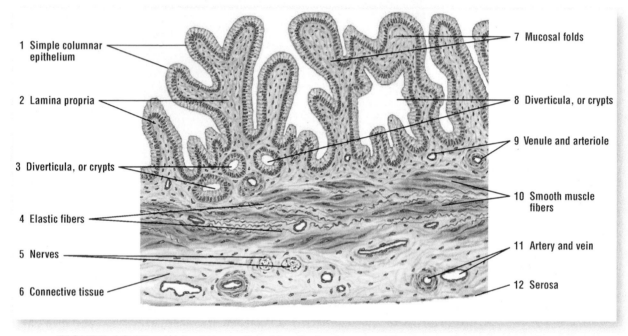

1 Simple columnar epithelium
2 Lamina propria
3 Diverticula, or crypts
4 Elastic fibers
5 Nerves
6 Connective tissue

7 Mucosal folds
8 Diverticula, or crypts
9 Venule and arteriole
10 Smooth muscle fibers
11 Artery and vein
12 Serosa

FIGURE 16.17 ■ Wall of the gallbladder. Stain: hematoxylin and eosin. Low magnification.

FUNCTIONAL CORRELATIONS 16.4 ■ Gallbladder

The primary functions of the gallbladder are to collect, store, concentrate, and expel **bile** when needed for emulsification of fat. Bile is continually produced by liver hepatocytes and transported via the excretory ducts to the gallbladder for storage. The epithelial cells in the gallbladder contain organelles similar to those in cells that participate in transmembrane transport of molecules. Here, sodium pumps in the basolateral membranes actively transport sodium through the epithelium into the extracellular connective tissue, creating a strong osmotic pressure. Most of the water and chloride ions passively follow from the bile, producing a highly concentrated bile.

Release of bile into the duodenum is under hormonal control. In response to dietary fats in the proximal duodenum, the hormone **cholecystokinin** (**CCK**) is released by enteroendocrine cells in the intestinal mucosa. CCK is carried in the bloodstream to the gallbladder, causing strong contractions of the smooth muscle in its wall and relaxing the smooth **sphincter muscles** around the neck of gallbladder. These two actions force the bile into the duodenum via the common bile duct.

Chapter 16 Summary

Digestive System Part IV: Accessory Digestive Organs

LIVER

- Located outside the digestive tube in strategic position
- All absorbed nutrients pass through liver via portal vein and hepatic sinusoids
- Has dual blood supply: portal vein and hepatic artery
- Is organized into repeating liver lobules, with central vein in the center of lobule
- Plates of liver cells (hepatocytes) radiate to lobule periphery from central vein
- Portal vein, hepatic artery, and bile duct in lobule periphery are portal areas
- Venous and arterial blood mix in sinusoids and flow toward central vein
- Hepatic sinusoids lined with discontinuous and fenestrated endothelium
- Substances in blood contact hepatocytes via subendothelial perisinusoidal space of Disse
- Phagocytic Kupffer cells and fat-storing hepatic stellate (Ito) cells are associated with sinusoids
- In liver damage, hepatic stellate (Ito) cells can differentiate into myofibroblasts and produce connective tissue matrix
- Performs more functions than any other organ
- In fetus, it is the site for hematopoiesis or blood cell formation
- Individual hepatocytes perform both exocrine and endocrine functions

Exocrine Functions

- Hepatocytes secrete bile into tiny channels, the bile canaliculi, which merge with canals of Hering
- From the canal of Hering, bile flows toward bile ducts in portal areas in opposite direction to blood
- Bile is stored in gallbladder, where water is removed and bile is concentrated
- Hormone cholecystokinin regulates the release of bile from liver and gallbladder
- Enteroendocrine cells in intestinal mucosa release cholecystokinin as fats in chyme enter duodenum
- Cholecystokinin causes gallbladder contraction and expulsion of bile
- Bile emulsifies fats for more efficient digestion by pancreatic lipases
- Fats are absorbed into lymphatic lacteals in the villi of small intestine
- Hepatocytes excrete bilirubin into bile and move antibodies from blood into bile

Endocrine Functions

- Take up, metabolize, accumulate, and store products from blood
- Synthesize and release most plasma proteins, including blood-clotting factors
- Store glycogen and release as glucose when needed

Phagocytic Functions

- Detoxify drugs and harmful substances that flow through sinusoids
- Specialized liver macrophages, Kupffer cells, line the sinusoids
- Kupffer cells filter and phagocytose debris and worn-out red blood cells

PANCREAS

Exocrine

- Head of organ lies in the duodenal loop and tail extends to the spleen
- Exocrine component forms majority of the organ and is composed of serous acini
- Acinar cells filled with granules that contain digestive enzymes
- Acini contain pale-staining centroacinar cells in their lumina from which excretory ducts start
- Centroacinar cells continuous with cells of short intercalated ducts
- Excretory ducts do not have striated cells, striated ducts, or myoepithelial cells
- Neural and hormones secretin and cholecystokinin regulate exocrine secretions
- Intestinal enteroendocrine cells release hormones when acidic chyme is present
- Secretin stimulates sodium bicarbonate production by centroacinar cells and intercalated duct cells
- Alkaline sodium bicarbonate fluid neutralizes acidic chyme for pancreatic enzymes
- Cholecystokinin released when fats and proteins are present in chyme

- Cholecystokinin stimulates production and release of numerous pancreatic digestive enzymes
- Enzymes produced and released in inactive form and activated first in duodenum
- Trypsinogen from pancreas converted to trypsin by intestinal mucosa hormone enterokinase
- Trypsin converts all pancreatic enzymes into active digestive enzymes

Endocrine

- Endocrine portion in the form of isolated pancreatic islets among exocrine acini
- Each pancreatic islet is surrounded and separated by fine reticular fibers
- Four cell types present in pancreatic islets: alpha, beta, delta, and pancreatic polypeptide cells
- Alpha cells produce glucagon in response to low sugar levels
- Glucagon elevates blood glucose by accelerating conversion of glycogen in liver
- Beta cells produce insulin during elevated glucose levels

- Insulin lowers blood glucose by inducing glucose transport into liver, muscle, and adipose cells
- Delta cells produce somatostatin, which inhibits the activity of both alpha and beta cells
- Delta cells also inhibit production of bicarbonate and enzymes by exocrine cells
- Pancreatic polypeptide cells inhibit bile production and enzymatic and alkaline pancreatic secretion and stimulates gastric chief (zymogen) cells

GALLBLADDER

- Hollow organ inferior to the liver designed to store and concentrate bile
- Bile produced by liver hepatocytes is delivered by major excretory ducts
- Sodium is actively transported out, water and chloride follow, and bile is concentrated
- Bile is released in response to fats in the duodenum because of the action of cholecystokinin
- Sphincter muscles relax and gallbladder contraction forces bile into the duodenum

Chapter 16 Review Questions

QUESTIONS

In the following multiple choice questions, choose the letter corresponding to the one best answer.

1. **During decreased glucose levels in the blood, what will bring the glucose levels back?**

   A. Increased levels of insulin
   B. Decreased levels of glucagon
   C. Decreased levels of somatostatin
   D. Increased levels of glucagon
   E. Increased secretions from all cells in pancreatic islets

2. **What cells in the pancreas reduce blood sugar levels after a meal?**

   A. Alpha cells
   B. Beta cells
   C. Delta cells
   D. Pancreatic polypeptide cells
   E. Centroacinar cells

3. **What hormone suppresses or inhibits the secretion of insulin and glucagon?**

   A. Somatostatin
   B. Secretin
   C. Cholecystokinin
   D. Pancreatic polypeptide
   E. Enterokinase

4. **What changes take place when bile is stored in the gallbladder?**

   A. It becomes more diluted.
   B. Sodium and chloride ions are added to bile.
   C. More water is added to bile.
   D. It becomes more concentrated.
   E. It remains unchanged.

5. **What hormone causes the gallbladder to contract and expel bile?**

   A. Secretin
   B. Enterokinase
   C. Pancreatic polypeptide
   D. Trypsinogen
   E. Cholecystokinin

ANSWERS

1. **Correct answer: D.** Increased levels of glucagon. This hormone increases elevation of glucose by accelerating the conversion of glycogen, amino acids, and fatty acids in the liver into glucose and its release into the blood stream.

2. **Correct answer: B.** Beta cells. These cells release insulin during elevated glucose levels, which then lowers glucose levels by its transport into hepatocytes, muscle cells, and fat cells.

3. **Correct answer: A.** Somatostatin. This hormone is produced by delta cells in the pancreatic islets. It has an inhibitory effect on cells that produce insulin (B cells) and glucagon (A cells).

4. **Correct answer: D.** Bile becomes more concentrated. Through transmembrane transport, sodium is actively transported from bile with water and chloride following, resulting in concentrated bile.

5. **Correct answer: E.** Cholecystokinin. Entrance of fatty foods into the duodenum induces the release of cholecystokinin that results in the contraction of the gallbladder muscular wall to expel bile.

ADDITIONAL HISTOLOGIC IMAGES

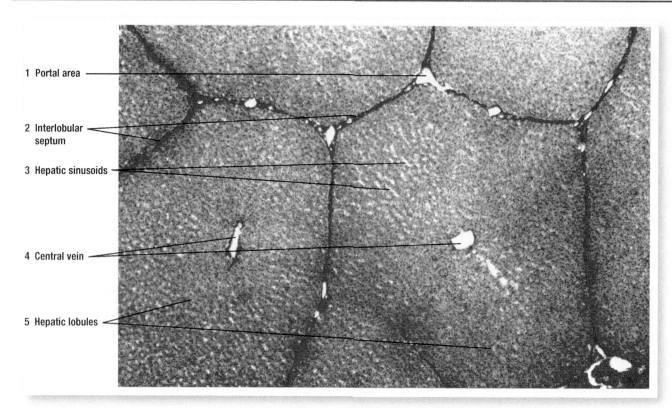

1 Portal area

2 Interlobular septum

3 Hepatic sinusoids

4 Central vein

5 Hepatic lobules

FIGURE 16.18 ■ Low magnification of a pig liver illustrating lobules separated by connective tissue septa. Stain: Mallory-Azan. ×17.

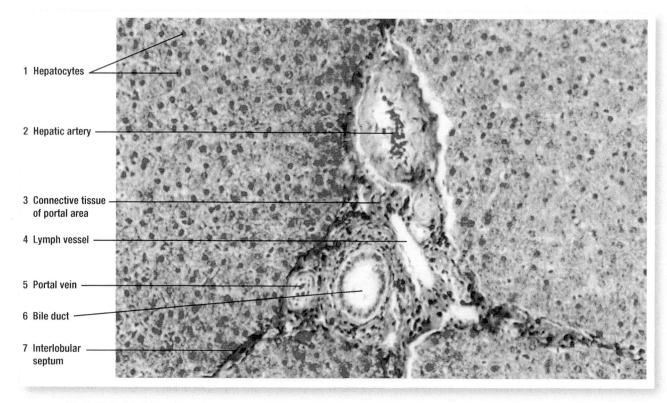

1 Hepatocytes

2 Hepatic artery

3 Connective tissue of portal area

4 Lymph vessel

5 Portal vein

6 Bile duct

7 Interlobular septum

FIGURE 16.19 ■ Portal area in a pig liver illustrating its contents. Stain: Mallory-Azan. ×100.

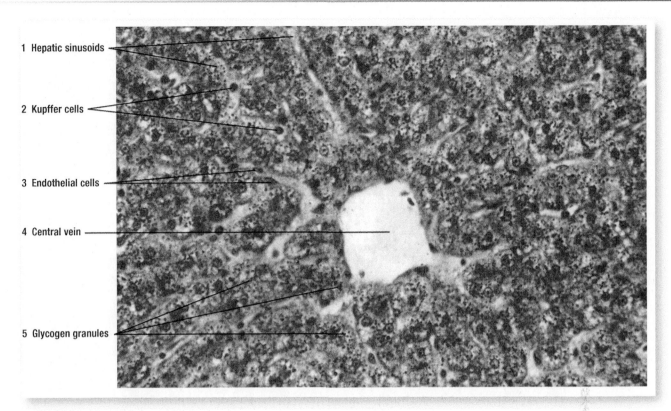

1 Hepatic sinusoids
2 Kupffer cells
3 Endothelial cells
4 Central vein
5 Glycogen granules

FIGURE 16.20 ■ Higher magnification of a liver lobule surrounding the central vein illustrating the glycogen granules in hepatocytes. Stain: periodic acid–Schiff. ×100.

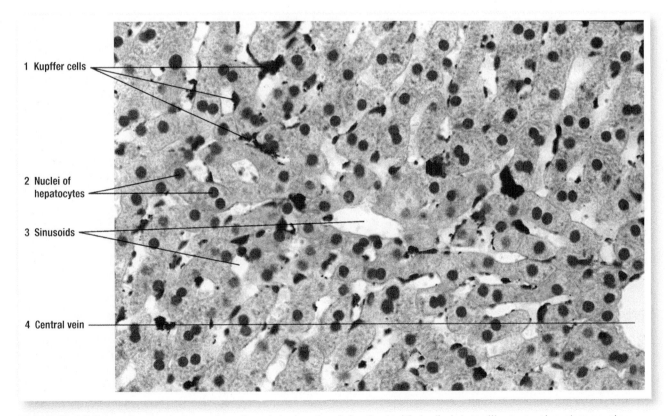

1 Kupffer cells
2 Nuclei of hepatocytes
3 Sinusoids
4 Central vein

FIGURE 16.21 ■ Section of a rodent liver lobule after injection with India ink to illustrate the phagocytic Kupffer cells. Stain: hematoxylin and eosin. ×100.

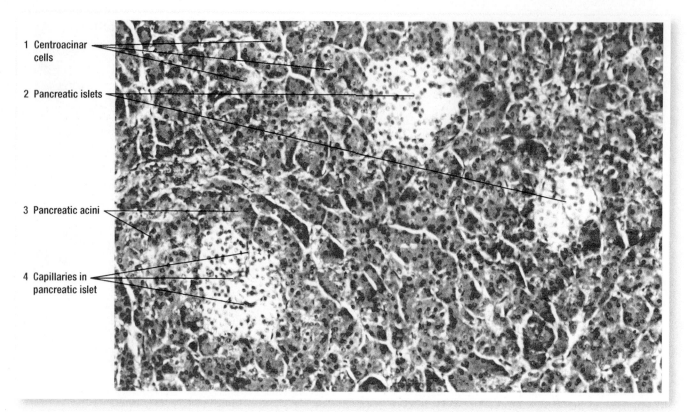

1 Centroacinar cells

2 Pancreatic islets

3 Pancreatic acini

4 Capillaries in pancreatic islet

FIGURE 16.22 ■ Low-power section of a primate pancreas illustrating the endocrine pancreatic islets and the surrounding exocrine acini. Stain: hematoxylin and eosin. ×50.

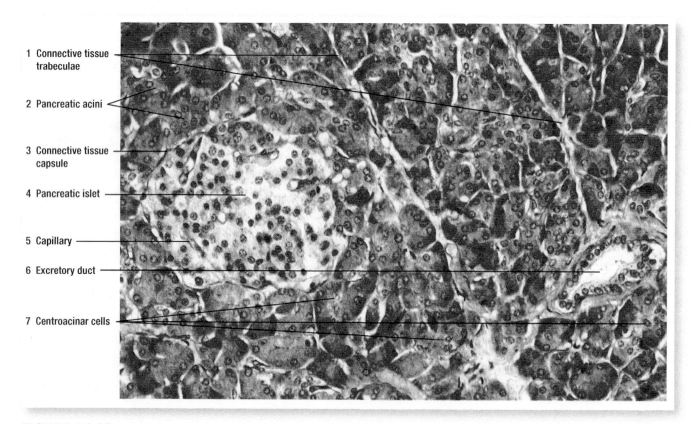

1 Connective tissue trabeculae

2 Pancreatic acini

3 Connective tissue capsule

4 Pancreatic islet

5 Capillary

6 Excretory duct

7 Centroacinar cells

FIGURE 16.23 ■ A higher-power section of a primate pancreatic islet, the excretory duct, and the surrounding acini. Stain: hematoxylin and eosin. ×80.

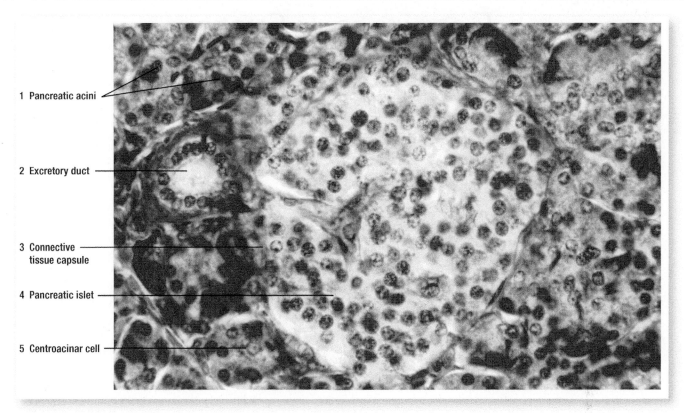

1 Pancreatic acini

2 Excretory duct

3 Connective tissue capsule

4 Pancreatic islet

5 Centroacinar cell

FIGURE 16.24 ■ More detailed image of a primate pancreatic islet, excretory duct, and the surrounding cells. Stain: Mallory-Azan. ×100.

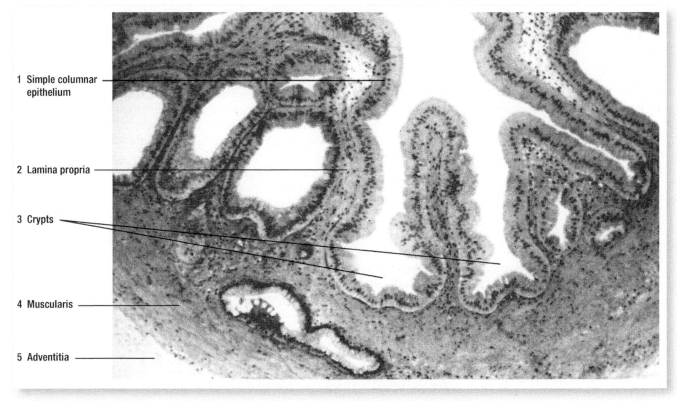

1 Simple columnar epithelium

2 Lamina propria

3 Crypts

4 Muscularis

5 Adventitia

FIGURE 16.25 ■ Low-power section of a primate gallbladder wall illustrating its contents. Stain: hematoxylin and eosin. ×17.

COMPONENTS OF RESPIRATORY SYSTEM

The respiratory system is made up of two parts, a conducting portion and a respiratory portion. Also located in the air passages of the nose are neuroepithelial sensory cells that detect odor or smell.

The **conducting portion** consists of passageways or tubes located outside (extrapulmonary) and inside (intrapulmonary) of the lungs that conduct air for gaseous exchange to and from the lungs. In contrast, the **respiratory portion** consists of passageways within the lungs that not only conduct the air but also allow **respiration** or gaseous exchange.

Such extrapulmonary passages as the trachea and different sizes of bronchi are lined with a **pseudostratified ciliated epithelium** with numerous **goblet cells**. As these bronchi enter the lungs, they undergo extensive branching, and their diameters become progressively smaller. There is also a gradual decrease in the height of the lining epithelium, the amount of cilia, and the number of goblet cells. The **bronchioles** represent the terminal portion of the conducting passageways. These give rise to the **respiratory bronchioles**, a **transition zone** between air conduction and respiratory or gaseous exchange regions.

The **respiratory portion** consists of respiratory bronchioles, alveolar ducts, alveolar sacs, and **alveoli** (Fig. 17.1). Gaseous exchange takes place in the alveoli, the very thin terminal air spaces of the respiratory system. In the alveoli, goblet cells are absent and the lining epithelium is thin **simple squamous**. The alveoli are in very close proximity to the capillaries.

RESPIRATORY EPITHELIUM

Most of the respiratory structures are lined by pseudostratified ciliated columnar epithelium. By examining this epithelium with both light and transmission electron microscopes, several different cell types are recognized. **Ciliated columnar cells** are the most abundant cells that extend the entire thickness of the epithelium. The cilia sweep the surface of the epithelium and protect the lungs by removing small inhaled particles.

Goblet cells are numerous in the more proximal airways and gradually decrease in number toward the distal parts of the respiratory tube. These cells contain and release mucus glycoproteins to form a protective layer on the epithelial surface.

Basal cells are located close to the basal lamina without their apices reaching the lumen of the epithelium. These cells serve as stem cells for continual replacement of other epithelial cells.

Brush cells are less numerous than the other cells. Because their basal surfaces contact afferent nerve endings, it is believed that these cells function as receptor cells.

Small granule cells (**Kulchitsky cells**) contain numerous membrane-bound granules and are analogous to the enteroendocrine cells of the diffuse neuroendocrine system (DNES).

Other cells are seen in the nasal cavity, in the bronchioles, and the alveoli.

OLFACTORY EPITHELIUM

Before entering the lungs, the air first passes through either the mouth or the nasal cavity. Located in the superior and lateral regions in the roof of the nose are the bony nasal shelves called **conchae**. Lining this selected region is a highly specialized sensory pseudostratified epithelium called the **olfactory epithelium** that detects and transmits odor sensations to the brain. This epithelium

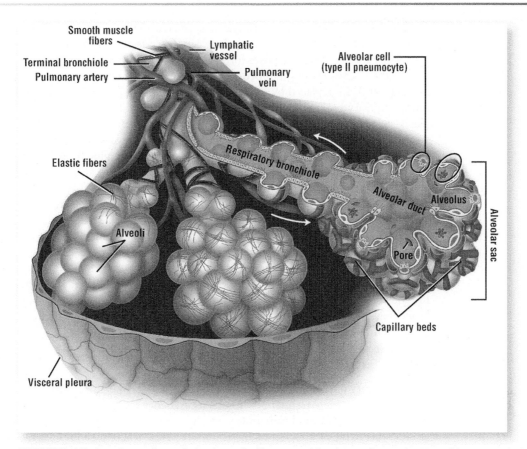

FIGURE 17.1 ■ A section of the lung is illustrated in three dimensions and in transverse section. Magnified versions of a bronchiole and a type II pneumocyte (both circled here) are illustrated in Figures 17.2 and 17.3, respectively.

consists of three major cell types: supportive (sustentacular), basal, and olfactory (sensory). Located inferior to the epithelium in the lamina propria are the **serous olfactory (Bowman) glands**. In contrast to the respiratory epithelium, the olfactory epithelium lacks goblet cells or motile cilia on its cells.

Olfactory cells are the **sensory bipolar neurons** that are distributed between the more **apical supportive cells** and the **basal cells**. The olfactory cells span the thickness of the olfactory epithelium and end at the surface as small, round bulbs called the **olfactory vesicles**. Radiating from each olfactory vesicle are long, **nonmotile olfactory cilia** that lie parallel to the epithelial surface. These cilia are nonmotile and function as sensory odor receptors. The bases of the olfactory cells connect to axons that leave the epithelium through the basement membrane, converge in the lamina propria below the epithelium to form bundle of nerve fibers that pass through the ethmoid bone of the skull, and synapse in the olfactory bulb of the brain (olfactory, or cranial nerve I).

In the olfactory epithelium are olfactory nerves, olfactory (Bowman) glands, blood vessels, lymphatic vessels, and other cellular components of the connective tissue. Olfactory (Bowman) glands produce a serous fluid that bathes the olfactory cilia and serves as a solvent to dissolve the odor molecules for stimulation of the olfactory cells for odor detection.

RESPIRATORY SYSTEM—CONDUCTING PORTION

The conducting portion of the respiratory system consists of the nasal cavities, the pharynx, the larynx, the trachea, the extrapulmonary bronchi, and a series of solid intrapulmonary bronchi and bronchioles with decreasing diameters that end as terminal **bronchioles. Hyaline cartilage** supports and keeps the larger air passageways always patent (open). Starting with the trachea, incomplete C-shaped **hyaline cartilage rings** encircle the tube. Elastic and smooth muscle fibers, the trachealis muscle, bridge the space between the ends of the hyaline cartilage. The ends of the C-shaped cartilage rings face posteriorly and are adjacent to the esophagus.

As the trachea divides into **bronchi** and the bronchi enter the lungs, the C-shaped hyaline cartilage rings are replaced by irregular **hyaline cartilage plates** that encircle the lumen of the intrapulmonary bronchi. As the bronchi continue to divide and decrease in size, the cartilage plates also decrease in size and number. When the diameters of bronchioles decrease to about 1 mm, cartilage plates disappear from conducting passageways. Terminal bronchioles represent the final solid conducting passageways with the diameters ranging from 0.5 to 1.0 mm. There are between 20 and 25 generations of branching of intrapulmonary bronchi before the passageways reach the size of terminal bronchioles.

The larger bronchioles are lined with a tall, **ciliated pseudostratified epithelium** similar to trachea and bronchi. As the tubular size decreases, the epithelial height is gradually reduced, and the epithelium becomes a **simple ciliated epithelium**. The epithelium of larger bronchioles also contains numerous **goblet cells**. The number of goblet cells, however, decreases with the decreasing tubule size; the goblet cells are absent from the epithelium of terminal bronchioles.

Small terminal bronchioles are lined only with a **simple cuboidal epithelium**. In place of the goblet cells, **Clara cells** are found mixed with the ciliated cells in the terminal and respiratory bronchioles. Clara cells are nonciliated, secretory cuboidal cells with dome-shaped apices that protrude into the lumen and increase in number as ciliated cells decrease.

RESPIRATORY SYSTEM—RESPIRATORY PORTION

The respiratory portion is the distal continuation of the conducting portion that starts with the air passageways where respiration or gaseous exchange can occur. Terminal bronchioles branch to give rise to **respiratory bronchioles**, which are characterized by thin-walled outpockets called alveoli. This is the first region of the respiratory tube where gaseous exchange can take place. The respiratory bronchioles represent the **transitional zone** where air conduction and gaseous exchange or respiration can take place.

Respiration occurs only in **alveoli** because the barrier between inspired air in the alveoli and the capillaries is extremely thin. Each alveolus is surrounded by capillary plexuses that bring

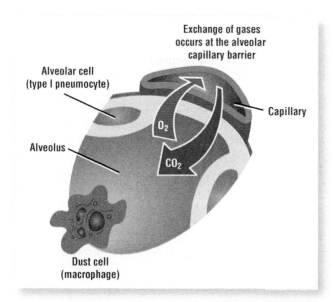

FIGURE 17.2 ■ Internal structure of the respiratory bronchiole in the lung illustrating the close proximity of air in the alveolus, the blood in the capillary, and the macrophage dust cell.

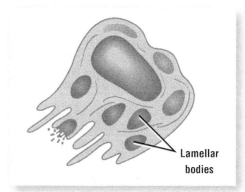

FIGURE 17.3 ■ High magnification of a type II alveolar cell in an alveolus.

venous blood close to the inspired air inside the alveoli for gaseous exchange (Fig. 17.2). Other intrapulmonary structures where respiration occurs are the **alveolar ducts** and **alveolar sacs**.

The alveoli contain two cell types with the most abundant cells being the squamous **type I alveolar cells**, or **type I pneumocytes**. These are extremely thin cells that line all alveolar surfaces. Interspersed among the squamous alveolar cells singly or in groups are the **type II alveolar cells**, or **type II pneumocytes** (Fig. 17.3). Lung **macrophages**, derived from circulating blood monocytes, are found both in the connective tissue of alveolar walls, or interalveolar septa (**alveolar macrophages**), and in the alveoli (**dust cells**). Present in the interalveolar septa are extensive capillary networks, pulmonary arteries, pulmonary veins, lymphatic ducts, and nerves.

thePoint® Supplemental micrographic images are available at **www.thePoint.com/Eroschenko13e** under Respiratory System.

FIGURE 17.4 | Olfactory Mucosa and Superior Concha (Panoramic View)

The olfactory mucosa is located in the roof of the nasal cavity, on each side of the dividing septum, and on the surface of the **superior concha** (**1**), one of the bony shelves in the nasal cavity.

The olfactory **epithelium** (**2, 6**) (see Figs. 17.4 to 17.6) is specialized for the reception of smell. As a result, its morphology appears different from the respiratory epithelium. The olfactory epithelium (2, 6) is a pseudostratified tall columnar epithelium without goblet cells and without motile cilia, in contrast to the respiratory epithelium.

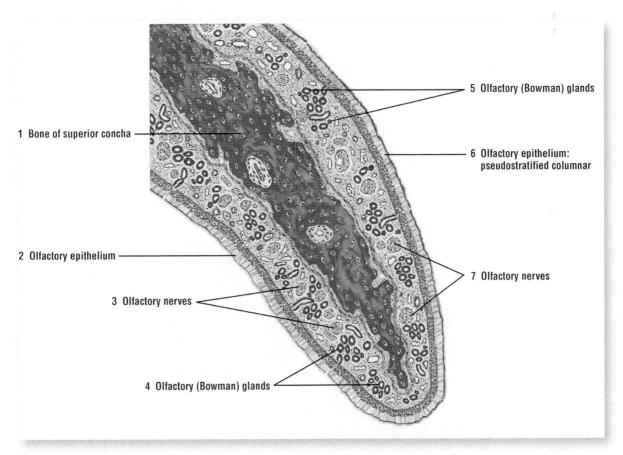

1 Bone of superior concha

2 Olfactory epithelium

3 Olfactory nerves

4 Olfactory (Bowman) glands

5 Olfactory (Bowman) glands

6 Olfactory epithelium: pseudostratified columnar

7 Olfactory nerves

FIGURE 17.4 ■ Olfactory mucosa and superior concha (panoramic view). Stain: hematoxylin and eosin. Low magnification.

The lamina propria contains the branched tubuloacinar **olfactory (Bowman) glands** (**4, 5**). These glands produce a serous secretion, in contrast to the mixed mucous and serous secretions produced by glands in the rest of the nasal cavity. Small nerves that are located in the lamina propria are the **olfactory nerves** (**3, 7**) and represent the afferent axons that leave the olfactory cells, continue into the cranial cavity, and synapse in the olfactory (cranial) nerves.

FIGURE 17.5 | Olfactory Mucosa: Details of Transitional Area

This illustration depicts a transition between the **olfactory epithelium** (**1**) and the **respiratory epithelium** (**9**). The olfactory epithelium (1) is a tall, pseudostratified columnar epithelium composed of three different cell types: supportive, basal, and neuroepithelial olfactory cells. The individual cell outlines are difficult to distinguish in a routine histologic preparation; however, the location and shape of nuclei allow identification of the cell types.

The supportive, or **sustentacular cells** (**3**), are elongated, with oval nuclei situated more apically (or superficially) in the epithelium. The **olfactory cells** (**4**) have oval or round nuclei that are located between the nuclei of the supportive cells (3) and the **basal cells** (**5**). The apices and bases of the olfactory cells (4) are slender. The apical surfaces of the olfactory cells (4) contain slender, nonmotile microvilli that extend into the **mucus** (**2**) that covers the epithelial surface. The basal cells (5) are short cells located at the base of the epithelium between the supportive (3) and olfactory cells (4).

Extending from the bases of the olfactory cells (4) are axons that pass into the **lamina propria** (**6**) as bundles of unmyelinated **olfactory nerves**, or **fila olfactoria** (**14**). The olfactory nerves (14) leave the nasal cavity and pass into the olfactory bulbs at the base of the brain.

The transition from the olfactory epithelium (1) to the respiratory epithelium (9) is abrupt. The respiratory epithelium (9) is a pseudostratified columnar epithelium with distinct motile **cilia** (**10**) and numerous **goblet cells** (**11**). Also, the height of the respiratory epithelium (9) is similar to that of the olfactory epithelium (1). In other regions of the tract, the respiratory epithelium (9) is reduced in comparison to the olfactory epithelium (1).

The lamina propria (6) contains capillaries, lymphatic vessels, arterioles (8), venules (13), and branched, tubuloacinar serous **olfactory (Bowman) glands** (**7**). The olfactory glands (7) deliver their secretions through narrow excretory **ducts** (**12**) that penetrate the olfactory epithelium (1). The secretions from the olfactory glands (7) moisten the epithelial surface, dissolve the molecules of odoriferous substances, and stimulate the olfactory cells (4).

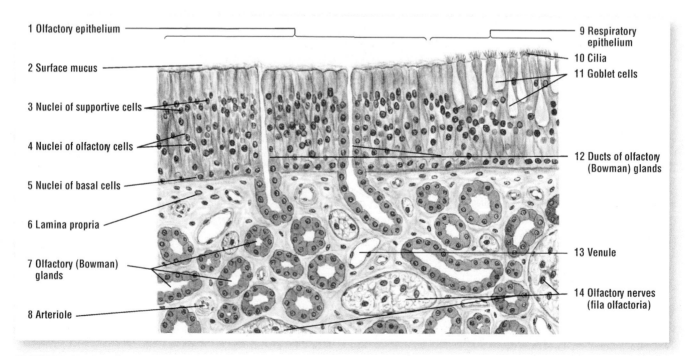

1 Olfactory epithelium
2 Surface mucus
3 Nuclei of supportive cells
4 Nuclei of olfactory cells
5 Nuclei of basal cells
6 Lamina propria
7 Olfactory (Bowman) glands
8 Arteriole
9 Respiratory epithelium
10 Cilia
11 Goblet cells
12 Ducts of olfactory (Bowman) glands
13 Venule
14 Olfactory nerves (fila olfactoria)

FIGURE 17.5 ■ Olfactory mucosa: details of a transitional area. Stain: hematoxylin and eosin. High magnification.

FIGURE 17.6 | Olfactory Mucosa in Nose: Transition Area

In the superior region of the nasal cavity, the **respiratory epithelium** changes abruptly into the olfactory epithelium, as shown in this higher-power photomicrograph.

The respiratory epithelium is lined with motile **cilia** (**1**) and contains **goblet cells** (**2**). The olfactory epithelium lacks cilia (1) and **goblet cells** (2). Instead, olfactory epithelium exhibits nuclei of **supportive cells** (**5**), located near the epithelial surface; nuclei of odor-receptive **olfactory cells** (**6**), located more in the center of the epithelium; and **basal cells** (**7**), located close to the **basement membrane** (**3**).

Below the olfactory epithelium in the lamina propria (4) are blood vessels (9), olfactory nerves (10), and olfactory (Bowman) glands (8).

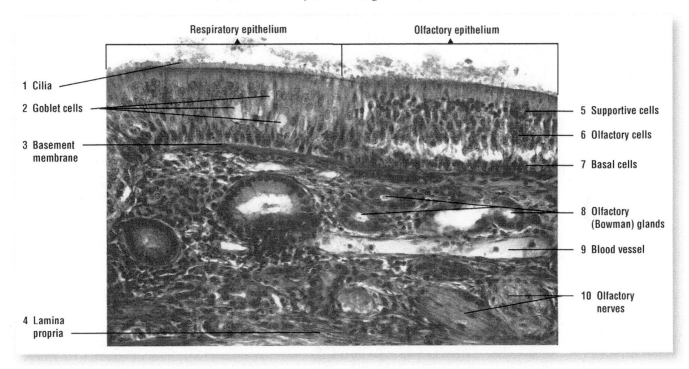

FIGURE 17.6 ■ Olfactory mucosa in the nose: transition area. Stain: Mallory-Azan. ×80.

FUNCTIONAL CORRELATIONS 17.1 ■ Olfactory Epithelium

To detect odors, the odorant (smell) substances are first dissolved in the serous fluid produced by the olfactory glands. The dissolved odorant molecules then bind to **odorant-binding proteins** present in the fluid secreted by the olfactory glands in the lamina propria. The odorant-binding proteins deliver the odorants to **olfactory receptors** present on the nonmotile olfactory cilia that stimulate the olfactory epithelium to conduct impulses. The unmyelinated afferent axons of olfactory cells leave the olfactory epithelium at the base to form small **olfactory nerve bundles** in the lamina propria. Impulses from olfactory cells are conducted in nerve bundles through the ethmoid bone in the skull and synapse in the **olfactory bulbs** of the brain located in the skull above the nasal cavity. From here, neurons relay

the information to the cortex of the brain for odor interpretation.

Olfactory epithelium is kept moist by a watery secretions produced by serous **olfactory** (**Bowman**) **glands** located below the epithelium in the lamina propria. This secretion, delivered via ducts through the olfactory epithelium, continually washes the surface of olfactory epithelium. In this manner, odor molecules are trapped, dissolved, and then washed away by the new fluid, allowing the receptor cells to detect and respond to new odorants.

The supportive cells form junctional complexes with the adjacent olfactory cells to provide structural support. Basal cells serve as stem cells and can give rise to new olfactory cells and supportive cells of the olfactory epithelium.

FIGURE 17.7 | **Epiglottis (Longitudinal Section)**

The epiglottis is the superior portion of the larynx that projects upward from the larynx's anterior wall. It has both a lingual and a laryngeal surface.

A central **elastic cartilage** forms the framework **of the epiglottis** (3). Its **lingual mucosa** (2) (anterior side) is lined with a **stratified squamous nonkeratinized epithelium** (1). The underlying lamina propria merges with the connective tissue **perichondrium** (4) of the elastic cartilage (3).

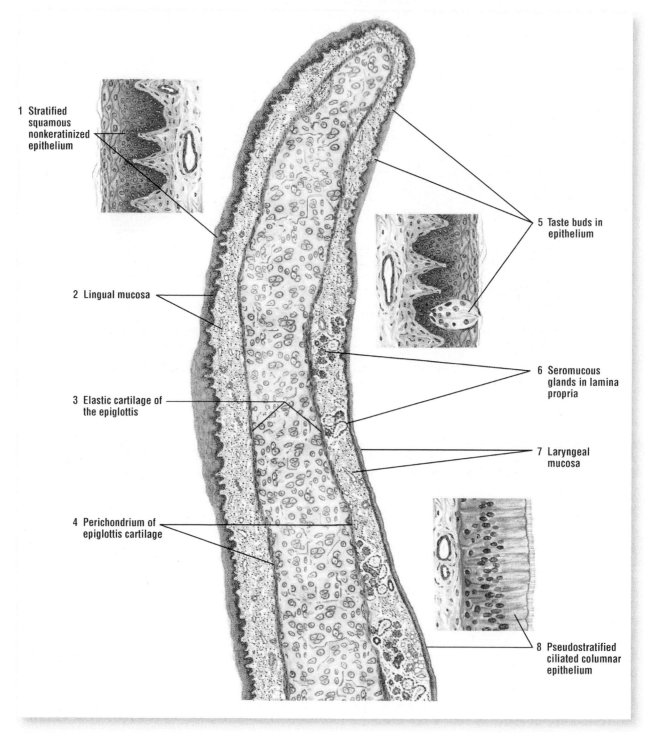

1 Stratified squamous nonkeratinized epithelium

2 Lingual mucosa

3 Elastic cartilage of the epiglottis

4 Perichondrium of epiglottis cartilage

5 Taste buds in epithelium

6 Seromucous glands in lamina propria

7 Laryngeal mucosa

8 Pseudostratified ciliated columnar epithelium

FIGURE 17.7 ■ Epiglottis (longitudinal section). Stain: hematoxylin and eosin. Low magnification. Insets: high magnification.

The lingual mucosa (2) with its stratified squamous epithelium (1) covers the apex of the epiglottis and about half of the **laryngeal mucosa** (7) (posterior side). Toward the base of the epiglottis on the laryngeal surface (7), the lining stratified squamous epithelium (1) changes to **pseudostratified ciliated columnar epithelium** (8). Located below the epithelium in the **lamina propria** (6) on the laryngeal side (7) of the epiglottis are tubuloacinar **seromucous glands** (6).

In addition to the tongue, **taste buds** (5) and solitary lymphatic nodules may be observed in the lingual epithelium (2) or laryngeal epithelium (7).

FIGURE 17.8 | Larynx (Frontal Section)

This image illustrates a vertical section through one half of the larynx.

The **false (superior) vocal fold** (9), also called the vocal cord, is covered by the mucosa that is continuous with the posterior surface of the epiglottis. As in the epiglottis, the false vocal fold (9)

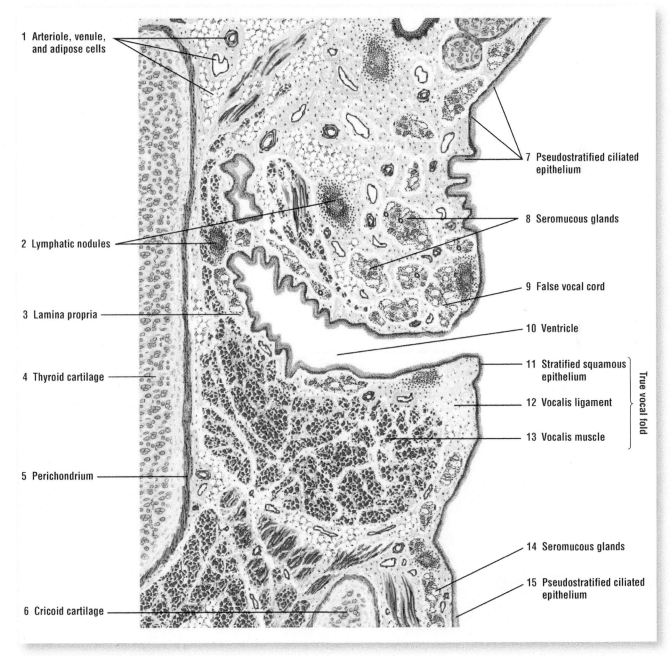

1 Arteriole, venule, and adipose cells

2 Lymphatic nodules

3 Lamina propria

4 Thyroid cartilage

5 Perichondrium

6 Cricoid cartilage

7 Pseudostratified ciliated epithelium

8 Seromucous glands

9 False vocal cord

10 Ventricle

11 Stratified squamous epithelium

12 Vocalis ligament

13 Vocalis muscle

True vocal fold

14 Seromucous glands

15 Pseudostratified ciliated epithelium

FIGURE 17.8 ■ Larynx (frontal section). Stain: hematoxylin and eosin. Low magnification.

is lined with a **pseudostratified ciliated columnar epithelium** (7) with goblet cells. In the lamina propria (3) are mixed **seromucous glands** (8) whose excretory ducts open onto the epithelial surface (7). Numerous **lymphatic nodules** (2), **blood vessels** (1), and **adipose cells** (1) are also located in the lamina propria (3) of the false vocal fold (9).

The **ventricle** (10) is a deep indentation that separates the false (superior) vocal fold (9) from the **true** (**inferior**) **vocal fold** (11–13). The mucosa in the wall of the ventricle (10) is similar to the false vocal fold (9). Lymphatic nodules (2) are more numerous in this area and are sometimes called the laryngeal tonsils. The lamina propria (3) blends with the **perichondrium** (5) of the hyaline **thyroid cartilage** (4). There is no distinct submucosa. The lower wall of the ventricle (10) makes the transition to the true vocal fold (11–13).

The mucosa of the true vocal fold (11–13) is lined with a nonkeratinized **stratified squamous epithelium** (11) and a thin, dense lamina propria devoid of glands, lymphatic tissue, or blood vessels. At the apex of the true vocal fold is the **vocalis ligament** (12) with dense elastic fibers that extend into the adjacent lamina propria and the skeletal **vocalis muscle** (13). The skeletal thyroarytenoid muscle and the thyroid cartilage (4) constitute the remaining wall.

The epithelium in the lower larynx changes to **pseudostratified ciliated columnar epithelium** (15), and the lamina propria contains mixed **seromucous glands** (14). The hyaline **cricoid cartilage** (6) is the lowermost cartilage of the larynx.

FIGURE 17.9 | Trachea (Panoramic View, Transverse Section)

The wall of the trachea consists of mucosa, submucosa, hyaline cartilage, and adventitia. The trachea is kept patent (open) by C-shaped **hyaline cartilage** (3) rings that are surrounded by **perichondrium** (9), which merges with the **submucosa** (4) on one side and the **adventitia** (1) on the other. **Nerves** (6), **blood vessels** (8), and **adipose tissue** (2) are located in the adventitia.

The gap between the posterior ends of the hyaline cartilage (3) is filled by the smooth **trachealis muscle** (7) that lies deep to the **elastic membrane** (14) of the mucosa. Most of the trachealis muscle (7) fibers insert into the perichondrium (9) that covers the hyaline cartilage (3).

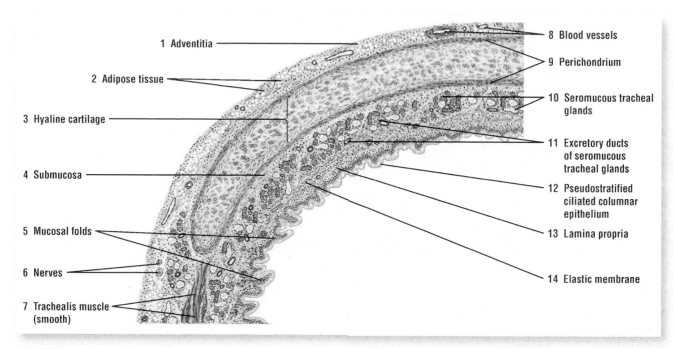

FIGURE 17.9 ■ Trachea (panoramic view, transverse section). Stain: hematoxylin and eosin. Low magnification.

The lumen of the trachea is lined with a **pseudostratified ciliated columnar epithelium (12)** with goblet cells. The underlying lamina propria (13) contains connective tissue fibers, diffuse lymphatic tissue, and occasional lymphatic nodules. Located deeper in the **lamina propria (13)** is the longitudinal elastic membrane (14) formed by elastic fibers. This membrane (14) divides the lamina propria (13) from the submucosa (4) in which are found the tubuloacinar **seromucous tracheal glands (10)** whose **excretory ducts (11)** pass through the lamina propria (13) to the tracheal lumen.

The mucosa exhibits **mucosal folds (5)** along the posterior wall of the trachea. The seromucous tracheal glands (10) that are present in the submucosa can be seen in the adventitia (1).

FIGURE 17.10 | Tracheal Wall (Sectional View)

A section of tracheal wall between the **hyaline cartilage (1)** and the **pseudostratified ciliated columnar epithelium (8)** with **goblet cells (10)** is illustrated at a higher magnification. A thin **basement membrane (9)** separates the lining epithelium (8) from the **lamina propria (11)**.

The **submucosa (6)** contains **seromucous tracheal glands (3)** with a **serous demilune (7)** surrounding a mucous acinus of the tracheal glands (3). The **excretory duct (5)** of the tracheal glands (3) is lined with a simple cuboidal epithelium and extends through the lamina propria (11) to the epithelial surface (8).

The hyaline cartilage (1) is surrounded by **perichondrium (2)**. The larger **chondrocytes in lacunae (4)** that are located in the interior of the hyaline cartilage (1) become flatter toward the perichondrium (2) that blends with the submucosa (6). An **arteriole** and a **venule (12)** supply the connective tissue of the submucosa (6) and the lamina propria (11).

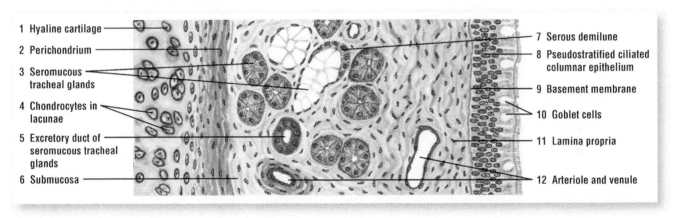

1 Hyaline cartilage
2 Perichondrium
3 Seromucous tracheal glands
4 Chondrocytes in lacunae
5 Excretory duct of seromucous tracheal glands
6 Submucosa
7 Serous demilune
8 Pseudostratified ciliated columnar epithelium
9 Basement membrane
10 Goblet cells
11 Lamina propria
12 Arteriole and venule

FIGURE 17.10 ■ Tracheal wall (sectional view). Stain: hematoxylin and eosin. Medium magnification.

FIGURE 17.11 | Lung (Panoramic View)

This low-magnification illustration shows the major structures in the lung for air conduction and gaseous exchange (respiration).

The histology of the intrapulmonary bronchi is similar to that of the trachea and extrapulmonary bronchi, except that in the intrapulmonary bronchi, the C-shaped cartilage rings of the trachea are replaced by cartilage plates. All cartilage in the trachea and lung is hyaline.

The wall of an **intrapulmonary bronchus** (**5**) can be identified by the presence of hyaline **cartilage plates** (**7**). The wall (**5**) also consists of lamina propria (**4**), a layer of **smooth muscle** (**3**), a **submucosa** (**2**) with **bronchial glands** (**6**), hyaline cartilage plates (**7**), and an **adventitia** (**1**). The surface of a bronchus (**5**) is also lined with a pseudostratified columnar ciliated epithelium with goblet cells.

As the intrapulmonary bronchus (**5**) branches into smaller bronchi and bronchioles, the epithelial height and the cartilage plates around the bronchi decrease until an occasional piece of cartilage is seen. Cartilage disappears from the bronchi walls when their diameters decrease to about 1 mm.

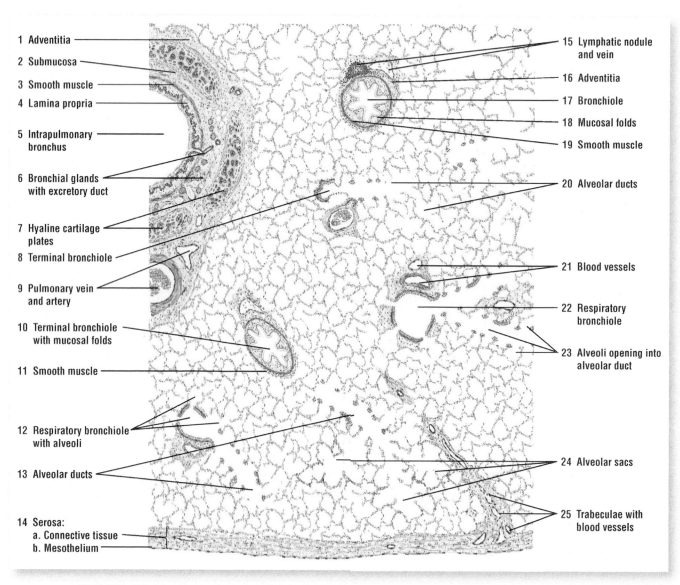

1 Adventitia
2 Submucosa
3 Smooth muscle
4 Lamina propria
5 Intrapulmonary bronchus
6 Bronchial glands with excretory duct
7 Hyaline cartilage plates
8 Terminal bronchiole
9 Pulmonary vein and artery
10 Terminal bronchiole with mucosal folds
11 Smooth muscle
12 Respiratory bronchiole with alveoli
13 Alveolar ducts
14 Serosa:
   a. Connective tissue
   b. Mesothelium

15 Lymphatic nodule and vein
16 Adventitia
17 Bronchiole
18 Mucosal folds
19 Smooth muscle
20 Alveolar ducts
21 Blood vessels
22 Respiratory bronchiole
23 Alveoli opening into alveolar duct
24 Alveolar sacs
25 Trabeculae with blood vessels

FIGURE 17.11 ■ Lung (panoramic view). Stain; hematoxylin and eosin. Low magnification.

In the **bronchiole** (**17**), pseudostratified columnar ciliated epithelium with occasional goblet cells lines the lumen. The lumen shows **mucosal folds** (**18**) caused by the contractions of the surrounding **smooth muscle** (**19**) layer. Bronchial glands and cartilage plates are not present, and the bronchiole (**17**) is surrounded by the adventitia (**16**). In this illustration, a lymphatic nodule (**15**) and a vein (**15**) adjacent to the adventitia (**16**) accompany the bronchiole (**17**).

The terminal **bronchioles** (**8, 10**) exhibit **mucosal folds** (**10**) and are lined with a columnar ciliated epithelium without goblet cells. A thin layer of lamina propria, **smooth muscle** (**11**), and adventitia surrounds the terminal bronchioles (**8, 10**).

The respiratory **bronchioles** (**12, 22**) with alveoli outpocketings are connected to the **alveolar ducts** (**13, 20**) and the **alveoli** (**23**). In these bronchioles (**12, 22**), the epithelium is low columnar, or cuboidal, and may be ciliated in the proximal portion of the tubules. A thin connective tissue layer supports the smooth muscle, the elastic fibers of the lamina propria, and the **blood vessels** (**21**). The **alveoli** (**12**) in the walls of the respiratory bronchioles (**12, 22**) appear as small evaginations, or outpockets.

Each respiratory bronchiole (**12, 22**) divides into several alveolar ducts (**13, 20**) that are lined with alveoli (**23**) that open into the alveolar duct. Clusters of alveoli (**23**) that surround and open into alveolar ducts (**13, 20**) are called alveolar sacs (**24**). In this illustration, a plane of section passes from a terminal bronchiole (**8**) to the respiratory bronchiole and into alveolar ducts (**20**).

The **pulmonary vein** (**9**) and **pulmonary artery** (**9**) branch as they accompany the bronchi and bronchioles into the lung. Small blood vessels are also seen in the connective tissue **trabeculae** (**25**) that separate the lungs into different segments.

The **serosa** (**14**) or visceral pleura surrounds the lungs. It (**14**) consists of a thin layer of pleural **connective tissue** (**14a**) and a simple squamous layer of pleural **mesothelium** (**14b**).

FIGURE 17.12 | **Intrapulmonary Bronchus (Transverse Section)**

The trachea divides outside the lungs and gives rise to primary, or extrapulmonary, bronchi. On entering the lungs, the primary bronchi divide and give rise to a series of smaller or intrapulmonary bronchi.

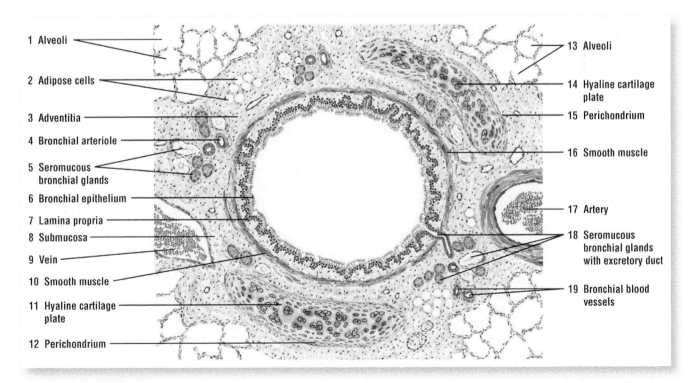

1 Alveoli
2 Adipose cells
3 Adventitia
4 Bronchial arteriole
5 Seromucous bronchial glands
6 Bronchial epithelium
7 Lamina propria
8 Submucosa
9 Vein
10 Smooth muscle
11 Hyaline cartilage plate
12 Perichondrium

13 Alveoli
14 Hyaline cartilage plate
15 Perichondrium
16 Smooth muscle
17 Artery
18 Seromucous bronchial glands with excretory duct
19 Bronchial blood vessels

FIGURE 17.12 ■ Intrapulmonary bronchus (transverse section). Stain: hematoxylin and eosin. Low magnification.

The intrapulmonary bronchi are lined with a pseudostratified columnar ciliated **bronchial epithelium** (6) supported by **lamina propria** (7) of fine connective tissue with elastic fibers (not illustrated) and a few lymphocytes. A thin layer of **smooth muscle** (10, 16) surrounds the lamina propria (7) and separates it from the **submucosa** (8) that contains numerous **seromucous bronchial glands** (5, 18). An **excretory duct** (18) from the bronchial gland (5, 18) passes through the lamina propria (7) to open into the bronchial lumen. In mixed seromucous bronchial glands (5, 18), serous demilunes may be seen.

In the lung, the surrounding hyaline cartilage rings of the trachea are replaced by **cartilage plates** (11, 14). A **perichondrium** (12, 15) covers each cartilage plate (11, 14) as they become smaller and farther apart as the bronchi continue to divide and decrease in size. Between the cartilage plates (11, 14), the submucosa (8) blends with the **adventitia** (3). Bronchial glands (5, 18) and **adipose cells** (2) are present in the submucosa (8) of larger bronchi.

Bronchial blood vessels (19) and a **bronchial arteriole** (4) are in the connective tissue around the bronchus. Accompanying the bronchus are also a larger **vein** (9) and an **artery** (17).

Surrounding the intrapulmonary bronchus, its connective tissue, and the hyaline cartilage plates (11, 14) are the lung **alveoli** (1, 13).

FIGURE 17.13 | Intrapulmonary Bronchus, Cartilage Plates, and Surrounding Alveoli of Lung

This medium-power micrograph of a small, intrapulmonary bronchus cut in cross section shows the **cartilage plates** (5, 9) around its **lumen** (2). The **respiratory epithelium** (1) of ciliated and goblet cells lines the lumen of bronchus (2). Surrounding each cartilage plate (5, 9) is the **perichondrium** (3). Located below the respiratory epithelium (1) is a layer of **smooth muscle** (7) that encircles the bronchus and controls its diameter during respiration. In the connective tissue below the epithelium are **seromucous tracheal glands** (8), some of which open into the lumen of the bronchus (1). Also present in the connective tissue is a **lymphatic nodule** (11) filled with lymphocytes. An **adventitia** (10) surrounds the bronchus and its associated tissue. Outside the adventitia of the intrapulmonary bronchus are thin-walled **alveoli** (4, 6).

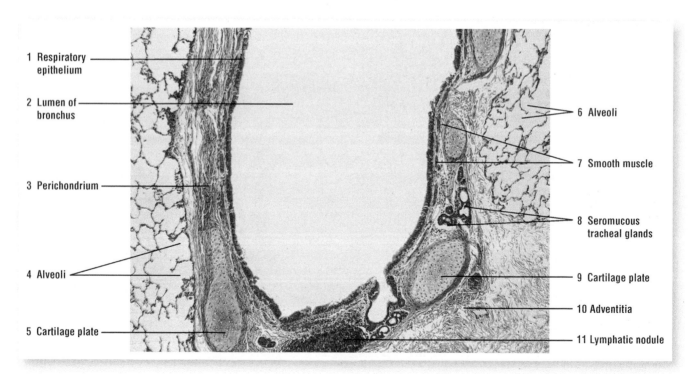

FIGURE 17.13 ■ Intrapulmonary bronchus, cartilage plates, and surrounding alveoli of the lung. Stain: hematoxylin and eosin. ×75. From: Gartner LP, Hiatt JM. *BRS Cell Biology & Histology*. 6th ed. Baltimore: Lippincott Williams & Wilkins, 2011.

FIGURE 17.14 | Terminal Bronchiole (Transverse Section)

The bronchioles subdivide into smaller terminal bronchioles, whose diameters are approximately 1 mm or less and their lumina lined with a **simple columnar epithelium** (3). In the smallest bronchioles, the epithelium may be simple cuboidal. The cartilage plates, bronchial glands, and goblet cells are absent from the terminal bronchioles. The terminal bronchioles represent the smallest conducting passageways for air.

Because of smooth muscle contractions, **mucosal folds** (7) are prominent in the bronchioles. A well-developed **smooth muscle** (5) layer surrounds the thin **lamina propria** (6), which, in turn, is surrounded by the **adventitia** (8).

Adjacent to the bronchiole is a branch of the **pulmonary artery** (2). The terminal bronchiole is surrounded by the lung **alveoli** (1). Surrounding the alveoli are the thin **interalveolar septa with capillaries** (4).

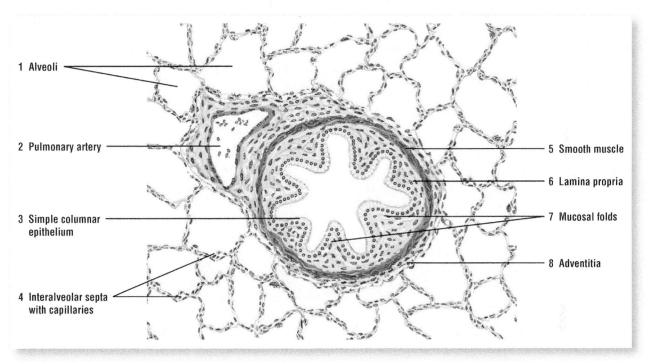

1 Alveoli

2 Pulmonary artery

3 Simple columnar
  epithelium

4 Interalveolar septa
  with capillaries

5 Smooth muscle

6 Lamina propria

7 Mucosal folds

8 Adventitia

FIGURE 17.14 ■ Terminal bronchiole (transverse section). Stain: hematoxylin and eosin. Low magnification.

FIGURE 17.15 | Respiratory Bronchiole, Alveolar Duct, and Lung Alveoli

The terminal bronchioles give rise to the respiratory bronchioles. The **respiratory bronchiole (2)** represents a transition zone between the conducting and respiratory portions of the respiratory system.

The wall of the respiratory bronchiole (2) is lined with a **simple cuboidal epithelium (3)**. Single **alveolar outpocketings (1, 6)** are found in the wall of each respiratory bronchiole (2). Cilia may be present in the epithelium of the proximal portion of the respiratory bronchiole (2) but disappear in the distal portion. A thin layer of **smooth muscle (7)** surrounds the epithelium. A small branch of the **pulmonary artery (4)** accompanies the respiratory bronchiole (2) into the lung.

Each respiratory bronchiole (2) gives rise to an **alveolar duct (9)** into which open numerous alveoli (8). In the lamina propria that surrounds the rim of alveoli (8) in the alveolar duct (9) are **smooth muscle bundles (5)** that appear as knobs between adjacent alveoli.

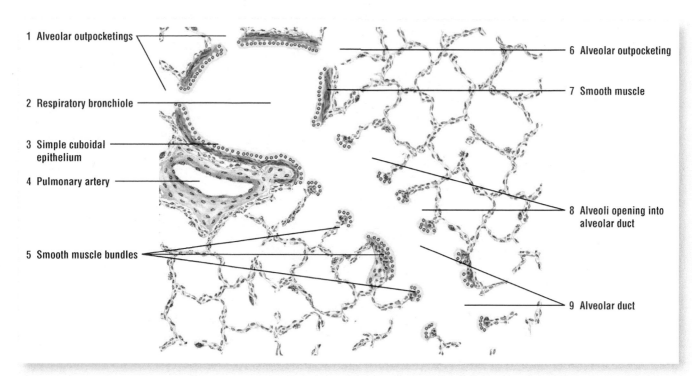

1 Alveolar outpocketings

2 Respiratory bronchiole

3 Simple cuboidal epithelium

4 Pulmonary artery

5 Smooth muscle bundles

6 Alveolar outpocketing

7 Smooth muscle

8 Alveoli opening into alveolar duct

9 Alveolar duct

FIGURE 17.15 ■ Respiratory bronchiole, alveolar duct, and lung alveoli. Stain: hematoxylin and eosin. Low magnification.

FIGURE 17.16 | Lung: Terminal Bronchiole, Respiratory Bronchiole, Alveolar Ducts, Alveoli, and Blood Vessel

This photomicrograph of the lung shows the smallest air-conducting passage, the **terminal bronchiole** (**7**) that gives rise to thinner **respiratory bronchioles** (**3**), characterized by numerous **alveoli** (**2**). Each respiratory bronchiole (**3**) gives rise to an **alveolar duct** (**1, 4, 8**) that continues into the **alveolar sacs** (**5**). The terminal bronchiole (**7**) and the adjacent **blood vessel** (**6**) are surrounded by the alveoli (**2**).

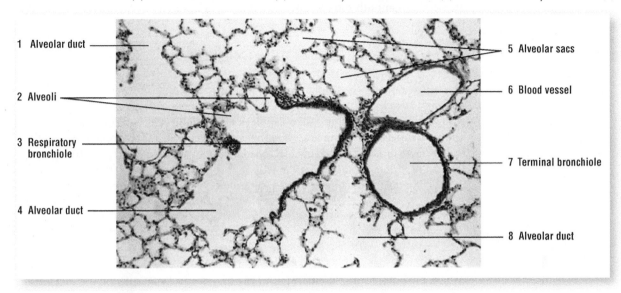

1 Alveolar duct
2 Alveoli
3 Respiratory bronchiole
4 Alveolar duct
5 Alveolar sacs
6 Blood vessel
7 Terminal bronchiole
8 Alveolar duct

FIGURE 17.16 ■ Lung: terminal bronchiole, respiratory bronchiole, alveolar ducts, alveoli, and a blood vessel. Stain: hematoxylin and eosin. ×40.

FIGURE 17.17 | Alveolar Walls and Alveolar Cells

The **alveoli** (**3**) are evaginations or outpocketings of the respiratory bronchioles, alveolar ducts, and alveolar sacs, the terminal ends of the alveolar ducts. The alveoli (**3**) are lined by thin, simple squamous **alveolar cells** (**type I pneumocytes**) (**7**). The adjacent alveoli (**3**) share an **interalveolar septum** (**4**), or alveolar wall.

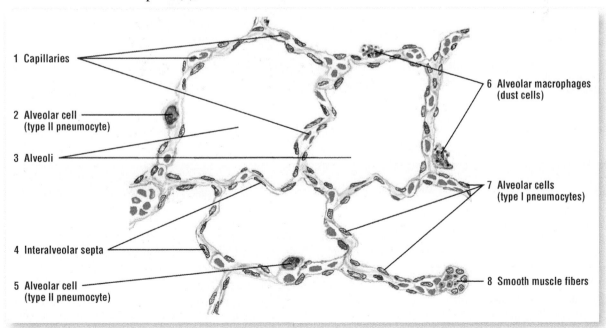

1 Capillaries
2 Alveolar cell (type II pneumocyte)
3 Alveoli
4 Interalveolar septa
5 Alveolar cell (type II pneumocyte)
6 Alveolar macrophages (dust cells)
7 Alveolar cells (type I pneumocytes)
8 Smooth muscle fibers

FIGURE 17.17 ■ Alveolar walls and alveolar cells. Stain: hematoxylin and eosin. High magnification. ×205.

The interalveolar septa (4) consist of simple squamous alveolar cells (7), fine connective tissue fibers and fibroblasts, and numerous **capillaries** (1) that are close to the alveolar cells (7) of the adjacent alveoli (3).

The alveoli (3) also contain **alveolar macrophages** (6) or dust cells that normally contain several carbon or dust particles in their cytoplasm. Also in the alveoli (3) are the **alveolar cells** (2, 5) or type II pneumocytes that are interspersed among the simple squamous alveolar cells (6) in the alveoli (3).

At the free ends of the interalveolar septa (4) and around the open ends of the alveoli (3) are bands of **smooth muscle fibers** (8) that are continuous with the muscle layer that lines the respiratory bronchioles.

FIGURE 17.18 | Section of Lung Alveoli Adjacent to Bronchiole Wall

This micrograph shows the different cells and structures of the lung at a higher magnification. One **alveolus** (2) is clear with air, whereas adjacent alveoli contain **alveolar macrophages (dust cells)** (1). Also visible are the very thin-walled **capillaries with blood cells** (3, 5) located adjacent to the alveoli. The inner surfaces of the alveoli are lined by simple squamous **alveolar cells (type I pneumocytes)** (4) and the more prominent and cuboidal **alveolar cells (type II pneumocytes)** (6). An elongated **alveolar duct** (8) exhibits some **smooth muscle** (7) in its wall. Adjacent to the alveoli is a section of a terminal/respiratory **bronchiole** with its clear **lumen** (9) lined with a simple cuboidal **epithelium** (10).

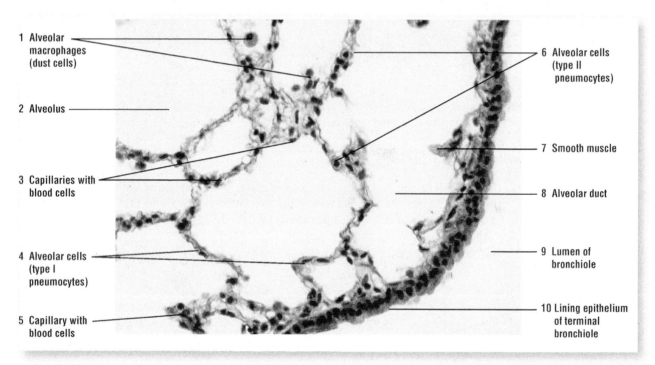

FIGURE 17.18 ■ A section of lung alveoli adjacent to a bronchiole wall. Stain: hematoxylin and eosin. ×205.

FUNCTIONAL CORRELATIONS 17.2 ■ Clara Cells

Clara cells are most numerous in the terminal bronchioles and become the predominant cell type in the distal part of the respiratory bronchioles as the ciliated cells decrease in number. Clara cells have several important functions. They secrete one of the **surfactant-like** lipoproteins that coat the bronchial epithelium and break down (via proteolytic enzymes) the luminal stickiness of mucus for more efficient respiration. These lipoproteins also serve as tension-reducing agents in the alveoli helping to reduce the collapse of the airway walls. Clara cells also function as **stem cells** that replace lost or injured bronchial ciliated and nonciliated epithelial cells. These cells also secrete proteins and lysozymes into the bronchioles to protect the lung from inhaled toxic substances, oxidative pollutants, or inflammation and transfer immunoglobulins into bronchiolar lumina.

FIGURE 17.19 | **Low-Power Ultrastructure of Lung Showing Portion of Bronchiole Wall and Adjacent Alveoli**

This lung was perfused with fixatives, and, as a result, the capillaries are empty and do not exhibit any blood cells. This low-power ultrastructure of the lung shows a section of the bronchiole wall and the alveoli. The **lumen of the bronchiole (14)** is lined with the secretory, dome-shaped **Clara cells (1, 8)** and **ciliated cells (2, 9)**. The cytoplasm of the Clara cells (1, 8) contains dense-staining secretory granules. The very thin **capillaries (5, 11)** with empty lumina are adjacent to the very thin **cytoplasm of alveolar cells (6, 13)** (type I pneumocytes) that line the lumina of alveoli (7, 12). Surrounding the wall of the bronchiole is a layer of **connective tissue (10)**, **smooth muscle cells (3)**, and a **blood vessel with a white blood cell (4)** in its lumen.

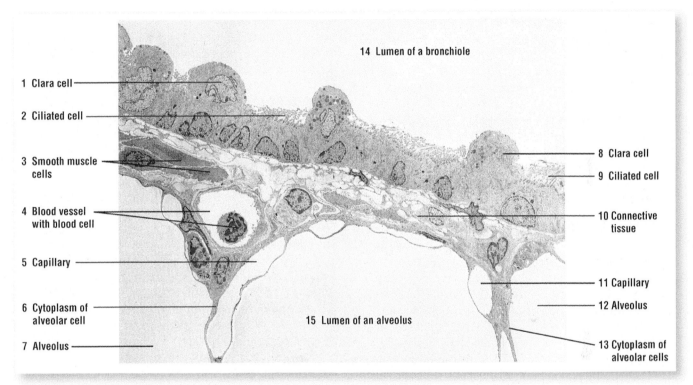

FIGURE 17.19 ■ A low-power ultrastructure of the lung, showing a portion of a bronchiole wall and adjacent alveoli. ×1,500. From: Gartner LP, Hiatt JM. *BRS Cell Biology & Histology*. 6th ed. Baltimore: Lippincott Williams & Wilkins, 2011.

FUNCTIONAL CORRELATIONS 17.3 ■ Cells in Lung

RESPIRATORY SYSTEM—CONDUCTING PORTION

The conducting portions of the respiratory system condition the inhaled air. **Mucus** that is produced by **goblet cells** in the pseudostratified ciliated respiratory epithelium and **mucous glands** in the lamina propria contain antimicrobial substances. The goblet cells and serous secretions from serous glands contain immunoglobulins, lysozymes, and enzymes that destroy bacteria. These secretions form the airway mucus layer that covers the luminal surfaces in conducting tubes. As a result, the **moist mucosa** in the conducting airways **humidifies** the air. The mucus and ciliated epithelium also filter and clean the air of particulate matter, infectious microorganisms, and other airborne matter. These secretions are moved toward the pharynx by the motility of cilia where they are either swallowed or expelled. In addition, an extensive **capillary network** beneath the epithelium in the lamina propria **warms** the inspired air in the conducting portion before it reaches the respiratory portion in the lungs.

CELLS OF LUNG ALVEOLI

The lung alveoli contain different cell types. **Type I alveolar cells**, or **type I pneumocytes**, are extremely thin simple squamous cells that line the alveoli and are the main sites for gaseous exchange. A thin **interalveolar septum** with reticular and elastic fibers that is located between adjacent alveoli contains a network of capillaries. Type I alveolar cells are in very close contact with the endothelial lining of capillaries, forming a very thin **blood–air barrier** for gaseous exchange. The blood–air barrier consists of a thin layer of the secreted material surfactant, cytoplasm of type I pneumocyte, the fused basal lamina of the pneumocyte and the endothelial cell, and the thin cytoplasm of the capillary endothelium.

Type II alveolar cells, also called **type II pneumocytes**, or **septal cells**, in comparison to type I alveolar cells are fewer in number and cuboidal in shape. They appear singly or in groups adjacent to the squamous type I alveolar cells within the alveoli. Their rounded apices project into the alveoli above the type I alveolar cells. These type II alveolar cells are secretory and contain dense-staining **lamellar bodies** in their apical cytoplasm. These cells synthesize and secrete a phospholipid-rich product called **pulmonary surfactant**. When released into the alveolus, surfactant spreads as a thin layer over the surfaces of type I alveolar cells, lowering the alveolar **surface tension** at the air–epithelium interface. The reduced surface tension in the alveoli decreases the force that is needed to inflate alveoli during inspiration. Surfactant stabilizes the alveolar diameters, facilitates their expansion, and prevents their collapse during respiration by minimizing the collapsing forces. During fetal development, the type II alveolar cells secrete sufficient amount of surfactant for respiration during the last 28 to 32 weeks of gestation. In addition to producing surfactant, the type II cells can divide and function as **stem cells** for type I squamous alveolar cell replacement in the alveoli during lung injury. Surfactant also has some **bactericidal** effects and induces immune responses in the alveoli to counteract inhaled pathogens, fungi, viruses, and bacteria.

Alveolar macrophages, or **dust cells**, are blood monocytes that have entered the pulmonary connective tissue septa and alveoli and function as phagocytes in both areas. The primary function of these macrophages is to clean the alveoli of invading microorganisms and inhaled particulate matter by **phagocytosis**. These cells are seen either in the individual alveoli or in the thin alveolar septa. They can be recognized in the alveoli or in the connective tissue septa by their phagocytosed particulate or carbon particles.

Chapter 17 Summary

Respiratory System

COMPONENTS OF RESPIRATORY SYSTEM—OVERVIEW

- Conducting portion consists of solid passageways that move air in and out of lungs
- Extrapulmonary passages include the trachea and bronchi
- Pseudostratified ciliated epithelium with numerous goblet cells lines the larger passageways
- As passageways branch and enter lung, there is a decrease in epithelium height and tubule size
- Terminal bronchioles represent the terminal portion of conducting portion
- Respiratory bronchioles represent the transition zone between conducting and respiratory zones

RESPIRATORY EPITHELIUM

- Ciliated cells are most common and extend the thickness of epithelium and sweep the surface
- Goblet cells are numerous in airways, secrete protective mucus, but decrease in distal parts
- Basal cells are close to basal lamina, do not reach the surface, and serve as stem cells
- Brush cells are less numerous, contact afferent axons, and may function as receptors cells
- Small granule cells contain granules and are analogous to enteroendocrine cells (DNES)

OLFACTORY EPITHELIUM

- Located in the roof of the nasal cavity and laterally on each side of the superior conchae
- Specialized pseudostratified epithelium consisting of three cell types without goblet cells
- Contains supportive, basal, and olfactory cells, the sensory bipolar neurons
- Olfactory cells are the sensory bipolar neurons that respond to smell
- Olfactory cells span the thickness of epithelium and end as olfactory vesicles
- Surface of vesicles shows radiating nonmotile olfactory cilia that contain olfactory receptors for odorants
- Olfactory cilia contain odorant-binding receptors that are stimulated by odor molecules

- Unmyelinated axons leave bases of olfactory cells to form nerve bundles
- Nerve bundles continue through skull bone to synapse in the olfactory bulbs of the brain
- Below epithelium, serous olfactory glands bathe olfactory cilia and provide odor solvents
- Dissolved odorant molecules bind to odorant-binding proteins in fluid produced by olfactory glands
- Supportive cells provide structural support, whereas basal cells serve as stem cells for the olfactory epithelium
- Transition from olfactory to respiratory epithelium is abrupt

RESPIRATORY SYSTEM—CONDUCTING PORTION

- Extrapulmonary structures are the nose, pharynx, larynx, trachea, and extrapulmonary bronchi
- Intrapulmonary structures include bronchi, bronchioles, and terminal bronchioles
- Conditions air by humidifying, warming, and filtering it because of cilia and mucus
- Secretions from glands contain immunoglobulins, lysozyme, and enzymes to kill bacteria
- Incomplete hyaline cartilage C rings encircle and keep trachea patent (open)
- In the lungs, hyaline cartilage plates replace C rings and encircle the larger bronchi
- Bronchioles of about 1 mm diameter no longer have cartilage plates
- As tubular size decreases, epithelium becomes simple ciliated and goblet cells disappear

Clara Cells

- Replace goblet cells and become predominant cells in terminal and respiratory bronchioles
- Are secretory, nonciliated cells that increase in number as ciliated cells decrease
- Secrete surfactant-like lipoprotein components that break down mucus stickiness and reduce surface tension
- Also function as stem cells to replace lost or injured bronchial epithelial cells
- Secrete proteins and lysozymes into bronchial tree to protect lung from inflammation or toxic pollutants

RESPIRATORY SYSTEM—RESPIRATORY PORTION

- Starts with a passageway where initial respiration can take place
- Terminal bronchioles give rise to respiratory bronchioles, a transition zone for respiration
- Respiratory bronchioles exhibit thin-walled alveoli, where gaseous exchange takes place
- Gaseous exchange can take place only when alveoli are present
- Alveoli are final airspaces and are surrounded by capillary plexus for gaseous exchange
- Consists of respiratory bronchioles, alveolar ducts, alveolar sacs, and alveoli
- Goblet cells are absent from alveoli and the lining is very thin where respiration occurs

Cells of Lung Alveoli

- Type I alveolar cells (type I pneumocytes) are very thin that line the lung alveoli
- Capillary endothelium and type I alveolar cells form the thin blood–air barrier
- Type II alveolar cells (type II pneumocytes) are adjacent to type I alveolar cells
- Type II alveolar cells are secretory cells whose apices project above type I alveolar cells
- Contain numerous secretory lamellar bodies
- Synthesize phospholipid surfactant for alveoli to reduce surface tension
- Surfactant reduces alveolar surface tension, allowing expansion and preventing collapse
- During fetal development, sufficient amount of surfactant produced for respiration
- Surfactant has bactericidal effects to counteract inhaled pathogens
- Type II alveolar cells also serve as stem cells to replace type I cells after injury to lung

Alveolar Macrophages

- Are blood monocytes that enter pulmonary connective tissue and alveoli

- Clean alveoli of invading organisms and phagocytose particular matter

Epiglottis

- Superior part of larynx that projects upward from larynx wall
- A central elastic cartilage forms core of the epiglottis
- Stratified squamous epithelium lines lingual (anterior) and part of laryngeal (posterior) surface
- Base of epiglottis lined with pseudostratified ciliated columnar epithelium
- Taste buds may be present in lingual or laryngeal epithelium

Larynx

- Pseudostratified ciliated columnar epithelium lines false vocal fold, as posterior epiglottis
- Mixed seromucous glands, blood vessels, lymphatic nodules, and adipose cells in lamina propria
- Ventricle, a deep indentation, separates false vocal fold from true vocal fold
- True vocal fold lined with stratified squamous nonkeratinized epithelium
- Vocalis ligament is at the apex of true vocal fold and skeletal vocalis muscle is adjacent
- Hyaline thyroid cartilage and cricoid cartilage provide support for the larynx
- Epithelium in lower larynx changes back to pseudostratified ciliated columnar epithelium

Trachea

- Wall consists of mucosa, submucosa, hyaline cartilage, and adventitia
- Cartilage C rings keep trachea open with gaps between rings filled with trachealis muscle
- Lining is pseudostratified ciliated columnar epithelium with goblet cells
- Submucosa contains seromucous tracheal glands with ducts opening into trachea lumen

Chapter 17 Review Questions

QUESTIONS

In the following multiple choice questions, choose the letter corresponding to the one best answer.

1. **What cells can serve as stem cells for replacing type I alveolar cells?**

   A. Goblet cells
   B. Septal cells
   C. Type II alveolar cells
   D. Blood monocytes
   E. Type I alveolar cells

2. **Which cells in the alveoli contain lamellar bodies in their cytoplasm?**

   A. Type I alveolar cells
   B. Type II alveolar cells
   C. Goblet cells
   D. Septal cells
   E. All alveolar cells

3. **What is the main function of surfactant?**

   A. To reduce air flow into the lung
   B. To increase air flow into the lung
   C. To reduce alveolar surface tension
   D. To reduce the alveolar lumina
   E. To decrease the blood–air barrier

4. **Which cells serve as stem cells for renewing the olfactory epithelium?**

   A. Goblet cells
   B. Sustentacular cells
   C. Ciliated cells
   D. Basal cells
   E. Connective tissue cells

5. **The serous secretory substance in which odorant molecules dissolve is produced by:**

   A. olfactory (Bowman) glands.
   B. olfactory vesicles.
   C. goblet cells.
   D. olfactory cilia.
   E. basal cells.

ANSWERS

1. **Correct Answer: C.** Type II alveolar cells. These cells not only produce surfactant material but also can serve as stem cells for replacing type I alveolar cells during lung injury.

2. **Correct Answer: B.** Type II alveolar cells. These cells synthesize and release the tension-reducing substance surfactant for alveoli.

3. **Correct Answer: C.** To reduce alveolar surface tension. This allows for easier alveolar expansion and prevention of alveolar collapse during respiration.

4. **Correct Answer: D.** Basal cells. These cells give rise to olfactory and supportive cells of the olfactory epithelium.

5. **Correct Answer: A.** Olfactory (Bowman) glands. The secretion from these glands contains odorant-binding proteins that bind with an odorant and is then presented to the odorant receptors on the surface of the nonmotile olfactory cilia.

ADDITIONAL HISTOLOGIC IMAGES

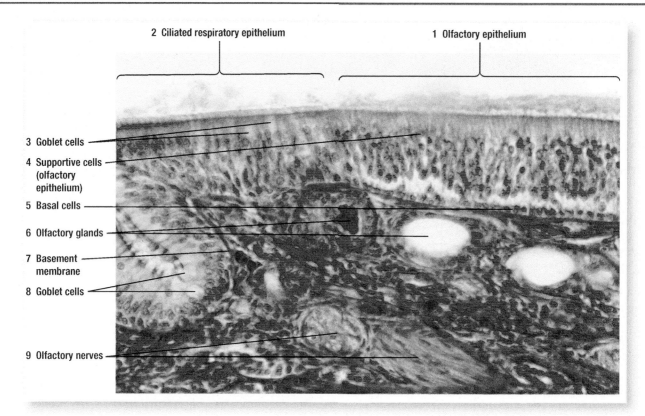

FIGURE 17.20 ■ A section of a human nasal cavity illustrating the transition and difference between ciliated respiratory epithelium (*left*) and olfactory epithelium (*right*). Stain: Mallory-Azan. ×80.

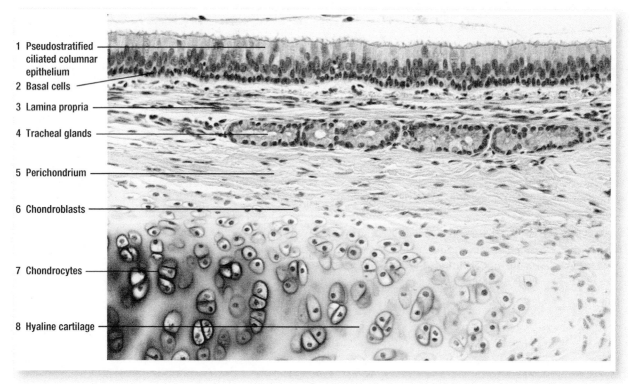

FIGURE 17.21 ■ A section of a primate trachea illustrating the pseudostratified ciliated columnar epithelium and the supportive hyaline cartilage. Stain: hematoxylin and eosin. ×50.

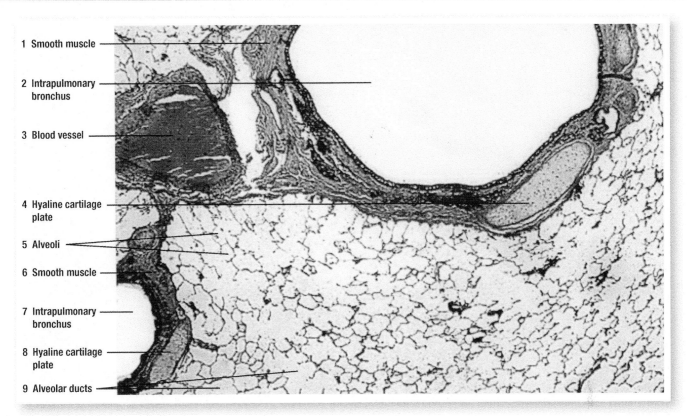

1 Smooth muscle

2 Intrapulmonary bronchus

3 Blood vessel

4 Hyaline cartilage plate

5 Alveoli

6 Smooth muscle

7 Intrapulmonary bronchus

8 Hyaline cartilage plate

9 Alveolar ducts

FIGURE 17.22 ■ A section of a primate intrapulmonary bronchi with surrounding lung tissues. Stain: hematoxylin and eosin. ×5.

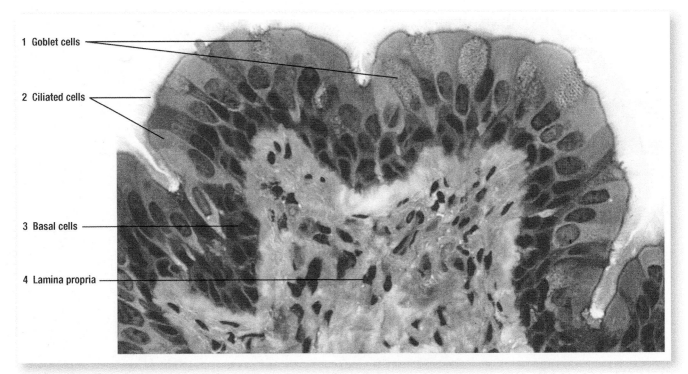

1 Goblet cells

2 Ciliated cells

3 Basal cells

4 Lamina propria

FIGURE 17.23 ■ A plastic section of the pseudostratified ciliated columnar epithelium from a human intrapulmonary bronchus. Stain: hematoxylin and eosin. ×165.

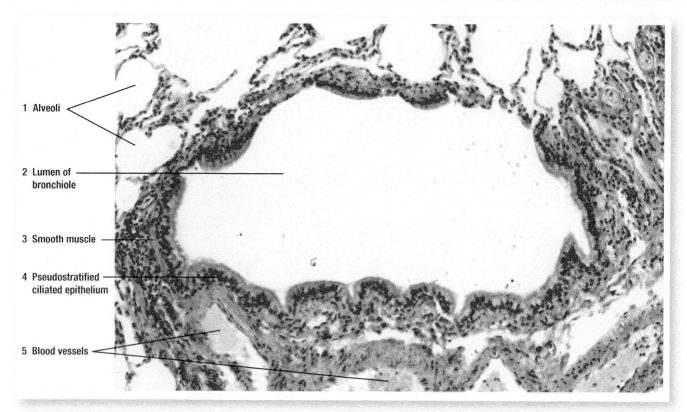

1 Alveoli

2 Lumen of bronchiole

3 Smooth muscle

4 Pseudostratified ciliated epithelium

5 Blood vessels

FIGURE 17.24 ■ A transverse section of a primate bronchiole with surrounding tissues. Stain: hematoxylin and eosin. ×45.

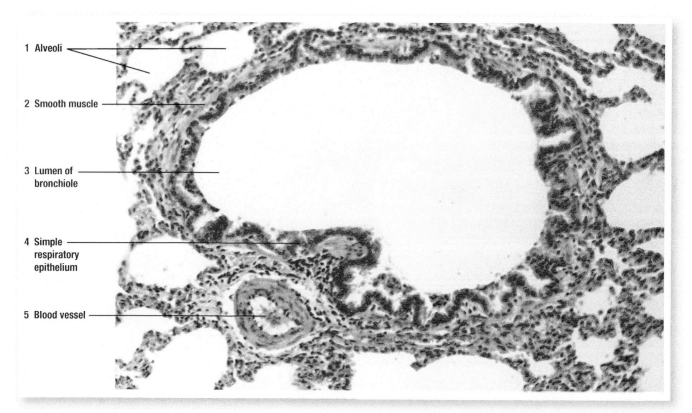

1 Alveoli

2 Smooth muscle

3 Lumen of bronchiole

4 Simple respiratory epithelium

5 Blood vessel

FIGURE 17.25 ■ A smaller bronchiole in a primate lung surrounded by alveoli. Stain: hematoxylin and eosin. ×45.

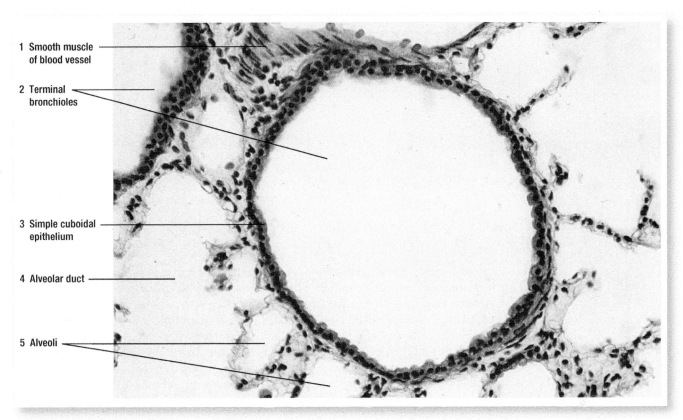

1 Smooth muscle of blood vessel

2 Terminal bronchioles

3 Simple cuboidal epithelium

4 Alveolar duct

5 Alveoli

FIGURE 17.26 ■ A solid terminal primate bronchiole surrounded by alveoli. Stain: hematoxylin and eosin. ×80.

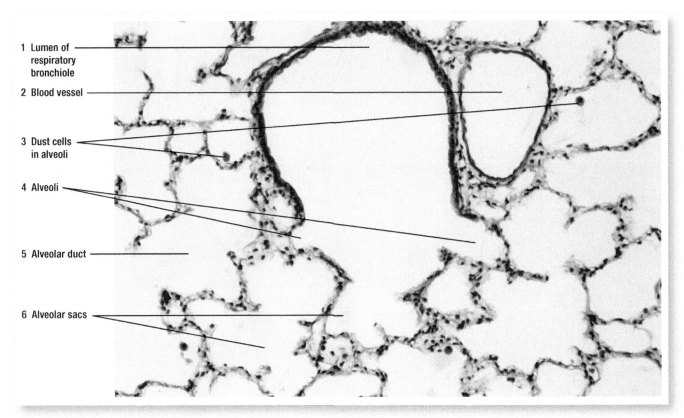

1 Lumen of respiratory bronchiole

2 Blood vessel

3 Dust cells in alveoli

4 Alveoli

5 Alveolar duct

6 Alveolar sacs

FIGURE 17.27 ■ A primate respiratory bronchiole with alveoli and surrounded by alveoli. Stain: hematoxylin and eosin. ×80.

Urinary System

KIDNEY

The urinary system consists of two **kidneys**, two **ureters** that lead to a single urinary **bladder**, and a single **urethra** that extends from the bladder through the penis to the exterior. The kidneys are large, bean-shaped organs located retroperitoneally adjacent to the posterior body wall. Superior to each kidney is the **adrenal gland** embedded in renal fat and connective tissue. The concave, medial border of the kidney is the **hilum**, which contains three structures: the **renal artery**, **renal vein**, and the funnel-shaped **renal pelvis** that narrows to become the ureter. Surrounding these structures is loose connective tissue and a fat-filled space called the **renal sinus**.

Each kidney is covered by a dense connective tissue capsule. A sagittal section through the kidney shows a darker outer **cortex** and a lighter inner **medulla**, which consists of cone-shaped renal pyramids (Fig. 18.1). The base of each pyramid faces the cortex and forms the

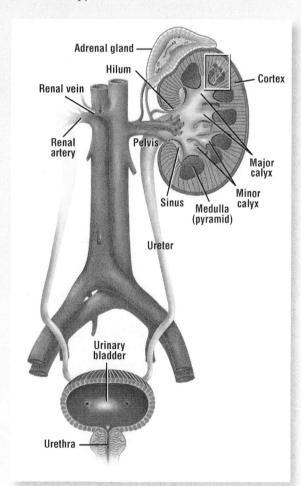

FIGURE 18.1 ■ A sagittal section of the kidney shows the cortex and medulla, with blood vessels and the excretory ducts, including the pelvis and the ureter.

corticomedullary boundary. The round apex of each pyramid extends downward to the renal pelvis to form the domelike **renal papilla**. A portion of the cortex also extends on each side of the renal pyramids to form the **renal columns**.

Each renal papilla is surrounded by a funnel-shaped **minor calyx** that collects urine from the papilla. The minor calyces join in the renal sinus to form a **major calyx** that, in turn, joins to form a single funnel-shaped renal pelvis. The renal pelvis leaves each kidney through the hilum, narrows to become a muscular **ureter**, and descends toward the bladder on each side of the posterior body wall.

Uriniferous Tubules

The functional unit of each kidney is the microscopic **uriniferous tubule**. It consists of a **nephron** and a **collecting duct** into which empty the filtered contents of the nephron. Nephrons produce urine, and the excretory collecting ducts conduct the urine from the kidneys. Millions of nephrons are present in each kidney cortex. The nephron, in turn, is subdivided into two components: a renal corpuscle and renal tubules.

Nephrons of Kidney

There are two types of nephrons, based on their location in the kidney. **Cortical nephrons** are located in the upper cortex of the kidney, whereas the **juxtamedullary nephrons** are situated near the junction of the cortex and medulla of the kidney. Although all nephrons participate in urine formation, juxtamedullary nephrons produce a hypertonic environment in the interstitium of the kidney medulla that produces concentrated (hypertonic) urine.

Renal Corpuscle

The renal corpuscle consists of a tuft of capillaries, called the **glomerulus**, surrounded by a double layer of epithelial cells called the **glomerular (Bowman) capsule**. The inner or **visceral layer** of the capsule consists of specialized branching epithelial cells called **podocytes**. These cells are adjacent to the capillaries, and their long cytoplasmic processes completely invest the fenestrated glomerular capillaries. From these cytoplasmic processes arise numerous smaller foot processes or **pedicles** that interdigitate with pedicles from adjacent podocytes and form tight-fitting **filtration slits**. A thin, semipermeable **filtration slit diaphragm** spans each filtration slit. The **outer, or parietal, layer** of the glomerular capsule consists of simple squamous epithelium.

The renal corpuscle is the initial segment of each nephron. The entry point of the afferent glomerular capillaries into and the exit of efferent vessels from the renal corpuscle is the **vascular pole**. On the opposite end of the vascular pole of the renal corpuscle is the **urinary pole**, where the filtrate produced by the glomerulus leaves the renal corpuscle.

Blood Filtration

Blood flowing through the kidneys is filtered in renal corpuscles through the glomerular capillaries. The produced filtrate then enters the **capsular (urinary) space** located between the parietal and visceral cell layers of the glomerular capsule of the renal corpuscle. The filtrate leaves each renal corpuscle at the urinary pole where the proximal convoluted tubule originates. The filtration barrier for blood in the renal corpuscles consists of three different components: the glomerular **capillary endothelium**, the underlying thicker glomerular **basement membrane**, and the visceral layer of the Bowman capsule, **podocytes**, and **pedicles**.

Filtration Barrier in Glomerulus

Blood filtration is facilitated by the glomerular endothelium of the capillaries, which is thin, porous (fenestrated), and permeable to many substances in the blood, except to the formed blood elements or large plasma proteins. Located between the capillary endothelium and the visceral podocytes is the denser **glomerular basement membrane** formed by the fusion of the endothelium and the visceral layer of podocytes. The glomerular basement membrane is a selective physical barrier that filters and restricts the movement of macromolecules such as albumin from the blood. The semipermeable slit diaphragms between the individual pedicles of the podocytes are highly specialized junctional complexes containing a transmembrane protein called **nephrin** that becomes the main structural and functional portion of the slit diaphragm. The protein nephrin connects or anchors firmly with the actin filaments in the adjacent pedicles of the podocytes forming filtration slits that act like a fine sieve in the renal corpuscle. Thus, although each component of the filtration barrier in the glomerulus contributes to blood filtration, the podocyte slit diaphragms are responsible for glomerular permeability and filtration because they function as **size-selective molecular filters**. Thus, the filtrate that enters the capsular (urinary) space in the renal corpuscle is not urine. Instead, it is an ultrafiltrate that is similar to plasma, except for the absence of proteins.

RENAL TUBULES

The glomerular ultrafiltrate that leaves the renal corpuscle first enters the **renal tubule**, which extends from the glomerular capsule to the collecting tubule. This renal tubule has several distinct histologic and functional regions (Fig. 18.2).

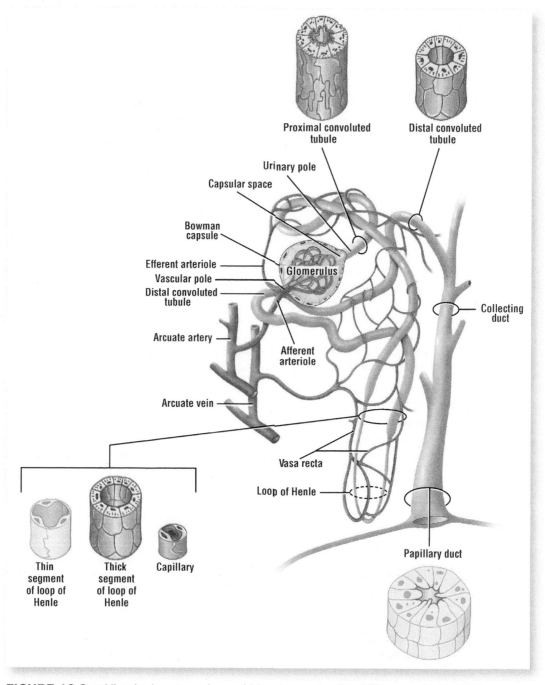

FIGURE 18.2 ■ Histologic comparison of blood vessels, the different tubules of the nephron, and the collecting ducts.

The renal tubule that starts at the renal corpuscle is highly twisted, or tortuous, and is therefore called the **proximal convoluted tubule**. Initially, this tubule is located in the cortex but then descends into the medulla to become continuous with another tubule, the loop of Henle. The **loop of Henle** consists of several parts: a thick descending portion of the proximal convoluted tubule, a thin descending and ascending segment, and a thick ascending portion called the **distal convoluted tubule**. The distal convoluted tubule is shorter and less convoluted than the proximal convoluted tubule, and it ascends back into the kidney cortex. Because the proximal convoluted tubule is longer than the distal convoluted tubule, it is more frequently observed near the renal corpuscles and in the renal cortex. The distal convoluted tubule then joins to the **collecting tubule**. In juxtamedullary nephrons, the loop of Henle is very long. It descends from the kidney cortex deep into the medulla and then loops back to ascend into the cortex.

The collecting tubule and the collecting duct are not part of the nephron. A number of short collecting tubules join to form several larger **collecting ducts**. As the collecting ducts become larger and descend further toward the papillae of the medulla, they are called papillary ducts. Smaller collecting ducts are lined with a cuboidal epithelium. Deeper in the medulla, the epithelium changes to columnar. At the tip of each papilla, the papillary ducts empty their contents into the minor calyx. The area on the papilla that exhibits openings of the numerous papillary ducts is the **area cribrosa**.

The kidney cortex also exhibits numerous, lighter-staining **medullary rays** that extend vertically from the bases of the pyramids into the cortex. Medullary rays consist of collecting ducts, blood vessels, and straight portions of a number of nephrons that penetrate the cortex from the base of the pyramids.

RENAL BLOOD SUPPLY

To understand the functional correlation of the kidney, it is important to understand the blood supply (see Fig. 18.1). Each kidney is supplied by a large **renal artery** that divides in the hilum into several segmental branches, which branch into several **interlobar arteries**. These arteries continue in the kidney between the pyramids toward the cortex. At the corticomedullary junction, the interlobar arteries branch into **arcuate arteries** that arch over the base of the pyramids and give rise to **interlobular arteries**. These arteries branch further into the **afferent arterioles**, which give rise to the **capillaries** in the **glomeruli** of renal corpuscles. **Efferent arterioles** leave the renal corpuscles and form a complex **peritubular capillary network** around the tubules in the cortex and long, straight capillary vessels, or **vasa recta**, in the medulla that loops back to the corticomedullary region. The vasa recta form loops that are parallel to the long loops of Henle that contain the urinary filtrate. The interstitium around these tubules and blood vessels is drained by interlobular veins that continue toward the arcuate veins.

the**Point** Supplemental micrographic images are available at **www.thePoint.com/Eroschenko13e** under Urinary System.

FIGURE 18.3 | Kidney: Cortex, Medulla, Pyramid, Renal Papilla, and Minor Calyx (Panoramic View)

In this sagittal section, the kidney exhibits an outer darker-staining **cortex** and an inner lighter-staining **medulla**. Externally, the cortex is covered with a dense irregular connective tissue **renal capsule** (1).

The cortex contains both distal and **proximal convoluted tubules** (4, 11), **glomeruli** (2), and **medullary rays** (3). Present also in the cortex are the **interlobular arteries** (12) and **interlobular veins** (13). The medullary rays (3) are formed by the straight portions of nephrons, blood vessels, and collecting tubules that join in the medulla to form the larger **collecting ducts** (6). The medullary rays do not extend to the kidney capsule (1) because of the **subcapsular convoluted tubules** (10).

The medulla comprises the renal pyramids. The **base** of each **pyramid** (5) is adjacent to the cortex, and its apex forms the pointed **renal papilla** (7) that projects into the surrounding

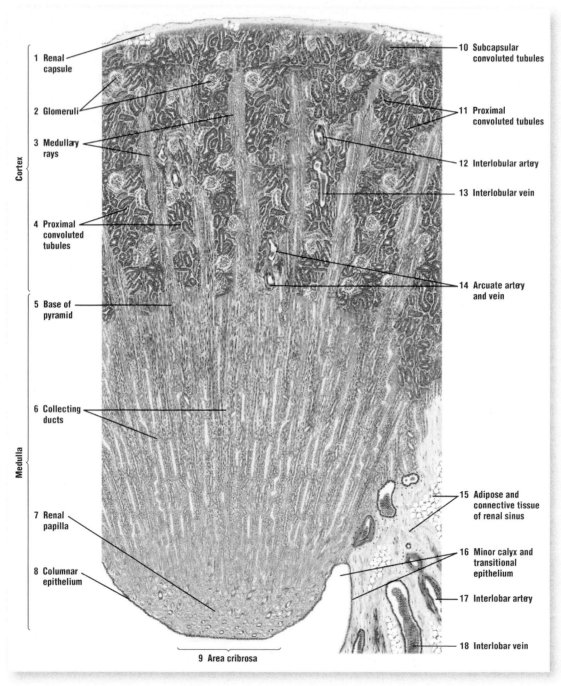

FIGURE 18.3 ■ Kidney: cortex, medulla, pyramid, renal papilla, and minor calyx (panoramic view). Stain: hematoxylin and eosin. Low magnification.

funnel-like structure, the **minor calyx (16)**, which represents the dilated portion of the ureter. The **area cribrosa (9)** is pierced by small holes, which represent the openings of the collecting ducts (6) into the minor calyx (16).

The tip of the renal papilla (7) is usually covered with a simple **columnar epithelium (8)**. As the columnar epithelium of the renal papilla (7) extends onto the outer wall of the minor calyx (16), it becomes a **transitional epithelium (16)**. A thin layer of connective tissue and smooth muscle (not illustrated) under this epithelium then merges with the connective tissue of the **renal sinus (15)**.

Present in the renal sinus (15) are branches of the renal artery and vein called the **interlobar artery (17)** and the **interlobar vein (18)**. The interlobar vessels (17, 18) enter the kidney and arch over the base of the pyramid (5) at the corticomedullary junction as the **arcuate artery and vein (14)**. The arcuate vessels (14) give rise to smaller interlobular arteries (12) and interlobular veins (13) that pass radially into the kidney cortex and give rise to the afferent glomerular arteries that give rise to the capillaries of the glomeruli (3).

FIGURE 18.4 | Kidney Cortex and Upper Medulla

A higher magnification of the kidney shows greater detail of the cortex. The **renal corpuscles (5, 9)** consist of a **glomerulus (5a)** and the **glomerular (Bowman) capsule (5b)**. The glomerulus (5a) is a tuft of capillaries formed from the afferent **glomerular arteriole (11)**, is supported by fine connective tissue, and is surrounded by the glomerular capsule (5b).

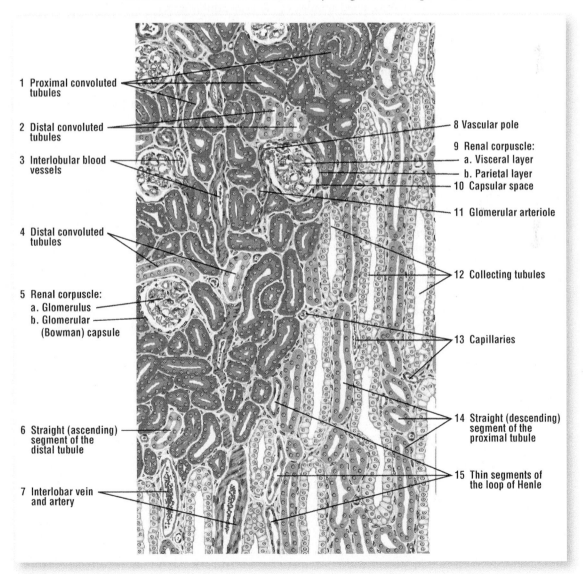

1 Proximal convoluted tubules

2 Distal convoluted tubules

3 Interlobular blood vessels

4 Distal convoluted tubules

5 Renal corpuscle:
   a. Glomerulus
   b. Glomerular (Bowman) capsule

6 Straight (ascending) segment of the distal tubule

7 Interlobar vein and artery

8 Vascular pole

9 Renal corpuscle:
   a. Visceral layer
   b. Parietal layer

10 Capsular space

11 Glomerular arteriole

12 Collecting tubules

13 Capillaries

14 Straight (descending) segment of the proximal tubule

15 Thin segments of the loop of Henle

FIGURE 18.4 ■ Kidney cortex and upper medulla. Stain: hematoxylin and eosin. Low magnification.

The internal or **visceral layer (9a)** of the glomerular capsule (5b) surrounds the glomerular capillaries with modified epithelial cells called **podocytes (9a)**. At the **vascular pole (8)** of the renal corpuscle (9), the epithelium of the visceral layer (9a) turns back to form the simple squamous parietal layer (9b) of the glomerular capsule (5b). The space between the visceral layer (9a) and the **parietal layer (9b)** of the renal corpuscle (9) is the **capsular space (10)**.

Two types of convoluted tubules, sectioned in various planes, surround the renal corpuscles (5, 9). These are the **proximal convoluted tubules (1)** and **distal convoluted tubules (2, 4)**. The convoluted tubules are the initial and terminal segments of the nephron. The proximal convoluted tubules (1) are longer than the distal convoluted tubules (2, 4) and are, therefore, more numerous in the cortex. The proximal convoluted tubules (1) exhibit a small, uneven lumen and a single layer of cuboidal cells with eosinophilic granular cytoplasm. A brush border (microvilli) lines the cells but is not always well preserved in the sections. Also, the cell boundaries in the proximal convoluted tubules (1) are not distinct because of the extensive basal and lateral cell membrane interdigitations with the neighboring cells.

The urinary capsular space (10) in the renal corpuscle (5, 9) is continuous with the lumen of the proximal convoluted tubule at the urinary pole (see Fig. 18.5). At the urinary pole, the squamous epithelium of the parietal layer (9b) of the glomerular capsule (5b) changes to the cuboidal epithelium of the proximal convoluted tubule (1).

The distal convoluted tubules (2, 4) are shorter and are fewer in number in the cortex. The distal convoluted tubules (2, 4) also exhibit larger lumina with smaller cuboidal cells. The cytoplasm stains less intensely than that in the proximal convoluted tubules (1), and the brush border is not present on the cells. Similar to the proximal convoluted tubules (1), the distal convoluted tubules (2, 4) show deep basal and lateral cell membrane infoldings and interdigitations.

Also seen in the cortex are the medullary rays. The medullary rays include the following three types of tubules: **straight (descending) segments of the proximal tubules (14)**, **straight (ascending) segments of the distal tubules (6)**, and **collecting tubules (12)**. The straight (descending) segments of the proximal tubules (14) are very similar to the proximal convoluted tubules (1), and the straight (ascending) segments of the distal tubules (6) are similar to distal convoluted tubules (2, 4). The collecting tubules (12) in the cortex are distinct because of their lightly stained cuboidal cells and distinct cell membranes.

The medulla contains only straight portions of the tubules and the segments of the loop of Henle (thick and thin descending segments and thin and thick ascending segments). The **thin segments of the loops of Henle (15)** are lined with a simple squamous epithelium and resemble the **capillaries (13)**. The distinguishing features of the thin loops of Henle (15) are the thicker epithelial lining and the absence of blood cells in their lumina. In contrast, most capillaries (13) have blood cells in the lumina.

Also visible in the cortex are the **interlobular blood vessels (3)** and the **larger interlobar vein and artery (7)**. The interlobular blood vessels (3) give rise to the afferent glomerular arteriole (11) that enters the glomerular capsule (5b) at the vascular pole (8) and forms the capillary tuft of the glomerulus (5a).

FUNCTIONAL CORRELATIONS 18.1 ■ Kidney Cells and Kidney Tubules

MESANGIAL CELLS

In addition to podocytes around the capillaries, there are other specialized cells in the glomerulus called **mesangial cells**. These cells are also attached to the capillaries and perform several important functions. Mesangial cells synthesize the extracellular matrix and provide structural support for the glomerular capillaries. As the blood is filtered through the glomerular capillaries, numerous proteinaceous macromolecules are trapped in the glomerular basement membrane and filtration slit diaphragms. Mesangial cells function as **macrophages** in the intraglomerular regions by removing the trapped material from filtration slits and glomerular basal membrane, thus preventing its clogging and keeping the glomerular filter free of debris. They also phagocytose antigen–antibody complexes and produce several interleukins in response to glomerular injury or damage. Mesangial cells are also contractile and regulate glomerular blood flow and pressure changes in the vascular pole region, between the afferent and efferent arterioles. Here, they are called the **extraglomerular mesangial cells**, also called lacis cells, and form part of the juxtaglomerular apparatus.

KIDNEY CELLS

The kidneys maintain body' s stable internal environment, or **homeostasis**. This function is performed by regulating the body's blood pressure; blood composition; and pH, fluid volume, and acid–base balance. The kidneys also produce urine, which is formed by three main functions: (1) **filtration** of blood in the glomeruli, (2) **reabsorption** of nutrients and other valuable substances from the ultrafiltrate that enters the proximal and distal convoluted tubules, and (3) **secretion**, or **excretion**, of metabolic waste products or unwanted chemicals or substances into the filtrate that become urine. Approximately 99% of the glomerular ultrafiltrate produced by the kidneys is reabsorbed into the system; the remaining 1% of the filtrate is voided as urine.

In addition, kidneys have endocrine functions by producing hormones **erythropoietin** and **renin**. Endothelial cells of the peritubular capillary network in the renal cortex produce the glycoprotein hormone erythropoietin, which is a growth factor that stimulates erythrocyte production in red bone marrow in response to **hypoxia**, a decrease in oxygen concentration in blood or tissues. Renin is produced by kidney cells to regulate blood pressure and to maintain proper filtration pressure in the glomeruli.

KIDNEY TUBULES

Proximal Convoluted Tubules

All nephrons participate in the formation of urine. As the ultrafiltrate from nephrons passes through the uriniferous and collecting tubules of the kidneys, it undergoes significant changes in its content and volume producing concentrated urine, containing metabolic waste products. The cells of the proximal convoluted tubules show deep **infoldings** of the basal cell membrane, between which are located elongated mitochondria and lateral membrane **interdigitations** with neighboring cells. These features are characteristic of cells involved in active transport of molecules and electrolytes from the filtrate across the cell membrane into the interstitium. The mitochondria supply the necessary ATP (energy) for active transport of sodium by **Na$^+$/K$^+$ ATPase** (sodium pump) that is located in the basolateral regions of the cell membrane.

Reabsorption that is both active and passive of most of the substances from the glomerular filtrate takes place in the proximal convoluted tubules, which receive the glomerular ultrafiltrate from the capsular (urinary) space of the Bowman capsule. As the glomerular filtrate enters the proximal convoluted tubules, all **glucose**, **proteins**, and **amino acids**; almost all carbohydrates; and about 75% to 85% of water and sodium chloride ions are absorbed from the glomerular filtrate into the surrounding interstitium and **peritubular capillaries**. The presence of long and closely spaced **microvilli** (brush border) on proximal convoluted tubule cells greatly increases the surface area and facilitates absorption of the filtered material. In addition, the proximal convoluted tubules secrete certain metabolites, hydrogen, ammonia, dyes, and drugs such as penicillin from the body into the glomerular filtrate. The metabolic waste products urea and uric acid remain in the filtrate of the proximal convoluted tubules and are eliminated from the body in the urine.

Loops of Henle

The descending and ascending **loops of Henle** of the juxtaglomerular nephrons are long, extend deep into the medulla, and have different permeabilities and different functions. As a result, **hypertonic**

(continued)

urine is produced in the tubules by an osmotic gradient in the surrounding interstitium from the cortex of the kidney to the tips of the renal papillae. Sodium chloride and urea are transported and concentrated in the interstitial tissue of the kidney medulla by means of a complex **countercurrent multiplier system**, which creates a high interstitial osmolarity deep in the medulla. The descending loop of Henle is permeable to water but much less to sodium chloride, whereas the thin ascending limb is permeable to sodium chloride but not to water. The hypertonicity (high osmotic pressure) of the extracellular fluid in the medulla interstitium removes water from the glomerular filtrate as it flows through the descending thin tubules, thereby increasing its sodium and chloride concentration. In the ascending thin limb, water remains behind, whereas sodium chloride leaves the fluid and is concentrated in the interstitium. The countercurrent flow of ultrafiltrate in the descending and ascending thin loops of Henle produces a gradient of osmolarity in the interstitium of the medulla. The water that enters the interstitium is then removed by the countercurrent blood flow in the capillary loops of the **vasa recta**, thus maintaining the osmotic concentration gradient in the medulla, resulting in water conservation and urine concentration. These capillary loops are permeable to water and take up the water from the medullary interstitium to return it to the systemic circulation.

Distal Convoluted Tubules

The **distal convoluted tubules** are shorter, less convoluted than the proximal tubules, and less frequently observed in the cortex and near the renal corpuscles. In comparison with the proximal convoluted tubules, the distal convoluted tubules do not exhibit brush borders, the cells are smaller, and more nuclei are seen per tubule. The basolateral membranes of distal convoluted tubule cells also show increased cell membrane interdigitations and elongated mitochondria within these infoldings. The distal convoluted tubules actively **reabsorb sodium** ions from the tubular filtrate and excrete hydrogen, potassium, and ammonium ions into the tubular fluid. The **excretion** of hydrogen ions is connected with the absorption of bicarbonate ions and increasing the acidification of urine.

Sodium reabsorption in the distal convoluted tubules is controlled by the hormone **aldosterone** secreted by the adrenal cortex. Aldosterone hormone induces cells of the distal convoluted tubules to actively absorb sodium and chloride ions from the filtrate and transport them into the interstitium. From the interstitium, sodium chloride ions are quickly absorbed by the **peritubular capillaries** and returned back to the systemic circulation, thereby decreasing sodium loss in urine. These functions of the distal convoluted tubules are vital for maintaining the proper acid–base balance of body fluids and blood.

FIGURE 18.5 | Kidney Cortex: Juxtaglomerular Apparatus

A higher magnification of the kidney cortex illustrates the renal corpuscle, the surrounding convoluted tubules, and the juxtaglomerular apparatus.

In the middle is the renal corpuscle with **glomerular capillaries** (5), **parietal** (8a) and **visceral** (8b) **layers** (epithelium) of the **glomerular** (**Bowman**) **capsule** (8), and the **capsular space** (10) around the glomerulus. Surrounding the renal corpuscle are the **proximal convoluted tubules** (7) with brush borders and acidophilic cells. These tubules are distinguished from the **distal convoluted tubules** (1, 6) that exhibit smaller and less intensely stained cells that lack the brush borders. In contrast to the convoluted tubules, the cuboidal cells of the **collecting tubule** (11) exhibit pale cytoplasm and distinct cell outlines. **Basement membrane** (12) surrounds the collecting tubules (11).

Each renal corpuscle exhibits a vascular pole where the afferent **glomerular arteriole** (4) enters and the efferent glomerular arteriole exits the renal corpuscle. Inside the renal corpuscle, the glomerular arteriole forms a network of glomerular capillaries (5). On the opposite side of the vascular pole is the **urinary pole** (9). Here, the capsular space (10) becomes continuous with the lumen of the proximal convoluted tubule (7). The plane of section through both the vascular and urinary poles is only occasionally seen in the kidney cortex. This illustration shows the glomerular arteriole (4) on one end and the urinary pole (9) at the opposite end of the renal corpuscle.

At the vascular pole, modified epithelioid cells with cytoplasmic granules replace the smooth muscle cells in the tunica media of the afferent glomerular arteriole (4). These cells are the juxtaglomerular cells (3). In the adjacent distal convoluted tubule, the cells next to the **juxtaglomerular cells** (3) are narrow and more columnar and exhibit a more compact cell arrangement. This region in the distal convoluted tubule is called the macula densa (2). The juxtaglomerular cells (3) in the afferent glomerular arteriole (4) and the **macula densa** (2) cells in the distal convoluted tubule form the juxtaglomerular apparatus.

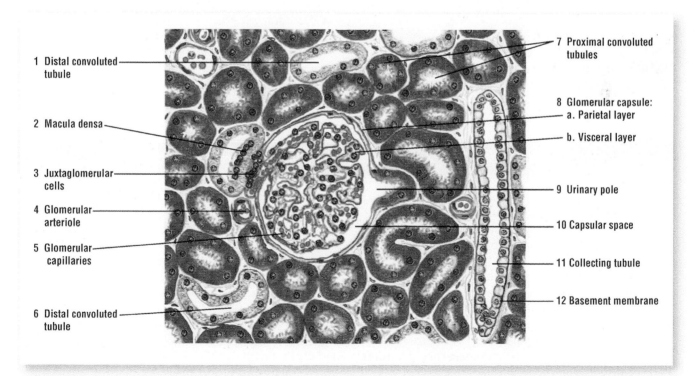

1 Distal convoluted tubule
2 Macula densa
3 Juxtaglomerular cells
4 Glomerular arteriole
5 Glomerular capillaries
6 Distal convoluted tubule
7 Proximal convoluted tubules
8 Glomerular capsule:
  a. Parietal layer
  b. Visceral layer
9 Urinary pole
10 Capsular space
11 Collecting tubule
12 Basement membrane

FIGURE 18.5 ■ Kidney cortex: juxtaglomerular apparatus. Stain: hematoxylin and eosin. Medium magnification.

FIGURE 18.6 | **Kidney: Renal Corpuscle, Juxtaglomerular Apparatus, and Convoluted Tubules**

This high-magnification photomicrograph shows a renal corpuscle with surrounding tubules. The renal corpuscle consists of the **glomerulus** (1) and the **glomerular capsule** (2) with a **parietal layer** (2a) and a **visceral layer** (2b). Between these layers is the **capsular space** (5), with **podocytes** (4, 7) located on the surface of the visceral layer (2b). At the vascular pole of the renal corpuscle, blood vessels enter and leave the renal corpuscle. Adjacent to the vascular pole is the **juxtaglomerular apparatus** (3). The juxtaglomerular apparatus (3) consists of modified smooth muscle cells of the afferent arteriole in the vascular pole, the **juxtaglomerular cells** (3a), and the **macula densa** (3b) of the **distal convoluted tubule** (6, 9). Surrounding the renal corpuscle are the darker-staining **proximal convoluted tubules** (8) and the distal convoluted tubules (6, 9).

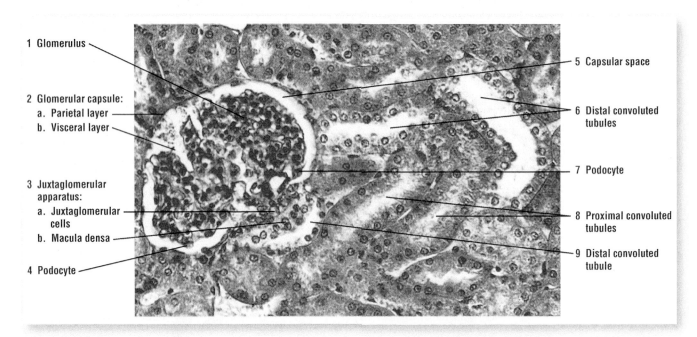

1 Glomerulus

2 Glomerular capsule:
  a. Parietal layer
  b. Visceral layer

3 Juxtaglomerular apparatus:
  a. Juxtaglomerular cells
  b. Macula densa

4 Podocyte

5 Capsular space

6 Distal convoluted tubules

7 Podocyte

8 Proximal convoluted tubules

9 Distal convoluted tubule

FIGURE 18.6 ■ Kidney cortex: renal corpuscle, juxtaglomerular apparatus, and convoluted tubules. Stain: hematoxylin and eosin. ×130.

FUNCTIONAL CORRELATIONS 18.2 ■ Juxtaglomerular Apparatus

Adjacent to the renal corpuscles and distal convoluted tubules lies the **juxtaglomerular apparatus** consisting of three components: the juxtaglomerular cells, the macula densa, and the extraglomerular mesangial cells (or lacis cells).

Juxtaglomerular cells are modified **smooth muscle cells** located in the wall of the **afferent arteriole** of the vascular pole of the renal corpuscle before it penetrates the glomerular capsule to form the glomerulus. The cytoplasm of juxtaglomerular cells contains membrane-bound **secretory granules** of the enzyme **renin**, which is synthesized, stored, and released into the bloodstream when needed. Opposite the afferent arteriole is the **macula densa**,

a group of modified distal convoluted tubule cells that form a dense cluster. The macula densa cells and juxtaglomerular cells are close to each other and are separated only by a thin basement membrane allowing the juxtaglomerular cells and the macula densa closer integration of their functions.

The main function of the juxtaglomerular apparatus is to maintain the necessary blood pressure, blood flow, and proper glomerular filtration in the kidney. The cells of this apparatus act as both baroreceptors and chemoreceptors. The juxtaglomerular cells monitor the **systemic blood pressure** by responding to stretching in the walls of the afferent arterioles. The cells in the macula densa monitor **sodium chloride**

FUNCTIONAL CORRELATIONS 18.2 ■ Juxtaglomerular Apparatus (*Continued*)

concentrations in the tubular fluid. A decrease in the blood pressure results in a decreased glomerular filtrate and decreased sodium ion concentration in the filtrate as it flows past the macula densa.

A decrease in systemic blood pressure or in sodium concentration in the filtrate induces the juxtaglomerular cells to release the enzyme renin into the bloodstream. Renin, in turn, converts the blood plasma protein **angiotensinogen** to **angiotensin I**, which, in turn, is converted to **angiotensin II** by angiotensin-converting enzyme located in the **endothelial cells** of lung capillaries. Angiotensin II is an active hormone and a powerful **vasoconstrictor** that initially produces arterial constriction, thereby increasing the systemic blood pressure. In addition,

angiotensin II stimulates the release of the hormone **aldosterone** from the zona glomerulosa of the adrenal gland cortex.

Aldosterone influences some cells of distal convoluted tubules, but mainly the cells of the collecting ducts to increase their reabsorption of sodium and chloride ions from the glomerular filtrate. Water follows sodium chloride by osmosis and increases fluid volume in the circulatory system raising the systemic blood pressure, increasing glomerular filtration rate, and decreasing the secretion of renin by juxtaglomerular cells. Aldosterone also facilitates the elimination of potassium and hydrogen ions and is an essential hormone for maintaining electrolyte balance in the body.

FIGURE 18.7 | **Ultrastructure of Cells in Proximal Convoluted Tubule of Kidney**

This medium-power ultrastructure image shows cells of the proximal convoluted tubules in the kidney. The very long and closely packed **microvilli** (1) that line the apices are recognized as the brush border in the light microscopic images. The apices also exhibit a number of clear **pinocytotic vesicles** (6) and dense-staining **lysosomes** (2, 5). Note that the cytoplasm of these cells is packed with **mitochondria** (4, 7) that provide the energy to transport the nutrients from the ultrafiltrate. In the center of these cells is a **nucleus** (3).

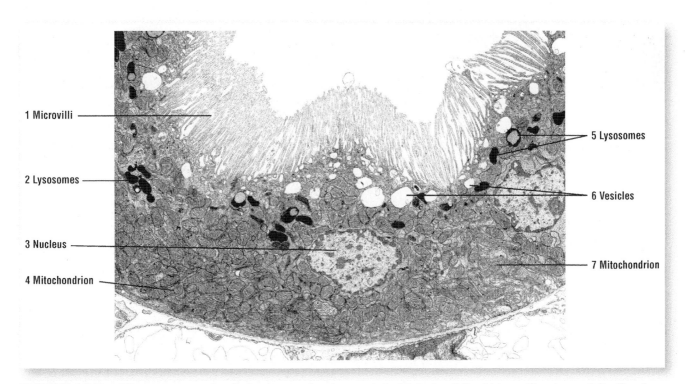

1 Microvilli
2 Lysosomes
3 Nucleus
4 Mitochondrion
5 Lysosomes
6 Vesicles
7 Mitochondrion

FIGURE 18.7 ■ Ultrastructure of cells in the proximal convoluted tubule of the kidney. Courtesy of Dr. Rex A. Hess, Professor Emeritus, Comparative Biosciences, College of Veterinary Medicine, University of Illinois, Urbana, IL. ×55,000.

FIGURE 18.8 | Ultrastructure of Apical Cell Surface in Proximal Convoluted Tubule of Kidney

This high-power ultrastructure image shows the apical cell surface of the proximal convoluted tubules of the kidney. The long and closely packed **microvilli** (**1, 6**) of the brush border extend into the lumen. In the cytoplasm are also clear **pinocytotic vesicles** (**2, 7**). A tight **junctional complex** (**3**) is visible as a dark strip near the base of the microvilli or the apical region of the cell. However, individual cell boundaries in the proximal tubules are not seen because of the complex interdigitations of the lateral cell walls. Also visible in the apical cytoplasm are numerous dense-staining **lysosomes** (**4, 8**), which will break down the substances that are brought into the cytoplasm by the pinocytotic vesicles (2, 7). The apical cytoplasm also exhibits numerous **mitochondria** (**5**) and a section of the **nucleus** (**9**).

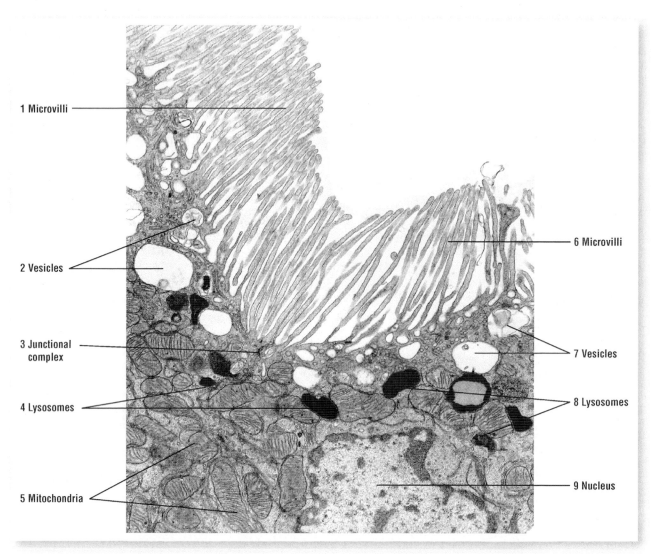

FIGURE 18.8 ■ Ultrastructure of the apical cell surface in the proximal convoluted tubule of the kidney. Courtesy of Dr. Rex A. Hess, Professor Emeritus, Comparative Biosciences, College of Veterinary Medicine, University of Illinois, Urbana, IL. ×8,000.

FIGURE 18.9 | Kidney: Scanning Electron Micrograph of Podocytes

This scanning electron micrograph illustrates the unique appearance of the visceral epithelium of the glomerular capsule and the podocytes, which surround all the capillaries in the kidney glomeruli. The flattened **cell body** of the **podocyte (6)** extends thicker **primary processes (1, 3)** that surround the capillary walls. The primary processes (1, 3) give rise to the smaller **pedicles (2, 7)**, which interdigitate with pedicles from other podocytes around the capillaries. Between the pedicles (2, 6) are the tiny **filtration slits (5)**. Also visible are remnants of **proteinaceous debris (4)** that became lodged in the filtration slits (5) during blood filtration. Surrounding the podocytes in the renal corpuscle is the dark-appearing capsular space that would contain the glomerular filtrate in a functioning kidney.

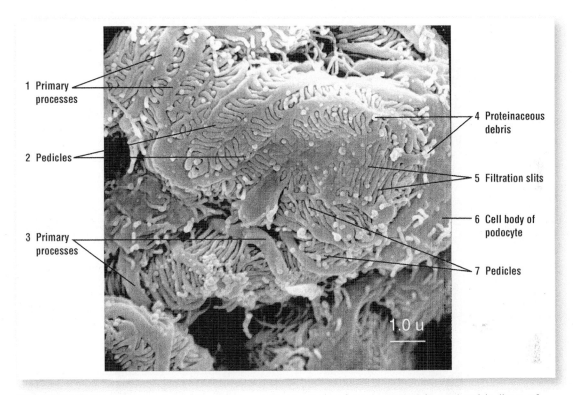

FIGURE 18.9 ■ Kidney: scanning electron micrograph of podocytes (visceral epithelium of the glomerular [Bowman] capsule) surrounding the glomerular capillaries.

FIGURE 18.10 | Kidney: Transmission Electron Micrograph of Podocyte and Glomerular Capillary

This transmission electron micrograph shows the association of a podocyte with glomerular capillaries in the renal corpuscle of kidney. The **nucleus** (3) and **cytoplasm** of the **podocyte** (**11**) are separated from the adjacent **basement membrane** of the **capillary** (**13**). The larger **primary process** of the **podocyte** (**12**) extends from the podocyte cytoplasm (11) to surround the wall of the capillary. The smaller **pedicles** (**2, 5**) from the primary process of the podocyte (12) are attached to the basement membrane of the capillary (13). Between the individual pedicles (2, 5) are the **filtration slits** (**1**). Separating the podocyte (3, 11) from the capillaries and adjacent podocytes is the clear **capsular space** (**4**). In the **lumen of the capillary** (**6, 8**) are the **nucleus of an endothelial cell** (**10**) and sections of an **erythrocyte** (**7**) and a **leukocyte** (**9**). In the lumen of the capillary (6, 8) are also visible tiny **fenestrations** in the endothelium (*arrowheads*).

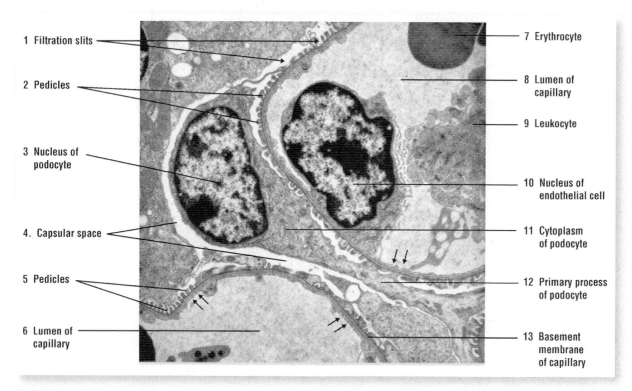

1 Filtration slits

2 Pedicles

3 Nucleus of podocyte

4. Capsular space

5 Pedicles

6 Lumen of capillary

7 Erythrocyte

8 Lumen of capillary

9 Leukocyte

10 Nucleus of endothelial cell

11 Cytoplasm of podocyte

12 Primary process of podocyte

13 Basement membrane of capillary

FIGURE 18.10 ■ Kidney: transmission electron micrograph of a podocyte and adjacent capillaries in the renal corpuscle. ×6,500.

FIGURE 18.11 | **Kidney Medulla: Papillary Region (Transverse Section)**

The papilla in the kidney faces the minor calyx and contains the terminal portions of the collecting tubules, now called the **papillary ducts (3)**. The papillary ducts (3) exhibit large diameters and wide lumina and are lined with tall, pale-staining columnar cells. Also present in the papilla are the **straight (ascending) segments of the distal tubules (7, 10)** and the **straight (descending) segments of the proximal tubules (1, 6, 11)**. The straight segments in the medulla are very similar to the convoluted tubules in the cortex. Interspersed among the ascending (7, 10) and descending straight tubules (1, 6, 11) are the transverse sections of the **thin segments of the loop of Henle (5, 8)** that resemble the **capillaries (4, 9)** or small **venules (2)**. The capillaries (4, 9) and the small venules (2) differ from the thin segments of the loop of Henle (5, 8) by thinner walls and by blood cells in their lumina.

The **connective tissue (12)** surrounding the tubules is more abundant in the papillary region of the kidney, and the papillary ducts (3) are spaced further apart.

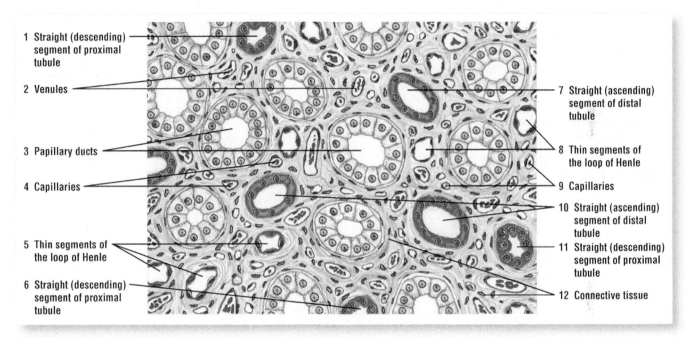

1 Straight (descending) segment of proximal tubule

2 Venules

3 Papillary ducts

4 Capillaries

5 Thin segments of the loop of Henle

6 Straight (descending) segment of proximal tubule

7 Straight (ascending) segment of distal tubule

8 Thin segments of the loop of Henle

9 Capillaries

10 Straight (ascending) segment of distal tubule

11 Straight (descending) segment of proximal tubule

12 Connective tissue

FIGURE 18.11 ■ Kidney medulla: papillary region (transverse section). Stain: hematoxylin and eosin. Medium magnification.

FIGURE 18.12 | **Kidney Medulla: Terminal End of Papilla (Longitudinal Section)**

Collecting ducts merge in the papilla of the kidney medulla to form large **papillary ducts** (6), which are lined with a simple cuboidal or columnar epithelium. Openings of the papillary ducts (6) at the tip of the papilla produce a sievelike appearance called the area cribrosa. The contents from the papillary ducts (6) continue into the minor calyx that is adjacent to and surrounds the tip of each papilla.

In this illustration, the papilla tip is lined with a stratified **covering epithelium** (7). At the area cribrosa, the covering epithelium (7) is usually a tall simple columnar type that is continuous with the papillary ducts (6).

Thin segments of the loops of Henle (3, 5) descending deep into the papilla are identifiable as thin ducts with empty lumina. **Venules** (1) and the **capillaries** (4) of the vasa recta are identified by blood cells in their lumina. Surrounding the blood vessels (1, 4) and the papillary ducts (6) is the **renal interstitium** (**connective tissue**) (2).

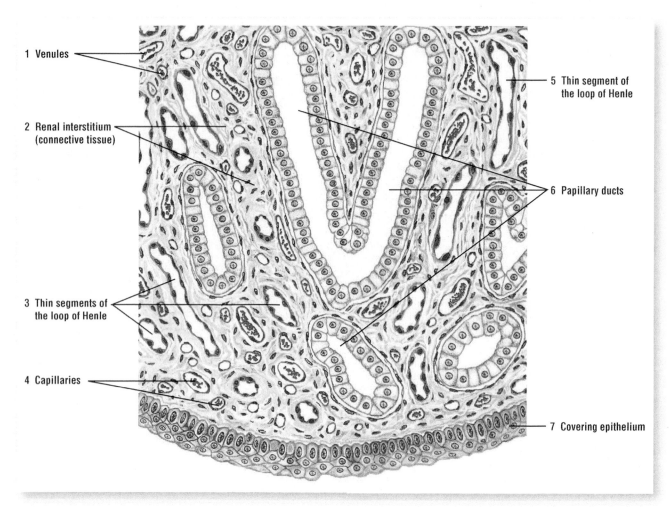

1 Venules

2 Renal interstitium (connective tissue)

3 Thin segments of the loop of Henle

4 Capillaries

5 Thin segment of the loop of Henle

6 Papillary ducts

7 Covering epithelium

FIGURE 18.12 ■ Kidney medulla: terminal end of a papilla (longitudinal section). Stain: hematoxylin and eosin. Medium magnification.

FUNCTIONAL CORRELATIONS 18.3 ■ **Collecting Tubules, Collecting Ducts, and Antidiuretic Hormone**

Glomerular filtrate flows from the distal convoluted tubules to the **collecting tubules** and collecting ducts. Under normal conditions, these tubules are not permeable to water, and the urine remains dilute or hypotonic. However, during excessive water loss or dehydration, **antidiuretic hormone** (**ADH**) is released from the posterior lobe (neurohypophysis) of the **pituitary gland**. The ADH induces the epithelium of collecting tubules and collecting ducts to become highly permeable to water passage. The water-permeable cells in the collecting ducts contain integral transmembrane pore proteins called **aquaporins** that function as channels for water molecules. Aquaporins, also known as water channels, increase water permeability and selectively conduct water molecules in and out of the cells. The functions of aquaporins

are regulated by the ADH that binds to the receptors on the duct cells and activates aquaporins, resulting in increased water absorption from the filtrate. As a result, water freely leaves the filtrate in the collecting ducts and enters the hypertonic interstitium established by the thin loops of Henle and the surrounding capillary network, the vasa recta. Water in the interstitium is then collected or absorbed and returned to the general circulation via the peritubular capillaries and vasa recta, and the glomerular filtrate in the collecting ducts becomes hypertonic (concentrated) urine.

In the absence of ADH, the cells of the collecting tubules and ducts remain impermeable to water. Consequently, increased amount of water remains in the glomerular filtrate of the collecting ducts, resulting in dilute urine.

FIGURE 18.13 | **Kidney: Ducts of Medullary Region (Longitudinal Section)**

The medullary region of the kidney consists of various sized tubules, larger ducts, and blood vessels of the vasa recta. In this photomicrograph, different kidney tubules and blood vessels have been sectioned in a longitudinal plane. The tubules with large, light-staining cuboidal cells are the **collecting tubules** (**1**). Adjacent to the collecting tubules (1) are tubules with darker-staining cuboidal cells. These are the **thick segments of the loop of Henle** (**2**). Between the tubules are blood vessels of the **vasa recta** (**4**) and the **thin segments of the loop of Henle** (**3**). Blood vessels of the vasa recta (4) can be distinguished from the thin segments of the loop of Henle (3) by the presence of blood cells in their lumina.

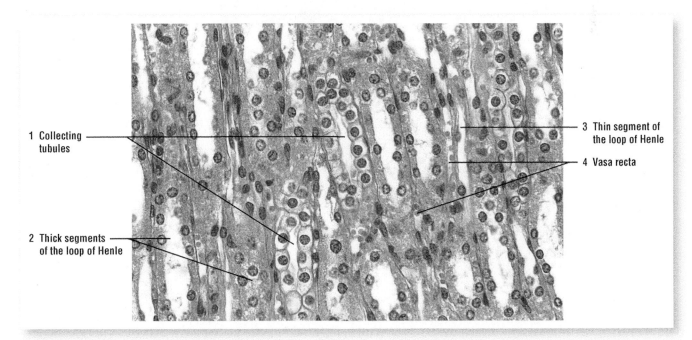

1 Collecting tubules

2 Thick segments of the loop of Henle

3 Thin segment of the loop of Henle

4 Vasa recta

FIGURE 18.13 ■ Kidney: ducts of the medullary region (longitudinal section). Stain: hematoxylin and eosin. ×130.

FIGURE 18.14 | Urinary System: Ureter (Transverse Section)

An undistended **lumen of the ureter** (4) exhibits longitudinal mucosal folds formed by the muscular contractions. The wall of the ureter consists of mucosa, muscularis, and adventitia.

The ureter mucosa consists of **transitional epithelium** (7) and a wide **lamina propria** (5). The transitional epithelium has several cell layers, the outermost layer characterized by large cuboidal cells. The intermediate cells are polyhedral in shape, whereas the basal cells are low columnar or cuboidal.

The lamina propria (5) contains fibroelastic connective tissue that is denser with more fibroblasts under the epithelium and looser near the muscularis. Diffuse lymphatic tissue and small lymphatic nodules may be observed in the lamina propria.

In the upper ureter, the muscularis consists of two muscle layers: an inner **longitudinal smooth muscle layer** (3) and a middle **circular smooth muscle layer** (2); these layers are not always distinct. An additional third outer longitudinal layer of smooth muscle is found in the lower third of the ureter near the bladder.

The **adventitia** (9) blends with the surrounding fibroelastic connective tissue and **adipose tissue** (1, 10), which contains numerous **arterioles** (6), **venules** (8), and small nerves.

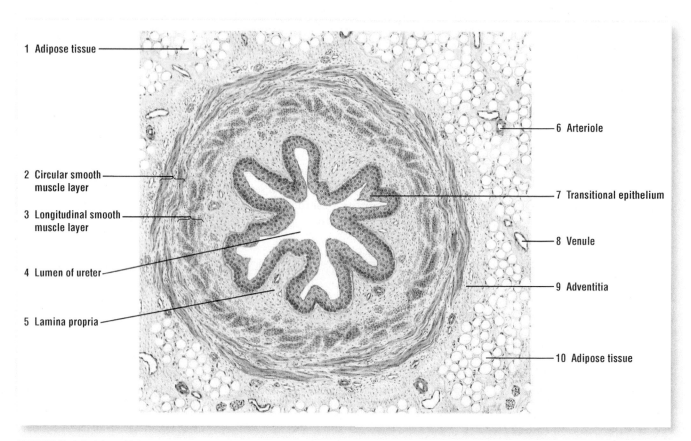

1 Adipose tissue

2 Circular smooth muscle layer

3 Longitudinal smooth muscle layer

4 Lumen of ureter

5 Lamina propria

6 Arteriole

7 Transitional epithelium

8 Venule

9 Adventitia

10 Adipose tissue

FIGURE 18.14 ■ Urinary system: ureter (transverse section). Stain: hematoxylin and eosin. Low magnification.

FIGURE 18.15 | **Section of Ureter Wall (Transverse Section)**

This illustration shows a higher magnification of a ureter wall. The **transitional epithelium** (7) in an undistended ureter shows numerous **mucosal folds** (6). The superficial cells of the transitional epithelium (7) have a special **surface membrane** (5) that serves as an osmotic barrier between the urine and the underlying tissue. A thin basement membrane separates the epithelium from the loose **lamina propria** (9).

The **muscularis** (2, 8) appears as loosely arranged smooth muscle bundles surrounded by connective tissue. The upper ureter has an inner **longitudinal smooth muscle layer** (8) and a middle **circular smooth muscle layer** (2). A third longitudinal smooth muscle layer is found in the lower third of the ureter.

The **adventitia** (4) with **adipose cells** (3) merges with the connective tissue of the posterior abdominal wall to which the ureter is attached.

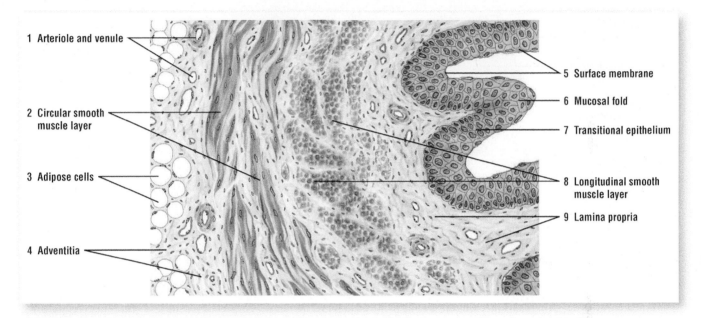

1 Arteriole and venule

2 Circular smooth muscle layer

3 Adipose cells

4 Adventitia

5 Surface membrane

6 Mucosal fold

7 Transitional epithelium

8 Longitudinal smooth muscle layer

9 Lamina propria

FIGURE 18.15 ■ Section of a ureter wall (transverse section). Stain: hematoxylin and eosin. Medium magnification.

FIGURE 18.16 | Ureter (Transverse Section)

The ureter conveys urine from the kidneys to the bladder by the contractions of the thick, smooth muscle layers in its wall. This low-magnification photomicrograph shows a ureter in transverse section. The mucosa is highly folded and lined with a thick **transitional epithelium** (1) below which is the **lamina propria** (2). The muscularis exhibits an **inner longitudinal layer** (3) and a **middle circular muscle layer** (4). A third outer longitudinal layer (not shown) is added to the wall in the lower third of the ureter, near the bladder. A connective tissue **adventitia** (6), with **blood vessels** (5) and **adipose tissue** (7), surrounds the ureter.

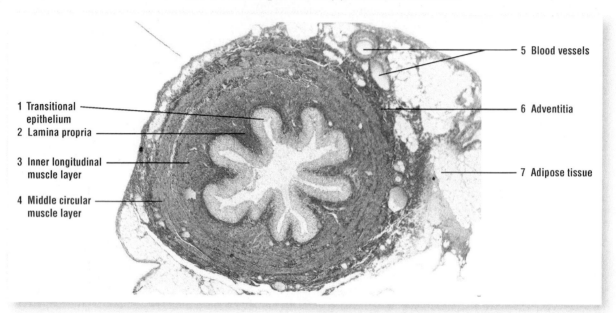

FIGURE 18.16 ■ Ureter (transverse section). Stain: iron hematoxylin and Alcian blue. ×10.

FIGURE 18.17 | Urinary Bladder: Wall (Transverse Section)

The bladder has a thick muscular wall that is similar to that of the lower third of the ureter. In the wall are found three loosely arranged layers of smooth muscle, the inner longitudinal, middle circular, and the outer longitudinal layers. However, as in the ureter, the distinct muscle

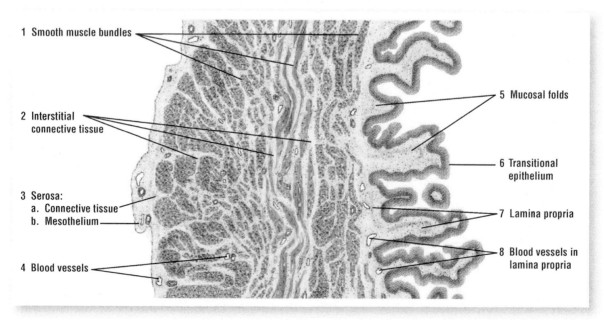

FIGURE 18.17 ■ Urinary bladder: wall (transverse section). Stain: hematoxylin and eosin. Low magnification.

layers are difficult to distinguish. The three layers are arranged in anastomosing **smooth muscle bundles** (**1**) between which is found the **interstitial connective tissue** (**2**). In this illustration, the muscle bundles are sectioned in various planes (1), and the three distinct muscle layers are not distinguishable. The interstitial connective tissue (2) merges with the connective tissue of the **serosa** (**3**). **Mesothelium** (**3b**) covers the **connective tissue of the serosa** (**3a**) and is the outermost layer. Serosa (3) lines the superior surface of the bladder, whereas its inferior surface is covered by the connective tissue adventitia, which merges with the connective tissue of adjacent structures.

The mucosa of an empty bladder exhibits **mucosal folds** (**5**) that disappear during bladder distension. The **transitional epithelium** (**6**) is thicker than in the ureter and consists of about six layers of cells. The **lamina propria** (**7**), inferior to the epithelium, is wider than in the ureters. The loose connective tissue in the deeper zone contains more elastic fibers. Numerous **blood vessels** (**4**, **8**) are found in the serosa (3), between the smooth muscle bundles (1), and in the lamina propria (8).

FIGURE 18.18 | Urinary Bladder: Contracted Mucosa (Transverse Section)

The mucosa from an empty and contracted urinary bladder wall is illustrated at a higher magnification. The superficial cells of the **transitional epithelium** (**4**) are low cuboidal, or columnar, and appear dome shaped. Also, some superficial cells may be **binucleate** (**6**) (contain two nuclei). The outer **plasma membrane** (**5**) of the superficial cells is prominent. The deeper cells in the epithelium are round (4) and the basal cells more columnar (see also Fig. 4.7).

The subepithelial **lamina propria** (**3**) contains connective tissue fibers, numerous fibroblasts, and the blood vessels, a **venule and arteriole** (**2**). The muscularis consists of three indistinct muscle layers that are visible as **smooth muscle bundles** (**1**) sectioned in longitudinal and transverse planes.

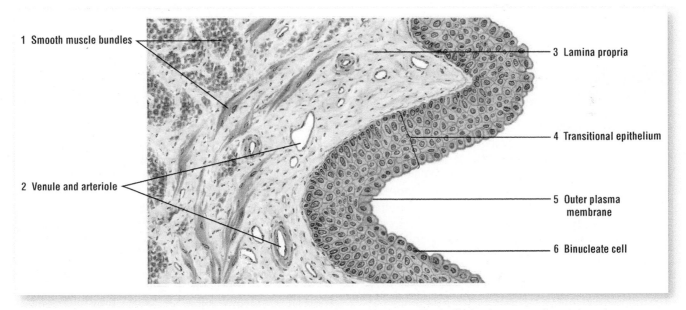

FIGURE 18.18 ■ Urinary bladder: contracted mucosa (transverse section). Stain: hematoxylin and eosin. Medium magnification.

FIGURE 18.19 | **Urinary Bladder: Stretched Mucosa (Transverse Section)**

When fluid fills the bladder, the **transitional epithelium** (**1**) changes its shape. Increased volume reduces the number of cell layers, the **surface cells** (**5**) appear squamous, and the thickness of the epithelium (**1**) is reduced to about three layers. This is because the surface cells (**5**) flatten to accommodate the increasing surface area. In the stretched condition, the transitional epithelium (**1**) may resemble stratified squamous epithelium found in other regions of the body. Folds in the bladder wall also disappear, and the **basement membrane** (**2**) is not folded. As in an empty bladder (Fig. 18.18), the underlying **connective tissue** (**6**) contains **venules** (**3**) and **arterioles** (**7**). Below the connective tissue (**6**) are **smooth muscle fibers** (**4, 8**), sectioned in cross (**4**) and longitudinal (**8**) planes.

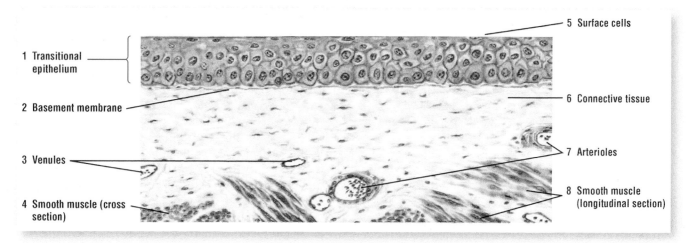

1 Transitional epithelium

2 Basement membrane

3 Venules

4 Smooth muscle (cross section)

5 Surface cells

6 Connective tissue

7 Arterioles

8 Smooth muscle (longitudinal section)

FIGURE 18.19 ■ Urinary bladder: stretched mucosa (transverse section). Stain: hematoxylin and eosin. Medium magnification.

FUNCTIONAL CORRELATIONS 18.4 ■ Urinary Bladder

The **urinary bladder** is a hollow organ with a thick muscular wall whose main function is to store urine. Because the lumen of the bladder is lined with a transitional epithelium, the wall of the organ can stretch or enlarge (change shape) as the bladder fills with urine. When the bladder is empty, the thick **transitional epithelium** may exhibit five or six layers of cells. The superficial cells in the epithelium are cuboidal, large, dome shaped, and bulge into the lumen. When the bladder fills with urine, however, the transitional epithelium is stretched, and the cells in the epithelium appear thinner and squamous to accommodate the increased volume of urine.

The changes in the appearance and cell shapes in the transitional epithelium are due to the thickened rigid regions in the integral plasma membrane of superficial cells called **plaques** that are connected to thinner, shorter, and more flexible **interplaque regions**. These structures act like "hinges," and, in an empty bladder, the interplaque regions allow the cell membrane to fold at the hinge regions by confining or compartmentalizing the folded plaques in fusiform-shaped vesicles. When the bladder is filled with urine, the apical membrane expands as the contents of the vesicles become part of the apical membrane. The interplaque regions allow the epithelium to expand during full stretch, changing the cell's shape from cuboidal to squamous shape.

The exposed or apical cell membrane of superficial cells in the transitional epithelium is also thicker. In addition, **desmosomes** and **occluding junctions** attach the lateral borders of the cells to each other. The plaques are impermeable to water, salts, and urine even when the epithelium is fully stretched. These unique properties of transitional epithelium in the urinary passages provide an effective **osmotic barrier** between concentrated urine and the underlying connective tissue.

Chapter 18 Summary

Urinary System

KIDNEY

- System consists of two kidneys, two ureters, a bladder, and a urethra
- Hilum contains renal artery, renal vein, and renal pelvis surrounded by renal sinus
- Darker outer region of kidney is cortex; lighter inner region is medulla
- Medulla contains numerous pyramids, which face the cortex at corticomedullary junction
- Round apex of each pyramid extends toward renal pelvis as renal papilla
- Cortex that extends on each side of renal pyramid constitutes the renal columns
- Each papilla is surrounded by a minor calyx that joins to form a major calyx
- Major calyces join to form funnel-shaped renal pelvis that narrows into muscular ureter
- Urine is formed as a result of blood filtration and absorption from and excretion into the filtrate
- Almost all filtrate is reabsorbed into the systemic circulation and about 1% is voided as urine
- Produces renin that regulates filtration pressure and erythropoietin for erythrocyte production

Uriniferous Tubules

- Functional unit of kidney is uriniferous tubule
- Consist of nephron and collecting duct

Nephrons of Kidney

- Two types of nephrons: cortical nephrons in cortex and juxtamedullary nephrons in medulla
- Nephron is subdivided into renal corpuscle and renal tubules

Renal Corpuscle

- Blood is filtered in the glomerular capillaries of the corpuscle to form ultrafiltrate
- Consists of capillaries called glomerulus and double-layered glomerular (Bowman) capsule
- Visceral layer of capsule contains podocytes that invest fenestrated glomerular capillaries
- Podocytes exhibit primary processes from which arise smaller pedicles

- Pedicles form filtration slits around capillaries that are spanned by filtration slit diaphragm
- Parietal layer is lined with simple squamous epithelium of the glomerular capsule
- Between parietal and visceral layers is the capsular (urinary) space for glomerular filtrate
- At vascular pole, afferent and efferent arterioles enter and exit the renal corpuscle
- At opposite urinary pole, ultrafiltrate enters the proximal convoluted tubule

Blood Filtration

- In renal corpuscle, it is through glomerular capillaries
- Consists of capillary endothelium, basement membrane, and podocytes/pedicles
- Glomerular filtrate enters capsular space between parietal and visceral layers

Filtration Barrier in Glomerulus

- Glomerular endothelium is fenestrated and permeable except for blood cells and large proteins
- Basement membrane restricts molecules the size of albumin
- Slit diaphragms between pedicles contain the transmembrane protein nephrin
- Filtration slits responsible for glomerular permeability because of size-selective molecular filters

Renal Tubules

- From capsular space, glomerular filtrate enters renal tubules that extend to collecting ducts
- Initial tubule is the proximal convoluted tubule that starts at the urinary pole of renal corpuscle
- Loop of Henle consists of thick descending tubules, a thin loop, and thick ascending tubules
- Distal convoluted tubule ascends into kidney cortex and joins the collecting tubule
- Juxtamedullary nephrons have very long loops of Henle
- Collecting tubules are not part of nephron but join larger collecting ducts to form papillary ducts
- Deep in medulla, papillary ducts are lined with columnar epithelium and exit in area cribrosa
- Medullary rays in cortex are collecting ducts, blood vessels, and straight portions of nephrons

Renal Blood Supply

- Renal artery divides in the hilus into segmental arteries that become interlobar arteries
- At corticomedullary junction, interlobar arteries branch into arcuate arteries
- Arcuate arteries form interlobular arteries from which arise afferent glomerular arterioles
- Glomerular arterioles form capillaries of glomeruli that exit renal corpuscles as efferent arterioles
- Efferent arterioles form peritubular capillaries and vasa recta in the medulla around kidney tubules

KIDNEY CELLS

Mesangial Cells

- Attached to capillaries in the renal corpuscle and serve important functions
- Produce extracellular matrix and provide structural support for glomerular capillaries
- Serve as phagocytes in glomerulus and phagocytose antigen–antibody complexes
- Produce interleukins in response to glomerular injury or damage
- Regulate blood pressure as a result of their contractile function
- Extraglomerular cells form part of the juxtaglomerular apparatus

Kidney Cells

- Responsible for homeostasis of the body
- Involved in forming urine through filtration, absorption, and excretion
- Produce enzyme renin to regulate blood pressure and maintain proper filtration pressure in glomeruli
- Synthesize erythropoietin to stimulate erythrocyte production in red bone marrow in response to hypoxia

KIDNEY TUBULES

Proximal Convoluted Tubules

- Proximal convoluted tubules lined with brush border and absorb most of filtrate
- Basal infoldings of cell membrane contain numerous mitochondria and sodium pumps
- Mitochondria supply energy for ionic transport across cell membrane into the interstitium
- Absorb all glucose, proteins, and amino acids, almost all carbohydrates, and 75% to 85% of water
- Secrete metabolic waste, hydrogen, ammonia, dyes, and drugs into the filtrate for voiding
- Longer than distal convoluted tubules and more frequently seen in cortex near renal corpuscles

Loop of Henle

- In juxtamedullary nephrons, it produces hypertonic urine owing to the countercurrent multiplier system
- Countercurrent flow of ultrafiltrate in descending and ascending loops of Henle produces osmotic gradient in the interstitium
- High interstitial osmolarity draws water from the filtrate as it flows through the loop
- Vasa recta capillaries take up water from interstitium and return it to systemic circulation

Distal Convoluted Tubules

- Shorter than proximal convoluted tubules, less frequent in cortex, and lack brush border
- Basolateral membrane shows infoldings and contains numerous mitochondria
- Under the influence of aldosterone, sodium ions actively absorbed from the filtrate
- Peritubular capillaries return ions to systemic circulation to maintain vital acid–base balance

Juxtaglomerular Apparatus

- Located adjacent to renal corpuscle and distal convoluted tubule
- Consists of juxtaglomerular cells, macula densa, and extraglomerular mesangial cells
- Juxtaglomerular cells are modified smooth muscle cells in afferent arteriole before entering glomerular capsule
- Main function is to maintain proper blood pressure for blood filtration in renal corpuscles
- Juxtaglomerular cells respond to stretching in the wall of afferent arterioles, as baroreceptors
- Macula densa is a group of modified distal convoluted tubule cells
- Macula densa responds to changes in sodium chloride concentration in glomerular filtrate
- Decreased blood pressure and ionic content causes release of enzyme renin by juxtaglomerular cells
- Renin release eventually causes plasma proteins to convert to angiotensin II, a powerful vasoconstrictor
- Angiotensin II stimulates release of aldosterone, which acts mainly on cells in collecting ducts
- Collecting ducts absorb NaCl with water, increasing blood volume and pressure
- Collecting ducts also eliminates hydrogen and potassium to maintain acid–base balance

Collecting Tubules, Collecting Ducts, and Antidiuretic Hormone

- Glomerular filtrate flows from distal convoluted tubules to collecting tubules and ducts

- During excessive water loss or dehydration, ADH is released from the pituitary gland
- ADH causes epithelium of collecting duct to become highly permeable to water
- Water-permeable cells contain transmembrane pore protein aquaporins that function as channels for water passage
- Aquaporin regulated by the ADH that binds to receptors and activates aquaporins
- Water that is retained in interstitium is collected by peritubular capillaries and vasa recta
- In the absence of ADH, increased water is retained in collecting ducts and urine is diluted

URETER

- Lined with transitional epithelium and consists of mucosa, muscularis, and adventitia
- Upper part lined with inner longitudinal and middle circular smooth muscle layers
- Third longitudinal smooth muscle layer added in the lower third of the ureter
- Connective tissue adventitia surrounds the ureter

Bladder

- Thick muscular wall with three indistinct layers of smooth muscle
- Serosa lines superior surface and adventitia covers the inferior surface
- Transitional epithelium in empty bladder exhibits about six layers of cells
- When stretched, transitional epithelium appears stratified squamous
- Changes in epithelium caused by thicker plasma membrane of superficial cells and folded plaques
- In relaxed bladder, plaques confined to vesicles
- Plaques act like hinges and allow apical cells to expand during stretching; cells become squamous
- Thicker plasma membrane and transitional epithelium provide osmotic barrier to urine

Chapter 18 Review Questions

QUESTIONS

In the following multiple choice questions, choose the letter corresponding to the one best answer.

1. The enzyme renin is released as a result of:

A. increased filtration volume and high blood pressure.

B. release of aldosterone and high sodium concentration in filtrate.

C. decreased systemic blood pressure and sodium concentration in filtrate.

D. strong vasoconstriction in afferent arterioles.

E. the influence of the hormone aldosterone.

2. The main effects of angiotensin II on kidney function are:

A. dilation of afferent arterioles and reduction of blood pressure.

B. increased absorption of water and antidiuretic hormone release.

C. inhibition of aldosterone release and decreased sodium absorption.

D. vasoconstriction and release of the hormone aldosterone.

E. increased release of the enzyme renin and decreased sodium absorption.

3. Which kidney structures respond to the effects of antidiuretic hormone (ADH)?

A. Collecting tubules and collecting ducts

B. Proximal convoluted tubules

C. Distal convoluted tubules

D. Thin tubules in the loop of Henle

E. Vasa recta

4. What unique features in the bladder wall allow it to stretch or enlarge to increased volume?

A. Thicker smooth muscle layers in the wall

B. Thicker connective tissue in the lamina propria

C. The presence of membrane plaques in the superficial cells

D. Increased numbers of desmosomes and junctional complexes

E. Denser connective tissue surrounding the bladder wall

5. What are some of the unique properties of the transitional epithelium?

A. It forms an osmotic barrier against concentrated urine.

B. It absorbs fluids and electrolytes.

C. It produces mucus to lubricate the interior of the bladder wall.

D. It becomes permeable to water when urine is dilute.

E. It continues to concentrate urine.

ANSWERS

1. **Correct Answer: C.** Decreased systemic blood pressure and sodium concentration in filtrate. Renin converts the protein angiotensin I, which is converted to angiotensin II, a powerful vasoconstrictor that constricts the blood vessels and increases blood pressure.

2. **Correct Answer: D.** Vasoconstriction and release of the hormone aldosterone. This action increases the reabsorption of sodium chloride and raises the systemic blood pressure and glomerular filtration rate.

3. **Correct Answer: A.** Collecting tubules and collecting ducts. The cells of these ducts contain aquaporins that function as water channels in these cells. The functions of aquaporins are regulated by ADH that results in increased water absorption from the filtrate.

4. **Correct Answer: C.** The presence of membrane plaques in the superficial cells. The plaques are folded in an empty bladder and are internalized in vesicles. When the bladder is stretched, the apical membranes expand as the vesicular compartment becomes part of the apical membrane.

5. **Correct Answer: A.** It forms an osmotic barrier against concentrated urine. The apical membrane is thicker and the plaques are impermeable to bladder contents.

ADDITIONAL HISTOLOGIC IMAGES

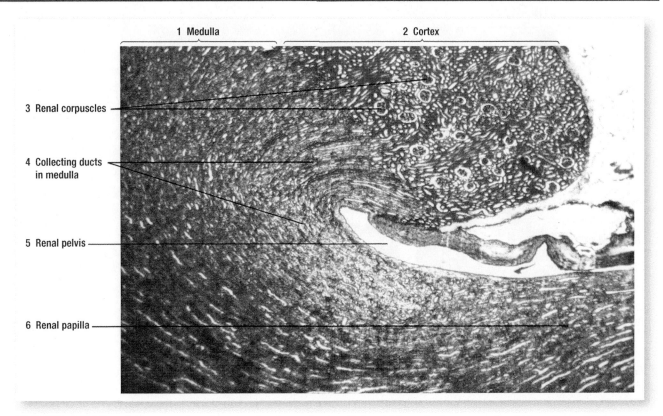

FIGURE 18.20 ■ A low-power micrograph of a rodent unilobar kidney (in humans, the kidney is multilobar). Stain: periodic acid–Schiff. ×10.

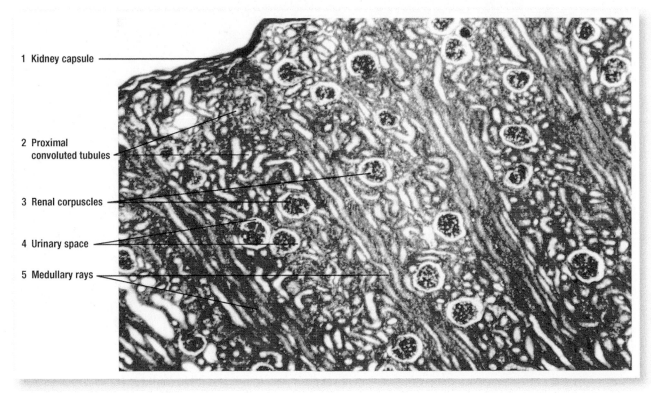

FIGURE 18.21 ■ A higher-power section of rodent kidney cortex illustrating its contents. Stain: periodic acid–Schiff. ×40.

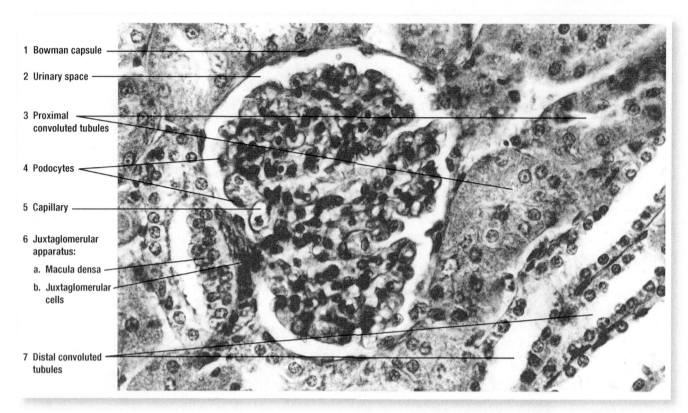

1 Bowman capsule

2 Urinary space

3 Proximal
   convoluted tubules

4 Podocytes

5 Capillary

6 Juxtaglomerular
   apparatus:
   a. Macula densa
   b. Juxtaglomerular
      cells

7 Distal convoluted
   tubules

FIGURE 18.22 ■ A section through a human kidney cortex illustrating the renal corpuscle and the surrounding ducts. Stain: hematoxylin and eosin. ×130.

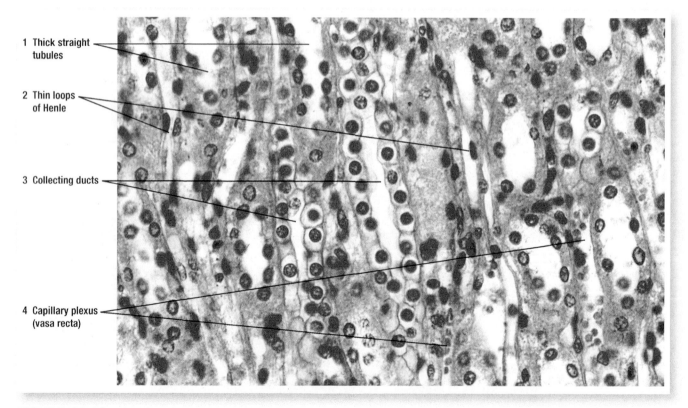

1 Thick straight
   tubules

2 Thin loops
   of Henle

3 Collecting ducts

4 Capillary plexus
   (vasa recta)

FIGURE 18.23 ■ Longitudinal section of the medullary region of a primate kidney with different tubules and blood vessels. Stain: hematoxylin and eosin. ×130.

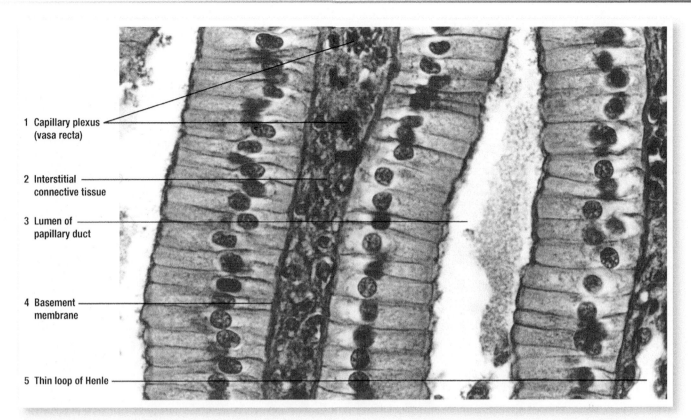

1 Capillary plexus (vasa recta)

2 Interstitial connective tissue

3 Lumen of papillary duct

4 Basement membrane

5 Thin loop of Henle

FIGURE 18.24 ■ Longitudinal section of papillary ducts in the papilla of a primate kidney illustrating simple columnar epithelium and the surrounding tissue. Stain: hematoxylin and eosin. ×205.

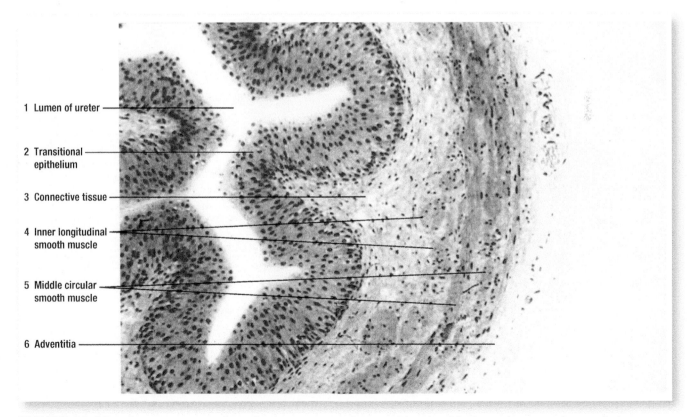

1 Lumen of ureter

2 Transitional epithelium

3 Connective tissue

4 Inner longitudinal smooth muscle

5 Middle circular smooth muscle

6 Adventitia

FIGURE 18.25 ■ A transverse section of primate ureter, its transitional epithelium, the smooth muscle layers, and the surrounding tissues. Stain: hematoxylin and eosin. ×40.

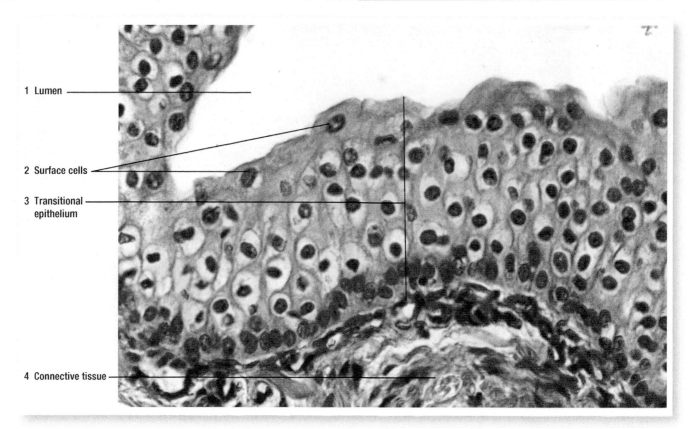

1 **Lumen**

2 **Surface cells**

3 **Transitional epithelium**

4 **Connective tissue**

FIGURE 18.26 ■ A section of the wall from an empty primate bladder and the appearance of the transitional epithelium. Stain: hematoxylin and eosin. ×130.

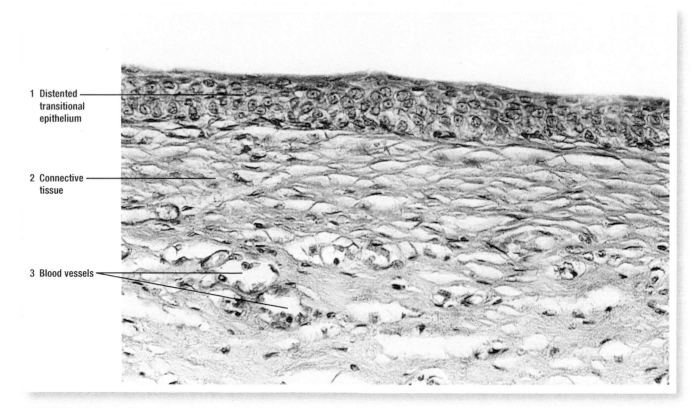

1 **Distended transitional epithelium**

2 **Connective tissue**

3 **Blood vessels**

FIGURE 18.27 ■ A section of a distended primate bladder wall and the appearance of the transitional epithelium. Stain: hematoxylin and eosin. ×100.

CHAPTER 19

Endocrine System

SECTION 1 Hormones and Pituitary Gland

The endocrine system consists of cells, tissues, and organs that synthesize and secrete **hormones** that are then released into the interstitial connective tissue from which they pass into the blood or lymph circulation. As a result, endocrine cells, tissues, glands, and organs are called **ductless** glands because there are no excretory ducts for the hormone release. Furthermore, the cells in most endocrine tissues and organs are arranged into **cords** and **clumps** and surrounded by a **capillary network** for more efficient transport of the hormones.

Hormones produced by endocrine cells include polypeptides, proteins, steroids, amino acid derivatives, and catecholamines. Because hormones act at a distance from the site of their release, the circulatory system delivers them to their **target organs**. Here, they influence the structure and the programmed function of the target organ cells by binding to and interacting with specific hormone receptors.

Hormone receptors are located on the cell membrane, in the cytoplasm, or in the nucleus of target cells. These receptors are specific for certain hormones. Nonsteroid receptors for protein and peptide hormones are usually located on cell surfaces because these hormones do not penetrate the cell membrane. The interaction with the hormone produces molecules called **second messengers**, which is **cyclic adenosine monophosphate (cAMP)** for most hormones. cAMP then activates a specific sequence of enzymes and cellular events in the cytoplasm and/or nucleus for a hormone-specific response.

Other receptors are **intracellular**, are localized in the **nucleus**, and are activated by hormones that penetrate the cellular and nuclear membranes. Steroid and thyroid hormones are lipid soluble and cross these membranes. Once inside the target cells, these steroid hormones combine with specific receptor molecules. The resulting hormone–receptor complex enters the nucleus and binds to a particular DNA sequence that either activates or inhibits specific genes. The activated genes then initiate the synthesis of messenger RNA that enters the cytoplasm to initiate production of hormone-specific proteins and induce cellular changes specifically associated with the particular hormone. The hormones that combine with the intracellular receptors do not use the second messenger. Instead, they directly influence **gene expression** of the affected cell.

Numerous organs in the body contain individual endocrine cells or endocrine tissues mixed with other tissues. Individual endocrine cells, such as those in the digestive organs, are part of the **diffuse neuroendocrine system (DNES)**. Mixed (endocrine–exocrine) organs are the pancreas, kidneys, reproductive organs of both sexes, and placenta. Endocrine cells and endocrine tissues are discussed with the specific exocrine organs in their respective chapters.

There are also complete endocrine organs or glands (Fig. 19.1). These include the **hypophysis**, or **pituitary gland** (described below), **thyroid gland**, **adrenal (suprarenal) glands**, and **parathyroid glands** (described in Section 2).

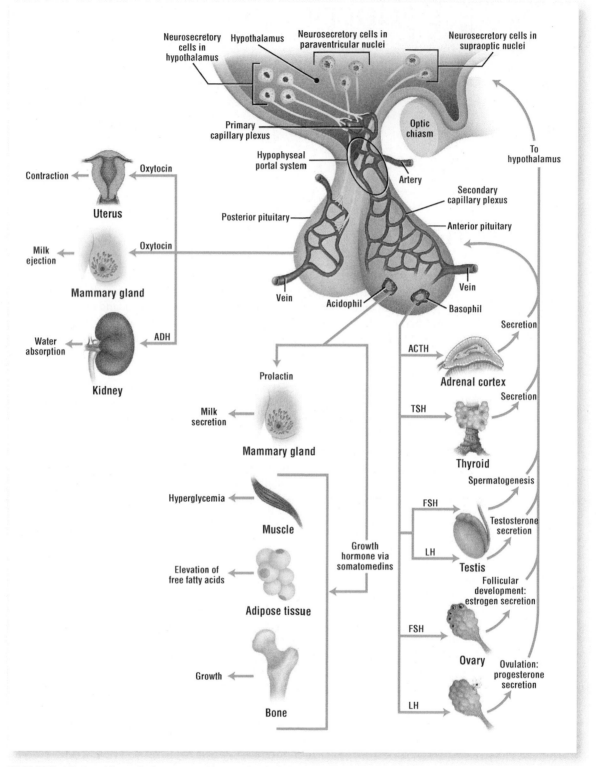

FIGURE 19.1 ■ Hypothalamus and hypophysis (pituitary gland). A section of hypothalamus and hypophysis illustrates the neuronal, axonal, and vascular connections between the hypothalamus and the hypophysis. Also illustrated are the major target cells, tissues, and organs that respond to the hormones that are produced by both the anterior (adenohypophysis) and posterior (neurohypophysis) pituitary gland. ACTH, adrenocorticotropic hormone; TSH, thyroid-stimulating hormone; FSH, follicle-stimulating hormone; LH, luteinizing hormone.

EMBRYOLOGIC DEVELOPMENT OF HYPOPHYSIS (PITUITARY GLAND)

The pituitary gland or hypophysis secretes numerous hormones that influence the action of peripheral tissues or organs. However, the pituitary gland is controlled by the **hypothalamus** of the brain from which regulatory hormones are transported to the pituitary gland.

The structure and function of the hypophysis are directly related to its dual embryologic origin. During embryonic development, the epithelium of the **pharyngeal roof** (oral cavity) forms an upward outpocketing called the **hypophyseal (Rathke) pouch**. As development proceeds, the hypophyseal pouch detaches from the oral cavity to become the cellular or glandular portion of the hypophysis, the **adenohypophysis (anterior pituitary)**. At the same time, the downward growth from the developing brain (diencephalon) forms the neural portion of the hypophysis, the **neurohypophysis (posterior pituitary)**. The two separately developed structures unite to form a single pituitary gland, the hypophysis. The hypophysis remains attached to a ventral extension of the brain called the **hypothalamus**. A short neural stalk, the **infundibulum**, becomes the neural pathway that attaches and connects the hypophysis to the hypothalamus. The neurons in the hypothalamus control the release of hormones from the adenohypophysis as well as secrete hormones that are then transported to and stored in the neurohypophysis until needed.

After development, the hypophysis rests in a bony depression of the sphenoid bone of the skull called the **sella turcica** located inferior to the hypothalamus at the base of the brain.

SUBDIVISIONS OF HYPOPHYSIS

The epithelial-derived adenohypophysis has three subdivisions: pars distalis, pars tuberalis, and pars intermedia. The **pars distalis** is the largest part of the hypophysis. The **pars tuberalis** surrounds the neural stalk, or infundibulum. The **pars intermedia** is a thin cell layer between the pars distalis and the neurohypophysis. It represents the remnant of the hypophyseal (Rathke) pouch that becomes rudimentary in humans but prominent in other mammals.

The neurohypophysis, situated posterior to the adenohypophysis, also consists of three parts: median eminence, infundibulum, and pars nervosa. The **median eminence** is located at the base of the hypothalamus of the brain from which extends the pituitary stalk, or **infundibulum**. In the infundibulum is found a multitude of unmyelinated axons that extend from the neurons in the hypothalamus. The large portion of the neurohypophysis is the **pars nervosa**. This region contains the terminal ends of unmyelinated axons for the storage of hormones that have been secreted by the neurons in the hypothalamus. Surrounding the axons are the nonsecretory **pituicytes** that function in supporting roles for the axons.

VASCULAR AND NEURAL CONNECTIONS OF HYPOPHYSIS

Adenohypophysis

The adenohypophysis does not develop from the neural tissue and is connected to the **hypothalamus** of the brain via a vascular network. **Superior hypophyseal arteries** from the internal carotid artery supply the pars tuberalis, median eminence, and infundibulum. These arteries form a **primary capillary plexus** in the median eminence at the base of the hypothalamus. Secretory neurons located in the hypothalamus synthesize hormones that have a direct influence on cell functions in the adenohypophysis. The axons from these neurons in the hypothalamus terminate on the fenestrated capillaries of the primary capillary plexus and into which they release their hormones.

Small **hypophyseal portal venules** drain the primary capillary plexus into the hypophyseal portal veins and deliver the blood with the hormones to a **secondary capillary plexus** that surrounds the cells in the pars distalis of the adenohypophysis. The venules that connect the primary capillary plexus of the hypothalamus with the secondary capillary plexus in the adenohypophysis form the **hypothalamohypophyseal** portal system. To ensure efficient transport of hormones from the blood to the cells, the capillaries in the primary and secondary capillary plexuses are **fenestrated** (contain small pores).

Cells of Adenohypophysis

The cells of the adenohypophysis were initially classified as **chromophobes** and **chromophils** based on the affinity of their cytoplasmic granules for specific stains. The pale-staining chromophobes either are believed to be cells that depleted their hormones or are undifferentiated stem cells. The chromophils were further subdivided into **acidophils** and **basophils** because of their staining properties. Immunocytochemical techniques now identify these cells on the basis of their specific hormones. The adenohypophysis contains two types of acidophils, the **somatotrophs** and **lactotrophs** (**mammotrophs**), as well as three types of basophils: **gonadotrophs**, **thyrotrophs**, and **corticotrophs**.

The hormones from these cells are carried in the bloodstream to the target organs, where they bind to specific receptors that influence the structure and function of the target cells. After activation of target cells and release of their secretory products, a **feedback mechanism** (positive or negative) controls the synthesis and further release of these hormones. This is accomplished by direct action on cells in the adenohypophysis and/or neurons in the hypothalamus that produced these hormones.

Neurohypophysis

In contrast to the adenohypophysis, the neurohypophysis has a direct neural connection with the brain. There are no neurons or hormone-producing cells in the neurohypophysis, and it remains connected to the brain by unmyelinated axons supported by pituicytes. The **neurons** (cell bodies) of these axons are located in the **supraoptic** and **paraventricular nuclei** (a collection of neurons) in the hypothalamus. The unmyelinated axons that extend from the hypothalamus into the neurohypophysis form the **hypothalamohypophyseal tract** and the bulk of the neurohypophysis. These axons terminate near the fenestrated capillaries in the pars nervosa.

Neurons in the hypothalamus first synthesize the hormones that are then released from the neurohypophysis. The released hormones bind to the carrier glycoprotein **neurophysin** and are transported from the hypothalamus down the axons by **axonal transport** to the neurohypophysis. Here, the hormones accumulate and are stored in the distended terminal ends of unmyelinated axons as **Herring bodies**. When needed, hormones from the neurohypophysis are released and enter the adjacent fenestrated capillaries in the pars nervosa. Thus, the neurohypophysis functions as a storage site for neuroendocrine secretions that were synthesized in and transported from the supraoptic and paraventricular nuclei of the hypothalamus.

thePoint®   Supplemental micrographic images are available at **www.thePoint.com/Eroschenko13e** under Endocrine System.

FIGURE 19.2 | Hypophysis (Panoramic View, Sagittal Section)

The hypophysis (pituitary gland) consists of the adenohypophysis and neurohypophysis. The adenohypophysis is further subdivided into the **pars distalis (anterior lobe) (5)**, **pars tuberalis (7)**, and **pars intermedia (9)**. The neurohypophysis is divided into the **pars nervosa (11)**, **infundibulum (6)**, and the median eminence (not illustrated). The pars tuberalis (7) surrounds the infundibulum (6) and is visible in a sagittal section. The infundibulum (6) connects the hypophysis with the hypothalamus at the base of the brain.

The pars distalis (5) contains two main cell types: chromophobe cells and chromophil cells. The chromophils are subdivided into **acidophils (alpha cells) (4)** and **basophils (beta cells) (2)**, illustrated at a higher magnification in Figure 19.3.

The pars intermedia (9) and pars nervosa (11) form the posterior lobe of the hypophysis. The pars nervosa (11) consists primarily of unmyelinated axons and supporting pituicytes. A **connective tissue capsule (1, 10)** surrounds the pars distalis (5) and pars nervosa (11) portions of the gland.

The pars intermedia (9) is situated between the pars distalis (5) and the pars nervosa (11) and represents the residual lumen of the hypophyseal (Rathke) pouch. The pars intermedia (9) normally contains **colloid-filled vesicles (9a)** that are surrounded by the cells of the pars intermedia (9).

Both the pars distalis (5) and pars nervosa (11) are supplied by **blood vessels (8)** and **capillaries (3)**.

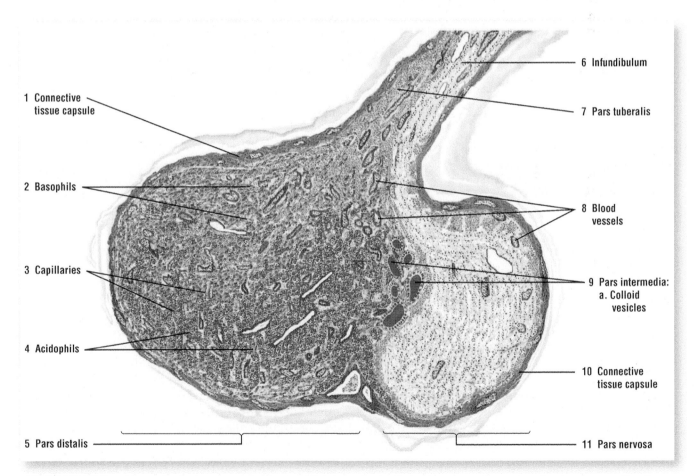

1 Connective tissue capsule

2 Basophils

3 Capillaries

4 Acidophils

5 Pars distalis

6 Infundibulum

7 Pars tuberalis

8 Blood vessels

9 Pars intermedia: a. Colloid vesicles

10 Connective tissue capsule

11 Pars nervosa

FIGURE 19.2 ■ Hypophysis (panoramic view, sagittal section). Stain: hematoxylin and eosin. Low magnification.

FIGURE 19.3 | Hypophysis: Sections of Pars Distalis, Pars Intermedia, and Pars Nervosa

At a higher magnification, **sinusoidal capillaries** (1) and different cell types are visible in the **pars distalis. Chromophobe cells** (2) have a light-staining, homogeneous cytoplasm and are smaller than the chromophils. The cytoplasm of chromophils stains reddish in the **acidophils** (3) and bluish in the **basophils** (4).

The **pars intermedia** contains **follicles** (6) and colloid-filled **cystic follicles** (7). Follicles lined with basophils (8) are often present in the pars intermedia.

The **pars nervosa** is characterized by unmyelinated axons and the supportive **pituicytes** (5) with oval nuclei.

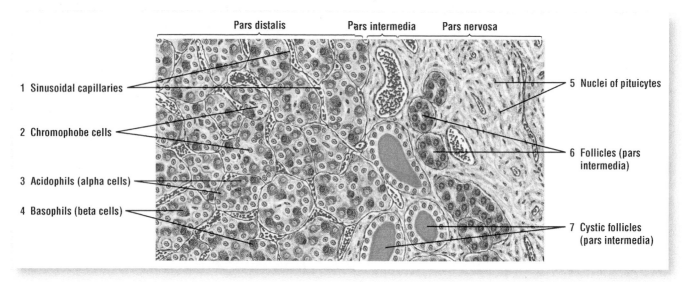

FIGURE 19.3 ■ Hypophysis: sections of pars distalis, pars intermedia, and pars nervosa. Stain: hematoxylin and eosin. Medium magnification.

FUNCTIONAL CORRELATIONS 19.1 ■ Hormones of Hypophysis

Hormones produced by neurons in the **hypothalamus** control the synthesis and release of six specific hormones from the adenohypophysis by specific **releasing hormones**. The releasing hormones are produced by the hypothalamic neurons for each hormone that is released from the adenohypophysis. These releasing hormones are thyrotropin-releasing hormone, gonadotropin-releasing hormone, corticotropin-releasing hormone, and growth hormone–releasing hormone. For two hormones, growth hormone (GH), also called somatotropin, and prolactin, **inhibitory hormones** are also produced. The inhibitory hormones are somatostatin, which inhibits the release of GH, and **dopamine** (prolactin-inhibiting hormone), which inhibits the secretion of prolactin.

The releasing and inhibitory hormones are carried from the primary capillary plexus of the median eminence of the hypothalamus to the second capillary plexus in the adenohypophysis via the **hypothalamo-hypophyseal portal system**. On reaching the cells of the adenohypophysis, the hormones bind to specific receptors and either stimulate the cells to secrete and release a specific hormone into the circulation or inhibit this function.

In contrast, the cells in the neurohypophysis do not secrete hormones. Instead, the neurohypophysis stores and releases only two hormones, **oxytocin** and **vasopressin** (antidiuretic hormone [ADH]), which were synthesized in the hypothalamus by the neurons in the **paraventricular nuclei** and **supraoptic nuclei**. These hormones are then transported along unmyelinated axons and stored as tiny dilations in the axon terminals of the neurohypophysis as **Herring bodies** from which they are released near the capillaries of the par nervosa (Herring bodies are visible with a light microscope).

FIGURE 19.4 | **Hypophysis: Pars Distalis (Sectional View)**

This illustration shows the two main populations of cells in the pars distalis of the adenohypophysis. The cells here are arranged in clumps. Between the clumps are seen the **capillaries** (5), **blood vessels** (3), and thin **connective tissue fibers** (6) that separate the clumps. Cell types in the pars distalis can be identified by the staining affinity of the cytoplasmic granules.

The **chromophobes** (4) exhibit pale nuclei and pale cytoplasm with poorly defined cell outlines. The aggregation of chromophobes in groups or clumps is seen in this illustration.

The **acidophils** (2) are numerous and can be distinguished by red-staining granules in the cytoplasm and blue nuclei.

The **basophils** (1) are less numerous and contain blue-staining granules in their cytoplasm. The degree of granularity and the stain density vary in different cells.

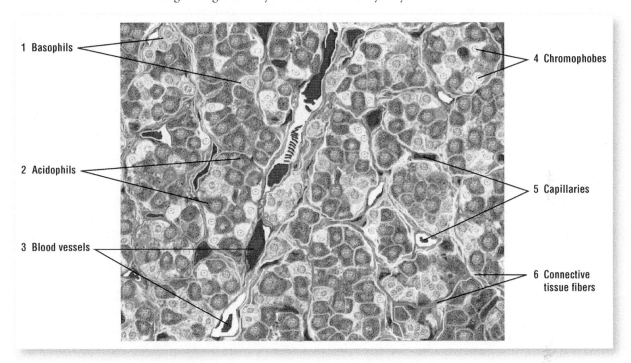

FIGURE 19.4 ■ Hypophysis: pars distalis (sectional view). Stain: Azan. High magnification.

FIGURE 19.5 | **Cell Types in Hypophysis**

Different cell types of the hypophysis are illustrated at a higher magnification after modified Azan staining. The nuclei of all cells are stained orange-red.

The **chromophobes** (a) exhibit a clear and light orange cytoplasm indicating that the cells do not have granules, and their cell boundaries are indistinct.

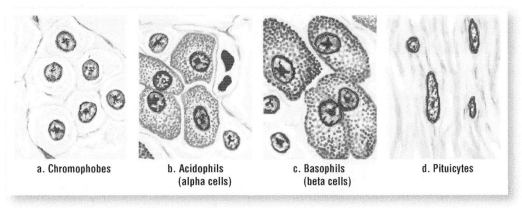

a. Chromophobes   b. Acidophils   c. Basophils   d. Pituicytes
                        (alpha cells)   (beta cells)

FIGURE 19.5 ■ Cell types in the hypophysis. Stain: modified Azan. Oil immersion.

The cytoplasmic granules of **acidophils** (**b**) stain intensely red, and the cell outlines are distinct. A sinusoid capillary surrounds the acidophils.

The **basophils** (**c**) exhibit variable cell shapes and granules that vary in size.

The **pituicytes** (**d**) of the pars nervosa have variable cell shape and cell size. The small, orange-stained cytoplasm is diffuse and barely visible.

FIGURE 19.6 | Hypophysis: Pars Distalis, Pars Intermedia, and Pars Nervosa

This higher-power photomicrograph illustrates the cellular pars distalis and pars intermedia of the adenohypophysis and the light-staining pars nervosa of the neurohypophysis. With this stain, different cell types can be identified. The red-staining, or eosinophilic, cells are the **acidophils** (**5**). The cells with bluish cytoplasm are the **basophils** (**4**). The light, unstained cells scattered among the acidophils (**5**) and basophils (**4**) are the **chromophobes** (**7**). The pars intermedia exhibits small cysts, or **vesicles** (**6**), filled with colloid.

The pars nervosa is filled with the unmyelinated, light-staining axons of secretory cells, whose cell bodies are located in the hypothalamus. Most of the red-staining nuclei in the pars nervosa are the supportive **pituicytes** (**2**). Accumulations of the neurosecretory material at the end of the axon terminals in the pars nervosa are the irregular-shaped, red-staining **Herring bodies** (**3**) that are closely associated with fenestrated capillaries and **blood vessels** (**1**).

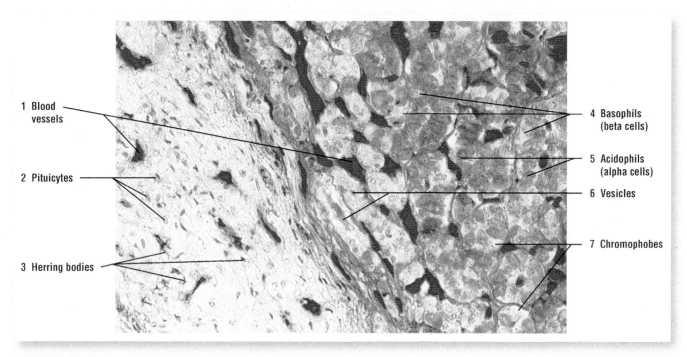

1 Blood vessels

2 Pituicytes

3 Herring bodies

4 Basophils (beta cells)

5 Acidophils (alpha cells)

6 Vesicles

7 Chromophobes

FIGURE 19.6 ■ Hypophysis: pars distalis, pars intermedia, and pars nervosa. Stain: Mallory-Azan and orange G. ×80.

FUNCTIONAL CORRELATIONS 19.2 ■ **Cells and Hormones of Adenohypophysis**

ACIDOPHILS

Somatotrophs secrete **somatotropin**, also called growth hormone, or GH. This hormone targets the whole body and its general growth. It stimulates cellular metabolism, uptake of amino acids, protein synthesis, and the liver to produce **somatomedins**, also called insulin-like growth factor 1 (IGF-1). These hormones increase proliferation of cartilage cells

(chondrocytes) in the **epiphyseal plates** of developing or growing long bones to increase the bone length. There is also an increase in the growth of the skeletal muscle and increased release of fatty acids from the adipose cells for energy production by body cells. GH-inhibiting hormone, also called **somatostatin**, has an inhibitory effect on the release of GH from somatotrophs in the pituitary gland.

FUNCTIONAL CORRELATIONS 19.2 ■ Cells and Hormones of Adenohypophysis (Continued)

Mammotrophs produce the lactogenic hormone **prolactin** that stimulates the development of mammary glands during pregnancy. After parturition (birth) and during lactation, prolactin stimulates secretion of nutrients and milk production in the developed mammary glands. The release of prolactin from mammotrophs is inhibited by a prolactin release inhibitory hormone, also called **dopamine**.

BASOPHILS

Thyrotrophs secrete **thyroid-stimulating hormone** (**thyrotropin** or **TSH**). This hormone stimulates follicular cells in the thyroid gland to synthesize and secrete thyroglobulin and the production and release of thyroid hormones. TSH also stimulates the release of prolactin.

Gonadotrophs secrete **follicle-stimulating hormone** (**FSH**) and **luteinizing hormone** (**LH**). In females, FSH promotes growth and maturation of ovarian follicles and **estrogen** secretion by developing follicles. In males, FSH promotes **spermatogenesis** in the testes and secretion of **androgen-binding protein** into seminiferous tubules by Sertoli cells. The androgen-binding protein maintains the needed concentration of testosterone in the seminiferous tubules to ensure proper spermatogenesis.

In females, LH in association with FSH induces ovulation, promotes the final maturation of ovarian follicles, and stimulates the formation of the **corpus luteum** after ovulation. LH also promotes the secretion of estrogen and progesterone from the corpus luteum. In males, LH maintains and stimulates the **interstitial cells** (of Leydig) in the testes to produce the hormone **testosterone**. LH is also called interstitial cell–stimulating hormone (ICSH). Both hormones, FSH and LH, are essential for reproductive functions in both sexes.

Corticotrophs secrete **adrenocorticotropic hormone** (**ACTH**). ACTH stimulates the cells in **adrenal cortex** to synthesize and release glucocorticoids and steroids (adrenal androgens) from the zona fasciculata and zona reticularis of adrenal cortex.

PARS INTERMEDIA

In lower vertebrates (amphibians and fishes), the pars intermedia is developed and produces **melanocyte-stimulating hormone** (**MSH**). MSH increases skin pigmentation by causing the dispersion of melanin granules. In humans and most mammals, the pars intermedia is rudimentary.

FUNCTIONAL CORRELATIONS 19.3 ■ Cells and Hormones of Neurohypophysis

OXYTOCIN

The two hormones, oxytocin and antidiuretic hormone (ADH), that are released from the neurohypophysis are synthesized in the supraoptic and paraventricular nuclei of the hypothalamus. Oxytocin release is stimulated by vaginal and cervical distension before birth and nursing of the infant after birth. **Oxytocin** targets the smooth muscles of the pregnant uterus. During labor, oxytocin induces strong contractions of smooth muscles in the uterus, resulting in childbirth (parturition). After parturition, the suckling action of the infant on the nipple stimulates and activates the **milk ejection reflex** in the lactating mammary glands. Afferent impulses from the nipple stimulate neurons in the hypothalamus, causing oxytocin release. Oxytocin then stimulates the contraction of **myoepithelial cells** around the alveoli and ducts in the lactating mammary glands, ejecting milk into the excretory ducts and the nipple.

ANTIDIURETIC HORMONE (VASOPRESSIN)

The main action of ADH is to increase **water permeability** in the **distal convoluted tubules** and **collecting ducts** of the kidney. As a result, more water is reabsorbed from the filtrate into the interstitium and retained in the body, creating more concentrated urine. In addition, an increase in blood tonicity or a decrease in blood volume stimulates the osmoreceptor cells in the hypothalamus to activate the release of ADH from the neurons in the neurohypophysis. Increased water retention/absorption through ADH action on the kidney tubules increases fluid volume and restores the osmotic balance of body fluids.

Chapter 19 Summary

SECTION 1 • Hormones and Pituitary Gland

- Consists of cells, tissues, and organs that produce blood-borne chemicals
- Consists of ductless glands, arranged in cords and clumps, and surrounded by capillaries
- Hormones enter connective tissue and then blood or lymphatic circulation
- Hormones interact with target organs that have specific receptors
- Hormone receptors located on cell membrane, in cytoplasm, or in nucleus
- Nonsteroid hormone receptors located on cell surface
- Proteins and polypeptide hormones use second messenger (cAMP) to activate responses
- Steroid and thyroid hormones enter cells and influence gene expression in nucleus
- There are complete endocrine organs and mixed organs with endocrine cells and tissues

EMBRYOLOGIC DEVELOPMENT OF HYPOPHYSIS (PITUITARY GLAND)

- Has dual embryologic origin, epithelial and neural
- Epithelial portion develops from pharyngeal roof and Rathke pouch
- Pouch detaches and becomes the cellular portion, adenohypophysis (anterior pituitary)
- Downgrowth of brain forms the neural portion, neurohypophysis (posterior pituitary)
- Neurohypophysis remains attached to hypothalamus by a neural stalk, infundibulum
- Neurons in hypothalamus control release of hormones from adenohypophysis

SUBDIVISIONS OF HYPOPHYSIS

- Adenohypophysis (anterior pituitary) has three subdivisions
- Pars distalis is the largest part
- Pars intermedia is remnant of the pouch and rudimentary in humans
- Pars tuberalis surrounds the neural stalk
- Neurohypophysis (posterior pituitary) consists of three parts

- Median eminence is located at the base of hypothalamus
- Infundibulum is the neural stalk that connects neurohypophysis to hypothalamus
- Pars nervosa is the largest portion that consists of unmyelinated axons and pituicytes

VASCULAR AND NEURAL CONNECTIONS OF HYPOPHYSIS

Adenohypophysis

- Connection between hypothalamus of brain and adenohypophysis is vascular
- Superior hypophyseal arteries form fenestrated primary capillary plexus in median eminence
- Secretory neurons in hypothalamus terminate on capillary plexus and release hormones
- Hypophyseal venules connect to secondary capillary plexus in the adenohypophysis, forming a hypothalamohypophyseal portal system
- Hypothalamus produces both releasing hormones and inhibitory hormones for cells in adenohypophysis
- Releasing or inhibitory hormones are carried via the portal system to cells in pars distalis
- Releasing hormones bind to specific receptors in cells of pars distalis

Cells and Hormones of Adenohypophysis

- Based on stains, there are three cell types: acidophils, basophils, and chromophobes
- Acidophils are subdivided into somatotrophs and mammotrophs
- Basophils are subdivided into thyrotrophs, gonadotrophs, and corticotrophs

Somatotrophs

- Secrete somatotropin or growth hormone for cell metabolism and general body growth
- Somatotropin also stimulates liver to produce somatomedins
- Somatomedins influence cartilage cells in epiphyseal plates to increase growth in length
- Somatostatin inhibits release of growth hormone from somatotrophs

Mammotrophs

- Produce prolactin that stimulates mammary gland development during pregnancy
- Prolactin maintains milk production after parturition
- Release of prolactin inhibited by inhibitory hormone called dopamine

Thyrotrophs

- Release thyroid-stimulating hormone that stimulates thyroid gland hormones
- Thyroid cells produce thyroglobulin, thyroxin, and triiodothyronine

Gonadotrophs

- Secrete both follicle-stimulating hormone and luteinizing hormone
- In females, follicle-stimulating hormone stimulates follicular development, maturation, and estrogen production
- In males, follicle-stimulating hormone promotes spermatogenesis and androgen-binding protein secretion by Sertoli cells
- In females, luteinizing hormone induces follicular maturation, ovulation, and corpus luteum formation
- Corpus luteum secretes estrogen and progesterone
- In males, luteinizing hormone stimulates interstitial cells in testes to produce testosterone (androgens)

Corticotrophs

- Secrete adrenocorticotropic hormone to regulate adrenal cortex functions
- Feedback mechanism controls further synthesis and release of specific hormones
- Pars intermedia in humans is rudimentary and in lower vertebrates produces melanocyte-stimulating hormone

Neurohypophysis

- Does not have any secretory cells; secretory neurons are located in hypothalamus of brain
- Has a direct neural connection to hypothalamus via multitude of unmyelinated axons
- Contains axonal hypothalamohypophyseal tract and supportive cells, pituicytes
- Neurons of axons located in supraoptic and paraventricular nuclei of hypothalamus
- Neurons synthesize hormones that are transported in and stored at axon terminals as Herring bodies
- Carrier glycoprotein neurophysin binds to hormones for transport to axon terminals
- Releases two hormones from axon terminals, oxytocin and antidiuretic hormone (vasopressin)

Oxytocin

- Release stimulated by vaginal and cervical distension during labor and nursing infant
- Stimulates contraction of smooth uterine muscles during childbirth
- Activates milk ejection in lactating glands by stimulating contraction of myoepithelial cells

Antidiuretic Hormone

- Increases permeability to water in distal convoluted tubules and collecting ducts of kidney
- Creates more concentrated urine after water is reabsorbed from glomerular filtrate
- Is also released during decreased blood volume and increase in blood tonicity
- Increased osmotic pressure stimulates osmoreceptors to activate the release of ADH
- Increased water retention restores osmotic balance of body fluids

Chapter 19 Review Questions: Section 1

QUESTIONS

In the following multiple choice questions, choose the letter corresponding to the one best answer.

1. **Releasing hormones for the cells in the adenohypophysis are produced in the:**

   A. pars distalis.
   B. pars tuberalis.
   C. pars intermedia.
   D. hypothalamus.
   E. pars nervosa.

2. **The releasing hormones reach the target cells in the adenohypophysis (anterior pituitary) via:**

   A. axonal transport.
   B. superior hypophyseal arteries.
   C. the hypothalamohypophyseal tract.
   D. the hypothalamohypophyseal portal system.
   E. the posterior pituitary.

3. **What do Herring bodies contain?**

   A. Releasing hormones
   B. Oxytocin and vasopressin (ADH)
   C. Inhibitory hormones
   D. Secretory neurons
   E. Capillary plexuses

4. **The hormone that affects total body growth and energy production is:**

   A. adrenocorticotropic hormone.
   B. dopamine.
   C. somatostatin.
   D. somatotropin.
   E. somatomedin.

5. **Gonadotrophs create hormones that:**

   A. promote growth and maturation of follicles and spermatogenesis.
   B. induce retention of body fluids in the system.
   C. stimulate milk production and ejection from the mammary gland.
   D. cause release of hormones from the adrenal gland.
   E. inhibit the release of prolactin.

ANSWERS

1. **Correct Answer: D.** The hypothalamus. The hormones are then brought to the cells of the adenohypophysis via the hypothalamohypophyseal portal system.

2. **Correct Answer: D.** The hypothalamohypophyseal portal system. This system connects the neurons of the hypothalamus with the cells in the adenohypophysis.

3. **Correct Answer: B.** Oxytocin and vasopressin (ADH). These hormones are stored in the axon terminals until needed by the organism.

4. **Correct Answer: D.** Somatotropin. This is the growth hormone that affects the entire body's development and growth.

5. **Correct Answer: A.** Promote growth and maturation of follicles and spermatogenesis. The hormones from these cells affect the growth and development of sex organs in both sexes.

SECTION 2 Thyroid Gland, Parathyroid Glands, and Adrenal Gland

THYROID GLAND

The **thyroid gland** is located in the anterior neck inferior to the larynx. It is a single gland that consists of large right and left lobes, connected to an isthmus. Most endocrine cells, tissues, or organs are arranged in cords or clumps and store their secretory products within their cytoplasm. In the thyroid gland, the cells are arranged into spherical structures, called **follicles**, in which the thyroid hormones are stored. Each follicle is lined with a single layer of follicular cells and surrounded by reticular fibers. A vascular capillary network surrounds the follicles for entrance of thyroid hormones into the bloodstream. The follicular epithelium can be simple squamous, cuboidal, or low columnar, depending on gland activity.

Follicles are the structural and functional units of the thyroid gland. The surrounding **follicular cells**, also called principal cells, synthesize, release, and store their product extracellularly in the lumen of the follicles as a gelatinous substance called **colloid**. The apices of the follicular cells come in contact with the colloid, which is composed of **thyroglobulin**, an inactive iodinated glycoprotein compound for storage of the thyroid hormones. Thyroglobulin, by itself, does not have any hormonal activity.

The thyroid gland also contains larger, pale-staining parafollicular cells or **C cells**. These cells are found either peripherally in the follicular epithelium within the follicle basal lamina or as clusters between follicular cells.

PARATHYROID GLANDS

Mammals generally have four **parathyroid glands**. These small oval glands are embedded on the posterior surface of the thyroid gland but are separated from the thyroid gland by a thin connective tissue **capsule**. Normally, one parathyroid gland is located on the superior pole and one on the inferior pole of each lobe of the thyroid gland. In contrast to the thyroid gland, the cells of the parathyroid glands are arranged into cords or clumps, surrounded by a rich capillary network and normally without follicles that are seen in the adjacent thyroid gland.

There are two types of cells in the parathyroid glands: functional **principal**, or **chief cells** and **oxyphil cells** (Fig. 19.7). Oxyphil cells are larger than the principal (chief cells) but are less

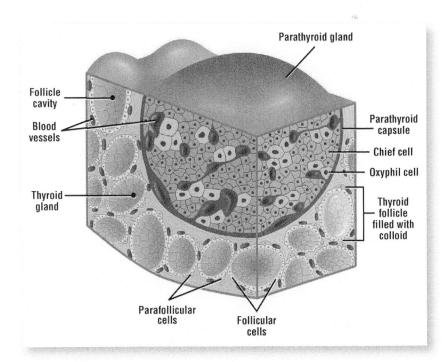

FIGURE 19.7 ■ The microscopic organization of the parathyroid and thyroid gland is illustrated.

numerous and appear as single cells or in small groups. In histologic sections, oxyphil cells stain acidophilic. Occasionally, small colloid-filled follicles may be seen in the parathyroid glands.

ADRENAL (SUPRARENAL) GLANDS

The **adrenal glands** are endocrine organs situated near the superior pole of each kidney. Each adrenal gland is surrounded by a dense irregular connective tissue capsule and embedded in the adipose tissue around the kidneys. The secretory portion of each adrenal gland consists of an outer **cortex** and an inner **medulla**. Although these two regions of the adrenal gland are located in one organ and are linked by a common blood supply, they have separate and distinct embryologic origins, structures, and functions.

Cortex

The adrenal cortex exhibits three concentric zones: the zona glomerulosa, zona fasciculata, and zona reticularis (Fig. 19.8).

The **zona glomerulosa** is a thin zone inferior to the adrenal gland capsule. It consists of cells arranged in small clumps.

The **zona fasciculata** is intermediate and the thickest zone of the adrenal cortex. This zone exhibits vertical columns of one-cell thickness adjacent to straight capillaries and is characterized by pale-staining cells because of the presence of numerous lipid droplets.

The **zona reticularis** is the innermost zone that is adjacent to the adrenal medulla. The cells in this zone are arranged in cords or clumps.

In all three zones, the secretory endocrine cells are adjacent to fenestrated capillaries. The cells of the adrenal cortex produce steroid hormones: **mineralocorticoids**, **glucocorticoids**, and **sex hormones**.

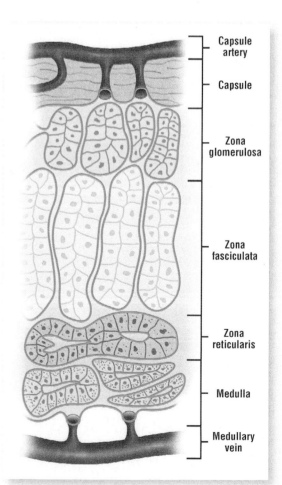

FIGURE 19.8 ■ The microscopic organization of the adrenal gland is illustrated.

Medulla

The medulla is in the center of the adrenal gland with its cells also arranged in small cords. The medullary cells, called **chromaffin cells**, are modified postganglionic sympathetic neurons that lost their axons and dendrites during development have become secretory cells that synthesize and secrete **catecholamines** (primarily epinephrine and norepinephrine). Preganglionic axons of the sympathetic neurons innervate the adrenal medulla cells. Ganglion cells are also present in the adrenal medulla.

thePoint®) Supplemental micrographic images are available at **www.thePoint.com/Eroschenko13e** under Endocrine System.

FIGURE 19.9 | Thyroid Gland: Canine (General View)

The thyroid gland is characterized by variable-sized **follicles** (1, 10) filled with an acidophilic **colloid** (1, 10). The follicles are lined with a simple cuboidal epithelium of **follicular (principal) cells** (5, 6). The **follicles** (6, 9) sectioned peripherally or tangentially do not exhibit follicular content and appear as cell clumps (6, 9). The follicular cells (5, 6) synthesize and secrete the colloid and the thyroid hormones. In routine preparations, colloid often retracts from the follicular wall of the follicle (10).

Within the thyroid gland are also found **parafollicular cells** (11) or C cells. These cells occur as single cells or in clumps on the periphery of the follicles. The parafollicular cells (11) stain lighter than the follicular cells (5) and are clearly visible in the canine thyroid. Parafollicular cells (11) (C cells) synthesize and secrete the hormone calcitonin.

Connective tissue **septa** (8) from the thyroid gland capsule extend into the gland's interior and divide the gland into lobules. Numerous blood vessels—**arterioles** (3), **venules** (4), and **capillaries** (2)—are seen in the connective tissue septa (8) and around individual follicles (2). A small amount of **interfollicular connective tissue** (7) is found between individual follicles.

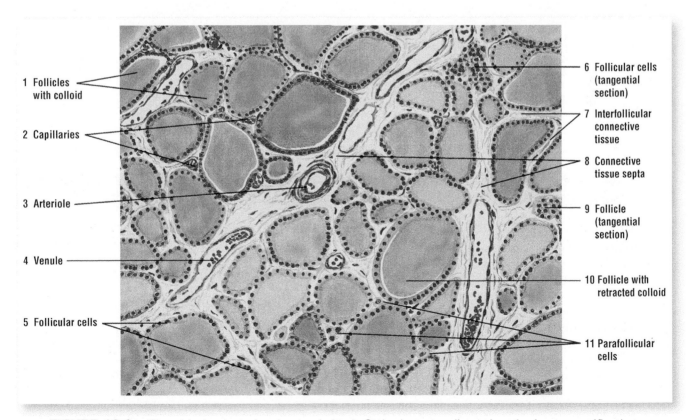

1 Follicles with colloid
2 Capillaries
3 Arteriole
4 Venule
5 Follicular cells
6 Follicular cells (tangential section)
7 Interfollicular connective tissue
8 Connective tissue septa
9 Follicle (tangential section)
10 Follicle with retracted colloid
11 Parafollicular cells

FIGURE 19.9 ■ Thyroid gland: canine (general view). Stain: hematoxylin and eosin. Low magnification.

FIGURE 19.10 | Thyroid Gland Follicles: Canine (Sectional View)

This higher magnification of the thyroid gland shows individual **thyroid follicles** (7) with secretory colloid material. The height of the **follicular cells** (2, 6, 10) depends on the function of the individual follicles. In active follicles, the epithelium is cuboidal (2, 10). In less active follicles, the epithelial cells appear flattened. All thyroid follicles (7) are filled with the **colloid** (7), some of which show **retraction** (1) from the follicular wall or **distortion** (1) as a result of chemicals used in slide preparation.

The **parafollicular cells** (3, 11) (C cells) are adjacent to the follicular cells (2, 10) or in small clumps (3) adjacent to the thyroid follicles (7). These cells (3, 11) are larger than the follicular cells (2, 10) with an oval shape and lighter-staining cytoplasm.

Surrounding the thyroid follicles (7), the follicular cells (2, 10), and the parafollicular cells (3, 11) (C cells) is a thin **interfollicular connective tissue** (9) with numerous **blood vessels** (5) and **capillaries** (4, 8) that are very close to the individual follicles.

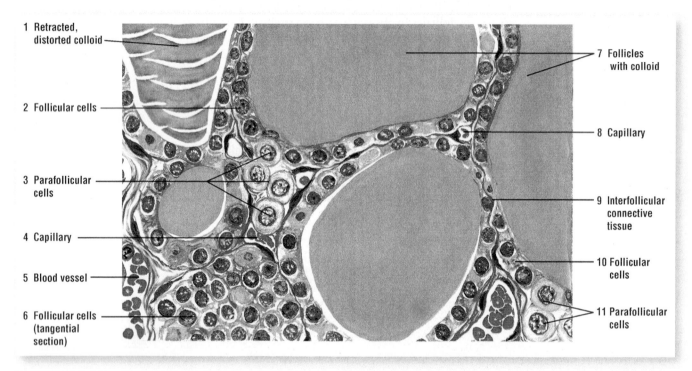

1 Retracted, distorted colloid
2 Follicular cells
3 Parafollicular cells
4 Capillary
5 Blood vessel
6 Follicular cells (tangential section)
7 Follicles with colloid
8 Capillary
9 Interfollicular connective tissue
10 Follicular cells
11 Parafollicular cells

FIGURE 19.10 ■ Thyroid gland follicles: canine (sectional view). Stain: hematoxylin and eosin. High magnification.

FUNCTIONAL CORRELATIONS 19.4 ■ Thyroid Gland

FORMATION OF THYROID HORMONES

The **follicular cells** that produce the thyroid hormones in the thyroid gland are controlled by **thyroid-stimulating hormone** (**TSH**) from the adenohypophysis. **Iodide** is an essential element for the production of the active thyroid hormones **triiodothyronine** (T_3) and **tetraiodothyronine**, or **thyroxine** (T_4).

Low levels of thyroid hormones in the blood stimulate the release of TSH from the adenohypophysis. In response to TSH stimulus, the follicular cells in the thyroid gland synthesize thyroglobulin and take up **iodide** from the blood into their cytoplasm via the iodide pump in the follicular basal cell membrane. Iodide is then oxidized to iodine within the follicular cells and transported into the follicular lumen containing colloid material. In the follicular lumen, iodine combines with amino acid tyrosine groups to form **iodinated thyroglobulin**, of which T_3 and T_4 are the principal products. T_3 and T_4 remain bound to the iodinated thyroglobulin in thyroid follicles in an inactive form until needed. TSH released from the adenohypophysis stimulates the thyroid gland cells to release the thyroid hormones into the systemic circulation.

FUNCTIONAL CORRELATIONS 19.4 ■ Thyroid Gland (*Continued*)

RELEASE OF THYROID HORMONES

The release of thyroid hormones involves endocytosis (uptake) of thyroglobulin by follicular cells, hydrolysis of the iodinated thyroglobulin by lysosomal proteases, and release of the principal **thyroid hormones** (**T₃** and **T₄**) at the base of follicular cells into the surrounding capillaries. Most of the released thyroid hormones are tightly bound to specific thyroxin-binding protein. The thyroid secretes greater quantities of T₄ than T₃ into the circulation; however, T₃ is much more potent than T₄ and is primarily responsible for the physiologic activity in the organism. The thyroid hormones accelerate the metabolic rate of the body and increases its cell metabolism, growth, differentiation, and development. In addition, thyroid hormones increase the rate of protein, carbohydrate, and fat metabolism.

PARAFOLLICULAR CELLS (C CELLS)

The thyroid gland also contains **parafollicular cells**. These cells are on the periphery of the follicular epithelium, visible as single cells or as cell clusters between the follicles. Parafollicular cells are not part of thyroid follicles and are not in contact with colloid in the follicular lumen. These cells are most prominent in canine thyroid glands.

The parafollicular cells synthesize and secrete the hormone **calcitonin** (**thyrocalcitonin**), which regulates calcium metabolism in the body in lower animals. The function of calcitonin is to lower blood calcium levels by inhibiting the resorptive action of **osteoclasts**, reducing calcium release, and increasing calcium deposition in bones. Calcitonin also promotes excretion of calcium and phosphate ions from the kidneys into the urine. The release of calcitonin by the parafollicular cells depends on increased blood calcium levels and is **independent** of the pituitary gland hormones. Thus, the release of calcitonin is regulated by calcium levels through a simple **feedback** mechanism.

FIGURE 19.11 | Thyroid and Parathyroid Glands: Canine (Sectional View)

The **follicles** (**1**) with the secretory material colloid of the **thyroid gland** (**7**) are closely associated with the cell types of the **parathyroid gland** (**9**). Thin **connective tissue** (**3**, **8**) septa from the glandular capsule extend into the thyroid gland to separate the parathyroid gland (**9**) cells

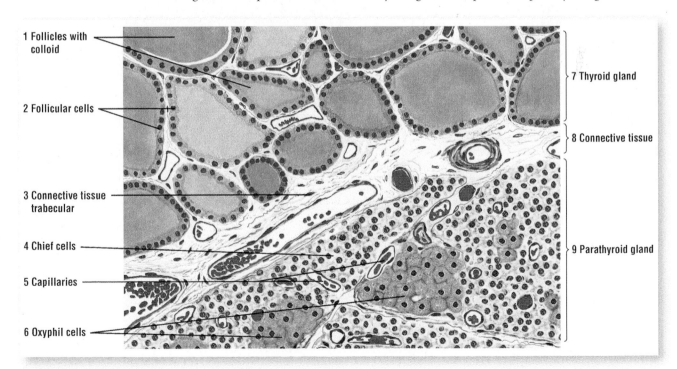

1 Follicles with colloid

2 Follicular cells

3 Connective tissue trabecular

4 Chief cells

5 Capillaries

6 Oxyphil cells

7 Thyroid gland

8 Connective tissue

9 Parathyroid gland

FIGURE 19.11 ■ Thyroid and parathyroid glands: canine (sectional view). Stain: hematoxylin and eosin. Low magnification.

from the thyroid gland (7) follicles. In the connective tissue (3, 8) are blood vessels that branch into **capillaries** (5) to surround the parathyroid cells (9) as well as the follicles (1) in the thyroid gland (7).

The parathyroid gland (9) cells are arranged into anastomosing cords and clumps, instead of the follicles (1) filled with colloid surrounded by **follicular cells** (2). However, an isolated small follicle with colloid material may be observed in the parathyroid gland. The parathyroid gland (9) contains two cell types: the **chief (principal) cells** (4) and the **oxyphil cells** (6). The chief cells (4) are the most numerous cells and exhibit a pale, slightly acidophilic cytoplasm. In contrast, the oxyphil cells (6) are larger and less numerous and exhibit an acidophilic cytoplasm with dark nuclei (6). The oxyphil cells (6) are found as single cells or small clumps in the parathyroid gland (9); these cells increase in number with increasing age.

FIGURE 19.12 | Thyroid Gland and Parathyroid Gland

This photomicrograph shows parathyroid gland adjacent to the thyroid gland. A **connective tissue septum** (3) separates the two glands. Different size **follicles with colloid** (1) and **follicular cells** (2) characterize the thyroid gland.

The parathyroid gland contains the smaller **chief cells** (4) and **oxyphil cells** (5) that are larger and less numerous and exhibit an eosinophilic cytoplasm. Numerous **blood vessels** (6) surround the secretory cells in both organs.

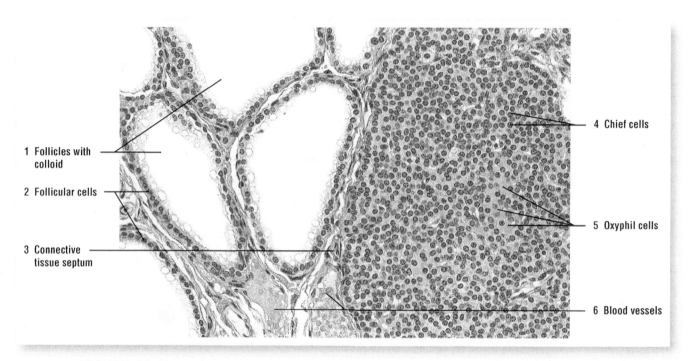

FIGURE 19.12 ■ Thyroid gland and parathyroid gland. Stain: hematoxylin and eosin. ×80.

FUNCTIONAL CORRELATIONS 19.5 ■ Parathyroid Glands

The **chief cells** of the parathyroid glands produce **parathyroid hormone** (**parathormone**). The function of this hormone is to maintain proper calcium and phosphate levels in the extracellular body fluids by elevating calcium levels in the blood. This action is opposite, or antagonistic, to that of calcitonin, produced by parafollicular cells (C cells) in the thyroid glands.

The release of parathyroid hormone indirectly stimulates differentiation and increases the activity of the **osteoclasts** in bones. However, because parathyroid hormone receptors are found on osteoprogenitor cells, osteoblasts, and osteocytes, but not on osteoclasts, the osteoclasts are indirectly activated by the osteoblasts. Parathyroid hormone initially targets **osteoblasts** that produce **receptor activator of nuclear factor k B ligand** (**RANKL**). Also, osteoclast precursors express receptor molecules called **receptor activator of nuclear factor k B** (**RANK**). The RANKL of osteoblasts binds to osteoclasts RANK (receptors) that activate and stimulate osteoclast differentiation. Thus, the activation of the osteoclast–osteoblast/RANK–RANKL pathway induces differentiation, proliferation, and osteoclast functions. This action leads to increased bone resorption and release

of calcium and phosphates into the bloodstream, thereby raising and maintaining proper calcium levels. As the calcium concentration in the bloodstream increases, further production of parathyroid hormone is suppressed.

Parathyroid hormone also targets the kidneys and intestines. In kidneys, there is an increased tubular reabsorption of calcium from the glomerular filtrate and an increased elimination of phosphate, sodium, and potassium ions into urine. Parathyroid hormone also influences the kidneys to produce the hormone **calcitriol**, the active form of vitamin D, which increases calcium absorption from the gastrointestinal tract.

The release of parathyroid hormone depends on the concentration of blood calcium levels and not on any pituitary hormones. Thus, the release of parathyroid hormone is regulated by calcium levels through a simple **feedback** mechanism. Because parathyroid hormone maintains optimal levels of calcium in the blood, parathyroid glands are essential to life because calcium is essential for many vital functions.

The function of **oxyphil cells** in the parathyroid glands is presently not clear.

FIGURE 19.13 | Adrenal (Suprarenal) Gland

The adrenal (suprarenal) gland consists of an outer **cortex** (**1**) and an inner **medulla** (**5**), surrounded by a connective tissue **capsule** (**6**) with branches of adrenal blood vessels, veins, nerves (largely unmyelinated), and lymphatics. A **connective tissue septum** with a blood vessel (**2**) passes from the capsule (**6**) into the cortex and to the medulla (**5**). Fenestrated sinusoidal **capillaries** (**8**, **10**) and large **blood vessels** (**14**) are found throughout the cortex (**1**) and medulla (**5**).

The adrenal cortex (**1**) is subdivided into three concentric zones. Inferior to the connective tissue capsule (**6**) is the outer **zona glomerulosa** (**7**) in which the **cells** (**7**) are arranged into ovoid

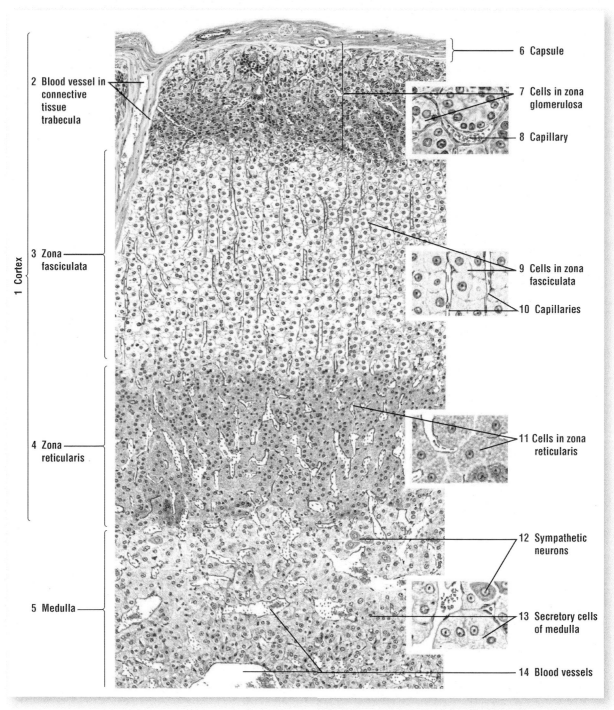

FIGURE 19.13 ■ Adrenal (suprarenal) gland. Stain: hematoxylin and eosin. Low magnification.

groups or clumps and surrounded by sinusoidal capillaries (8). The cytoplasm of these cells (7) stains pink and contains few lipid droplets.

The middle and the widest cell layer is the **zona fasciculata** (3, 9) with the cells arranged in vertical columns, or radial plates. Because of the high content of lipid in their cytoplasm, the **cells of the zona fasciculata** (9) appear light or vacuolated after a normal slide preparation. Sinusoidal capillaries (10) between the cell columns follow a similar vertical or radial course.

The third and the innermost cell layer is the **zona reticularis** (4, 11), which borders on the adrenal medulla (5). The **cells** (11) of the zona reticularis (4) form anastomosing cords surrounded by sinusoidal capillaries.

The medulla (5) is not sharply demarcated from the cortex with the **secretory cells of the medulla** (13) appearing clear. After tissue fixation in potassium bichromate, called the chromaffin reaction, fine brown granules are visible in the cells of the medulla, indicating the presence of the catecholamines epinephrine and norepinephrine.

The medulla also contains **sympathetic neurons** (12) seen singly or in small groups with a vesicular nucleus, prominent nucleolus, and a small amount of peripheral chromatin.

Sinusoidal capillaries drain the contents of the medulla (5) into the medullary blood vessels (14).

FIGURE 19.14 | **Adrenal (Suprarenal) Gland: Cortex and Medulla**

This lower-magnification photomicrograph illustrates a section of the adrenal gland. The cortex is surrounded by a connective tissue **capsule** (1). Inferior to the capsule (1) is the **zona glomerulosa** (2) with ovoid clumps of cells. The intermediate and widest zone is the zona fasciculata (3) with light-staining, narrow cords of cells, between which are capillaries and connective tissue fibers. The innermost zone of the adrenal cortex is the **zona reticularis** (4), in which the cells are arranged into groups of branching cords and clumps.

The adrenal **medulla** (5) is located adjacent to the zona reticularis (4). In the medulla (5), the cells are larger and also arranged into clumps. Large **blood vessels** (6) (veins) drain the medulla (5).

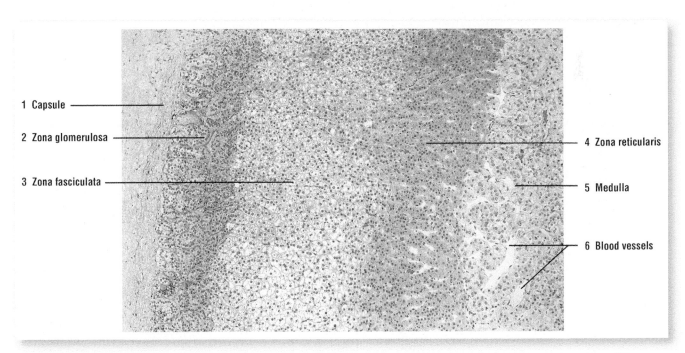

1 Capsule

2 Zona glomerulosa

3 Zona fasciculata

4 Zona reticularis

5 Medulla

6 Blood vessels

FIGURE 19.14 ■ Adrenal (suprarenal) gland: cortex and medulla. Stain: hematoxylin and eosin. ×25.

FUNCTIONAL CORRELATIONS 19.6 ■ Adrenal Gland Cortex and Medulla

ADRENAL GLAND CORTEX

The adrenal gland cortex is controlled by the anterior pituitary gland hormone adrenocorticotropic hormone (ACTH). Cells of the adrenal gland cortex synthesize and release three types of steroids: mineralocorticoids, glucocorticoids, and androgens.

The cells of the **zona glomerulosa** produce **mineralocorticoid aldosterone**. Its release is initiated via the kidney **renin–angiotensin** pathway because of decreased arterial filtration blood pressure and low sodium levels in the glomerular filtrate. These changes are detected by the **juxtaglomerular apparatus** (juxtaglomerular cells in the afferent arteriole and macula densa in the distal convoluted tubule) in the kidney cortex near the renal corpuscles.

Aldosterone has a major influence on fluid and electrolyte balance in the body, with the main target being the distal convoluted tubules in the kidneys. Aldosterone increases **sodium reabsorption** from the glomerular filtrate in the distal convoluted tubules of the kidney and increases potassium excretion into urine. As water follows sodium, fluid volume in the circulation increases. Restoration of the blood pressure, blood volume, and electrolyte balance decreases the release of renin from the juxtaglomerular apparatus.

The cells of the zona fasciculata secrete **glucocorticoids**, of which **cortisol** and **cortisone** are the most important, and some small amounts of weak androgens. Glucocorticoids are released response to stress, which then stimulate protein, fat, and carbohydrate metabolism, especially by gluconeogenesis to increase the concentration of blood **glucose**. Glucocorticoids (cortisol) also suppress the immune system and have an anti-inflammatory effect by reducing the number of circulating lymphocytes, thereby decreasing antibody production and suppressing the tissue response to injury.

The cells of the zona reticularis produce sex steroids, mainly weak androgens that can be converted to testosterone and estrogen to influence the development of secondary sex characteristics in both sexes. Glucocorticoid secretions and the secretory functions of zona fasciculata and zona reticularis are regulated by feedback control from the pituitary gland and ACTH.

ADRENAL GLAND MEDULLA

The functions of the adrenal medulla are controlled by the hypothalamus through the sympathetic division of the autonomic nervous system. Cells in the adrenal medulla are called the **chromaffin cells** because they stain with chromium salts. These cells arise from neural crest, just like the postganglionic neurons of sympathetic and parasympathetic ganglia, and can, therefore, be considered as postganglionic neurons that lack dendrites and axons. They are innervated and activated by preganglionic sympathetic axons in response to fear or acute emotional stress, causing them to release the catecholamines **epinephrine** and **norepinephrine**. The release of these chemicals prepares the individual for a "fight-or-flight" response, resulting in increased heart rate and respiratory rate, increased cardiac output and blood flow, and a surge of glucose into the bloodstream from the liver for added energy. Catecholamines produce the maximal use of energy and physical effort to overcome the stress.

Chapter 19 Summary

Section 2 • Thyroid Gland, Parathyroid Glands, and Adrenal Gland

THYROID GLAND

- Located in anterior neck region and consists of two large, connected lobes
- Consists of follicles surrounded by follicular cells that fill the lumen with colloid
- Colloid contains thyroglobulin, an iodinated inactive storage form of thyroid hormones
- Follicular cells controlled by thyroid-stimulating hormone (TSH)
- Iodide is an essential element in the production of thyroid hormones
- Low levels of thyroid hormones stimulate the release of TSH from adenohypophysis
- Iodide is taken from blood, oxidized to iodine, and transported into follicular lumen
- Iodine combines with tyrosine groups to form iodinated thyroglobulin
- Triiodothyronine (T_3) and tetraiodothyronine (T_4) are main thyroid gland hormones
- Release of thyroid hormones involves endocytosis of thyroglobulin and hydrolysis of thyroglobulin
- Thyroid hormones bound to thyroxin-binding protein
- T_4 is produced, but T_3 is physiologically more potent than T_4
- Thyroid hormones increase metabolic rate, growth, differentiation, and body development
- Parafollicular cells (C cells) are located in follicular peripheries of thyroid gland
- Parafollicular cells (C cells) secrete calcitonin to lower blood calcium by inhibiting osteoclasts
- Parafollicular cells (C cells) act independent of pituitary gland hormones but depend on calcium levels

PARATHYROID GLANDS

- Mammals have four parathyroid glands on the posterior surface of thyroid
- Instead of follicles, cells arranged in cords or clumps surrounded by capillary clumps
- Two cell types: principal or chief cells and oxyphil cells
- Chief cells produce parathyroid hormone (parathormone) to maintain proper calcium
- Parathyroid hormone counterbalances calcitonin action

- Parathyroid hormone initially targets osteoblasts that contain RANKL
- RANKL of osteoblasts binds to osteoclasts and stimulates osteoclasts bone absorption activity
- Parathyroid hormone induces kidney and intestines to absorb and retain more calcium
- Release of hormone depends on calcium levels and not pituitary hormones
- Are essential to life owing to maintenance of proper calcium levels
- Function of oxyphil cells is presently not clear

ADRENAL GLANDS

- Located near superior pole of each kidney
- Have separate and distinct embryologic origin, structure, and function
- Covered with a connective tissue capsule and consist of outer cortex and inner medulla
- Fenestrated capillaries and large vessels throughout both regions
- Cortex shows three zones: zona glomerulosa, zona fasciculata, and zona reticularis

Cortex

- Under direct influence of adrenocorticotropic hormone (ACTH) from anterior pituitary gland
- Releases three steroid hormones: mineralocorticoids, glucocorticoids, and androgens
- Cells in zona glomerulosa secrete mineralocorticoids, primarily aldosterone
- Aldosterone release is caused by decreased arterial blood pressure and low sodium levels
- Juxtaglomerular apparatus in kidney initiates the renin–angiotensin pathway to increase blood pressure
- Aldosterone increases sodium reabsorption and increased water retention by distal convoluted tubules
- Increased fluid volume increases blood pressure and inhibits further release of aldosterone
- Cells of zona fasciculata secrete glucocorticoids, of which cortisol and cortisone are important
- Glucocorticoids are released in response to stress, increase metabolism and glucose levels, and suppress inflammatory responses
- Cells of zona reticularis produce weak androgens that influence development of secondary sex characteristics

Medulla

- Cells are modified postganglionic sympathetic neurons that became secretory
- Stain with chromium salts and are called chromaffin cells
- Medulla cells can be considered as ganglion cells without dendrites and axons

- Action controlled by sympathetic division of autonomic nervous system, not pituitary gland
- Cells contain catecholamines (epinephrine and norepinephrine) and respond to stress
- Prepares the individual for flight-or-fight response
- Cells activate maximal use of energy and physical effort

Chapter 19 Review Questions: Section 2

QUESTIONS

In the following multiple choice questions, choose the letter corresponding to the one best answer.

1. **What important role do the parafollicular (C) cells perform in the system?**

   A. They secrete and release the hormone calcitonin.
   B. They stimulate osteoclast activity.
   C. They feed back on the pituitary gland to decrease its stimuli.
   D. They secrete parathyroid hormone.
   E. The function of these cells is not known.

2. **What directly activates the osteoclasts to absorb bone?**

   A. High calcium levels in the blood
   B. Increased levels of calcitonin
   C. Release of osteoclast-stimulating factor from osteoblasts
   D. Thyroid-stimulating hormone from the pituitary gland
   E. Release of parathyroid-stimulating hormone

3. **What physiological changes in the body induce the release of aldosterone?**

   A. Increased blood pressure
   B. Increased calcium levels
   C. Decreased secretion of adrenocorticotropic hormone
   D. Decreased filtration pressure in the kidneys
   E. Increased volume of concentrated urine

4. **What secretory products are released from the adrenal medulla?**

   A. Cortisol and cortisone
   B. Epinephrine and norepinephrine
   C. Aldosterone and sodium
   D. Adrenocorticotropic hormone and sodium
   E. Androgens

5. **The function and release of secretory products from the adrenal medulla is controlled by:**

   A. the adrenal cortex.
   B. the pituitary gland.
   C. the autonomic nervous system.
   D. adrenocorticotropic hormone.
   E. blood pressure.

ANSWERS

1. **Correct Answer: A.** They secrete and release the hormone calcitonin. This hormone regulates calcium concentration in the system by lowering calcium blood levels.

2. **Correct Answer: C.** Release of osteoclast-stimulating factor from osteoblasts. This activates osteoclasts to increase bone resorption and release more calcium into the blood.

3. **Correct Answer: D.** Decreased filtration pressure in the kidney. Also, the decreased sodium concentration in glomerular filtrate is detected by the juxtaglomerular apparatus, which activates the eventual release of aldosterone.

4. **Correct Answer: B.** Epinephrine and norepinephrine. The release of these chemicals is in response to stress and prepares the organism for a flight-or-fight situation.

5. **Correct Answer: C.** The autonomic nervous system. The cells of the adrenal medulla are activated by the sympathetic nervous system to overcome stressful situations.

ADDITIONAL HISTOLOGIC IMAGES

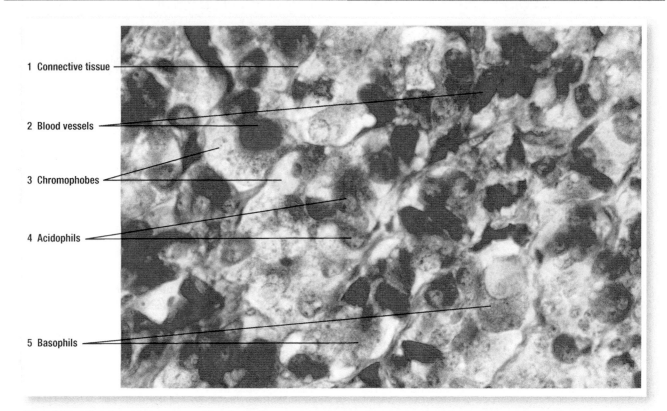

1 Connective tissue

2 Blood vessels

3 Chromophobes

4 Acidophils

5 Basophils

FIGURE 19.15 ■ Higher magnification of a section from a human pars distalis illustrating different cell types. Mallory-Azan and orange G. ×165.

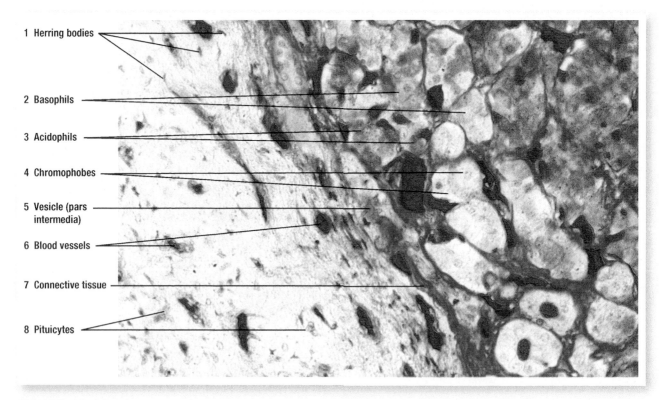

1 Herring bodies

2 Basophils

3 Acidophils

4 Chromophobes

5 Vesicle (pars intermedia)

6 Blood vessels

7 Connective tissue

8 Pituicytes

FIGURE 19.16 ■ A section of human hypophysis illustrating the pars nervosa (left), pars intermedia (middle), and pars distalis (right). Mallory-Azan and orange G. ×80.

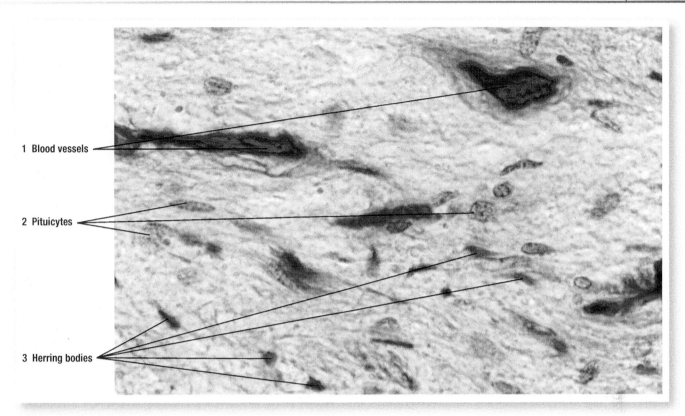

1 Blood vessels

2 Pituicytes

3 Herring bodies

FIGURE 19.17 ■ High magnification of a human pars nervosa illustrating the supportive pituicytes and Herring bodies surrounded by unmyelinated axons. Mallory-Azan and orange G. ×205.

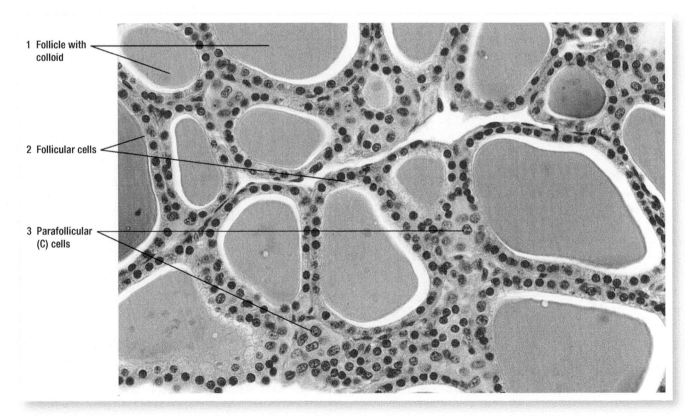

1 Follicle with
   colloid

2 Follicular cells

3 Parafollicular
   (C) cells

FIGURE 19.18 ■ A section of canine thyroid gland illustrating follicles with retracted colloid and interspersed parafollicular (C) cells. Stain: hematoxylin and eosin. ×130.

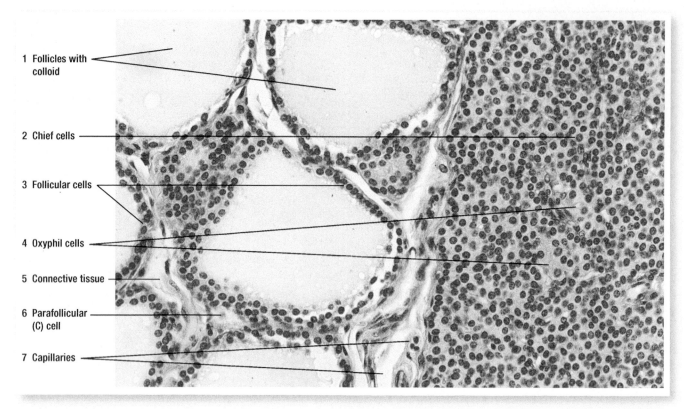

1 Follicles with colloid

2 Chief cells

3 Follicular cells

4 Oxyphil cells

5 Connective tissue

6 Parafollicular (C) cell

7 Capillaries

FIGURE 19.19 ■ A section of primate thyroid gland with colloid follicles adjacent to the parathyroid gland with oxyphil cells. Stain: hematoxylin and eosin. ×100.

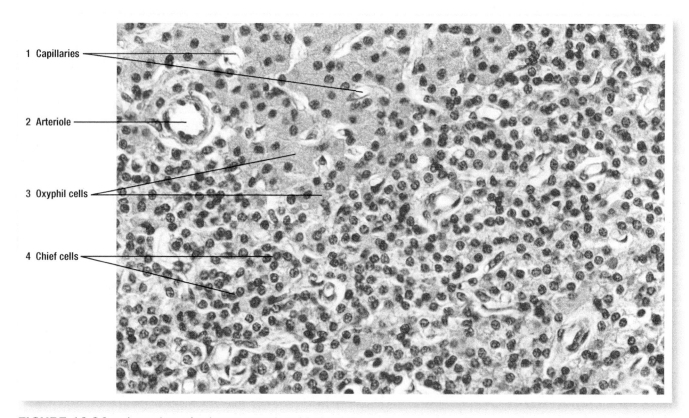

1 Capillaries

2 Arteriole

3 Oxyphil cells

4 Chief cells

FIGURE 19.20 ■ A section of primate parathyroid gland illustrating clumps of oxyphil cells among the chief cells. Stain: hematoxylin and eosin. ×100.

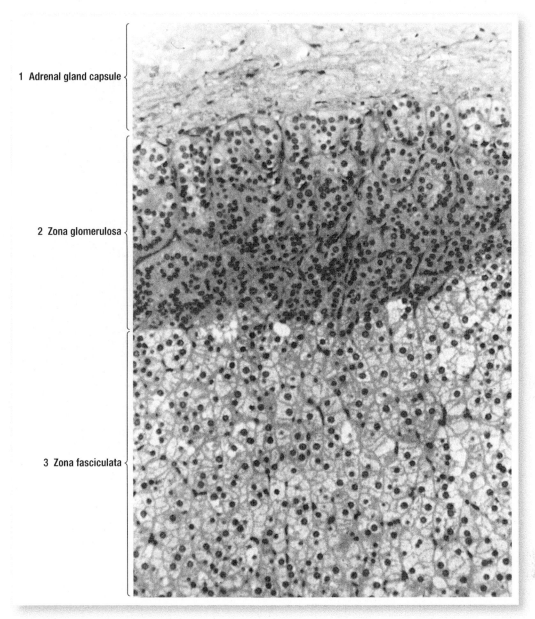

1 Adrenal gland capsule

2 Zona glomerulosa

3 Zona fasciculata

FIGURE 19.21 ■ Upper portion of a primate adrenal gland cortex illustrating the two top zones. Stain: hematoxylin and eosin. ×50.

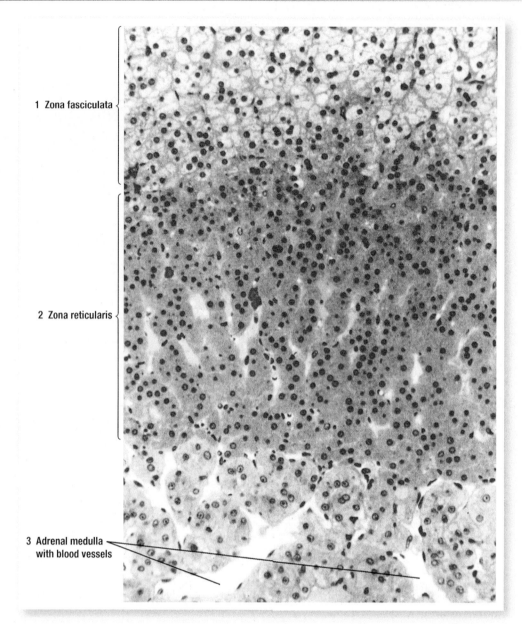

1 Zona fasciculata

2 Zona reticularis

3 Adrenal medulla
with blood vessels

FIGURE 19.22 ■ A section of primate adrenal cortex illustrating the lower two zones and a section of adrenal medulla. Stain: hematoxylin and eosin. ×50.

Male Reproductive System

SECTION 1 Testis

The male reproductive system consists of a pair of testes, numerous excurrent ducts, and accessory glands that produce secretions that are added to sperm to form semen. The **testis** (plural, testes) contains spermatogenic **stem cells** that continuously divide to produce new generations of cells that form **spermatozoa**, or **sperm**. From the testes, the sperm move through excurrent ducts to the **epididymis** for storage and maturation. During sexual excitation and ejaculation, sperm leave the epididymis via the **ductus (vas) deferens** and exit the reproductive system through the penile **urethra**.

The **accessory glands**—prostate gland, seminal vesicles, and bulbourethral glands—of the male reproductive system are discussed and illustrated in detail in Section 2.

SCROTUM

The testes are located outside the body cavity in the **scrotum** where the temperature of the testes is about 2°C to 3°C lower than the normal body temperature. This lower temperature is necessary for the normal functioning of the testes and **spermatogenesis**, or sperm production. In addition to the external location, perspiration and evaporation of sweat from the scrotal surface maintain the testes in a cooler environment. However, this lower temperature is not essential for hormone production by the testes.

Maintaining lower testicular temperature is also due to the arrangement of blood vessels that supply the testes. Testicular arteries that descend into the scrotum are surrounded by a plexus of veins that ascend from the testes and form the **pampiniform plexus**. Blood returning from the testes in the pampiniform plexus is cooler than the blood flowing in the arteries toward the testes. This **countercurrent heat-exchange mechanism** cools the arterial blood before it enters the testes and maintains a lower temperature in the testes.

TESTES

A thick connective tissue capsule, the **tunica albuginea**, surrounds each testis (Fig. 20.1). On the posterior side, the tunica albuginea thickens and extends inward into each testis to form the **mediastinum testis**. A thin connective tissue **septum** extends from the mediastinum testis and subdivides each testis into about 250 incomplete compartments or **testicular lobules**, each containing one to four highly coiled **seminiferous tubules**. Each seminiferous tubule is lined with a stratified **germinal epithelium**, containing proliferating **spermatogenic (germ) cells** and nonproliferating **supporting (sustentacular)**, or **Sertoli**, **cells**. The seminiferous tubules are the site of spermatogenic cell division, maturation, and transformation into sperm.

Surrounding each seminiferous tubule are fibroblasts, muscle-like cells, nerves, blood vessels, and lymphatic vessels. In addition, between the seminiferous tubules are clusters of epithelioid cells, the **interstitial cells (of Leydig)**. These cells are steroid-secreting cells that produce the male sex hormone **testosterone**.

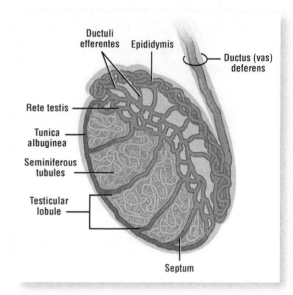

FIGURE 20.1 ■ Internal organization of the testis.

FORMATION OF SPERM: SPERMATOGENESIS

The process of sperm formation is called **spermatogenesis**. This process includes mitotic divisions of spermatogenic cells located at the base of the seminiferous tubules. Spermatogenic cells are subdivided into type A spermatogonia and type B spermatogonia. Dark type A spermatogonia are stem cells that continue to divide and give rise to other dark and pale type A spermatogonia. Pale type A spermatogonia replicate themselves and give rise to type B cells. Type B cells proliferate by mitosis and give rise to **primary spermatocytes**, which undergo the **first meiotic division** to produce **secondary spermatocytes**. The secondary spermatocytes complete the **second meiotic division** right away and produce round **spermatids**. During these meiotic divisions, there is a reduction in the number of chromosomes and the amount of DNA in each cell. After the completion of the second meiotic division, the spermatids now contain 23 single chromosomes (22 + X or 22 + Y). Spermatids do not continue to divide but instead undergo **spermiogenesis**, an extensive and complex morphological transformation of a round cell into an elongated sperm with a nucleus and a motile tail (flagellum). Upon fertilization of the egg by the sperm, the total normal number of chromosomes is restored to 46.

Once the spermatogenic cells in the germinal epithelium start to differentiate and begin to mature, they are held together by thin **intercellular or cytoplasmic bridges** during further development and differentiation. These intercellular bridges are broken when the developed spermatids are released (spermiation) into the fluid-filled seminiferous tubules as fully formed sperm from the luminal regions of the supportive Sertoli cells.

TRANSFORMATION OF SPERMATIDS: SPERMIOGENESIS

During spermiogenesis, the size and shape of the spherical spermatids are altered, the nuclear chromatin condenses, and the heads become elongated (Fig. 20.2). In the initial **Golgi phase**, small granules accumulate in the Golgi apparatus of the spermatids and form an **acrosomal granule** within a membrane-bound **acrosomal vesicle** next to the nuclear envelope. The location of the acrosomal vesicle indicates the anterior region of the developing sperm. During the **acrosomal phase**, both the acrosomal vesicle and the acrosomal granule spread over the anterior two thirds of the condensing spermatid nucleus as an **acrosome cap**. Also during this phase, centrioles migrate to the opposite or posterior pole of the spermatid and assemble the microtubules to form the sperm tail, or flagellum. The fully formed acrosome contains several hydrolytic enzymes, such as hyaluronidase, acid phosphatase, and protease with trypsin-like activity. The release of acrosomal enzymes assists the sperm in penetrating the cells (corona radiata) and the membrane (zona pellucida) that surrounds the ovulated oocyte and allows fertilization. During the **maturation phases**, the elongated spermatid heads are embedded in the cytoplasm of supportive Sertoli

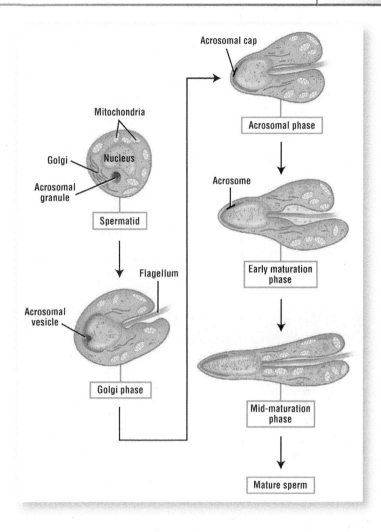

FIGURE 20.2 ■ The different phases of spermiogenesis.

cells. Also, the plasma membrane of the spermatid moves posterior from the nucleus to cover the developing **flagellum** (sperm tail), which now extends into the lumen of the seminiferous tubule. The mitochondria also migrate to and form a tight sheath around the middle piece of the developed flagellum. The final maturation phase is characterized by the shedding of the excess or **residual cytoplasm** of the spermatid and release of the sperm into the lumen of the seminiferous tubule. The supportive Sertoli cells then phagocytose the residual cytoplasm.

The mature sperm cell is composed of a **head** and an acrosome that surrounds the anterior portion of the nucleus, a **neck**, a **middle piece** characterized by the presence of a compact mitochondrial sheath, and a main or **principal piece** (Fig. 20.3).

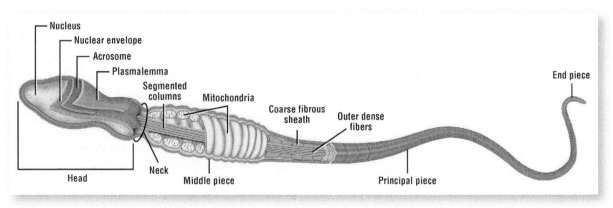

FIGURE 20.3 ■ The structure of a mature sperm.

EXCURRENT DUCTS

Newly released sperm are not motile and pass from the fluid in the seminiferous tubules into the fluid-filled intertesticular excurrent ducts that connect each testis with the overlying epididymis. These excurrent ducts consist of the **straight tubules** (tubuli recti) and the **rete testis**, the epithelial-lined channels in the mediastinum testis. From the rete testis, the sperm enter approximately 12 short tubules, the **ductuli efferentes** (efferent ducts), which conduct sperm from the rete testis to the initial segment or the head of the **epididymis**. The straight tubules are lined only by Sertoli cells, the rete testis lined by simple cuboidal/low columnar epithelium, and the ductuli efferentes lined by epithelium containing cuboidal nonciliated alternating with tall ciliated cells.

The extratesticular duct that conducts the sperm to the penile urethra is the **ductus epididymis**, which is continuous with the **ductus (vas) deferens** and **ejaculatory ducts** in the prostate gland. During sexual excitation and ejaculation, strong contractions of the **smooth muscle** that surrounds the **ductus epididymis** expel the sperm.

thePoint° Supplemental micrographic images are available at **www.thePoint.com/Eroschenko13e** under Male Reproductive System.

FUNCTIONAL CORRELATIONS 20.1 ■ Testes

SPERMATOGONIA

The two primary functions of the testes are the production of **sperm** (spermatogenesis) and the synthesis of the male sex hormone **testosterone**. Testosterone is an essential hormone for the development and maintenance of male sexual characteristics and normal functioning of the accessory reproductive glands.

The spermatogenic cells in the seminiferous tubules divide, differentiate, and produce sperm by a process called **spermatogenesis**. This process involves the following:

• Mitotic divisions of spermatogonia to form stem cells

• Formation of **primary** and **secondary spermatocytes** from spermatogenic cells

• **Meiotic divisions** of both primary and secondary spermatocytes to reduce the somatic chromosome numbers by one-half and formation of **spermatids** with only 23 single chromosomes (22 + X or 22 + Y)

• Morphologic transformation of round spermatids into mature, elongated sperm by a process called **spermiogenesis**

SUPPORTIVE SERTOLI CELLS

Sertoli cells are the supportive cells of the testes that are located among the spermatogenic cells in the seminiferous tubules. They adhere to the basal lamina in the tubules with their apices extending into the lumen. They perform numerous important functions in the testes, among which are the following:

• Physical support, protection, and nutrition of the developing spermatogenic cells.

• Phagocytosis of excess cytoplasm (residual bodies) from the developing spermatids as well as degenerating germ cells.

• Facilitate release of mature sperm, called spermiation, into the lumen of seminiferous tubules containing fluid produced by Sertoli cells.

• Secretion of fructose-rich testicular fluid for the nourishment and transport of sperm to the excurrent ducts.

• Production and release of androgen-binding protein (ABP) that binds to testosterone and increases the concentration of testosterone in the lumen of the seminiferous tubules necessary for spermatogenesis; ABP secretion is under the control of follicle-stimulating hormone (FSH) from the pituitary gland to which Sertoli cells respond.

• Secretion of the hormone inhibin, which suppresses the release of FSH from the pituitary gland.

• Production and release of the anti-Müllerian hormone, also called Müllerian-inhibiting hormone, that suppresses the development of Müllerian ducts in the male and inhibits the development of female reproductive organs.

BLOOD–TESTIS BARRIER

The adjacent cytoplasm of Sertoli cells is joined by occluding **tight junctions** (zonula occludens) producing a **blood–testis barrier** that subdivides each seminiferous tubule into a **basal compartment** and an **adluminal compartment**. This important barrier segregates the spermatogonia from all successive stages of spermatogenesis in the adluminal

FUNCTIONAL CORRELATIONS 20.1 ■ Testes (*Continued*)

compartment and excludes plasma proteins and bloodborne antibodies from the lumen of seminiferous tubules. The more advanced spermatogenic cells can be recognized by the body as foreign and cause an immune response. The blood–testis barrier protects developing cells from the immune system by restricting the passage of membrane **antigens** from developing sperm into the bloodstream. Thus, the blood–testis barrier prevents an autoimmune response to the individual's own sperm, antibody formation, and eventual destruction of spermatogenesis and induction of sterility. The blood–testis barrier also keeps harmful substances in the blood from entering the developing germinal epithelium.

FIGURE 20.4 | Peripheral Section of Testis (Sectional View)

Each testis is enclosed in a thick, connective tissue capsule called **tunica albuginea** (**1**), internal to which is a vascular layer of loose connective tissue called **tunica vasculosa** (**2, 8**). The connective tissue from the tunica vasculosa (2, 8) extends into the testis and forms the **interstitial connective tissue** (**3, 12**) that surrounds, binds, and supports the **seminiferous tubules** (**4, 6, 9**). Extending from the mediastinum testis (see Fig. 20.10) toward the tunica albuginea (1) are thin fibrous **septa** (**7, 10**) (singular, septum) that divide the testis into compartments called lobules containing one to four seminiferous tubules (4, 6, 9). The septa (7, 10) are not solid, allowing intercommunication between lobules.

Within the interstitial connective tissue (3, 12) are **blood vessels** (**13**), loose connective tissue cells, and clusters of endocrine **interstitial cells (of Leydig)** (**5, 11**) that secrete the male sex hormone testosterone.

The seminiferous tubules (4, 6, 9) are long, convoluted tubules that are normally observed cut in transverse (4), longitudinal (6), or tangential (9) planes of section. These tubules (4, 6, 9) are lined with a stratified epithelium called the **germinal epithelium** (**14**) that contains two major cell types: the spermatogenic cells that produce sperm and the supportive Sertoli cells that nourish them. The germinal epithelium (14) rests on the basement membrane of the seminiferous tubules (4, 6, 9) with its cells illustrated in greater detail in Figures 20.5 to 20.8.

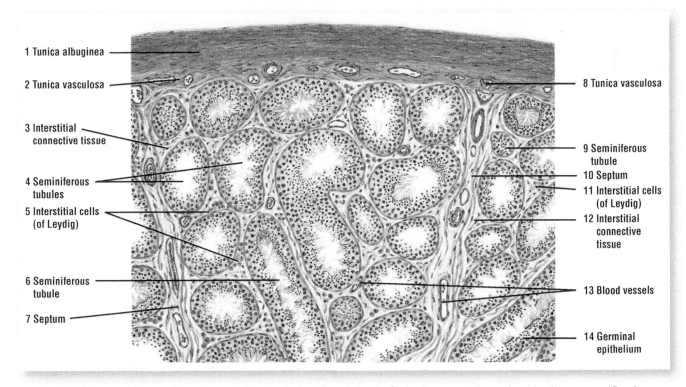

1 Tunica albuginea
2 Tunica vasculosa
3 Interstitial connective tissue
4 Seminiferous tubules
5 Interstitial cells (of Leydig)
6 Seminiferous tubule
7 Septum

8 Tunica vasculosa
9 Seminiferous tubule
10 Septum
11 Interstitial cells (of Leydig)
12 Interstitial connective tissue
13 Blood vessels
14 Germinal epithelium

FIGURE 20.4 ■ Peripheral section of the testis (sectional view). Stain: hematoxylin and eosin. Low magnification.

FIGURE 20.5 | Testis: Seminiferous Tubules (Transverse Section)

This photomicrograph illustrates a **seminiferous tubule** (5) and adjacent seminiferous tubules lined by a thick germinal epithelium.

The **dark type A** (1a) and the **pale type B** (1b) **spermatogonia** (1) are located at the base of the tubule. The **primary spermatocytes** (2) and **spermatids** (7) in different stages of maturation are embedded in the germinal epithelium closer to the lumen. The tails of the developing spermatids (7) protrude into the lumen of the seminiferous tubules (5). The supportive **Sertoli cells** (6) are prominent and located throughout the germinal epithelium.

Each seminiferous tubule (5) is surrounded by a fibromuscular interstitial **connective tissue** (3) that also contains the testosterone-secreting **interstitial cells** (4).

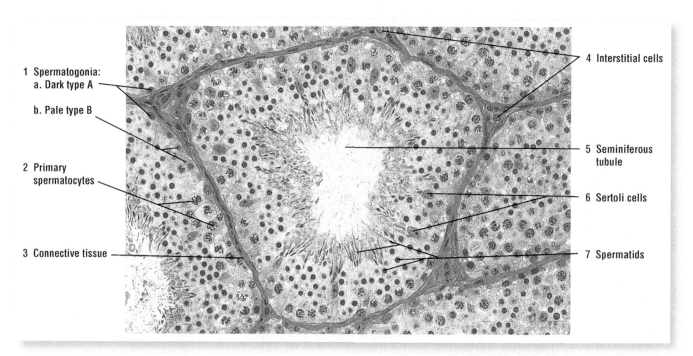

1 Spermatogonia:
  a. Dark type A
  b. Pale type B

2 Primary spermatocytes

3 Connective tissue

4 Interstitial cells

5 Seminiferous tubule

6 Sertoli cells

7 Spermatids

FIGURE 20.5 ■ Testis: seminiferous tubules (transverse section). Stain: hematoxylin and eosin (plastic section). ×80.

A higher magnification of a **seminiferous tubule** (8) allows identification of different cell types. Each seminiferous tubule (8) is surrounded by a layer of connective tissue with **fibrocytes** (11) and an inner **basement membrane** (3). Between each seminiferous tubules (8) are interstitial fibrocytes (11), **blood vessels** (5), nerves, lymphatic vessels, and the testosterone-producing **interstitial cells (of Leydig)** (1, 12).

The stratified germinal epithelium consists of supporting or **Sertoli cells** (6, 10) and different **spermatogenic cells** (7). Sertoli cells (6, 10) are elongated cells with irregular outlines that extend from the basement membrane (3) to the lumen of the seminiferous tubule (8). The nuclei of Sertoli cells (6, 10) are ovoid, or elongated, and contain fine, sparse chromatin. A distinct and dense-staining nucleolus distinguishes Sertoli cells (6, 10) from the spermatogenic cells (7).

The immature spermatogenic cells, the **spermatogonia** (7), are adjacent to the basement membrane (3) and divide mitotically to produce two types of spermatogonia: The **pale type A spermatogonia** (7b) have a light-staining cytoplasm and a round or ovoid nucleus with pale, finely granular chromatin; and the **dark type A spermatogonia** (7a) with darker chromatin.

Type A spermatogonia (7a) serve as stem cells for the germinal epithelium and give rise to type A and type B spermatogonia. The final mitotic division of type B spermatogonia produces **primary spermatocytes** (2, 9).

The primary spermatocytes (2, 9) are the largest germ cells in the seminiferous tubules (8) and occupy the middle region of the germinal epithelium. Their cytoplasm contains large nuclei with coarse clumps or thin threads of chromatin. The first meiotic division of the primary spermatocytes (Fig. 20.8, I, 5) produces smaller secondary spermatocytes with less-dense nuclear

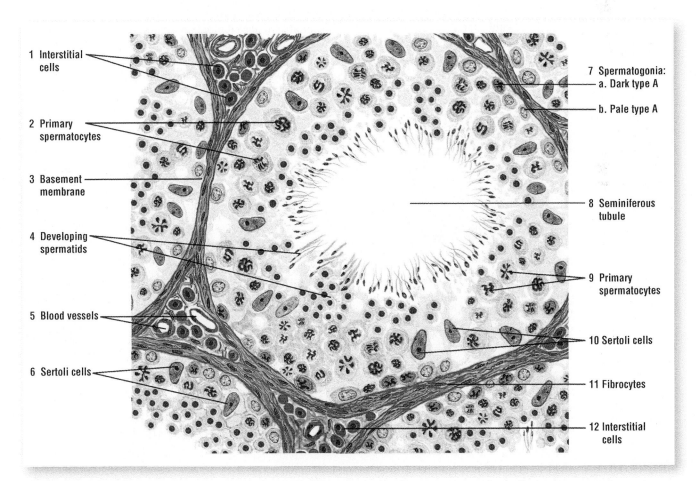

FIGURE 20.6 ■ Testis: spermatogenesis in seminiferous tubules (transverse section). Stain: hematoxylin and eosin. Medium magnification.

chromatin (Fig. 20.8, I, 3). Because the secondary spermatocytes undergo a second meiotic division shortly after their formation, they are infrequently seen in the seminiferous tubules (8).

The second meiotic division produces smaller **spermatids** (**4**) (Fig. 20.8, I, 2) that are grouped in the adluminal compartment of the seminiferous tubule (8) and closely associated with supportive Sertoli cells (6, 10). The more mature spermatids (4, *upper leader*) are located in the periphery of the germinal epithelium with their nuclei condensed and elongated and their tails extending into the lumen of the seminiferous tubule (8). The more immature spermatids (4, *lower leader*) are round cells with dense-staining round nuclei that are located deeper in the germinal epithelium. All developing spermatids (4) are embedded in the Sertoli cell (6, 10) cytoplasm and are grouped in the adluminal compartment of the seminiferous tubule (8). Here, the spermatids (4) differentiate through spermiogenesis and are released into seminiferous tubules (8) as sperm.

FIGURE 20.7 | **Cross Section of Seminiferous Tubules Showing Supportive Sertoli Cells, Spermatogonia, and Spermatids in Different Stages of Development**

This higher-magnification photomicrograph shows in greater detail the cells in and around the seminiferous tubules. In the central tubule, the germinal epithelium exhibits the largest cells, the **primary spermatocytes** (**3**). In the right tubule are the developing early **spermatids** (**10**) with dense, round nuclei. The central tubule contains the elongated and dense-staining nuclei of **late spermatids** (**6**) with their tails extending into the **lumen of the seminiferous tubule** (**5**). At the base of the germinal epithelium are the **dark type A** (**4**) and **pale type A spermatogonia** (**7**). Also visible are the very distinct **Sertoli cells** (**9, 12**) with oval nucleus and a characteristic dense-staining nucleolus. Sertoli cell cytoplasm extends from the base of the germinal epithelium to the lumen of the seminiferous tubule (5). Embedded within the Sertoli cell (9, 12) cytoplasm are the developing spermatocytes (3) and spermatids (6, 10). Surrounding the seminiferous tubules is a **basement membrane** (**11**) and the flattened **fibrocytes** (**8**). Located also between the seminiferous tubules are the testosterone-secreting **interstitial cells** (**of Leydig**) (**1, 13**), some of which are located adjacent to a **capillary** (**2**).

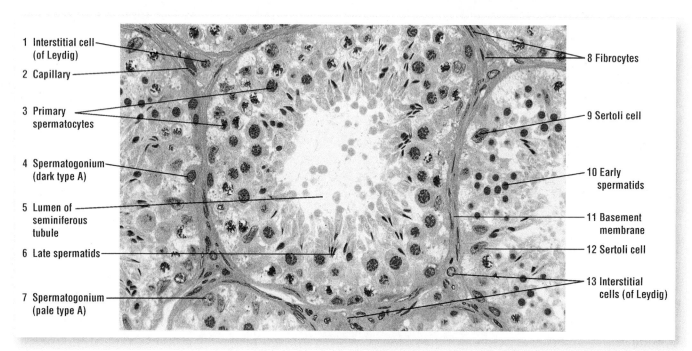

1 Interstitial cell (of Leydig)
2 Capillary
3 Primary spermatocytes
4 Spermatogonium (dark type A)
5 Lumen of seminiferous tubule
6 Late spermatids
7 Spermatogonium (pale type A)
8 Fibrocytes
9 Sertoli cell
10 Early spermatids
11 Basement membrane
12 Sertoli cell
13 Interstitial cells (of Leydig)

FIGURE 20.7 ■ Cross section of seminiferous tubules showing supportive Sertoli cells, spermatogonia, and spermatids in different stages of development. Stain: hematoxylin and eosin. Plastic section. ×125.

FIGURE 20.8 | Primate Testis: Different Stages of Spermatogenesis

Three stages of spermatogenesis are illustrated. In the left illustration (I), the large **primary spermatocytes (5)** divide to form smaller **secondary spermatocytes (3)**, which undergo rapid meiotic division to produce the **spermatids (1, 2)**. Both the early spermatids (2) and the mature spermatids (1) become embedded deep in the **Sertoli cell (4)** cytoplasm. Located at the base of the seminiferous tubule are the **dark** and **pale type A spermatogonia (6)**.

In the middle illustration (II), the **spermatids (7)** are near the lumen of the seminiferous tubule before their release. Also the early, round **spermatids (8)** and the large **primary spermatocytes (9)** are associated with the **Sertoli cells (10)**. Near the base of the seminiferous tubule are the **spermatogonia (11)**.

In the right illustration (III), the mature spermatids have been released as sperm (spermiation) into the seminiferous tubule, and the germinal epithelium contains only early **spermatids (8)**, **primary spermatocytes (9)**, **spermatogonia (11)**, and the supporting **Sertoli cells (10)**.

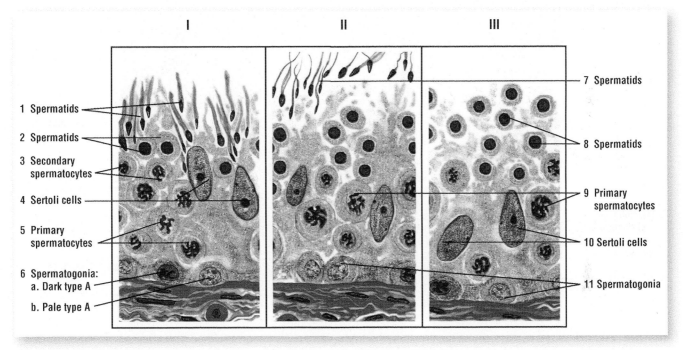

FIGURE 20.8 ■ Primate testis: different stages of spermatogenesis. Stain: hematoxylin and eosin. High magnification.

FIGURE 20.9 | Ultrastructure of Sertoli Cell and Surrounding Cells

In the center of this ultrastructure image is the **Sertoli cell cytoplasm** (1), the distinctive **Sertoli cell nucleus** (2), and the dense **Sertoli cell nucleolus** (9). A section of an **early spermatid** (7) with the **Golgi complex** (8) is seen on the right of the Sertoli cell. A distinct **junctional complex** (3, 10) between adjacent Sertoli cells forms the blood–testis barrier that separates the germinal epithelium into basal and adluminal compartments. Located below the Sertoli cell (1, 2, 9) is a thin **basal lamina** (4) adjacent to the thicker basement membrane (11). On the other side of the basement membrane (11) is the **interstitial cell of Leydig** (5) filled with **smooth endoplasmic reticulum** and **mitochondria** (12) with round cristae. At the bottom left-hand corner is a section of cytoplasm and nucleus of what appears to be a **spermatogonium** (6) of an adjacent seminiferous tubule.

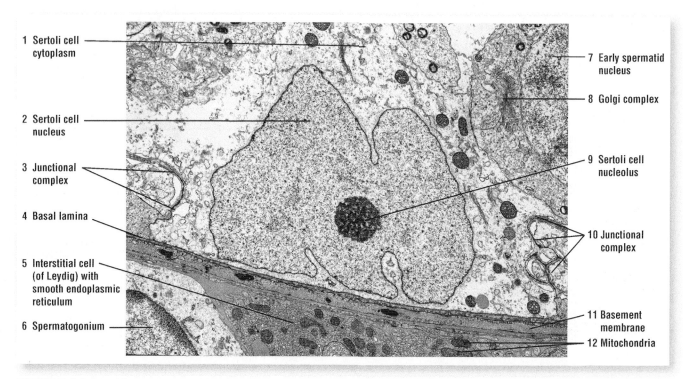

1 Sertoli cell cytoplasm
2 Sertoli cell nucleus
3 Junctional complex
4 Basal lamina
5 Interstitial cell (of Leydig) with smooth endoplasmic reticulum
6 Spermatogonium
7 Early spermatid nucleus
8 Golgi complex
9 Sertoli cell nucleolus
10 Junctional complex
11 Basement membrane
12 Mitochondria

FIGURE 20.9 ■ Ultrastructure of a Sertoli cell and surrounding cells. Courtesy of Dr. Rex A. Hess, Professor Emeritus, Comparative Biosciences, College of Veterinary Medicine, University of Illinois, Urbana, IL. ×8,100.

FIGURE 20.10 | Seminiferous Tubules, Straight Tubules, Rete Testis, and Ductuli Efferentes (Efferent Ductules)

In the posterior region of the testis, the tunica albuginea extends into the testis as the **mediastinum testis** (**10, 16**). In this illustration, the plane of section passes through the **seminiferous tubules** (**3, 5**), the connective tissue and blood vessels of the mediastinum testis (10, 16), and the excretory ducts, the **ductuli efferentes** (**efferent ductules**) (**9, 13**).

A few seminiferous tubules (3, 5) are visible on the left side. The tubules (3, 5) are lined with spermatogenic epithelium and sustentacular Sertoli cells. The **interstitial connective tissue** (**4**) is continuous with the mediastinum testis (10, 16) and contains the steroid (testosterone)-producing **interstitial cells** (**of Leydig**) (**1**). In the mediastinum testis (10, 16), the seminiferous tubules (3, 5) terminate in the **straight tubules** (**2, 6**) that are short, narrow ducts lined with a cuboidal or low columnar epithelium that are lined only by Sertoli cells.

The straight tubules (2, 6) continue into the **rete testis** (**7, 8, 12**) of the mediastinum testis (10, 16). The rete testis (7, 8, 12) is an anastomosing network of tubules with wide lumina lined with a simple cuboidal/low columnar epithelium. The rete testis (7, 8, 12) widens near the ductuli efferentes (efferent ductules) (9, 13) into which they empty. The ductuli efferentes (9, 13) are initially straight but become convoluted in the head of the ductus epididymis. The ductuli efferentes (9, 13) connect the rete testis (7, 8, 12) to the epididymis (see Fig. 20.11). Some tubules in the rete testis (12) and ductuli efferentes (9, 13) contain accumulations of **sperm** (**11, 14**).

The epithelium of the ductuli efferentes (9, 13) consists of columnar ciliated cells that alternate with shorter cuboidal cells with microvilli. Because of the alternating cell heights, the lining epithelium of the ductuli efferentes appears uneven.

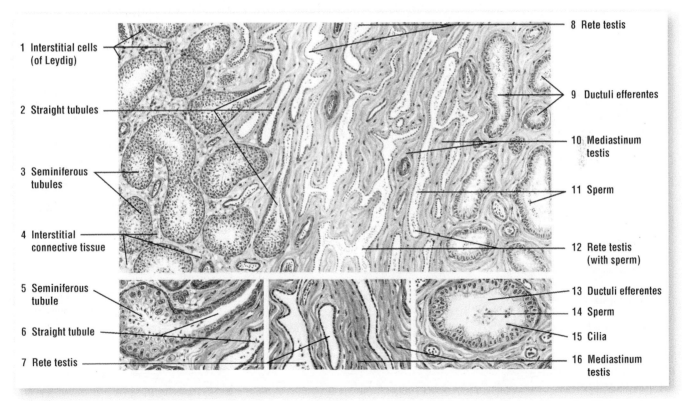

1 Interstitial cells (of Leydig)
2 Straight tubules
3 Seminiferous tubules
4 Interstitial connective tissue
5 Seminiferous tubule
6 Straight tubule
7 Rete testis
8 Rete testis
9 Ductuli efferentes
10 Mediastinum testis
11 Sperm
12 Rete testis (with sperm)
13 Ductuli efferentes
14 Sperm
15 Cilia
16 Mediastinum testis

FIGURE 20.10 ■ Seminiferous tubules, straight tubules, rete testis, and efferent ductules (ductuli efferentes). Stain: hematoxylin and eosin. Low magnification (*inset:* high magnification).

FUNCTIONAL CORRELATIONS 20.2 ■ Hormones of Male Reproductive Organs

Normal maintenance of spermatogenesis in adult testes depends on two hormones: **follicle-stimulating hormone** (**FSH**) and **luteinizing hormone** (**LH**), also called **interstitial cell–stimulating hormone** (**ICSH**). The neurons in the hypothalamus secrete **gonadotropin-releasing hormone** (GnRH) that stimulates the **gonadotrophs** in the adenohypophysis of the pituitary gland to synthesize and release LH. Normal spermatogenesis depends on LH, which binds to LH receptors on **interstitial cells** (**of Leydig**) and stimulates the synthesis of **testosterone**. FSH is also produced by gonadotrophs in the pituitary gland. FSH stimulates **Sertoli cells** to synthesize and release **androgen-binding protein** (**ABP**) into the seminiferous tubules, where it combines with and increases testosterone concentration in the vicinity of the developing spermatogenic cells, which then stimulates normal spermatogenesis. An increased concentration of testosterone in the seminiferous tubules is essential for spermatogenesis. In addition, the structure and function of the accessory reproductive glands, as well as the development and maintenance of male secondary sexual characteristics, are dependent on proper testosterone levels.

An excessive level of testosterone produces an **inhibitory effect** on the hypothalamic neurons and the hypophyseal cell release of additional FSH by the hormone **inhibin** that is also secreted by the Sertoli cells. Sertoli cells also produce **activin** that exerts an opposite and positive effect on FSH release.

FIGURE 20.11 | Ductuli Efferentes and Tubules of Ductus Epididymis

The **ductuli efferentes** (**1**), or efferent ductules, emerge from the mediastinum on the postero-superior surface of the testis and connect the rete testis with the ductus epididymis. The ductuli efferentes are located in the **connective tissue** (**2**, **12**) and form a portion of the head of the epididymis.

The lumen of the ductuli efferentes (**1**) exhibits an irregular contour because the epithelium consists of alternating groups of columnar **ciliated** and cuboidal **nonciliated cells** with microvilli. Located inferior to the basement membrane is a layer of connective tissue (**2**) with a **smooth muscle layer** (**5**, **11**). As the ductuli efferentes (**1**) terminate in the ductus epididymis, the lumina are lined with the **pseudostratified columnar epithelium** (**6**, **8**).

The **ductus epididymis** (**3**, **4**) illustrated in both **cross** (**3**) and **longitudinal sections** (**4**) is a long, convoluted tubule surrounded by connective tissue (**2**) and a thin smooth muscle layer (**5**, **11**). Some parts of the ductus contain mature **sperm** (**7**).

The pseudostratified columnar epithelium (**6**, **8**) consists of columnar **principal cells** (**9**) with long, modified nonmotile microvilli called **stereocilia** (**8**) and small **basal cells** (**10**).

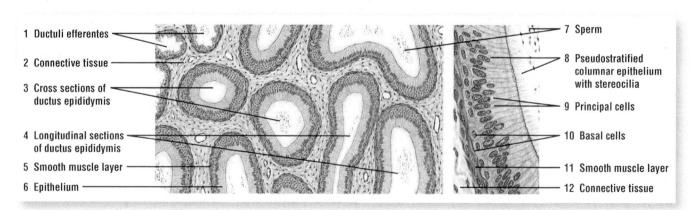

1 Ductuli efferentes
2 Connective tissue
3 Cross sections of ductus epididymis
4 Longitudinal sections of ductus epididymis
5 Smooth muscle layer
6 Epithelium
7 Sperm
8 Pseudostratified columnar epithelium with stereocilia
9 Principal cells
10 Basal cells
11 Smooth muscle layer
12 Connective tissue

FIGURE 20.11 ■ Ductuli efferentes and tubules of the ductus epididymis. Stain: hematoxylin and eosin. *Left*, low magnification; *right*, high magnification.

FIGURE 20.12 | Tubules of Ductus Epididymis (Transverse Section)

This photomicrograph illustrates the tubules of the ductus epididymis, some of which are filled with **sperm** (1). The tubules are lined with a **pseudostratified epithelium** (2). The **principal cells** (**2a**) are tall columnar epithelium and are lined with **stereocilia** (5). The **basal cells** (**2b**) are small, spherical, and situated near the base of the epithelium. A thin layer of **smooth muscle** (3) surrounds each tubule with adjacent cells and fibers of the **connective tissue** (4).

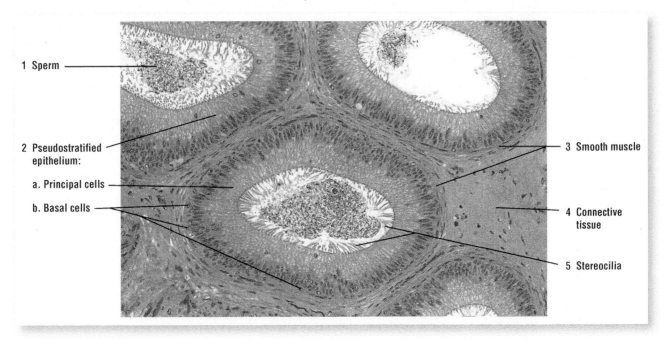

FIGURE 20.12 ■ Tubules of the ductus epididymis (transverse section). Stain: hematoxylin and eosin (plastic section). ×50.

FIGURE 20.13 | Ductus (Vas) Deferens (Transverse Section)

The ductus (vas) deferens exhibits a narrow and irregular lumen with **longitudinal mucosal folds** (6), a thin mucosa, a thick muscularis, and an adventitia.

The lumen of the ductus deferens is lined with a **pseudostratified columnar epithelium** (8) with stereocilia. The epithelium of the ductus deferens is lower than in the ductus epididymis.

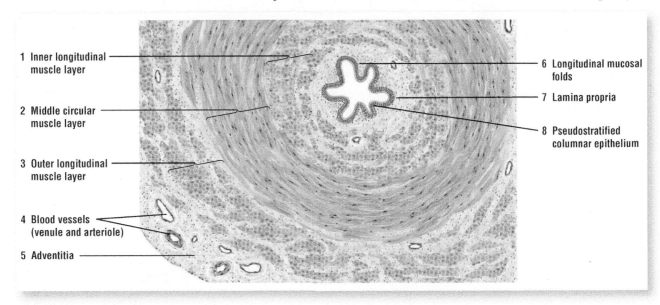

FIGURE 20.13 ■ Ductus (vas) deferens (transverse section). Stain: hematoxylin and eosin. Low magnification.

The underlying thin **lamina propria** (**7**) consists of compact collagen fibers and a network of elastic fibers.

The thick muscularis consists of three smooth muscle layers: a thinner **inner longitudinal layer** (**1**), a thick **middle circular layer** (**2**), and a thinner **outer longitudinal layer** (**3**). The muscularis is surrounded by **adventitia** (**5**) in which are found abundant **blood vessels** (**venule and arteriole**) (**4**) and nerves. The adventitia (**5**) of the ductus deferens merges with the connective tissue of the spermatic cord.

FIGURE 20.14 | Ampulla of Ductus (Vas) Deferens (Transverse Section)

The terminal portion of the ductus deferens enlarges into an ampulla that differs from the ductus deferens in the structure of its mucosa.

The **lumen** (**3**) of the ampulla is larger than that of the ductus deferens. The mucosa exhibits irregular, branching **mucosal folds** (**4**) and deep **glandular diverticula** or **crypts** (**1**) located between the folds that extend to the surrounding muscle layer. The secretory epithelium that lines the lumen (**3**) and the glandular diverticula (**1**) is simple columnar or cuboidal. Below the epithelium is the **lamina propria** (**6**).

The smooth muscle layers in the muscularis are similar to those in the ductus deferens. These consist of a thin **inner longitudinal muscle layer** (**7**), a **thick middle circular muscle layer** (**8**), and a thin **outer longitudinal muscle layer** (**9**). Surrounding the ampulla is the connective tissue **adventitia** (**5**).

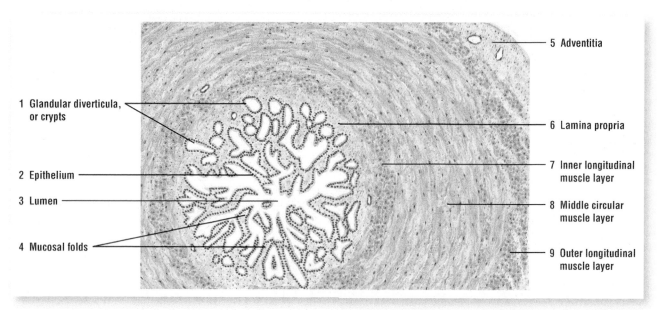

FIGURE 20.14 ■ Ampulla of the ductus (vas) deferens (transverse section). Stain: hematoxylin and eosin. Low magnification.

FUNCTIONAL CORRELATIONS 20.3 ■ **Excurrent Ducts of Testes**

DUCTULI EFFERENTES (EFFERENT DUCTULES)

The sperm leave the straight tubules and enter the rete testis. The motility of cilia in the **ductuli efferentes** creates a current that assists in transporting the fluid and sperm from the seminiferous tubules of the testes to the **ductus epididymis**. In addition, the contractility of the smooth muscle fibers that surround the ductules efferentes assists movement of the sperm into the ductus epididymis. The nonciliated cuboidal cells in the ductuli efferentes absorb most of the testicular fluid that was produced in the seminiferous tubules by Sertoli cells.

DUCTUS EPIDIDYMIS

The coiled ductus epididymis is the site for **accumulation**, **storage**, and further **maturation** of sperm. Upon entering the epididymis, the sperm are nonmotile and incapable of fertilizing an oocyte. However, during their passage through the tubules of the ductus epididymis, the sperm acquire motility, maturation of the acrosome, and the ability to fertilize an oocyte. The maturation process of the sperm is dependent on the proper levels of testosterone.

The **principal cells** in the ductus epididymis are lined with long microvilli, or **stereocilia**, that absorb testicular fluid that was not absorbed in the ductuli efferentes during sperm passage from the testes. In addition, the principal cells phagocytose abnormal or degenerating sperm cells and residual bodies that were not removed by the Sertoli cells in the seminiferous tubules. The principal cells in the ductus epididymis also produce a glycolipid **decapacitation factor** that binds to the surface of the sperm membrane. Decapacitation factor **inhibits capacitation**, or the fertilizing ability of the sperm, until the sperm are deposited into the female reproductive tract and this factor is removed.

The sperm are activated within the female reproductive tract by a process called **capacitation**. This action increases the sperm's affinity for fertilizing an oocyte by allowing the sperm to bind with sperm receptors on the zona pellucida of the ovulated oocyte. This produces an **acrosomal reaction** that releases the acrosomal enzymes, which disperse the cells that surround the ovulated oocyte, digest and penetrate the zona pellucida around the oocyte, and fertilize the ovum.

Chapter 20 Summary

SECTION 1 • Testis

- Consists of two testes that contain spermatogenic cells, which produce sperm
- Numerous excurrent ducts move sperm for storage and maturation into ductus epididymis
- During ejaculation, sperm leave system via ductus (vas) deferens and penile urethra
- Accessory glands include prostate, seminal vesicles, and bulbourethral glands

SCROTUM

- Testes located outside the body cavity in scrotum whose temperature is 2°C to 3°C lower than the body temperature
- Lower temperature in scrotum because of sweat evaporation and pampiniform plexus
- Countercurrent heat-exchange mechanism cools arterial blood as it enters the testes

TESTES

- Thick connective tissue tunica albuginea surrounds testes and forms mediastinum testis
- Thin connective tissue septa from mediastinum testis separate testis into testicular lobules
- Testicular lobules contain coiled seminiferous tubules lined with germinal epithelium
- Germinal epithelium contains spermatogenic cells and Sertoli (supportive) cells
- Between seminiferous tubules are testosterone-secreting interstitial cells (of Leydig)

FORMATION OF SPERM: SPERMATOGENESIS

- Includes mitotic divisions of spermatogenic cells to form type A and type B stem cells
- Type B spermatogenic cells give rise to primary spermatocytes, the largest cells in tubules
- Primary spermatocytes give rise to smaller secondary spermatocytes
- Meiotic divisions of spermatocytes reduce number of chromosomes and amount of DNA
- Secondary spermatocytes divide to form spermatids
- Spermatids do not divide and contain 23 single chromosomes (22 + X or 22 + Y)
- Spermatids undergo a morphologic transformation called spermiogenesis
- Spermatids connected by intercellular bridges until released as mature sperm into the tubules

TRANSFORMATION OF SPERMATIDS: SPERMIOGENESIS

- Size and shape of round spermatids altered, with condensation of nuclear chromatin
- On one side, acrosome granules in vesicle spread over the condensing nucleus as acrosome
- Acrosome contains hydrolytic enzymes needed to penetrate cells that surround the oocyte
- On the opposite side of acrosome, flagellum (tail) forms with mitochondria aggregating at middle piece
- Residual cytoplasm shed from spermatids and phagocytosed by Sertoli cells
- Mature sperm consists of head, neck, middle piece, and principal piece

EXCURRENT DUCTS

- Released nonmotile sperm enter straight tubules and rete testis to ductuli efferentes
- Ductuli efferentes in mediastinum conduct sperm to head of ductus epididymis
- Epithelium lining ductuli efferentes is ciliated and nonciliated
- Cilia in ductuli efferentes move sperm and fluid from seminiferous tubules to ductus epididymis
- Nonciliated cells absorb much of the testicular fluid as it passes to ductus epididymis
- Ductus epididymis is continuous with ductus (vas) deferens that conducts sperm to penile urethra
- Smooth muscles around ductuli efferentes, ductus epididymis, and vas deferens contract to move sperm
- Pseudostratified epithelium with principal and basal cells lines ductuli efferentes and epididymis
- Stereocilia line the surface of cells in ductus epididymis and vas deferens
- Stereocilia absorb testicular fluid, and the principal cells phagocytose residual cytoplasm
- Principal cells in the ductus epididymis also produce glycolipid decapacitation factor
- Decapacitation inhibits the fertilizing ability of sperm until removed in the female reproductive tract

- Activation of sperm is capacitation, allowing sperm to bind to the ovulated oocyte and fertilize it
- Acrosomal reaction releases acrosomal enzymes to assist sperm penetration of the ovum

SERTOLI CELLS

- Physical support, protection, nutrition, and release of mature sperm into tubules
- Secretion of fluid for sperm nutrition and transport of sperm to excurrent ducts
- Phagocytosis of residual cytoplasm of spermatids
- Secretion of androgen-binding protein to concentrate testosterone in tubules and testicular fluid for sperm transport
- Secretion of hormones inhibin, activin, and anti-Müllerian hormone

BLOOD–TESTIS BARRIER

- Formed by tight junctions of adjacent Sertoli cells
- Separates seminiferous tubules in basal and adluminal compartments

- Protects developing sperm from autoimmune response and harmful materials

MALE HORMONES

- Spermatogenesis dependent on luteinizing and follicle-stimulating hormones produced by the pituitary gland
- Luteinizing hormone binds to receptors on interstitial cells and stimulates testosterone secretion
- Follicle-stimulating hormone stimulates Sertoli cells to produce androgen-binding hormone into seminiferous tubules to bind testosterone
- Testosterone in seminiferous tubules is vital for spermatogenesis and accessory gland function
- Sertoli cells produce inhibin to inhibit FSH production and activin to release FSH from pituitary gland via negative feedback

Chapter 20 Review Questions: Section 1

QUESTIONS

In the following multiple choice questions, choose the letter corresponding to the one best answer.

1. What cells form the blood–testis barrier?

A. Spermatogonia
B. Spermatocytes
C. Capillary endothelial cells
D. Sertoli cells
E. Interstitial cells (of Leydig)

2. What important role does the blood–testis barrier perform in the male reproductive system?

A. It prevents the passage of testosterone into the seminiferous tubules.
B. It prevents an autoimmune response to sperm and induction of infertility.
C. It separates spermatocytes from Sertoli cells.
D. It separates the interstitial cells from the capillary network.
E. It forms tight junctions in the endothelial capillaries near the seminiferous tubules.

3. Which hormone is essential for maintaining accessory reproductive organs?

A. Testosterone
B. Androgen-binding protein
C. Inhibin
D. Luteinizing hormone
E. Sertoli cell hormone

4. When the sperm enter the epididymis:

A. they are motile and can fertilize an oocyte.
B. they undergo further spermiogenesis and development.
C. they are nonmotile and incapable of fertilizing an oocyte.
D. additional fluid is added to increase their motility.
E. stereocilia motility increases sperm motility.

5. Where do the sperm become activated and able to fertilize an oocyte?

A. In the testis
B. In the epididymis
C. In the efferent ducts
D. In the female reproductive tract
E. In the seminiferous tubules

ANSWERS

1. Correct Answer: D. Sertoli cells. Their tight junctions separate the seminiferous tubules into adluminal and basal compartments to protect the developing sperm from an autoimmune response.

2. Correct Answer: B. It prevents an autoimmune response to sperm and induction of infertility.

3. Correct Answer: A. Testosterone. This hormone is essential for spermatogenesis, maintenance of accessory reproductive organs, and secondary sex characteristics in males.

4. Correct Answer: C. They are nonmotile and incapable of fertilizing an oocyte. Further maturation is necessary in the epididymis before full maturity and fertilizing ability.

5. Correct Answer: D. In the female reproductive tract. Here, they are activated by a process of capacitation, at which time the decapacitation factor is removed and the sperm can fertilize the ovulated oocyte.

SECTION 2 Accessory Reproductive Sex Glands

The accessory glands of the male reproductive system consist of paired **seminal vesicles**, paired **bulbourethral glands**, and a single **prostate gland** (Fig. 20.15). These structures produce secretory products that mix with sperm to produce **semen**. The penis serves as the copulatory organ, and the penile urethra serves as a common passageway for urine or semen.

The seminal vesicles are located posterior to the bladder and superior to the prostate gland. The excretory duct of each seminal vesicle joins the dilated terminal part of each ductus (vas) deferens, the **ampulla**, to form the **ejaculatory ducts** that enter and continue through the prostate gland into the **prostatic urethra**.

The prostate gland is located inferior to the neck of the bladder. The urethra exits the bladder and passes through the prostate gland as the **prostatic urethra**. In addition to the ejaculatory ducts, excretory ducts from prostatic glands also open into the prostatic urethra.

The bulbourethral glands are small, pea-sized glands located at the root of the **penis** and embedded in the skeletal muscles of the urogenital diaphragm; their excretory ducts terminate in the proximal portion of the **penile urethra**.

The **penis** consists of **erectile tissues**, the paired dorsal **corpora cavernosa** and a single ventral **corpus spongiosum** that expands distally into the **glans penis**. Because the penile urethra extends through the entire length of the corpus spongiosum, this portion of the penis is also called the **corpus cavernosum urethrae**. Each erectile body in the penis is surrounded by the connective tissue layer **tunica albuginea**.

The erectile tissues in the penis consist of irregular vascular spaces lined with a vascular endothelium. The trabeculae between these spaces contain collagen and elastic fibers and smooth muscles. Blood enters the vascular spaces from the branches of the **dorsal artery** and **deep arteries of the penis** and is drained by peripheral veins.

thePoint® Supplemental micrographic images are available at **www.thePoint.com/Eroschenko13e** under Male Reproductive System.

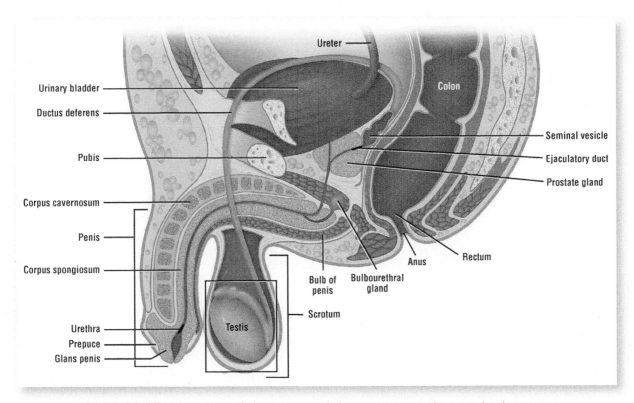

FIGURE 20.15 ■ Location of the testes and the accessory male reproductive organs.

FIGURE 20.16 | Prostate Gland and Prostatic Urethra

The prostate gland is an encapsulated organ situated inferior to the neck of the bladder. The urethra that leaves the bladder and passes through the prostate gland is the **prostatic urethra** (**1**). A **transitional epithelium** (**6**) lines the lumen of the crescent-shaped prostatic urethra (1). Most of the prostate gland consists of branched tubuloacinar **prostatic glands** (**5, 11**) with some exhibiting solid secretory aggregations called prostatic concretions (11) that appear as small red dots in this illustration. A characteristic **fibromuscular stroma** (**10**) with **smooth muscle bundles** (**4**) mixed with collagen and elastic fibers surrounds the prostatic glands (5, 11) and the prostatic urethra (1).

A longitudinal urethral crest of fibromuscular stroma without glands widens in the prostatic urethra (1) to form a domelike structure called the **colliculus seminalis** (**7**) that protrudes into and gives the prostatic urethra (1) a crescent shape. On each side of the colliculus seminalis (7) are the **prostatic sinuses** (**2**) into which open the excretory **ducts** of the **prostatic glands** (**9**).

In the middle of the colliculus seminalis (7) is a cul-de-sac called the **utricle** (**8**) with a dilation at its distal end before it opens into the prostatic urethra (1). The epithelium is simple secretory or pseudostratified columnar type. Two **ejaculatory ducts** (**3**) open at the colliculus, one on each side of the utricle (8).

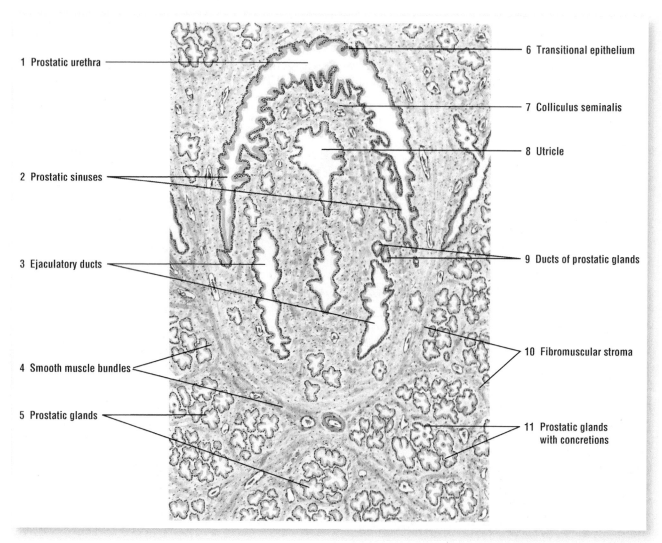

1 Prostatic urethra
2 Prostatic sinuses
3 Ejaculatory ducts
4 Smooth muscle bundles
5 Prostatic glands
6 Transitional epithelium
7 Colliculus seminalis
8 Utricle
9 Ducts of prostatic glands
10 Fibromuscular stroma
11 Prostatic glands with concretions

FIGURE 20.16 ■ Prostate gland and prostatic urethra. Stain: hematoxylin and eosin. Low magnification.

FIGURE 20.17 | Prostate Gland: Glandular Acini and Prostatic Concretions

A small section of the prostate gland from Figure 20.16 is illustrated at a higher magnification.

The **glandular acini (1)** in the prostate gland are highly variable with normally wide and typically irregular lumina because of the protrusion of the epithelium-covered **connective tissue folds (10)**. Some glandular acini (1) contain proteinaceous **prostatic secretions (9)**. Other acini (1) contain **prostatic concretions (4, 6, 8)** that are formed by condensed prostatic secretions and become the characteristic features of the prostate gland. The number of prostatic concretions (4, 6, 8) increases with the age of the individual, and they may become calcified.

Although the **glandular epithelium (5)** is usually simple columnar or pseudostratified, there is considerable variation where the epithelium may be squamous or cuboidal.

The **excretory ducts of the prostatic glands (2)** resemble the glandular acini (1), and in the terminal portions, the ductal epithelium (2) is usually columnar and stains darker before entering the urethra.

The **fibromuscular stroma (7)** also characterizes the prostate gland with **smooth muscle bundles (3)** and the connective tissue fibers blending together in the stroma (7).

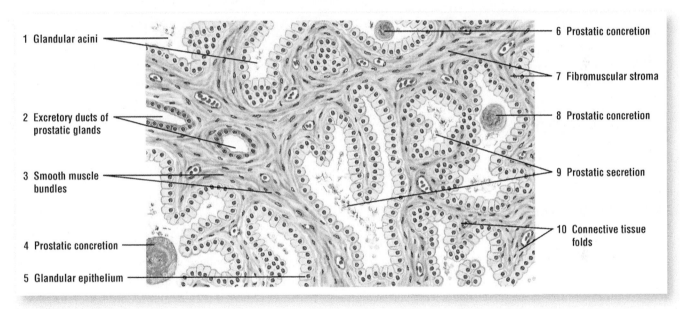

1 Glandular acini
2 Excretory ducts of prostatic glands
3 Smooth muscle bundles
4 Prostatic concretion
5 Glandular epithelium
6 Prostatic concretion
7 Fibromuscular stroma
8 Prostatic concretion
9 Prostatic secretion
10 Connective tissue folds

FIGURE 20.17 ■ Prostate gland: glandular acini and prostatic concretions. Stain: hematoxylin and eosin. Medium magnification.

FIGURE 20.18 | Prostate Gland: Prostatic Glands with Prostatic Concretions

The prostate gland consists of **prostatic glands** (3) with variable size and shape. The glandular epithelium also varies from simple cuboidal or **columnar** (2) to pseudostratified epithelium. In older individuals, the secretory material in the prostatic glands (3) precipitates to form **prostatic concretions** (1, 5). In this photomicrograph, the **smooth muscle fibers** (4a) in the characteristic fibromuscular stroma (4) are stained red, and the **connective tissue fibers** (4b) are stained blue.

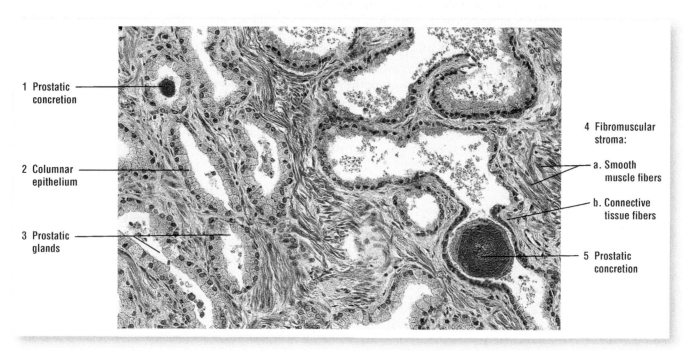

1 Prostatic concretion

2 Columnar epithelium

3 Prostatic glands

4 Fibromuscular stroma:
   a. Smooth muscle fibers
   b. Connective tissue fibers

5 Prostatic concretion

FIGURE 20.18 ■ Prostate gland: prostatic glands with prostatic concretions. Stain: Masson trichrome. ×64.

FIGURE 20.19 | Seminal Vesicle

The paired seminal vesicles are elongated glands located on the posterior side of the bladder. The excretory duct from each seminal vesicle joins the ampulla of each ductus deferens to form the ejaculatory duct, which runs through the prostate gland to open into the prostatic urethra.

FUNCTIONAL CORRELATIONS 20.4 ■ **Accessory Male Reproductive Glands**

The secretory products from the seminal vesicles, prostate gland, and bulbourethral glands mix with sperm and form fluid **semen**. Semen provides the sperm with a transport medium and nutrients. Semen also neutralizes the acidity of the male urethra and vaginal canal and activates the sperm after ejaculation.

The **seminal vesicles** produce a yellowish, viscous fluid with high concentration of **fructose**, the main carbohydrate component of semen. Fructose is metabolized by sperm and serves as the **energy** source for sperm motility. Seminal vesicles also produce most of the fluid found in semen including fibrinogen that coagulates semen after ejaculation and prostaglandins.

The **prostate gland** produces a thin, watery, slightly acidic fluid, rich in citric acid, prostatic acid phosphatase, amylase, and prostate-specific antigen (PSA). PSA is a very useful diagnostic tool for diagnosing prostatic cancer because its concentration often increases in the blood during malignancy. The enzyme fibrinolysin, also produced by prostate gland, liquefies the congealed semen after its ejaculation.

The **bulbourethral glands** produce a clear, viscid, mucus-like secretion that, during sexual stimulation, is released to lubricate the penile urethra and to neutralize its urine acidity. During ejaculation, secretions from the bulbourethral glands precede other components of the semen.

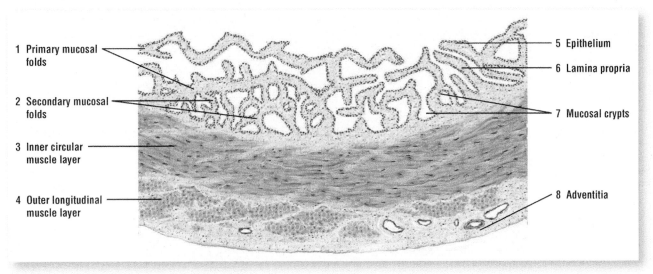

1 Primary mucosal folds

2 Secondary mucosal folds

3 Inner circular muscle layer

4 Outer longitudinal muscle layer

5 Epithelium

6 Lamina propria

7 Mucosal crypts

8 Adventitia

FIGURE 20.19 ■ Seminal vesicle. Stain: hematoxylin and eosin. Low magnification.

The seminal vesicle exhibits convoluted and irregular lumina. A cross section through the gland illustrates the complexity of the **primary mucosal folds** (1) that branch into **secondary mucosal folds** (2) and frequently anastomose to form irregular cavities, chambers, or **mucosal crypts** (7). The **lamina propria** (6) projects into and forms the core of the larger primary folds (1) and the smaller secondary folds (2) that extend into the lumen of the seminal vesicle.

The glandular **epithelium** (5) of the seminal vesicles varies but is usually low pseudostratified and low columnar or cuboidal.

The muscularis consists of an **inner circular muscle layer** (3) and an **outer longitudinal muscle layer** (4). This arrangement of the smooth muscles is often difficult to observe because of the complex folding of the mucosa. The **adventitia** (8) surrounds the muscularis and blends with the connective tissue.

FIGURE 20.20 | Bulbourethral Gland

The paired bulbourethral glands are compound tubuloacinar glands. The fibroelastic **capsule** contains **connective tissue** (3), smooth muscle fibers, and **skeletal muscle fibers** (2, 7) in the interlobular **connective tissue septum** (5). Because of their location in the urogenital diaphragm, the skeletal muscle fibers (2, 7) from the diaphragm are present in the bulbourethral glands. Connective tissue septa (5) from the capsule (3) divide the gland into several lobules.

The secretory units vary in structure and size and resemble mucous glands, exhibiting either **acinar** (6) or **tubular secretory units** (1). The secretory cells are cuboidal, low columnar, or squamous and light staining with the height of the epithelial cells depending on the function of the gland. The secretory product of the bulbourethral glands is primarily mucus.

Smaller **excretory ducts** (4) may be lined with secretory cells, whereas the larger ducts exhibit pseudostratified or stratified columnar epithelium.

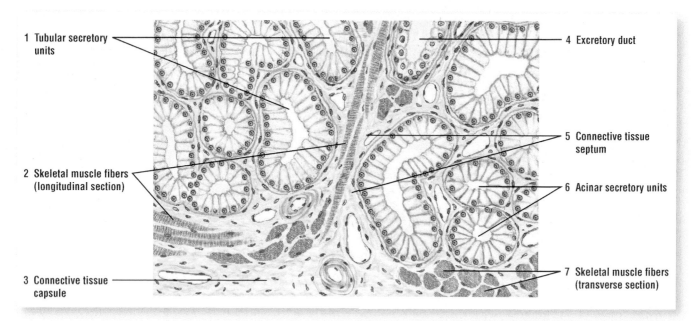

1 Tubular secretory units

4 Excretory duct

5 Connective tissue septum

2 Skeletal muscle fibers (longitudinal section)

6 Acinar secretory units

3 Connective tissue capsule

7 Skeletal muscle fibers (transverse section)

FIGURE 20.20 ■ Bulbourethral gland. Stain: hematoxylin and eosin. High magnification.

FIGURE 20.21 | **Human Penis (Transverse Section)**

A cross section of the human penis illustrates the two dorsal **corpora cavernosa** (**15**) (singular, corpus cavernosum) and a single ventral **corpus spongiosum** (**21**) that form the body of the organ. The **urethra** (**9**) passes through the length of the penis in the corpus spongiosum (21). A thick connective tissue capsule, **tunica albuginea** (**4**), surrounds the corpora cavernosa (15) and forms a **median septum** (**17**) between the two bodies. A thinner **tunica albuginea** (**8**) with smooth muscle fibers and elastic fibers surrounds the corpus spongiosum (21).

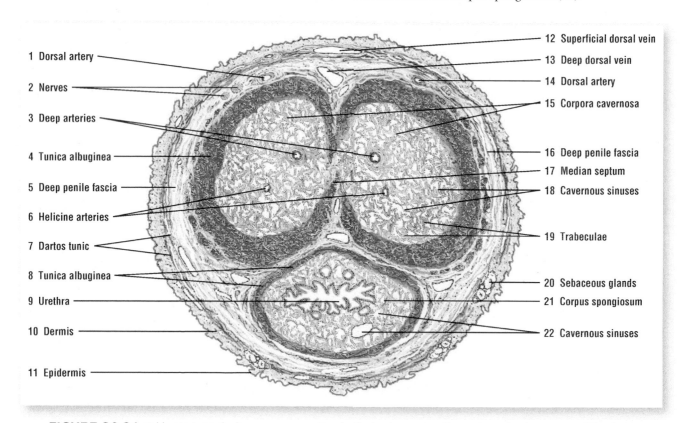

1 Dorsal artery

2 Nerves

3 Deep arteries

4 Tunica albuginea

5 Deep penile fascia

6 Helicine arteries

7 Dartos tunic

8 Tunica albuginea

9 Urethra

10 Dermis

11 Epidermis

12 Superficial dorsal vein

13 Deep dorsal vein

14 Dorsal artery

15 Corpora cavernosa

16 Deep penile fascia

17 Median septum

18 Cavernous sinuses

19 Trabeculae

20 Sebaceous glands

21 Corpus spongiosum

22 Cavernous sinuses

FIGURE 20.21 ■ Human penis (transverse section). Stain: hematoxylin and eosin. Low magnification.

All three cavernous bodies (15, 21) are surrounded by loose connective tissue called the deep **penile** (Buck) **fascia** (**5, 16**), which, in turn, is surrounded by the connective tissue of the **dermis** (**10**) located below the epithelium of the **epidermis** (**11**). Strands of smooth muscle of the **dartos tunic** (**7**), **nerves** (**2**), **sebaceous glands** (**20**), and peripheral blood vessels are present in the dermis (10).

Trabeculae (**19**) with collagenous, elastic, nerve, and smooth muscle fibers surround and form the core of the **cavernous sinuses** (veins) (**18, 22**) in the corpora cavernosa (15) and corpus spongiosum (21). The cavernous sinuses (18) of the corpora cavernosa (15) are lined with endothelium and receive blood from the **dorsal arteries** (**1, 14**) and **deep arteries** (**3**) of the penis. The deep arteries (3) branch in the corpora cavernosa (15) and form the **helicine arteries** (**6**), which empty directly into the cavernous sinuses (18). The cavernous sinuses (22) in the corpus spongiosum (21) receive blood from the bulbourethral artery, a branch of the internal pudendal artery. Blood leaving the cavernous sinuses (18, 22) exits mainly through the **superficial vein** (**12**) and the **deep dorsal vein** (**13**).

As the urethra (9) passes the base of the penis, it is lined with a pseudostratified or stratified columnar epithelium. As the urethra exits the penis, the epithelium is altered to stratified squamous. In the urethra (9) are invaginations called urethral lacunae (of Morgagni) with mucous cells. Branched tubular urethral glands (of Littre) located below the epithelium open into these recesses. These glands are shown at a higher magnification in Figure 20.22.

FIGURE 20.22 | Penile Urethra (Transverse Section)

This illustration shows a transverse section through the **lumen of the penile urethra** (**3**) and the surrounding **corpus spongiosum** (**9**). The lining of this portion of the urethra is a pseudostratified or stratified **columnar epithelium** (**2**). A thin underlying **lamina propria** (**5**) merges with the surrounding connective tissue of the corpus spongiosum (9).

Numerous outpockets or **urethral lacunae** (**4**) with mucous cells are located in the penile urethra (3) and are also connected with the mucous **urethral glands** (**of Littre**) (**6, 7**) in the connective tissue of the corpus spongiosum (9). The ducts from the urethral glands (6) open into the lumen of the penile urethra (3) throughout its length.

The corpus spongiosum (9) consists of **cavernous sinuses** (**1, 10**) lined with endothelial cells and separated by connective tissue **trabeculae** (**8**) with smooth muscle and collagen fibers. Numerous **blood vessels** (**arteriole and venule**) (**11**) supply the corpus spongiosum. The internal structure of the corpus spongiosum (9) is similar to that of the corpora cavernosa described in Figure 20.21.

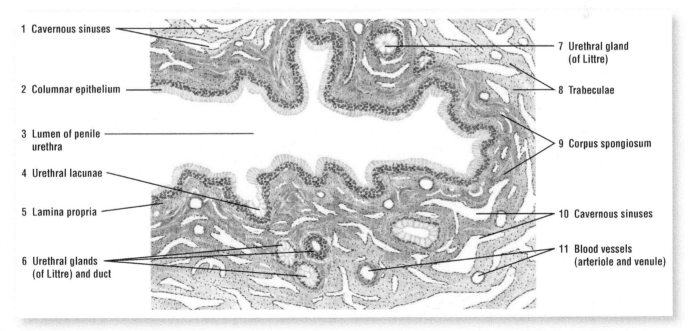

1 Cavernous sinuses

2 Columnar epithelium

3 Lumen of penile urethra

4 Urethral lacunae

5 Lamina propria

6 Urethral glands (of Littre) and duct

7 Urethral gland (of Littre)

8 Trabeculae

9 Corpus spongiosum

10 Cavernous sinuses

11 Blood vessels (arteriole and venule)

FIGURE 20.22 ■ Penile urethra (transverse section). Stain: hematoxylin and eosin. Low magnification.

Chapter 20 Summary

SECTION 2 • Accessory Reproductive Glands

SEMINAL VESICLES

- Located posterior to the bladder and superior to prostate gland
- Excretory ducts join with the ampulla of vas deferens to form ejaculatory ducts
- Ejaculatory ducts continue through prostate gland to open into prostatic urethra
- Produce fluid with sperm-activating fructose, the main energy source for sperm motility
- Produce most of the fluid found in semen, including fibrinogen to coagulate semen

PROSTATE GLAND

- Located inferior to the neck of the bladder
- Urethra exits bladder and passes through prostate as prostatic urethra
- Excretory ducts from the prostatic glands enter the prostatic urethra
- Transitional epithelium lines the prostatic urethra
- Characterized by fibromuscular stroma and prostatic concretions in the glands
- Produces watery secretions including prostate-specific antigen and fibrinolysin to liquefy semen

BULBOURETHRAL GLANDS

- Small glands located at the root of penis and in the skeletal muscle of urogenital diaphragm
- Excretory ducts enter the proximal part of penile urethra
- Produce mucus-like secretion that lubricates and neutralizes penile urethra

PENIS

- Consists of erectile tissue or vascular spaces lined with endothelium
- Erectile corpora cavernosa is located on dorsal side and corpus spongiosum on ventral side
- Tunica albuginea surrounds the erectile bodies
- Dorsal artery and deep artery supply erectile bodies with blood

Chapter 20 Review Questions: Section 2

QUESTIONS

In the following multiple choice questions, choose the letter corresponding to the one best answer.

1. **The ejaculatory ducts deliver their secretions into the:**
   A. prostatic urethra.
   B. penile urethra.
   C. seminal vesicles.
   D. prostate gland.
   E. ampulla of the vas deferens.

2. **Which accessory gland secretes fructose into the semen?**
   A. Prostate gland
   B. Seminal vesicles
   C. Bulbourethral glands
   D. Ampulla of the vas deferens
   E. None of the accessory glands

3. **What lubricates the penile urethra?**
   A. Secretions from the prostate gland
   B. Secretions from the seminal vesicles
   C. Semen
   D. Androgen-binding proteins
   E. Mucous secretions from the bulbourethral glands

4. **What precedes the semen during ejaculation?**
   A. Secretions from the prostate gland
   B. Secretions from the seminal vesicles
   C. Fructose secretion
   D. Mucous secretions from the bulbourethral glands
   E. Androgen-binding proteins

5. **What is the main source of energy for sperm in the ejaculate?**
   A. Testosterone
   B. Fructose
   C. Androgen-binding proteins
   D. Prostate-specific antigen
   E. Fibrinolysin

ANSWERS

1. **Correct Answer: A.** Prostatic urethra. The excretory ducts of seminal vesicles join the vas deferens to form the ejaculatory ducts that enter the prostate gland and empty their secretions into the prostatic urethra.

2. **Correct Answer: B.** Seminal vesicles. The sucrose becomes the main source of energy for sperm motility.

3. **Correct Answer: E.** Mucous secretions from the bulbourethral glands. Their secretion enters the penile urethra, lubricates the penile urethra, and neutralizes the acidity of the urethra.

4. **Correct Answer: D.** Mucous secretions from the bulbourethral glands.

5. **Correct Answer: B.** Fructose. This chemical is produced by the seminal vesicles that provides the energy for sperm motility.

ADDITIONAL HISTOLOGIC IMAGES

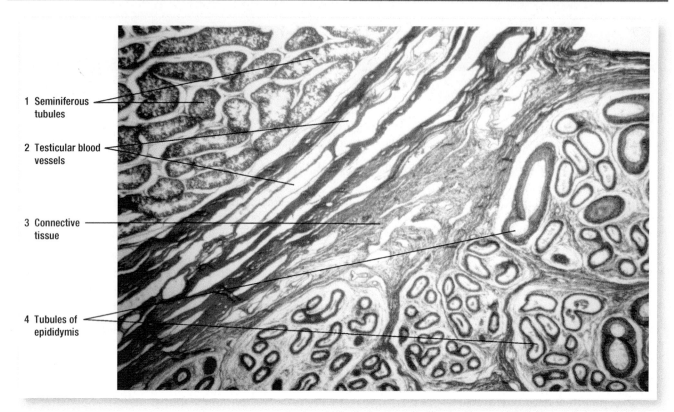

1 Seminiferous tubules

2 Testicular blood vessels

3 Connective tissue

4 Tubules of epididymis

FIGURE 20.23 ■ A low-power section of a canine testis, testicular blood vessels, and the ductules of the epididymis. Stain: hematoxylin and eosin. ×10.

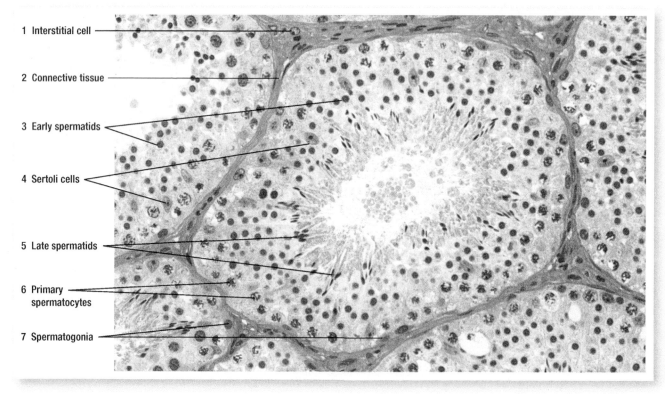

1 Interstitial cell

2 Connective tissue

3 Early spermatids

4 Sertoli cells

5 Late spermatids

6 Primary spermatocytes

7 Spermatogonia

FIGURE 20.24 ■ Cross sections of seminiferous tubules illustrating their contents. Stain: hematoxylin and eosin. Plastic section. ×125.

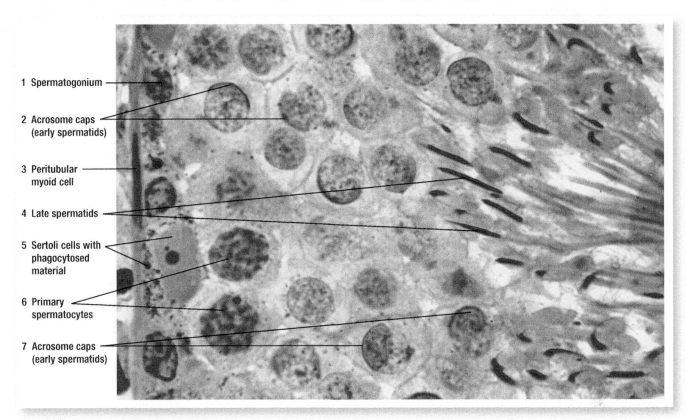

1 Spermatogonium

2 Acrosome caps
  (early spermatids)

3 Peritubular
  myoid cell

4 Late spermatids

5 Sertoli cells with
  phagocytosed
  material

6 Primary
  spermatocytes

7 Acrosome caps
  (early spermatids)

FIGURE 20.25 ■ A higher magnification of a section of rodent seminiferous tubule illustrating different cell types and their development. Stain: periodic acid–Schiff. ×403.

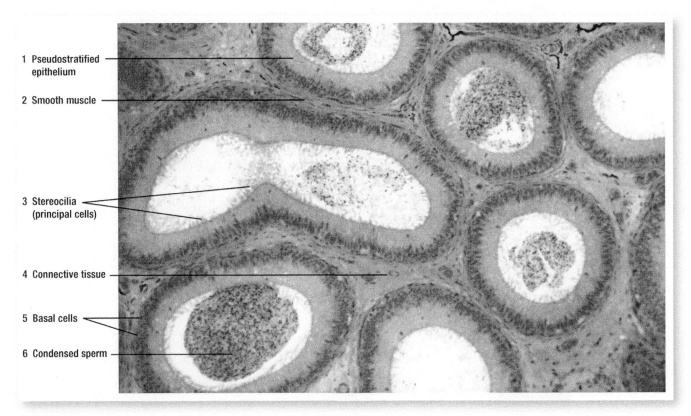

1 Pseudostratified
  epithelium

2 Smooth muscle

3 Stereocilia
  (principal cells)

4 Connective tissue

5 Basal cells

6 Condensed sperm

FIGURE 20.26 ■ Tubules of a primate ductus epididymis illustrating their structure and contents. Stain: hematoxylin and eosin. Plastic section. ×30.

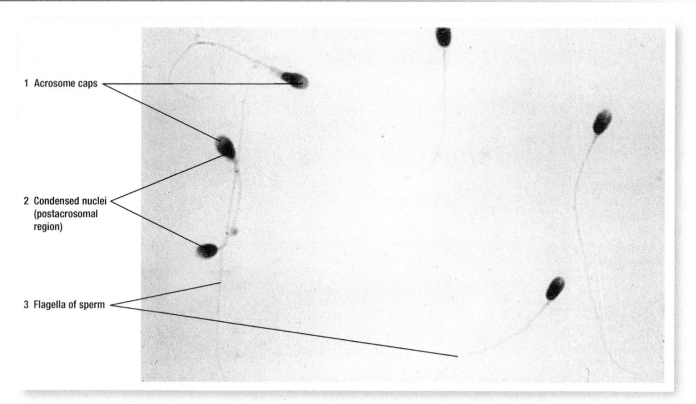

1 Acrosome caps

2 Condensed nuclei (postacrosomal region)

3 Flagella of sperm

FIGURE 20.27 ■ Smear of human semen illustrating the appearance of mature sperm with covering acrosome caps. Stain: hematoxylin and eosin. ×320.

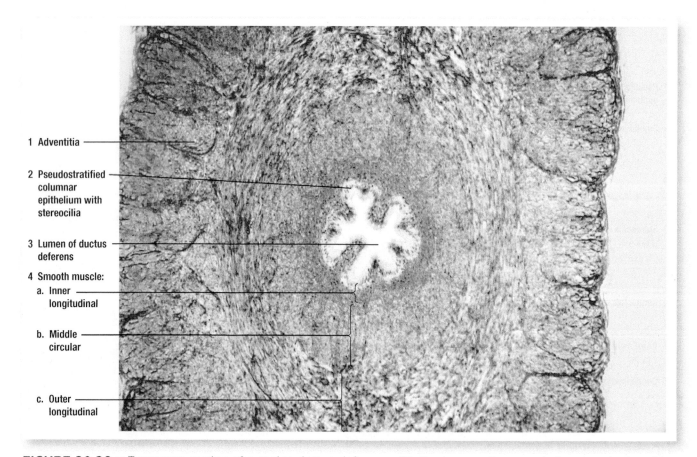

1 Adventitia

2 Pseudostratified columnar epithelium with stereocilia

3 Lumen of ductus deferens

4 Smooth muscle:
   a. Inner longitudinal

   b. Middle circular

   c. Outer longitudinal

FIGURE 20.28 ■ Transverse section of a canine ductus deferens with the surrounding muscle layers and adventitia. Stain: hematoxylin and eosin. ×20.

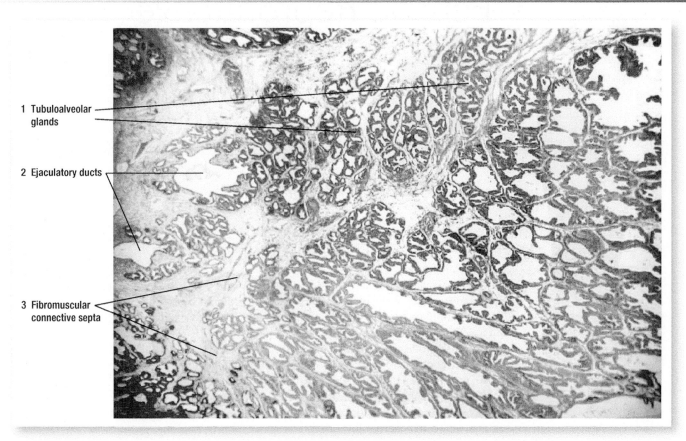

1 Tubuloalveolar
glands

2 Ejaculatory ducts

3 Fibromuscular
connective septa

FIGURE 20.29 ■ A section of canine prostate gland illustrating its glandular distribution and fibromuscular connective tissue. Stain: hematoxylin and eosin. ×6.5.

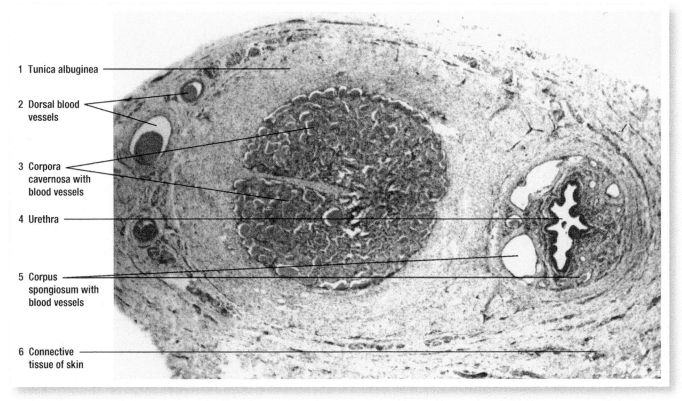

1 Tunica albuginea

2 Dorsal blood
vessels

3 Corpora
cavernosa with
blood vessels

4 Urethra

5 Corpus
spongiosum with
blood vessels

6 Connective
tissue of skin

FIGURE 20.30 ■ Transverse section of a primate penis illustrating the erectile tissues. Stain: hematoxylin and eosin. ×6.5.

Female Reproductive System

SECTION 1 Ovary and Uterus: Overview

The human female reproductive system consists of paired internal **ovaries**, paired **uterine (fallopian) tubes**, and a single **uterus**. Inferior to the uterus and separated by the cervix is the **vagina**. Because **mammary glands** are part of the female reproductive system, their histologic structure and function are included in this chapter.

During reproductive life, the human female reproductive organs exhibit cyclic monthly changes in structure and function that represent the **menstrual cycle**. The initial menstrual cycle is called **menarche**, and when these cycles eventually cease later in life, this phase represents the **menopause**.

The menstrual cycle is controlled by two hormones secreted by the adenohypophysis of the anterior pituitary gland, **follicle-stimulating hormone (FSH)** and **luteinizing hormone (LH)**, and by two ovarian steroid hormones, **estrogen** and **progesterone**, respectively. The release of FSH and LH from the pituitary gland is controlled by the **gonadotropin-releasing hormone (GnRH)** secreted by neurons in the hypothalamus (Fig. 21.1).

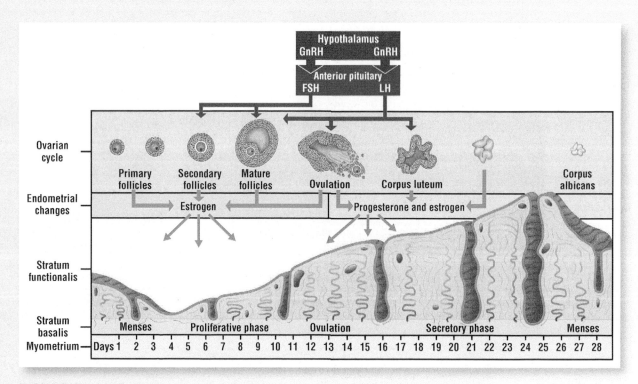

FIGURE 21.1 ■ The sequence of changes during follicular development, culminating in ovulation and corpus luteum formation. In addition, changes in the uterine wall during the menstrual cycle are correlated with pituitary hormones and ovarian functions. GnRH, gonadotropin-releasing hormone; FSH, follicle-stimulating hormone; LH, luteinizing hormone.

The female reproductive organs perform numerous functions. These include the secretion of female sex hormones (estrogen and progesterone) for the development of female sexual characteristics, production of oocytes, providing suitable environment for the fertilization of the oocytes in the uterine (fallopian) tube, transportation of the developing embryo to the uterus and its implantation, nutrition and development of the fetus during pregnancy, and nutrition of the newborn.

In humans, a mature ovarian follicle ovulates and releases an immature egg called the oocyte into the uterine tube approximately every 28 days. The oocyte remains viable in the female reproductive tract for about 24 hours, after which the oocyte degenerates if it is not fertilized. The transformation or maturation of the immature oocyte into a mature egg or ovum occurs at the time of **fertilization**. At the moment of contact between the sperm and the cells around the oocyte, the corona radiata, an acrosomal reaction takes place that causes the release of the hydrolytic enzymes from the acrosome on sperm head. This action dissolves the surrounding cell layers around the oocyte, and the sperm penetrates the zona pellucida of the oocyte to fertilize it.

OVARIES AND DEVELOPMENT OF FOLLICLES

Each ovary is a flattened, ovoid structure located deep in the pelvic cavity (Fig. 21.2). One section of the ovary is attached to the **broad ligament** by a peritoneal fold called the **mesovarium** and another section to the uterine wall by an **ovarian ligament**. The ovarian surface is covered by a single layer of cells called the **germinal epithelium** that overlies the dense connective tissue **tunica albuginea**. Inferior to the tunica albuginea is the ovarian cortex that contains the ovarian follicles. Deep to the cortex is the vascularized, connective tissue core of the ovary, the **medulla**. There is no distinct boundary line between the cortex and medulla, and these two regions blend together.

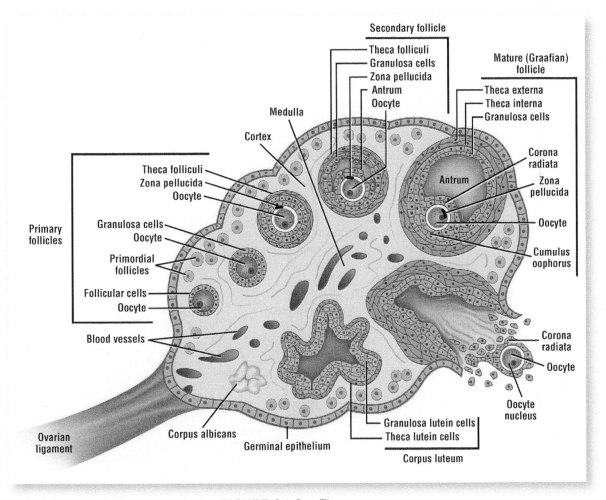

FIGURE 21.2 ▪ The ovary.

During embryonic development, **primordial germ cells** migrate from the yolk sac and colonize the embryonic gonadal ridges. Here, the germ cells differentiate into **oogonia** through the process of mitosis and then enter the first phase of **meiotic** division without completing it. The germ cells become arrested in this state of development and are now called **primary oocytes**. **Primordial follicles** are also formed during fetal life and consist of a primary oocyte surrounded by a single layer of squamous follicular cells. Beginning at puberty and under the influence of pituitary hormones, some selected primordial follicles grow and enlarge to become **primary, secondary**, and large **mature follicles**, which can span the ovarian cortex and extend into the medulla.

The cortex of a mature ovary is filled with ovarian follicles in various stages of development. In addition, a large **corpus luteum** of a previously ovulated follicle and a **corpus albicans** of a degenerated corpus luteum can be seen. Also, most ovarian follicles (primordial, primary, secondary, and maturate) may undergo degeneration called **atresia**, which are then phagocytosed by macrophages. Follicular atresia is common in an ovary. It starts before birth and continues throughout the reproductive period of the individual.

UTERINE (FALLOPIAN) TUBES

Each uterine tube is about 12 cm long and extends from the ovaries to the uterus (Fig. 21.3). One end of the uterine tube penetrates and opens into the uterus; the other end opens into the peritoneal cavity near the ovary. The uterine tubes are normally divided into four continuous regions. The region closest to the ovary is the funnel-shaped **infundibulum**. Extending from the infundibulum are finger-like processes called **fimbriae** (singular, fimbria) located close to the ovary. Continuous with the infundibulum is the second region, the **ampulla**, the widest and longest portion. The **isthmus** is short and narrow and joins each uterine tube to the uterus. The last portion of the uterine tube is the **interstitial** (**intramural**) **region**. It passes through the uterine wall to open into the uterine cavity.

UTERUS

The human uterus is pear shaped with a thick muscular wall (see Fig. 21.3). The **body** or **corpus** forms the major portion of the uterus. The rounded upper portion of the uterus located above the entrance of the uterine tubes is the **fundus**. The lower, narrower, and terminal portion of the uterus located below the body or corpus is the **cervix**. The cervix protrudes and opens into the vaginal canal.

The wall of the uterus is composed of three layers: an outer **perimetrium** lined with serosa or adventitia, a thick smooth muscle layer called the **myometrium**, and an inner **endometrium**. The endometrium is lined with a simple epithelium that descends into a lamina propria to form deep **uterine glands**.

The endometrium is subdivided into two functional layers, the luminal **stratum functionalis** and the basal **stratum basalis**. In a nonpregnant female, the functionalis layer with the uterine glands and blood vessels is sloughed off, or shed, during **menstruation**, leaving the intact deeper basalis layer with the basal remnants of the uterine glands whose cells regenerate a new

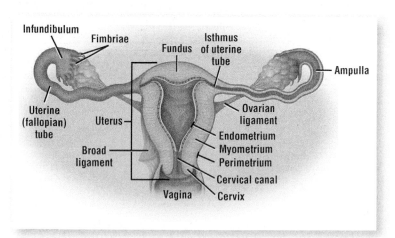

FIGURE 21.3 ■ The anatomy of the female reproductive organs.

functionalis layer. The arterial supply to the endometrium plays an important role during the menstrual phase of the menstrual cycle.

Uterine arteries in the broad ligament give rise to the **arcuate arteries** that penetrate and form a circumferential course in the myometrium. Arcuate vessels give rise to **straight** and **spiral arteries** that supply the endometrium of the uterus. The straight arteries are short and supply the basalis layer of the endometrium, whereas the spiral arteries are long and coiled and supply the functionalis layer of the endometrium. In contrast to the straight arteries, spiral arteries are highly sensitive to hormonal changes in the blood during menstrual cycles. Decreased blood levels of the estrogen and progesterone during the menstrual cycle results in the degeneration and then shedding of the stratum functionalis, resulting in menstruation.

thePoint® Supplemental micrographic images are available at **www.thePoint.com/Eroschenko13e** under Female Reproductive System.

FUNCTIONAL CORRELATIONS 21.1 ■ Ovaries, Follicles, and Their Development

Beginning at puberty and during the reproductive years, the ovaries exhibit structural and functional changes during each menstrual cycle, lasting an average of 28 days. Different follicles exhibit growth, and some mature. In other follicles, the developing oocyte completes the first meiotic division and is ovulated as a secondary oocyte from a mature dominant follicle. Following ovulation, a corpus luteum is formed, and, without fertilization and implantation of a developing embryo, the corpus luteum degenerates and forms a connective tissue corpus albicans. The initiation and activation of the developmental phase of primordial follicular growth in the ovaries is believed to be dependent on local growth factors and follicle-stimulating hormone (FSH) and luteinizing hormone (LH). These hormones are responsible for the later stages of follicular development, maturation, ovulation, and production of the hormones estrogen and progesterone. The first half of the menstrual cycle lasts about 14 days and involves the growth of some primordial ovarian follicles. At this time, FSH is the principal circulating gonadotropic hormone, and the growing follicles express receptors for FSH located on the surrounding granulosa cells. FSH controls the growth and maturation of ovarian follicles and stimulates the development of **theca interna cells** around the follicular peripheries. Theca interna cells exhibit numerous LH receptors and, after LH stimulation, secrete the estrogen precursors **androstenedione**, which diffuses into the follicles, where the **granulosa cells**, in response to FSH, convert it into **estrogen** with the **aromatase** enzyme. Estrogen then stimulates the granulosa cells to proliferate and increase the follicular size. As the follicles develop and mature, the circulating levels of estrogen in the blood rise. Under normal conditions, only one developing follicle becomes dominant and will reach maturity to ovulate an oocyte, whereas all the others will degen-

erate or become **atretic**. Increased levels of estrogen inhibit the release of gonadotropin-releasing hormone from the hypothalamus and decrease the release of FSH from the pituitary gland. This decreased level of FSH induces atresia in other follicles that started to develop.

At midcycle, or shortly before ovulation, estrogen levels reach a peak and produce a positive feedback on the pituitary gland. This peak causes a sharp surge of LH hormone from the adenohypophysis of the pituitary gland, with a concomitant smaller release of FSH hormone. Increased blood levels of both LH and FSH cause the following changes in the ovary:

- Completion of the first meiotic division of the oocyte before ovulation with the release of a secondary oocyte into the uterine tube.
- Final **maturation** of the mature ovarian follicle and **ovulation** (rupture) of a secondary oocyte at about the 14th day of the cycle.
- Before ovulation, blood flow ceases in the small area of the ovarian surface over the bulging mature follicle called stigma.
- Collapse of the ovulated mature follicle and the luteinization or modification of the granulosa lutein cells and theca lutein cells.
- Transformation of the postovulatory mature follicle into the corpus luteum, a temporary endocrine organ.
- Vascularization of the corpus luteum and, in response to LH, increased production of progesterone and estrogen by the luteal cells.

Final maturation, or the second meiotic division of the secondary oocyte, occurs at the time of fertilization by sperm. The liberated secondary oocyte remains viable in the female reproductive tract for about 24 hours before it begins to degenerate without completing the second meiotic division.

FIGURE 21.4 | **Ovary: Different Stages of Follicular Development (Panoramic View)**

This low-magnification image illustrates a sagittal section of an ovary and follicular developments that would normally be seen in different functional periods of the ovary.

The ovary is covered by a single layer of low cuboidal or squamous cells called the **germinal epithelium (11)**, which is continuous with the **mesothelium (13)** of the visceral peritoneum. Inferior to the germinal epithelium (11) is a dense, connective tissue layer called the **tunica albuginea (15)**.

The ovary contains a **cortex (10)** with follicles, fibrocytes, and collagen and reticular fibers. In the center is the **medulla (8)** with blood vessels, nerves, and lymphatics. The medulla (8) exhibits a typical dense irregular connective tissue that is continuous with the **mesovarium (23)** ligament that suspends the ovary. Larger **blood vessels from the medulla (8)** distribute smaller vessels to all parts of the ovarian cortex. The mesovarium (23) is covered by the germinal epithelium (11) and peritoneal mesothelium (13).

Numerous ovarian follicles are seen in various stages of development in the stroma (connective tissue) of the cortex (10). The most numerous follicles are the **primordial follicles (19)**,

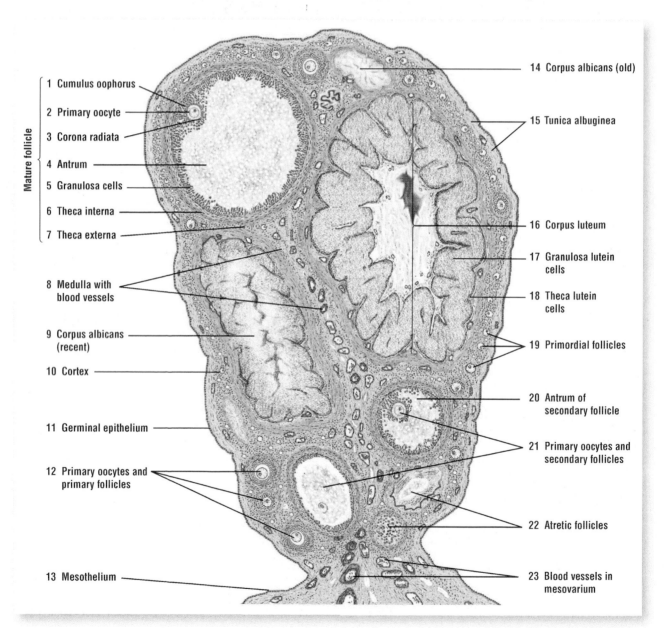

Mature follicle

1 Cumulus oophorus
2 Primary oocyte
3 Corona radiata
4 Antrum
5 Granulosa cells
6 Theca interna
7 Theca externa

8 Medulla with blood vessels

9 Corpus albicans (recent)

10 Cortex

11 Germinal epithelium

12 Primary oocytes and primary follicles

13 Mesothelium

14 Corpus albicans (old)

15 Tunica albuginea

16 Corpus luteum

17 Granulosa lutein cells

18 Theca lutein cells

19 Primordial follicles

20 Antrum of secondary follicle

21 Primary oocytes and secondary follicles

22 Atretic follicles

23 Blood vessels in mesovarium

FIGURE 21.4 ◾ Ovary: different stages of follicular development (panoramic view). Stain: hematoxylin and eosin. Low magnification.

located in the periphery of the cortex (10) and inferior to the tunica albuginea (15). The primordial follicles (19) are the smallest and simplest and are surrounded by a single layer of squamous follicular cells. The primordial follicles (19) contain the immature, small primary oocyte that gradually increases in size as the follicles develop into primary, secondary, and mature follicles. Before the ovulation of the mature follicle, all developing follicles contain a **primary oocyte (2, 12, 21)**.

Smaller follicles with cuboidal, columnar, or stratified cuboidal cells that surround the primary oocytes (12) are called **primary follicles (12)**. As the follicles increase in size, a fluid, called liquor folliculi (follicular liquid), begins to accumulate between the follicular cells, now called the **granulosa cells (5)**. The fluid areas eventually coalesce to form a fluid-filled cavity, called the **antrum (4, 20)**. Follicles with antral cavities are called **secondary (antral) follicles (21)**. They are larger and are situated deeper in the cortex (10). All larger follicles, including primary follicles (12), secondary follicles (21), and **mature follicles** exhibit a granulosa cell layer (5), a **theca interna (6)**, and an outer connective tissue layer, the **theca externa (7)**.

The largest ovarian follicle is the **mature follicle**. It exhibits a large antrum (4) filled with liquor folliculi (follicular fluid); **a cumulus oophorus (1)**, the mound on which the primary oocyte (2) is situated; a **corona radiata (3)**, the cell layer that is attached directly to the primary oocyte (2); **granulosa cells (5)** that surround the antrum (4); the inner layer theca interna (6); and the outer theca externa (7).

After ovulation, the large follicle collapses and transforms into a temporary endocrine organ, the **corpus luteum (16)**. The granulosa cells (5) of the follicle transform into light-staining **granulosa lutein cells (17)**, and the theca interna (6) cells become the darker-staining **theca lutein cells (18)** of the functioning corpus luteum (16). If fertilization and implantation do not occur, the corpus luteum (16) regresses, degenerates, and turns into a connective tissue scar called the **corpus albicans (9, 14)**. This illustration shows a recent larger corpus albicans (9) and an older smaller corpus albicans (14).

Most ovarian follicles do not attain maturity. Instead, they undergo degeneration (atresia) at all stages of follicular growth and become **atretic follicles (22)**, which eventually are replaced by the connective tissue.

FIGURE 21.5 | **Ovary: Longitudinal Section of Feline (Cat) Ovary Showing Numerous Follicles and Corpora Lutea**

This low-magnification photomicrograph shows a section of a feline (cat) ovary. The surface is covered with a low cuboidal, or squamous **germinal epithelium (1)**, that continues with the **mesothelium (6)** of the visceral peritoneum that covers the dense connective tissue of the

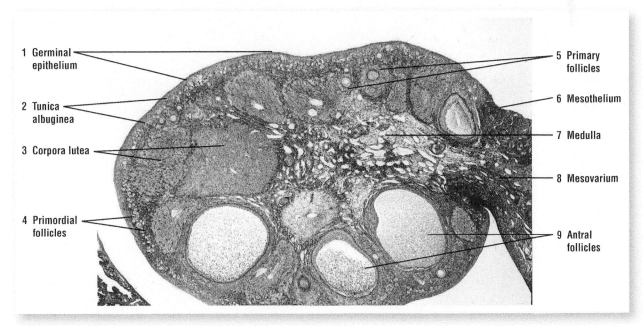

FIGURE 21.5 ■ Ovary: longitudinal section of a feline (cat) ovary showing numerous follicles and corpora lutea. Stain: Mallory-Azan. ×6.5.

suspensory ligament, the **mesovarium** (8). Blood vessels, lymphatic vessels, and nerves enter and supply the ovarian **medulla** (7) through the mesovarium (8). Located inferior to the germinal epithelium is the connective tissue tunica albuginea (2) that encloses the ovary. Inferior to the **tunica albuginea** (2) is the cortex of the ovary containing light-staining and small **primordial follicles** (4). Deeper in the cortex are the developing **primary follicles** (5) and larger **antral follicles** (9) filled with liquor folliculi (follicular fluid). The ovulated mature follicles have been transformed into temporary **corpora lutea** (3) in which the wall collapsed on the former antral cavity. The granulosa cells that surrounded the antral cavity are transformed into the granulosa lutein cells of the corpora lutea (3).

FIGURE 21.6 | Ovary: Section of Ovary Showing Ovarian Cortex with Developing Follicles

This higher-magnification photomicrograph illustrates a section of an ovarian cortex. Covering the ovarian surface is a thin layer of cuboidal cells of the **germinal epithelium** (1). Inferior to germinal epithelium (1) is the thicker layer of **tunica albuginea** (5). Inferior to the tunica albuginea (5) is the connective tissue of the **ovarian cortex** (8), which contains **primordial follicles** (2) surrounded by flat follicular cells. A larger **primary follicle** (4) with a **primary oocyte** (3) is surrounded by stratified cuboidal granulosa cells. Also visible are other **primary follicles** (6) with cuboidal follicular cells. On the right side is a larger follicle with disorganized granulosa cells in the antrum and with pyknotic nuclei; this appears to be an **atretic follicle** (7).

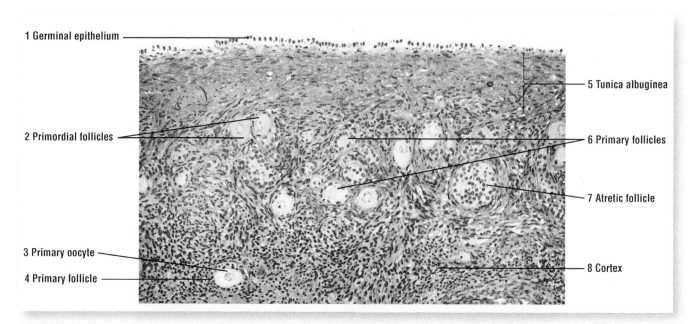

1 Germinal epithelium

5 Tunica albuginea

2 Primordial follicles

6 Primary follicles

7 Atretic follicle

3 Primary oocyte

4 Primary follicle

8 Cortex

FIGURE 21.6 ■ Ovary: a section of ovarian cortex and developing follicles. Stain: hematoxylin and eosin. ×64.

FIGURE 21.7 | Ovary: Ovarian Cortex and Primary and Primordial Follicles

The ovarian surface is covered by a cuboidal **germinal epithelium** (**10**) that overlies the **tunica albuginea** (**16**). **Primordial follicles** (**14, 17**) are located in the cortex inferior to the tunica albuginea (**16**), and each one is surrounded by a single layer of squamous **follicular cells** (**17**). As the follicles grow larger, the follicular cells (**17**) of the primordial follicles (**14, 17**) change to cuboidal, or low columnar, and the follicles now become **primary follicles** (**4, 11**). The developing oocytes (**4, 13**) in the follicles also have a large eccentric **nucleus** (**7, 13**) with a nucleolus.

In primary (growing) follicles (**4, 11**), the follicular cells proliferate by **mitosis** (**3**) and form layers of cuboidal cells called the **granulosa cells** (**8, 12**) that surround the primary oocytes (**4, 13**). A single layer of the granulosa cells around the oocyte forms the **corona radiata** (**5**).

Between the corona radiata (**5**) and the oocyte appears the noncellular glycoprotein layer called the **zona pellucida** (**6**). The stromal cells that surround the follicular cells now differentiate into the **theca interna** (**9**) layer located adjacent to the granulosa cells (**8, 12**). A thin basement membrane (not shown) separates the granulosa cells (**8, 12**) from the theca interna (**9**) cells.

Many primordial, developing, or mature follicles exhibit degeneration, die, and are lost through atresia. A degenerating **atretic follicle** (**1**) is illustrated in the upper left corner of the illustration. Numerous blood vessels (**2**) surround the developing follicles in the **connective tissue of the cortex** (**15**).

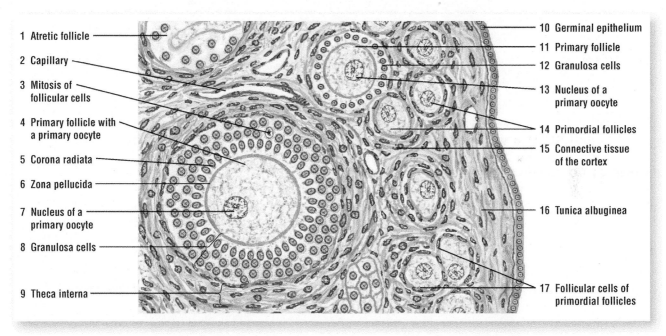

1 Atretic follicle
2 Capillary
3 Mitosis of follicular cells
4 Primary follicle with a primary oocyte
5 Corona radiata
6 Zona pellucida
7 Nucleus of a primary oocyte
8 Granulosa cells
9 Theca interna

10 Germinal epithelium
11 Primary follicle
12 Granulosa cells
13 Nucleus of a primary oocyte
14 Primordial follicles
15 Connective tissue of the cortex
16 Tunica albuginea
17 Follicular cells of primordial follicles

FIGURE 21.7 ■ Ovary: ovarian cortex and primordial and primary follicles. Stain: hematoxylin and eosin. Low magnification.

FIGURE 21.8 | Ovary: Primordial and Primary Follicles

This photomicrograph shows variety of follicles in the cortex of an ovary. The immature **primordial follicles** (2) consist of a primary **oocyte** (3) surrounded by a layer of simple squamous **follicular cells** (1, 7). As the primordial follicles (2) become **primary follicles** (4), the layer of simple squamous follicular cells around the oocyte changes to a cuboidal layer. In a larger **primary follicle** (8), the follicular cells have proliferated into a stratified layer called **granulosa cells** (11). A prominent layer of glycoprotein, the **zona pellucida** (10), develops between the granulosa cells (11) and the immature **oocyte** (9).

The cells around the larger follicles organize into the inner hormone-secreting **theca interna** (12) and the outer connective tissue layer **theca externa** (13). The theca interna (12) and theca externa (13) are separated from the granulosa cells (11) by a thin **basement membrane** (6). Surrounding the follicles in the cortex are the cells and fibers of the **connective tissue** (5).

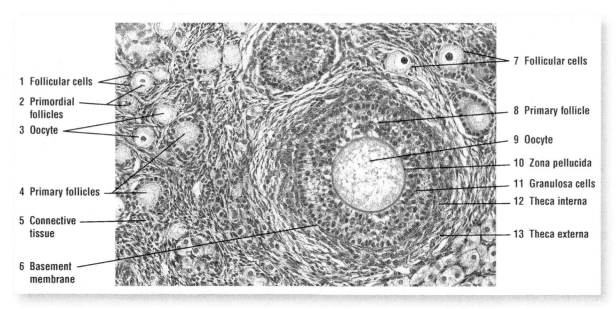

1 Follicular cells
2 Primordial follicles
3 Oocyte
4 Primary follicles
5 Connective tissue
6 Basement membrane

7 Follicular cells
8 Primary follicle
9 Oocyte
10 Zona pellucida
11 Granulosa cells
12 Theca interna
13 Theca externa

FIGURE 21.8 ■ Ovary: primordial and primary follicles. Stain: hematoxylin and eosin. ×64.

FIGURE 21.9 | Ovary: Maturing Ovarian Follicle in Feline (Cat) Ovary

This medium-magnification micrograph shows a maturing ovarian follicle in a feline ovary. An area filled with liquor folliculi is the **antrum** (3), displacing the **primary oocyte** (10) on one side of the follicle. Surrounding the oocyte is the **zona pellucida** (9). The primary oocyte (10) rests on

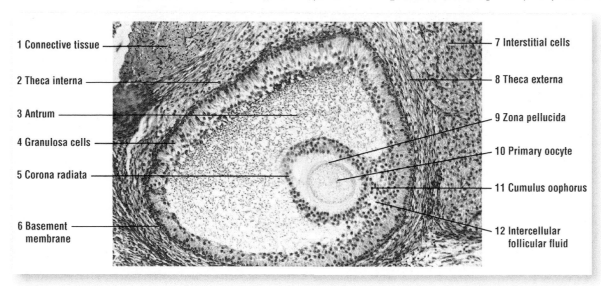

1 Connective tissue
2 Theca interna
3 Antrum
4 Granulosa cells
5 Corona radiata
6 Basement membrane

7 Interstitial cells
8 Theca externa
9 Zona pellucida
10 Primary oocyte
11 Cumulus oophorus
12 Intercellular follicular fluid

FIGURE 21.9 ■ Ovary: maturing ovarian follicle in a feline (cat) ovary. Stain: Mallory-Azan. ×45.

the **cumulus oophorus** (11), a mound of cells that also exhibits separation because of accumulation of **intercellular follicular fluid** (12). The cells that surround the oocyte form the **corona radiata** (5), although, in this image, the separation between the oocyte and the corona radiata is due to the fixation process. The cells around the antrum (3) are the **granulosa cells** (4). They are separated by a thin **basement membrane** (6) from the connective tissue that have been altered to form the inner secretory epithelioid cells, the **theca interna** (2) layer and the outer connective tissue layer, the **theca externa** (8). On the right side of the maturing follicle are the light-staining **interstitial cells** (7), which represent the remnants of the theca interna cells (2) that persist as individual cells or as a group of cells following follicular atresia. Also visible near the follicle is the **connective tissue** (1) of the cortex.

FIGURE 21.10 | Ovary: Primary Oocyte and Wall of Mature Follicle

This more detailed illustration of a mature follicle shows the primary oocyte, the surrounding cells, and the mound on which it is located. During the growth of the follicles, fluid accumulates between the granulosa cells around the oocyte, forming the antrum. The follicle becomes a secondary follicle when the antrum is present.

This figure illustrates the **cytoplasm** and **nucleus** of a **primary oocyte** (3) of a mature follicle. A thickening of the **granulosa cells** (5) on one side of the follicle surrounds the primary oocyte (3) and projects into the **antrum** (4, 7) in form a hillock (mound) called the **cumulus oophorus** (8). The single layer of granulosa cells (5) adjacent to the primary oocyte (3) forms the **corona radiata** (1). Between the corona radiata (1) and the cytoplasm of the primary oocyte (3) is the **zona pellucida** (2).

The granulosa cells (5) surround the antrum (4, 7) and secrete follicular fluid of the antrum cavity. Smaller isolated accumulation of the fluid among the granulosa cells (5) is the **intercellular follicular fluid** (6, 9).

The basal row of granulosa cells (5) rests on a thin **basement membrane** (10) that separates the granulosa cells (5) from the cells of the **theca interna** (11). Surrounding the cells of the theca interna (11) is the **theca externa** (12) layer that blends with the **connective tissue** (13) of the ovarian cortex.

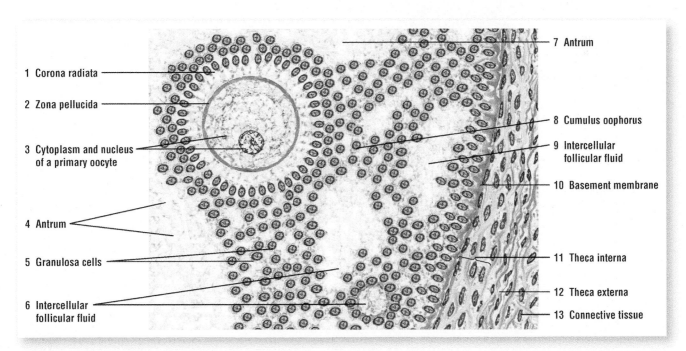

1 Corona radiata
2 Zona pellucida
3 Cytoplasm and nucleus of a primary oocyte
4 Antrum
5 Granulosa cells
6 Intercellular follicular fluid
7 Antrum
8 Cumulus oophorus
9 Intercellular follicular fluid
10 Basement membrane
11 Theca interna
12 Theca externa
13 Connective tissue

FIGURE 21.10 ■ Ovary: primary oocyte and the wall of a mature follicle. Stain: hematoxylin and eosin. High magnification.

FIGURE 21.11 | Corpus Luteum (Panoramic View)

At a higher magnification, the corpus luteum is a collapsed mass of glandular epithelium consisting of **theca lutein cells** (**5**) and **granulosa lutein cells** (**6**). Theca lutein cells (**5**) extend along the **connective tissue septa** (**3**) into the folds of the corpus luteum.

The **theca externa** (**2**) cells form a poorly defined capsule around the corpus luteum that also extends inward with the connective tissue septa (**3**) into folds.

The center of the corpus luteum or the **former follicular cavity** (**9**) contains remnants of follicular fluid, serum, blood cells, and loose **connective tissue with blood vessels** (**7**) from the theca externa that has extended into the glandular epithelium and then spread throughout the core of the corpus luteum. Some corpora lutea may contain a postovulatory **blood clot** (**8**) in the former follicular cavity (**9**).

The **connective tissue of the cortex** (**1**) that surrounds the corpus luteum contains numerous **blood vessels** (**4**).

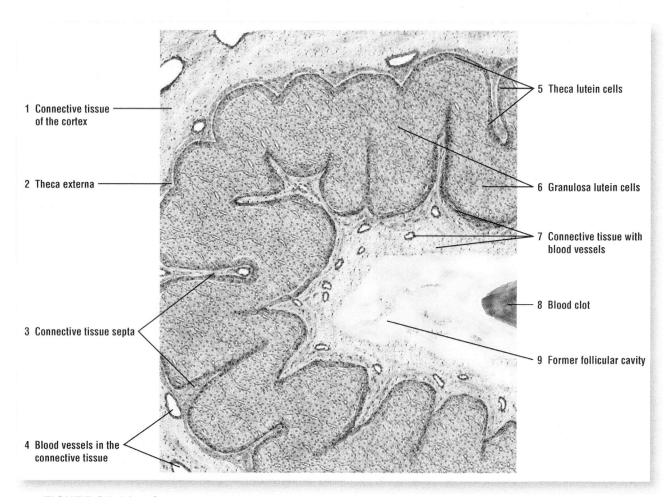

FIGURE 21.11 ■ Corpus luteum (panoramic view). Stain: hematoxylin and eosin. Low magnification.

FIGURE 21.12 | Corpus Luteum: Theca Lutein Cells and Granulosa Lutein Cells

The granulosa **lutein cells** (**6**) represent the hypertrophied former granulosa cells of the mature follicle and constitute the folded mass of the corpus luteum. The granulosa lutein cells (6) are large, have large vesicular nuclei, and stain lightly owing to lipid inclusions. The **theca lutein cells** (**1, 7**) (the former theca interna cells) are located external to the granulosa lutein cells (6) on the periphery of the glandular epithelium. The theca lutein cells (1, 7) are smaller than the granulosa lutein cells (6), stain darker, and their nuclei are smaller and darker.

The **theca externa** (**2**) with blood vessels, **venule and arteriole** (**4**), and **capillaries** (**5**) invades the granulosa lutein cells (6) and theca lutein cells (1, 7). A **connective tissue septum with fibrocytes** (**3**) penetrates the theca lutein cells (1, 7) with the fibrocytes (3) identified by their elongated and flattened appearance.

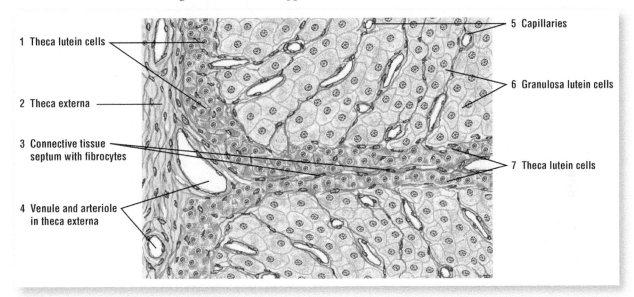

1 Theca lutein cells
2 Theca externa
3 Connective tissue septum with fibrocytes
4 Venule and arteriole in theca externa
5 Capillaries
6 Granulosa lutein cells
7 Theca lutein cells

FIGURE 21.12 ■ Corpus luteum: theca lutein cells and granulosa lutein cells. Stain: hematoxylin and eosin.

FIGURE 21.13 | Human Ovary: Section of Corpus Luteum and Corpus Albicans

This low-magnification micrograph shows a section of a human ovary. On the left side is a section of the folded wall of the corpus luteum with hypertrophied and lighter-staining **granulosa lutein cells** (**3, 5**) surrounded by darker-staining **theca lutein cells** (**1, 4**) located peripherally

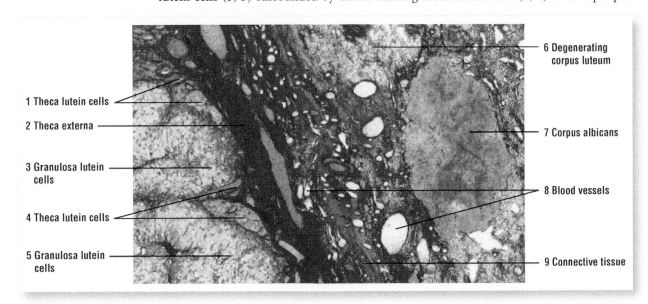

1 Theca lutein cells
2 Theca externa
3 Granulosa lutein cells
4 Theca lutein cells
5 Granulosa lutein cells
6 Degenerating corpus luteum
7 Corpus albicans
8 Blood vessels
9 Connective tissue

FIGURE 21.13 ■ Human ovary: a section of corpus luteum and corpus albicans. Stain: Mallory-Azan. ×10.5.

and between the folds of the granulosa lutein cells (3, 5). Surrounding the corpus luteum is the dense connective tissue layer **theca externa** (2). On the right side of the figure is the blue-staining connective tissue scar of the corpus luteum, the **corpus albicans** (7) with **degenerating corpus luteum** (6) above it. Between the corpus luteum and the corpus albicans (7) is the vascular **connective tissue** (9) with **blood vessels** (8).

FUNCTIONAL CORRELATIONS 21.2 ■ Corpus Luteum

After the mature follicle liberates the secondary oocyte into the infundibulum of the uterine tube, the wall of the ruptured mature follicle collapses, and the ovary enters the **luteal phase**. During this luteinization phase, luteinizing hormone (LH) secretion induces hypertrophy and transforms the granulosa cells and theca interna cells into **granulosa lutein cells** and **theca lutein cells**, respectively, forming a temporary endocrine tissue, the corpus luteum. In response to both follicle-stimulating hormone (FSH) and LH, the cells of the corpus lutein secrete **estrogen** and large amounts of **progesterone**. High levels of both hormones further stimulate the development of the **uterus** and mammary glands in anticipation of the implantation of a fertilized egg and pregnancy.

Rising levels of estrogen and progesterone produced by the corpus luteum eventually inhibit further release of FSH and LH, by its action on the neurons in the hypothalamus and gonadotrophs in the adenohypophysis. This effect prevents further ovulation.

If the ovulated secondary oocyte is not fertilized, the corpus luteum continues to secrete its hormones for about another 12 days and then begins to regress. After its regression, it is called the **corpus luteum of menstruation**, eventually becoming a **connective tissue scar corpus albicans**. With decreased functions of the corpus luteum, estrogen and progesterone levels decline, affecting the blood vessels in the endometrium of the uterus and inducing the shedding of the stratum functionalis of the endometrium in the menstrual flow.

As the corpus luteum ceases function, the inhibitory effects of estrogen, progesterone, and inhibin on the hypothalamus and pituitary gland cells are removed. As a result, FSH is again released from the adenohypophysis, initiating a new ovarian cycle of follicular development and maturation.

CORPUS LUTEUM AND PREGNANCY

If fertilization of the oocyte and implantation of the embryo occurs, the corpus luteum increases in size and becomes the **corpus luteum of pregnancy**. The hormone **human chorionic gonadotropin (hCG)**, secreted by the trophoblast cells of the developing placenta in the implanting embryo, continues to stimulate luteal functions of the corpus luteum and prevents its regression. The influence of hCG is similar to that by LH from the pituitary gland and extends its function of progesterone secretion. As a result, the corpus luteum of pregnancy persists for several months. As the pregnancy progresses, however, the function of the corpus luteum diminishes and is taken over by the **placenta** after about 6 weeks of pregnancy. During pregnancy, the placenta functions as a temporary endocrine organ and continues to secrete sufficient amounts of estrogen and progesterone to maintain the pregnancy until parturition.

FIGURE 21.14 | Uterine Tube: Ampulla with Mesosalpinx Ligament (Panoramic View, Transverse Section)

The paired, muscular uterine (fallopian) tubes extend from the ovaries to the uterus. On one end, the infundibulum opens into the peritoneal cavity adjacent to the ovary. The other end penetrates the uterine wall and opens into the uterus. The uterine tubes conduct the ovulated oocyte toward the uterus.

The ampulla is the longest part of the tube and is normally the site of fertilization. It exhibits the extensive **mucosal folds** (**8**) that form an irregular **lumen** (**7**) and produces deep grooves between the folds (**8**). These folds become smaller near the uterus.

The mucosa of the uterine tube consists of simple columnar ciliated and nonciliated **epithelium** (**6**) that overlies the **lamina propria** (**9**). The muscularis consists of two smooth muscle layers, an **inner circular layer** (**5**) and an **outer longitudinal layer** (**4**). The **interstitial connective tissue** (**10**) is abundant between the muscle layers, and as a result, the smooth muscle layers (**4, 5**)—especially the outer layer (**4**)—are not distinct. Numerous **venules** (**3**) and **arterioles** (**2**) are visible in the interstitial connective tissue (**10**). The **serosa** (**11**) of the visceral peritoneum forms the outermost layer on the uterine tube, which is connected to the **mesosalpinx ligament** (**1**) of the superior margin of the broad ligament.

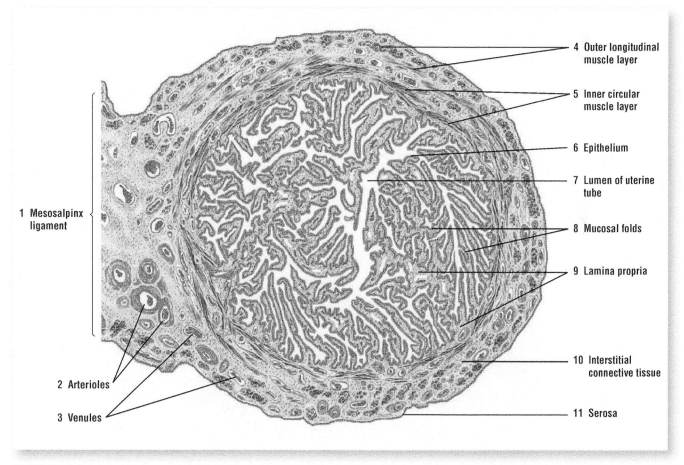

1 Mesosalpinx ligament
2 Arterioles
3 Venules
4 Outer longitudinal muscle layer
5 Inner circular muscle layer
6 Epithelium
7 Lumen of uterine tube
8 Mucosal folds
9 Lamina propria
10 Interstitial connective tissue
11 Serosa

FIGURE 21.14 ■ Uterine tube: ampulla with mesosalpinx ligament (panoramic view, transverse section). Stain: hematoxylin and eosin. Low magnification.

FIGURE 21.15 | Uterine Tube: Mucosal Folds

A higher magnification of the mucosal fold epithelium shows the **ciliated cells** (**3**) and nonciliated **peg** (**secretory**) **cells** (**1**). The ciliated cells (**3**) are most numerous in the infundibulum and ampulla of the uterine tube. The beat of the cilia is directed toward the uterus. Inferior to the epithelium is the **basement membrane** (**2**) and **lamina propria** (**4**) with **blood vessels** (**5**) and loose connective tissue. During the early proliferative phase of the menstrual cycle and under the influence of estrogen, the ciliated cells (**3**) undergo hypertrophy, exhibit cilia growth, and become predominant. In addition, the nonciliated peg cells (**1**) increase their secretory activity. The epithelium of the uterine tube shows cyclic changes, with the proportion of ciliated and nonciliated cells varying in the stages of the menstrual cycle.

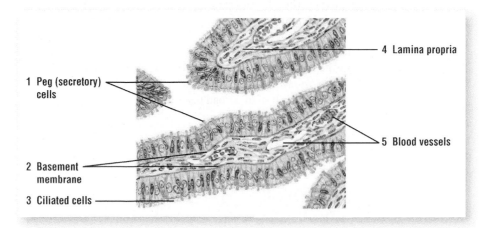

1 Peg (secretory) cells

4 Lamina propria

2 Basement membrane

5 Blood vessels

3 Ciliated cells

FIGURE 21.15 ■ Uterine tube: mucosal folds. Stain: hematoxylin and eosin. High magnification.

FIGURE 21.16 | Uterine Tube: Lining Epithelium

This high-magnification photomicrograph illustrates a section of the uterine tube with mucosal folds lined with a **simple columnar epithelium** (**2**).

The luminal epithelium consists of two cell types, the **ciliated cells** (**5**) and the nonciliated **peg cells** (**6**) with apical bulges that extend above the cilia. A **basement membrane** (**1**) separates

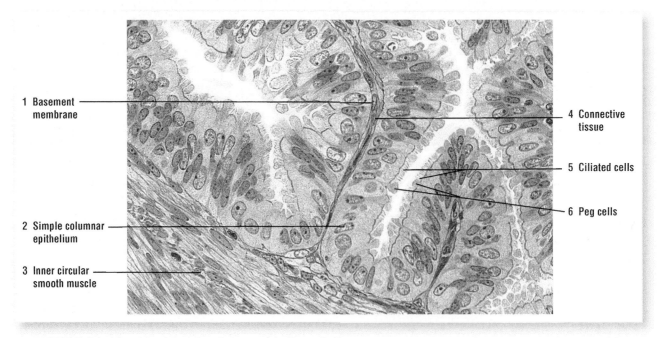

1 Basement membrane

2 Simple columnar epithelium

3 Inner circular smooth muscle

4 Connective tissue

5 Ciliated cells

6 Peg cells

FIGURE 21.16 ■ Uterine tube: lining epithelium. Stain: hematoxylin and eosin (plastic section). ×130.

the luminal epithelium (2) from the underlying **connective tissue** (4) that forms the core of the mucosal folds. A portion of the **inner circular smooth muscle** (3) layer that surrounds the uterine tube is visible on the left side of the illustration.

FUNCTIONAL CORRELATIONS 21.3 ■ **Uterine Tubes**

The uterine tubes perform important reproductive functions. Just before ovulation and rupture of the mature follicle, the finger-like **fimbriae** of the infundibulum that are close to the ovary begin to sweep its surface to capture the released oocyte. This function is accomplished by gentle **peristaltic contractions** of smooth muscles in the uterine tube wall and fimbriae. In addition, the ciliated cells on the fimbriae surfaces create a current toward the uterus that guides the released oocyte into the infundibulum of the uterine tube. The cilia action and the muscular contractions of the uterine tube transport the captured oocyte, or fertilized egg, through the uterine tube toward the uterus.

The uterine tubes also serve as the site of oocyte **fertilization**, which occurs in the **ampulla**. The nonciliated (peg) secretory cells in the uterine tube contribute nutritive material for the oocyte, the initial development of the fertilized ovum, and the embryo. The uterine secretions also maintain the viability of sperm in the uterine tubes and allow them to undergo **capacitation**, a complex biochemical and structural process that activates the sperm and enables them to bind to and fertilize the released oocyte. The fertilization triggers the ovulated

secondary oocyte to undergo the **second meiotic division** and produce an ovum that can be fertilized by the sperm.

When the sperm reaches the secondary oocyte, it must first penetrate the protective **corona radiata** layer around the oocyte. In order to fertilize the oocyte, the sperm must also penetrate the surrounding **zona pellucida** and bind to zona pellucida receptors to complete capacitation. This binding produces the **acrosome reaction**, which releases the hydrolytic enzymes from the acrosome on the sperm nucleus into the zona pellucida allowing its passage into the oocyte. As the sperm penetrates the oocyte, proteases released from the cortical granules present in the ovum cover the zona pellucida with a barrier and produce a block to **polyspermy** called the **cortical reaction**. This reaction allows the penetration of only one sperm to fertilize the egg.

The epithelium in the uterine tubes exhibits changes that are associated with the ovarian cycle. The height of the uterine tube epithelium is at its maximum during the follicular phase, at which time the ovarian follicles are maturing and circulating levels of estrogen are high.

FIGURE 21.17 | Uterus: Proliferative (Follicular) Phase

The surface of the **endometrium** is lined with a simple columnar **epithelium** (**1**) overlaying the **lamina propria** (**2**). The lining epithelium (1) extends down into the lamina propria (2) and forms long, tubular uterine glands (4). In the proliferative phase, the **uterine glands** (**4**) are usually straight in the superficial portion of the endometrium but may exhibit branching in the myometrium. As a result, numerous uterine glands (4) are seen in cross section.

The uterine wall consists of three layers: the inner endometrium (1 to 4), a middle layer of smooth muscle **myometrium** (**5, 6**), and the outer serous membrane perimetrium (not illustrated). The endometrium is further subdivided into a narrow, deep **basalis layer** (**8**) adjacent to the myometrium (5) and the **functionalis layer** (**7**), a wider, superficial layer above the basalis layer (8).

During the menstrual cycle, the endometrium exhibits morphologic changes that are correlated with ovarian functions. The cyclic changes in a nonpregnant uterus are divided into the proliferative (follicular) phase, the secretory (luteal) phase, and the menstrual phase.

In the proliferative phase and under the influence of increased levels of ovarian estrogen, the stratum functionalis (7) increases in thickness, and the uterine glands (4) elongate and follow a

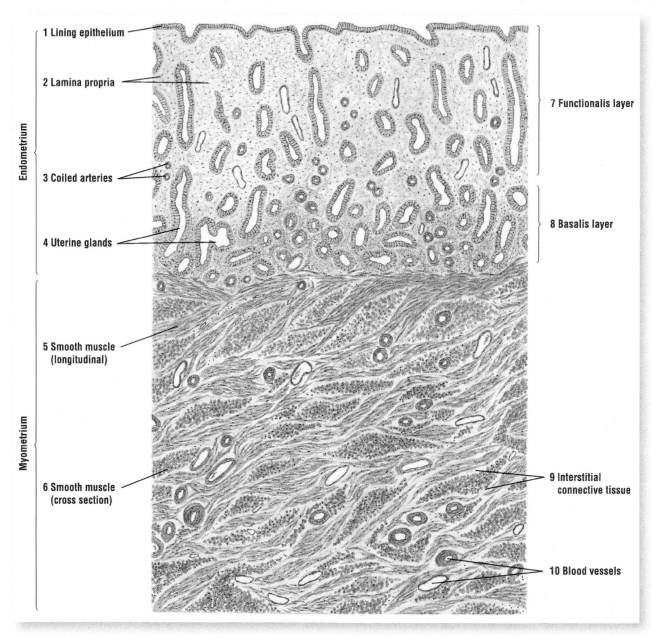

FIGURE 21.17 ■ Uterus: proliferative (follicular) phase. Stain: hematoxylin and eosin. Low magnification.

straight course to the surface. Also, the **coiled (spiral) arteries (3)** (in cross section) are primarily seen in the deeper regions of the endometrium. The lamina propria (2) in the upper regions of the endometrium resembles mesenchymal tissue. The connective tissue in the **basalis layer (8)** is more compact and appears darker in this illustration. The endometrium is situated above the myometrium (5, 6), which consists of compact bundles of **smooth muscle (5, 6)** separated by thin strands of **interstitial connective tissue (9)** with **blood vessels (10)**. As a result, the muscle bundles are seen in cross, oblique, and longitudinal sections.

FIGURE 21.18 | Uterus: Secretory (Luteal) Phase

The secretory (luteal) phase of the menstrual cycle starts after the ovulation of the mature follicle. The changes in the endometrium are now due to both estrogen and progesterone secreted by the functioning corpus luteum. As a result, the **functionalis layer (1)** and **basalis layer (2)** become thicker because of increased **glandular secretion (5)** and edema in the **lamina propria (6)**.

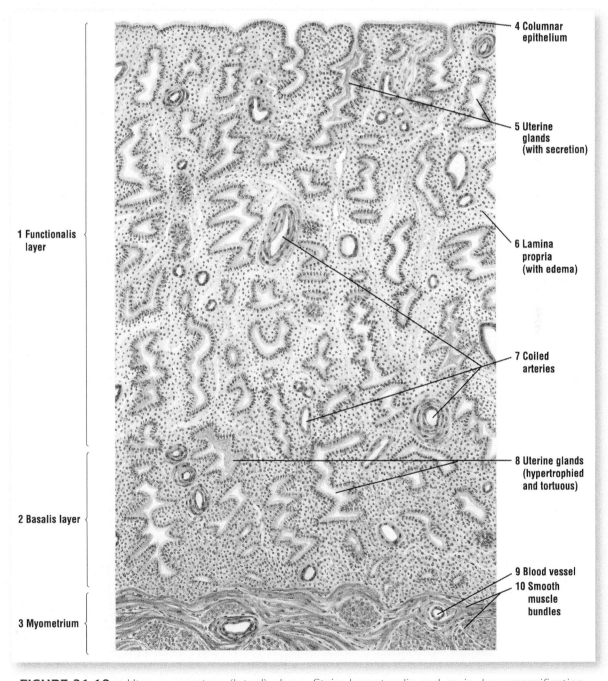

FIGURE 21.18 ■ Uterus: secretory (luteal) phase. Stain: hematoxylin and eosin. Low magnification.

The epithelium of the **uterine glands** (**5, 8**) undergoes hypertrophy (enlarges) because of increased accumulation of the secretory product (5, 8). The uterine glands (5, 8) also become highly coiled (tortuous), and their lumina dilated with **secretory material** (**5**) rich in carbohydrates. The **coiled arteries** (**7**) continue to extend into the upper portion of the endometrium (functionalis layer) (1) and become prominent because of thicker walls.

The alterations in the surface **columnar epithelium** (**4**), uterine glands (5), and lamina propria (6) characterize the functionalis layer (1) of the endometrium during the secretory or luteal phase of the menstrual cycle. The basalis layer (2) exhibits minimal changes. Below the basalis layer is the **myometrium** (**3**) with **smooth muscle bundles** (**10**), sectioned in different planes, and **blood vessels** (**9**).

FIGURE 21.19 | **Uterine Wall (Endometrium): Secretory (Luteal) Phase**

This low-magnification photomicrograph illustrates a section of the endometrium during the secretory (luteal) phase of the menstrual cycle. The thick and lighter area is the **stratum functionalis** (**1**). The darker and deeper endometrium is the **stratum basalis** (**2**). The **uterine glands** (**3**) are coiled (tortuous) and secrete glycogen-rich nutrients into their lumina.

Surrounding the uterine glands (3) is the **connective tissue** (**4**) with the light, empty spaces caused by increased edema. Below the stratum basalis (2) is the smooth muscle layer **myometrium** (**5**).

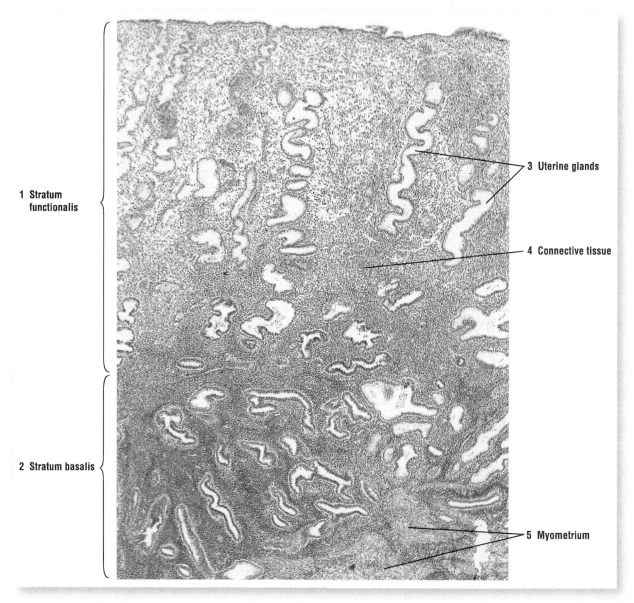

FIGURE 21.19 ■ Uterine wall (endometrium): secretory (luteal) phase. Stain: hematoxylin and eosin. ×10.

FIGURE 21.20 | Uterus: Early Menstrual Phase

If fertilization of the ovum and implantation of the embryo do not occur, the uterus enters the menstrual phase, and much of the preparatory changes made for implantation in the endometrium are lost. During the menstrual phase, the **functionalis layer (1)** degenerates and is sloughed off with fragments of disintegrated stroma, **blood clots (7)**, and uterine glands, some of which are filled with **blood (6)**. The deeper **basalis layer (4)** with the **bases of the uterine glands (9)** remains intact as the functionalis layer is shed during the menstrual flow.

The endometrial stroma of the functionalis layer also contains aggregations of erythrocytes (7) that have been extruded from the torn and disintegrating blood vessels. In addition, the endometrial stroma exhibits the infiltration of lymphocytes and neutrophils.

The basalis layer (4) of the endometrium remains unaffected during this phase. The distal (superficial) portions of the **coiled arteries (3, 8)** become necrotic, whereas the deeper parts of these vessels remain intact.

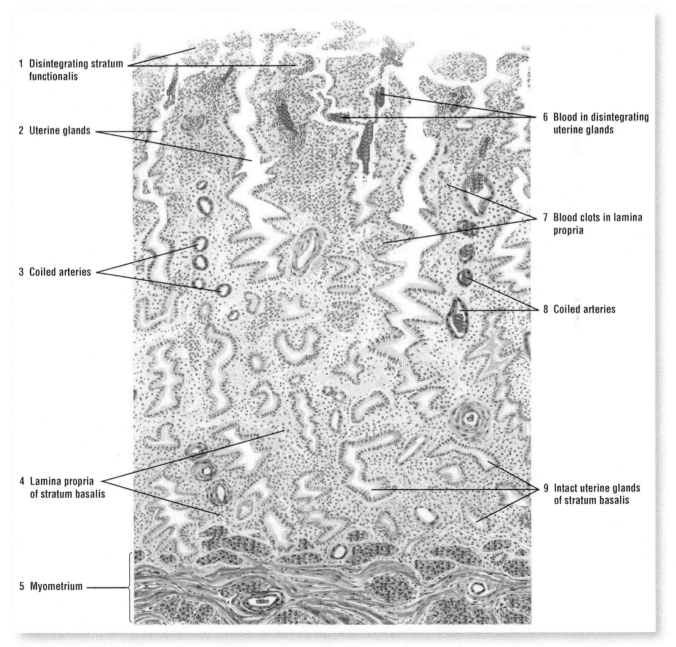

1 Disintegrating stratum functionalis

2 Uterine glands

3 Coiled arteries

4 Lamina propria of stratum basalis

5 Myometrium

6 Blood in disintegrating uterine glands

7 Blood clots in lamina propria

8 Coiled arteries

9 Intact uterine glands of stratum basalis

FIGURE 21.20 ■ Uterine wall: early menstrual phase. Stain: hematoxylin and eosin. Low magnification.

FUNCTIONAL CORRELATIONS 21.4 ■ Uterus

The endometrium exhibits cyclic changes in its structure and function in response to the ovarian hormones **estrogen** and **progesterone**. The uterine changes are associated with impending implantation and nourishment of the developing embryo. Secretion of progesterone by the functioning corpus luteum prepares the uterus for **implantation** of the embryo, formation of the placenta, and creation of a suitable environment for the development and maturation of the offspring. However, if fertilization of the oocyte and implantation of the embryo do not occur, the **functionalis layer** of endometrium is **shed** as part of the menstrual flow or discharge. With each menstrual cycle during the reproductive period, the endometrium passes through the proliferative, secretory, and menstrual phases, with each phase gradually passing into the next.

The **proliferative (preovulatory, follicular) phase** is characterized by rapid growth and development of the endometrium. The resurfacing and growth of the endometrium during the proliferative phase coincides with the growth of **ovarian follicles** and their production of **estrogen**. This phase starts at the end of the menstrual phase, or about day 5, and continues to about day 14 of the cycle. Increased mitotic activity of the connective tissue in the **lamina propria** and in basal remnants of the **uterine glands** in the **basalis layer** of the endometrium produces new cells and ground substance that begin to cover the raw surface of the uterine mucosa that was shed during menstruation. The resurfacing of the mucosa produces a new functionalis layer of the endometrium. As the functionalis layer thickens, the uterine glands proliferate, lengthen, become closely packed, and initiate secretory functions. The **spiral arteries** grow toward the endometrial surface and begin to show coiling.

The **secretory (postovulatory, luteal) phase** begins after ovulation on about day 15 and continues to about day 28 of the cycle. This phase is dependent on the functional corpus luteum formed after ovulation and the secretion of **progesterone** and **estrogen** by the lutein cells (granulosa lutein and theca lutein cells). During the postovulatory secretory phase, the endometrium thickens and accumulates fluid, becoming **edematous** (increased fluid reten-

tion). In addition, the uterine glands undergo hypertrophy, become tortuous, and their lumina are filled with **nutrient** secretions, especially **glycoproteins** and **glycogen**. The spiral arteries in the endometrium lengthen, become more coiled, and extend almost to the surface of the endometrium. These changes are due to hypertrophy of the glandular epithelium, increased vascularity, and edema in the endometrium.

The **menstrual (menses) phase** of the cycle begins when the ovulated oocyte is not fertilized, and no implantation occurs in the uterus. The corpus luteum begins to regress, resulting in reduced levels of progesterone (and estrogen) and initiating the menstrual phase. The spiral arteries in the endometrium are very sensitive to progesterone levels, and the decreased levels of this hormone cause intermittent constrictions of the spiral arteries and interruption of blood flow to the functionalis layer. These constrictions deprive the functionalis layer of oxygenated blood and produce **ischemia**, causing necrosis (degeneration) of blood vessels walls and the functionalis layer. After periods of vascular constriction, the spiral arteries dilate, rupturing their necrotic walls and causing hemorrhage (bleeding) into the stroma, leading to the detachment of the necrotic functionalis layer. Blood, uterine fluid, stromal cells, secretory material, and epithelial cells from the functionalis layer mix to form the **menstrual flow**, which lasts about 5 days. The basalis layer remains unaffected by these hormonal changes because it is supplied by straight arteries that are not dependent on or sensitive to the progesterone levels. As a result, the blood flow to basalis layer remains uninterrupted and unaffected by these cyclic changes.

The shedding of the functionalis layer continues until the raw surface of the basalis layer is left. At the end of the menstrual cycle, the stratum basalis consists of a thin layer of connective tissue and the basal parts of the uterine glands that will provide cells for regenerating the new functionalis layer. Rapid proliferation of cells in the glands of the basalis layer, influenced by rising estrogen levels during the proliferative phase, resurface and restore the lost stratum functionalis layer and prepare the uterus for the next phase of the menstrual cycle.

Chapter 21 Summary

SECTION 1 • Ovary and Uterus

FEMALE REPRODUCTIVE SYSTEM: OVERVIEW

- Consists of paired ovaries, uterine tubes, and a single uterus
- Uterus separated from vagina by cervix
- Organs exhibit cyclic monthly changes in the form of a menstrual cycle
- Start of first cycle is the menarche, and ending of cycles is the menopause
- Cycles controlled by follicle-stimulating hormone and luteinizing hormone and ovarian estrogen and progesterone
- Follicle-stimulating hormone and luteinizing hormone release controlled by gonadotropin-releasing hormone
- Immature oocyte released about every 28 days into uterine tube

OVARIES AND DEVELOPMENT OF FOLLICLES

- Germinal epithelium overlies connective tissue tunica albuginea
- Consist of an outer cortex and inner medulla, without distinct boundaries
- During embryonic development, oogonia divide by mitosis in gonadal ridges
- Oogonia enter first meiotic division and remain as primary oocytes in primordial follicles
- At puberty, primordial follicles can grow to become primary, secondary, and mature follicles
- Ovarian follicles can undergo degeneration or atresia at any stage of development
- Primordial follicles with primary oocyte are surrounded by squamous follicular cells
- Primordial follicles: initiation of development and activation dependent on local growth factors and gonadotropin stimulation
- Primary follicles exhibit simple cuboidal or stratified granulosa cell layers
- Secondary follicles exhibit liquid accumulations between granulosa cells or antrum
- Largest follicles are mature, span the cortex, and extend into medulla
- In maturing follicles, oocytes are located on the mound cumulus oophorus
- Theca interna and theca externa are visible in larger, developing follicles
- Primary oocytes are surrounded by zona pellucida and corona radiata cells in follicles
- Follicle-stimulating hormone (FSH) and luteinizing hormone (LH) are responsible for later development, maturation, and ovulation of follicles
- During the first half of the menstrual cycle and during follicular growth, FSH is the principal hormone
- FSH controls later growth of follicles and stimulates estrogen production from follicles
- LH stimulates theca interna cells that exhibit numerous LH receptors to secrete the estrogen precursor androstenedione
- Estrogenic steroid precursors converted to estrogen by aromatase enzyme in granulosa cells of the follicle
- Decreased follicle-stimulating hormone levels induce atresia in other developing follicles
- At midcycle, estrogen levels peak, induce a positive feedback, and cause the surge of LH
- FSH and LH release causes final maturation and ovulation of the dominant, mature follicle
- At ovulation, first meiotic division is completed, and a secondary oocyte is released
- Ovulation site on mature follicle is the thinned bulging area called stigma that is devoid of blood flow
- Ovulated follicle collapses, is vascularized, and becomes temporary corpus luteum
- Completion of second meiotic division occurs only when oocyte is fertilized by sperm
- Oocyte is viable for about 24 hours before it degenerates if not fertilized
- Interstitial cells in ovary are remnants of theca interna cells after follicular atresia

CORPUS LUTEUM

- Forms after ovulation and liberation of secondary oocyte
- LH induces hypertrophy and luteinization of granulosa cells and theca interna cells
- LH causes production of estrogen and increased amounts of progesterone
- Without fertilization, the corpus luteum is active for about 12 days before regression
- Regression leads to connective scar tissue corpus albicans
- After regression, inhibitory effects of estrogen and progesterone are removed

- FSH and LH are again released to start a new cycle of ovarian follicular development
- If fertilization occurs, corpus luteum becomes corpus luteum of pregnancy
- Human chorionic gonadotropin produced by trophoblasts stimulates corpus luteum
- Persists during pregnancy until the placenta produces estrogen and progesterone
- The placenta takes over corpus luteum functions and becomes temporary endocrine organ

UTERINE TUBES

- Extend from ovaries into the uterus and exhibit four continuous regions
- Infundibulum with fimbriae of the uterine tube located adjacent to the ovary
- Mucosa consists of extensive folds and forms irregular lumen
- Epithelium is simple columnar with ciliated and nonciliated secretory (peg) cells
- Ciliated cells create a current toward uterus and become predominant in proliferative phase
- Secretory cells provide nutrition for oocyte, fertilized ovum, and developing embryo
- Uterine tube secretions maintain sperm and enhance capacitation of sperm
- Smooth muscles provide peristaltic contractions to help capture ovulated oocyte
- Epithelium exhibits changes associated with ovarian cycle
- Sperm binds to receptors on zona pellucida, completes capacitation, and triggers acrosome reaction
- Acrosome reaction releases hydrolytic enzymes, and cortical reaction blocks polyspermy

UTERUS

- Consists of body, fundus, and cervix
- Wall consists of outer perimetrium, middle myometrium, and inner endometrium
- Endometrium is divided into stratum functionalis and stratum basalis
- During monthly menstrual cycles, stratum functionalis is shed with menstrual flow
- Endometrium morphology responds to estrogen and progesterone and ovarian functions
- Proliferative phase starts at the end of menstrual phase after estrogen release
- Ovarian estrogen induces endometrial growth and formation of a new stratum functionalis
- Secretory phase starts after ovulation and corpus luteum formation
- Estrogen and increased progesterone levels induce uterine gland secretion of nutrients
- Spiral arteries extend and reach the surface of endometrium
- Menstrual phase starts when the ovulated oocyte is not fertilized and no implantation occurs
- Spiral arteries are highly sensitive to declining hormone levels and constrict intermittently
- Ischemia destroys the walls of blood vessels and the stratum functionalis
- Dilation of spiral arteries ruptures walls, detaches functionalis, and causes menstruation
- Stratum basalis remains intact because straight arteries are not sensitive to progesterone levels
- Stratum basalis is not shed during menstruation, and blood flow is not interrupted
- Stratum basalis serves as the source of new cells for regenerating a new stratum functionalis

Chapter 21 Review Questions: Section 1

QUESTIONS

In the following multiple choice questions, choose the letter corresponding to the one best answer.

1. **What is main function of the acrosome reaction?**

   A. To activate the oocyte to undergo the first meiotic division
   B. To induce capacitation of sperm in the uterine tube
   C. To block polyspermy
   D. To release hydrolytic enzymes from sperm to penetrate the oocyte
   E. To increase sperm motility

2. **During the proliferative phase of the menstrual cycle, what changes are seen in the uterine wall?**

   A. Growth and resurfacing of the basalis layer to form a new functionalis layer
   B. Increased accumulation of fluid in the endometrium
   C. Constriction and expansion of the spiral arteries in the functionalis layer
   D. Increased accumulation of nutrients in glands
   E. Blood flow to the basalis layer is reestablished

3. **During the menstrual phase of the menstrual cycle, what changes take place in the endometrium?**

   A. The basalis layer exhibits increased connective tissue proliferation.
   B. The functionalis layer degenerates due to ischemia (lack of blood supply).

   C. The spiral arteries are coiled and highly dilated.
   D. The arteries in the basalis layer cut off blood supply to the endometrium.
   E. The basalis and functionalis layers become ischemic and are shed.

4. **After completing its function and regressing, the corpus luteum transforms into:**

   A. an atretic follicle.
   B. a new corpus luteum.
   C. interstitial cells.
   D. a corpus albicans.
   E. lutein cells.

5. **Decreasing levels of circulating hormones affect the endometrium by:**

   A. decreasing nutrient secretion of the uterine glands.
   B. interrupting the flow of blood to the functionalis layer.
   C. stopping the flow of blood to the basalis layer.
   D. increasing the edema of the endometrium.
   E. stopping the blood flow to the uterus.

ANSWERS

1. **Correct Answer: D.** To release hydrolytic enzymes from sperm to penetrate the oocyte. This reaction allows the sperm to penetrate the surrounding cells of the corona radiata and zona pellucida to fertilize the oocyte.

2. **Correct Answer: A.** Growth and resurfacing of the basalis layer to form a new functionalis layer. When the functionalis layer is shed during menstrual flow, the remnants of the uterine glands remain in the basalis layer that does not lose its blood supply. During proliferative phase, the hormones stimulate these cells to resurface the uterine wall and form a new functionalis layer.

3. **Correct Answer: B.** The functionalis layer degenerates due to ischemia (lack of blood supply). The spiral arteries in

the functionalis layer are sensitive to decreased hormonal levels and undergo constriction that induces degeneration of this layer and its shedding during menstruation.

4. **Correct Answer: D.** A corpus albicans. This is a connective tissue scar that forms after the functioning corpus luteum regresses and ceases to function.

5. **Correct Answer: B.** Interrupting the flow of blood to the functionalis layer. The spiral arteries are very sensitive to the circulating levels of progesterone and estrogen. When the circulating levels of these hormones declines, the functionalis layer is affected because the spiral arteries begin to constrict and eventually cause the functionalis layer to be shed.

ADDITIONAL HISTOLOGIC IMAGES

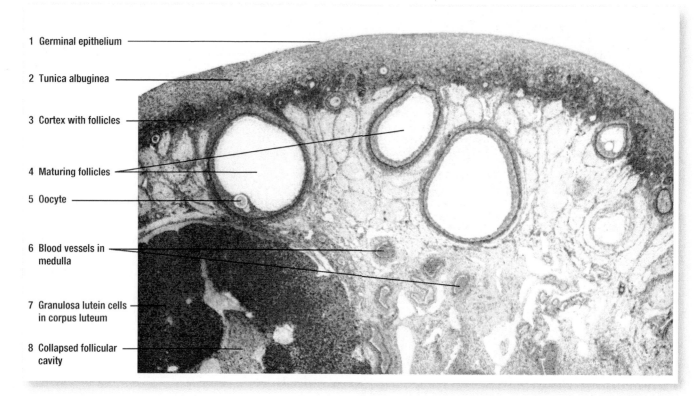

1 Germinal epithelium

2 Tunica albuginea

3 Cortex with follicles

4 Maturing follicles

5 Oocyte

6 Blood vessels in medulla

7 Granulosa lutein cells in corpus luteum

8 Collapsed follicular cavity

FIGURE 21.21 ■ Low-power section of a feline ovary with different stages of follicular development. Stain: hematoxylin and eosin. ×8.

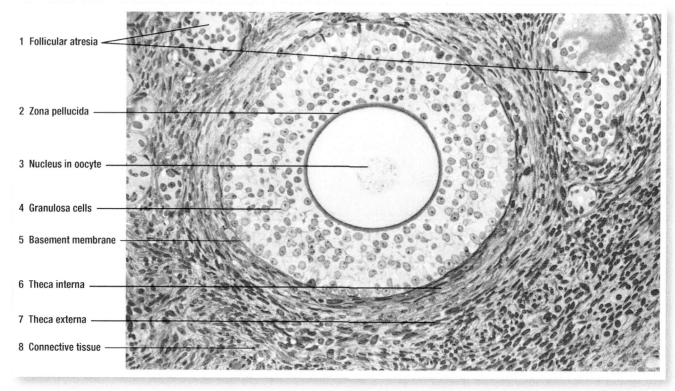

1 Follicular atresia

2 Zona pellucida

3 Nucleus in oocyte

4 Granulosa cells

5 Basement membrane

6 Theca interna

7 Theca externa

8 Connective tissue

FIGURE 21.22 ■ Structure of a developing primary follicle in the cortex with surrounding cells and an adjacent follicle undergoing atresia. Stain: hematoxylin and eosin. ×65.

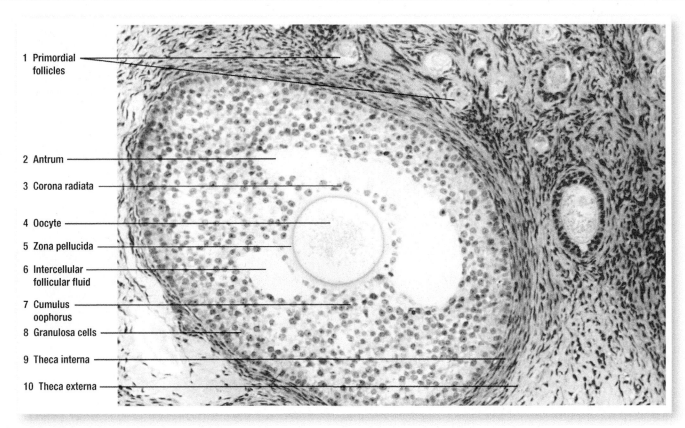

1 Primordial follicles

2 Antrum

3 Corona radiata

4 Oocyte

5 Zona pellucida

6 Intercellular follicular fluid

7 Cumulus oophorus

8 Granulosa cells

9 Theca interna

10 Theca externa

FIGURE 21.23 ■ Characteristic features of a maturing secondary ovarian follicle in the ovarian cortex. Stain: hematoxylin and eosin. ×65.

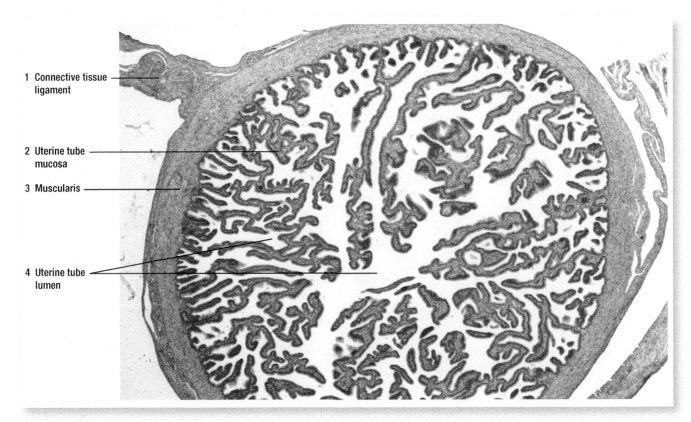

1 Connective tissue ligament

2 Uterine tube mucosa

3 Muscularis

4 Uterine tube lumen

FIGURE 21.24 ■ Ampullary region of a primate uterine tube illustrating the internal structure of the mucosa. Stain: hematoxylin and eosin. ×13.

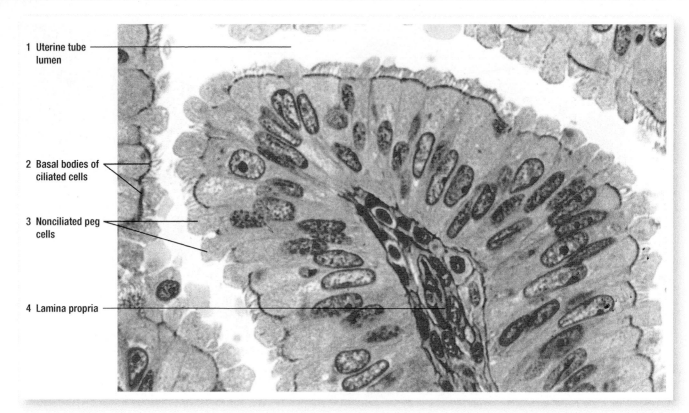

1 Uterine tube lumen

2 Basal bodies of ciliated cells

3 Nonciliated peg cells

4 Lamina propria

FIGURE 21.25 ■ A section of primate uterine mucosa illustrating the different cell types. Stain: hematoxylin and eosin. Plastic section. ×205.

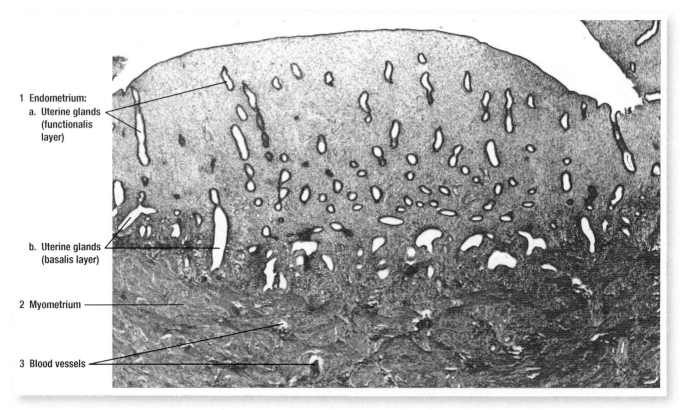

1 Endometrium:
  a. Uterine glands (functionalis layer)

  b. Uterine glands (basalis layer)

2 Myometrium

3 Blood vessels

FIGURE 21.26 ■ A section of human uterus during the proliferative phase. Stain: hematoxylin and eosin. ×6.5.

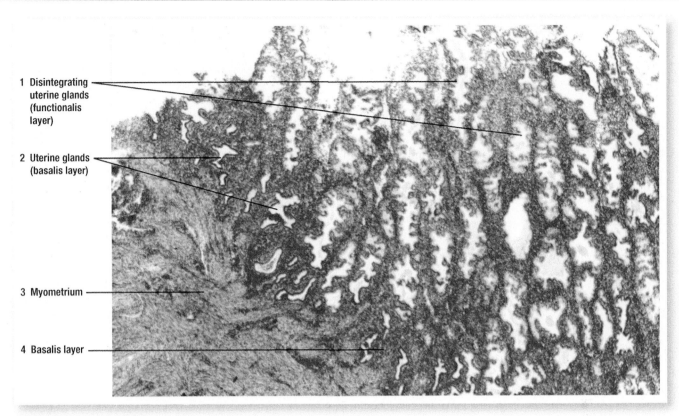

1 Disintegrating
  uterine glands
  (functionalis
  layer)

2 Uterine glands
  (basalis layer)

3 Myometrium

4 Basalis layer

FIGURE 21.27 ■ A section of human uterus during the menstrual phase. Stain: hematoxylin and eosin. ×6.5.

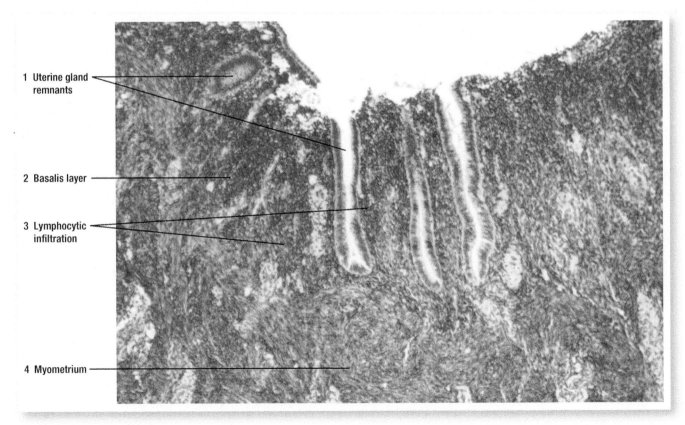

1 Uterine gland
  remnants

2 Basalis layer

3 Lymphocytic
  infiltration

4 Myometrium

FIGURE 21.28 ■ A section of human uterus in late menstrual phase showing the basalis layer and the remnants of uterine glands after the functionalis layer has been shed in menstrual flow. Stain: hematoxylin and eosin. ×6.5.

SECTION 2 Cervix, Vagina, Placenta, and Mammary Glands

CERVIX AND VAGINA

The cervix is located in the lower part of the uterus that projects into the vaginal canal as the **portio vaginalis**. A **cervical canal** passes through the cervix. The opening of the cervical canal that communicates with the uterus is the **internal os** and, with the vagina, the **external os**. The cervical mucosa is lined by simple columnar epithelium with branched mucus-secreting cervical glands. The mucosa undergoes minimal changes during the menstrual cycle and is not shed during menstrual flow. The **cervical glands** exhibit altered secretory activities during the different phases of the menstrual cycle. The amount and type of mucus that is secreted by the cervical glands change during the menstrual cycle because of varying levels of ovarian hormones.

The **vagina** is a fibromuscular structure that extends from the cervix to the vestibule of the external genitalia. Its wall has numerous folds and consists of an inner **mucosa**, a middle **muscular layer**, and an outer **adventitia**. The vagina does not have any glands in its wall, and its lumen is lined with a **nonkeratinized stratified squamous epithelium**. Mucus produced by cells in the **cervical glands** lubricates the vaginal lumen. Loose fibroelastic connective tissue and a rich vasculature constitute the lamina propria. Like the cervical epithelium, the vaginal lining is not shed during the menstrual flow.

PLACENTA

The **placenta** is a temporary organ that is formed when the developing embryo, now called a **blastocyst**, attaches to and implants in the endometrium of the uterus. The placenta consists of a **fetal portion**, formed by the **chorionic plate** and its **branching chorionic villi**, and a **maternal portion**, formed by the **decidua basalis** of the endometrium. Fetal and maternal blood comes into close proximity in the villi of the placenta. Exchange of nutrients, electrolytes, hormones, antibodies, gaseous products, and waste metabolites takes place as the blood passes over the villi. Fetal blood enters the placenta through a pair of **umbilical arteries**, passes into the villi, and returns through a single **umbilical vein**.

MAMMARY GLANDS

The adult mammary gland is a compound **tubuloalveolar gland** that consists of about 20 lobes connected to **lactiferous ducts** that open at the **nipple**. The lobes are separated by connective tissue partitions and adipose tissue.

The resting or inactive mammary glands are small, consist of **ducts**, and do not exhibit any developed or secretory alveoli. Inactive mammary glands also exhibit slight cyclic alterations during the menstrual cycle. Under estrogenic stimulation, the secretory cells increase in height, lumina appear in the ducts, and a small amount of secretory material is accumulated.

thePoint· Supplemental micrographic images are available at **www.thePoint.com/Eroschenko13e** under Female Reproductive System.

FIGURE 21.29 | Cervix, Cervical Canal, and Vaginal Fornix (Longitudinal Section)

The cervix is the lower part of the uterus. This figure illustrates a longitudinal section through the cervix, the endocervix or **cervical canal** (5), a portion of the **vaginal fornix** (8), and the **vaginal wall** (10).

The cervical canal (5) is lined with a tall, mucus-secreting simple columnar **epithelium** (2) that is different from the uterine epithelium, with which it is continuous. The cervical epithelium also lines the branched and tubular **cervical glands** (3) that extend at an oblique angle to the cervical canal (5) into the **lamina propria** (12). Some cervical glands may become occluded and develop small **glandular cysts** (4). The connective tissue in the lamina propria (12) of the cervix is more fibrous than in the uterus. Blood vessels, nerves, and occasional **lymphatic nodules** (11) may be seen.

The lower end of the cervix, the **os cervix** (6), bulges into the **vaginal canal** (13). The simple columnar epithelium (2) of the cervical canal (5) abruptly changes to nonkeratinized stratified squamous **epithelium** of the vaginal portion of the cervix called the **portio vaginalis** (7) and the external surface of the vaginal fornix (8). At the base of the fornix, the epithelium becomes the **vaginal epithelium** (9) of the vaginal wall (10).

The smooth muscles of the **muscularis** (1) extend into the cervix but are not as compact as the muscles in the body of the uterus.

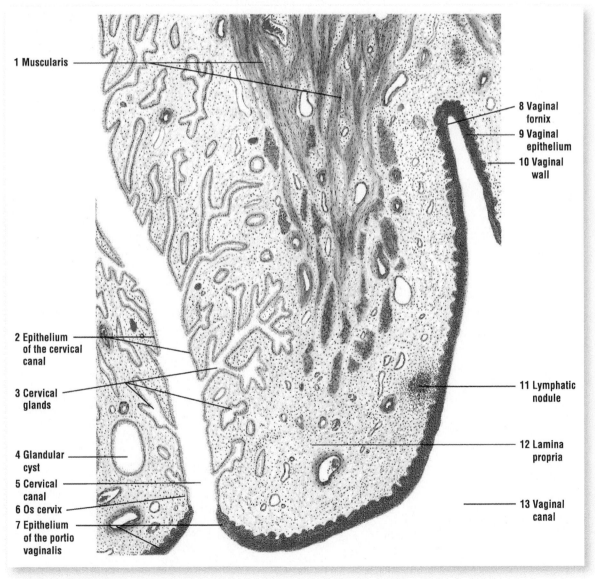

FIGURE 21.29 ■ Cervix, cervical canal, and vaginal fornix (longitudinal section). Stain: hematoxylin and eosin. Low magnification.

FUNCTIONAL CORRELATIONS 21.5 ■ Cervix

The cervical mucosa does not undergo extensive changes during the menstrual cycle. However, the cervical glands exhibit functional changes during the menstrual cycle that influence sperm passage through the cervical canal. During the **proliferative phase** of the menstrual cycle, the secretion from the cervical glands is thin and watery allowing for easier passage of sperm from the vagina through the cervical canal into the uterus. However, during the **secretory (luteal) phase** of the menstrual cycle and increased progesterone secretions, as well as during pregnancy, the cervical gland secretions change and become highly viscous, forming a **mucus plug** in the cervical canal. The mucus plug hinders the further passage of additional sperm and microorganisms from the vagina into the body of the uterus. Thus, the cervical glands in the cervical canal perform an important protective function initially in assisting the passage of sperm to fertilize the oocyte and later in protecting the developing embryo in the uterus.

FIGURE 21.30 | Vagina (Longitudinal Section)

The vaginal mucosa is irregular with **mucosal folds** (**1**) and covered by noncornified **stratified squamous** (**2**). The underlying connective tissue **papillae** (**3**) are prominent and indent the epithelium.

The **lamina propria** (**7**) contains dense, irregular connective tissue with elastic fibers that extend into the muscularis layer as **interstitial fibers** (**10**). Diffuse **lymphatic tissue** (**8**), **lymphatic nodules** (**4**), and small **blood vessels** (**9**) are in the lamina propria (**7**).

The muscularis of the vaginal wall consists predominantly of **longitudinal bundles** (**5a**) and oblique bundles of **smooth muscle** (**5**). The **transverse bundles** (**5b**) of the smooth muscle are less numerous but more frequently found in the inner layers. The interstitial connective tissue (**10**) is rich in elastic fibers. **Blood vessels** (**11**) and nerve bundles are abundant in the **adventitia** (**6, 12**).

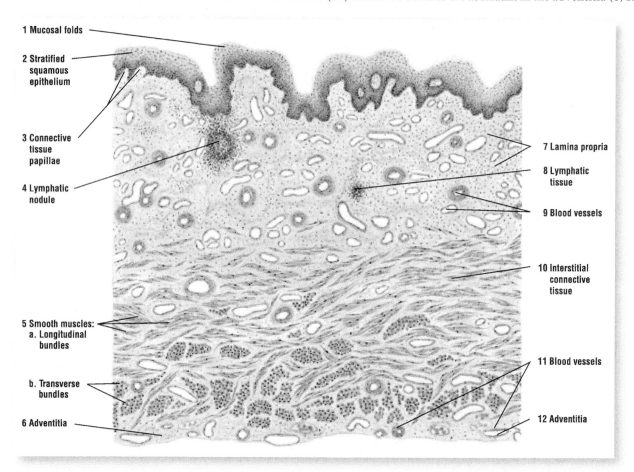

1 Mucosal folds

2 Stratified squamous epithelium

3 Connective tissue papillae

4 Lymphatic nodule

5 Smooth muscles:
a. Longitudinal bundles

b. Transverse bundles

6 Adventitia

7 Lamina propria

8 Lymphatic tissue

9 Blood vessels

10 Interstitial connective tissue

11 Blood vessels

12 Adventitia

FIGURE 21.30 ■ Vagina (longitudinal section). Stain: hematoxylin and eosin. Low magnification.

FIGURE 21.31 | **Glycogen in Human Vaginal Epithelium**

Glycogen is a prominent component of the vaginal epithelium, except in the deepest layers, where it is minimal or absent. During the follicular phase of the menstrual cycle, glycogen accumulates in the vaginal epithelium, reaching its maximum level before ovulation. Glycogen can be demonstrated by iodine vapor or iodine solution in mineral oil (Mancini method); glycogen stains a reddish purple.

The vaginal specimens in illustrations (a) and (b) were fixed in absolute alcohol and formaldehyde. The amount of glycogen in the vaginal epithelium is illustrated during the **interfollicular phase** (**a**). During the **follicular phase** (**b**), glycogen content increases in the intermediate and superficial cell layers.

The tissue sample in illustration (c) is from the same specimen as in (b) but was fixed by the Altmann-Gersh method (freezing and drying in a vacuum). This method produces less tissue shrinkage and illustrates more glycogen and its diffuse distribution in the vaginal epithelium during the **follicular phase** (**c**).

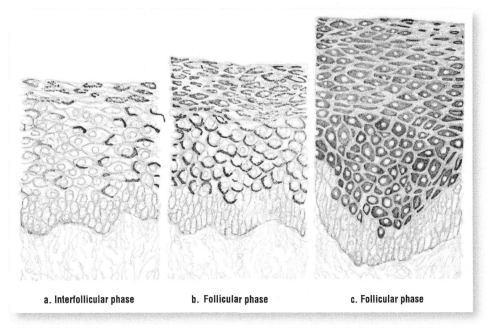

a. Interfollicular phase   b. Follicular phase   c. Follicular phase

FIGURE 21.31 ■ Glycogen in human vaginal epithelium. Stain: Mancini iodine technique. Medium magnification.

FUNCTIONAL CORRELATIONS 21.6 ■ Vagina

The wall of the vagina consists of the mucosa, a smooth muscle layer, and an adventitia without any glands. The surface of the vaginal canal is kept moist and lubricated by the mucus secretions produced by the **cervical glands**.

The vaginal epithelium exhibits minimal changes during each menstrual cycle. During the proliferative (follicular) phase of the menstrual cycle and increased estrogen stimulation, the vaginal epithelium increases in thickness. In addition, estrogen stimulates the vaginal cells to synthesize and accumulate **glycogen** as these cells migrate toward the vaginal lumen, into which they are shed, or desquamated. Bacterial flora in the vagina metabolizes glycogen into **lactic acid**, which increases acidity in the vaginal canal to protect the organ against microorganisms or pathogenic invasion.

Microscopic examination of cells collected (scraped) from the vaginal and cervical mucosae, called a **Pap smear**, provides valuable diagnostic information. Cervicovaginal Pap smears are routinely examined for early detection of pathologic changes in the epithelium of these organs that may lead to cervical cancer.

FIGURE 21.32 | Vaginal Exfoliate Cytology (Vaginal Smear) During Different Reproductive Phases

Vaginal exfoliate cytology (vaginal smear) is correlated with the ovarian cycle. The presence of certain cell types in the smear permits the recognition of the follicular activity during normal menstrual phases or after hormonal therapy. Also, exfoliate cytology together with cells from the endocervix provides information for the early detection of cervical or vaginal cancers.

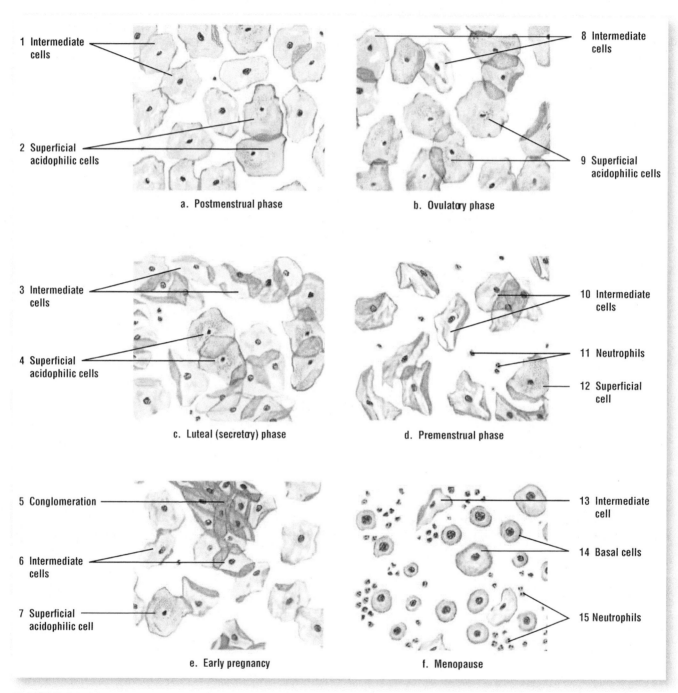

1 Intermediate cells
2 Superficial acidophilic cells

a. Postmenstrual phase

8 Intermediate cells
9 Superficial acidophilic cells

b. Ovulatory phase

3 Intermediate cells
4 Superficial acidophilic cells

c. Luteal (secretory) phase

10 Intermediate cells
11 Neutrophils
12 Superficial cell

d. Premenstrual phase

5 Conglomeration
6 Intermediate cells
7 Superficial acidophilic cell

e. Early pregnancy

13 Intermediate cell
14 Basal cells
15 Neutrophils

f. Menopause

FIGURE 21.32 ■ Vaginal exfoliate cytology (vaginal smear) during different reproductive phases. Stain: hematoxylin, orange G, and eosin azure. Medium magnification.

This figure illustrates cells in vaginal smears during different menstrual cycles, early pregnancy, and menopause. A combination of hematoxylin, orange G, and eosin azure facilitates the recognition of different cell types. In most phases, the surface squamous cells show small, dark-staining pyknotic nuclei and an increased amount of cytoplasm.

Figure (**a**) illustrates vaginal cells collected during the **postmenstrual phase** (5th day of the menstrual cycle). The **intermediate cells** (**1**) from the intermediate cell layers (precornified superficial vaginal cells) predominate including a few **superficial acidophilic** (**2**) cells and leukocytes.

Figure (**b**) represents a vaginal smear during the **ovulatory phase** (14th day) of the menstrual cycle. There is a scarcity of **intermediate cells** (**8**) and an absence of leukocytes, and the large superficial acidophilic cells (**9**) characterize this phase. This smear characterizes the high estrogenic stimulation prior to ovulation. The **superficial acidophilic cells** (**8**) mature during increased estrogen levels and become acidophilic. A similar type of smear is seen when a menopausal woman is treated with high estrogen doses.

Figure (**c**) represents a vaginal smear during the **luteal** (**secretory**) **phase** and represents the effects of increased progesterone. The large **intermediate cells** (**3**) with folded borders aggregate into clumps and characterize the smear. **Superficial acidophilic cells** (**4**) and leukocytes are scarce.

Figure (**d**) represents a vaginal smear during the **premenstrual phase**. This stage is characterized by a predominance of grouped **intermediate cells** (**10**) with folded borders, an increase in **neutrophils** (**11**), a scarcity of the **superficial acidophilic cells** (**12**), and an abundance of mucus.

Figure (**e**) illustrates a vaginal smear during **early pregnancy**. The cells exhibit dense groups or **conglomerations** (**5**) of **intermediate cells** (**6**) with folded borders. **Superficial acidophilic cells** (**7**) and neutrophils are scarce.

The vaginal smear during menopause in Figure (**f**) is different from all other phases. The **intermediate cells** (**13**) are scarce, whereas the predominant cells are the oval **basal cells** (**14**). Also, **neutrophils** (**15**) are in abundance. Menopausal smears are variable and depend on the stage of the menopause and the estrogen levels.

FUNCTIONAL CORRELATIONS 21.7 ■ Cellular Characteristics of Vaginal Cytology (Smear)

The superficial **acidophilic cells** of the vaginal epithelium appear flat and irregular in outline, measuring about 35 to 65 μm in diameter; exhibit small pyknotic nuclei; and contain cytoplasm that is stained light red (acidophilic) or orange.

The **intermediate cells** are flat like the superficial cell but are smaller, measuring 20 to 40 μm in diameter, and show a basophilic blue-green cytoplasm. The nuclei are larger than those of the superficial cells and are often vesicular. The intermediate cells are also elongated with folded borders and elongated, eccentric nuclei.

The larger **basal cells** are from the basal layers of the vaginal epithelium. All basal cells are oval, measure from 12 to 15 μm in diameter, and exhibit large nuclei with prominent chromatin. Most of these cells exhibit basophilic staining.

FIGURE 21.33 | Vagina: Surface Epithelium

This higher-magnification photomicrograph illustrates the vaginal epithelium and the underlying connective tissue. The surface epithelium is **stratified squamous nonkeratinized** (1). Most of the superficial cells in vaginal epithelium appear empty as a result of increased accumulation of glycogen in their cytoplasm. During histologic preparation, the glycogen was extracted by chemicals.

The **lamina propria** (2) contains dense, irregular connective tissue, lacks glands, but contains numerous **blood vessels** (4) and **lymphocytes** (3).

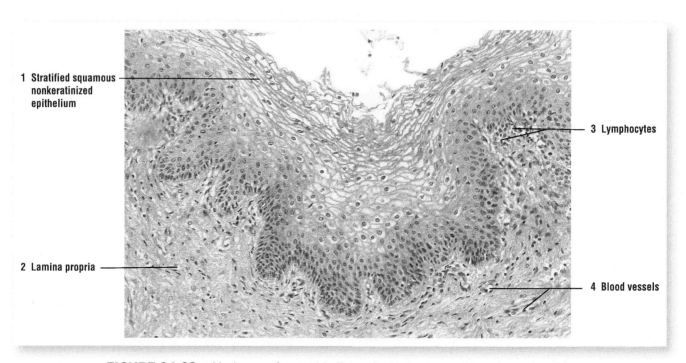

1 Stratified squamous nonkeratinized epithelium

2 Lamina propria

3 Lymphocytes

4 Blood vessels

FIGURE 21.33 ■ Vagina: surface epithelium. Stain: hematoxylin and eosin. ×50.

FIGURE 21.34 | Human Placenta (Panoramic View)

The upper region of the figure illustrates the fetal portion of the placenta, which includes the **chorionic plate** (1) and the **chorionic villi** (2, 10, 12, 14). The maternal part of the placenta is the **decidua basalis** (15) of the endometrium directly beneath the fetal placenta. The **amniotic surface** (8) is lined with a **simple squamous epithelium** (8), below which is the **connective tissue** (1) of the chorion (1). Inferior to the connective tissue (1) are the **trophoblast cells** (9) of the chorion (1). The trophoblasts (9) and the underlying connective tissue (1) form the chorionic plate (1).

The **anchoring chorionic villi** (2, 14) arise from the chorionic plate (1), extend to the uterine wall, and attach to the **decidua basalis** (15). The **floating villi (chorion frondosum)** (3, 10, 12), sectioned in various planes, extend in all directions from the anchoring villi (2). These villi "float" in the **intervillous space** (11) that is bathed in **maternal blood** (11).

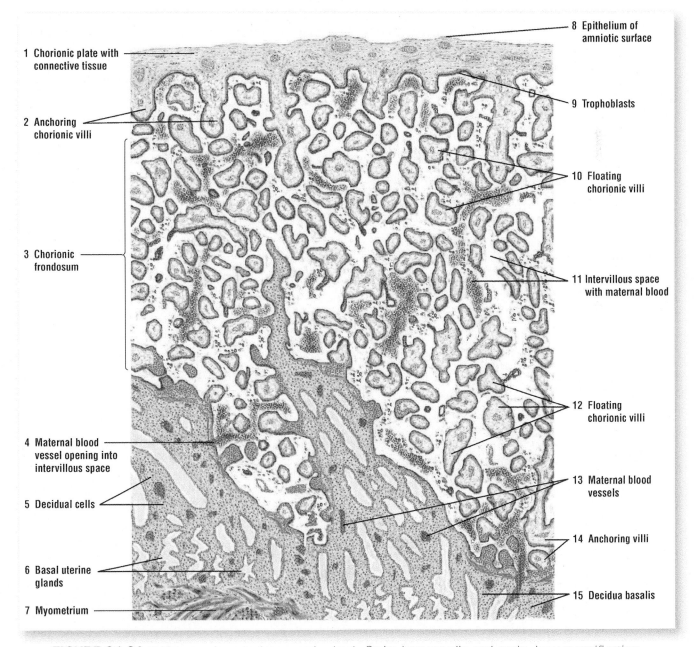

1 Chorionic plate with connective tissue

2 Anchoring chorionic villi

3 Chorionic frondosum

4 Maternal blood vessel opening into intervillous space

5 Decidual cells

6 Basal uterine glands

7 Myometrium

8 Epithelium of amniotic surface

9 Trophoblasts

10 Floating chorionic villi

11 Intervillous space with maternal blood

12 Floating chorionic villi

13 Maternal blood vessels

14 Anchoring villi

15 Decidua basalis

FIGURE 21.34 ■ Human placenta (panoramic view). Stain: hematoxylin and eosin. Low magnification.

The maternal portion of the placenta, the decidua basalis (15), contains anchoring villi (14), large **decidual cells** (5), and connective tissue stroma. The decidua basalis (15) also contains the basal portions of the **uterine glands** (6). The **maternal blood vessels** (13) in the decidua basalis (15) are recognized by their size or by the presence of blood cells in their lumina. A **maternal blood vessel** (4) is depicted as opening into the intervillous space (11).

A portion of the smooth muscle **myometrium** (7) of the uterine wall is visible in the left corner of the illustration.

FIGURE 21.35 | Chorionic Villi: Placenta During Early Pregnancy

The **chorionic villi** (6) from a placenta during early pregnancy are illustrated at a higher magnification. The embryonic trophoblast cells give rise to the embryonic portion of the placenta. The chorionic villi (6) arise from the chorionic plate and become surrounded by the trophoblast epithelium that consists of an outer layer of the darker-staining **syncytiotrophoblasts** (1, 10) and an inner layer of lighter-staining **cytotrophoblasts** (2, 9).

The core of each chorionic villus (6) contains mesenchyme, or embryonic connective tissue, and two cell types, the fusiform **mesenchyme cells** (8) and the darker-staining **macrophage** (Hofbauer cell) (4). The **fetal blood vessels** (3, 7), branches of the umbilical arteries and veins, are in the core of the chorionic villi (6) and contain fetal nucleated erythroblasts, although nonnucleated cells can also be seen. The **intervillous space** (11) is bathed by **maternal blood cells** (5) and nonnucleated erythrocytes.

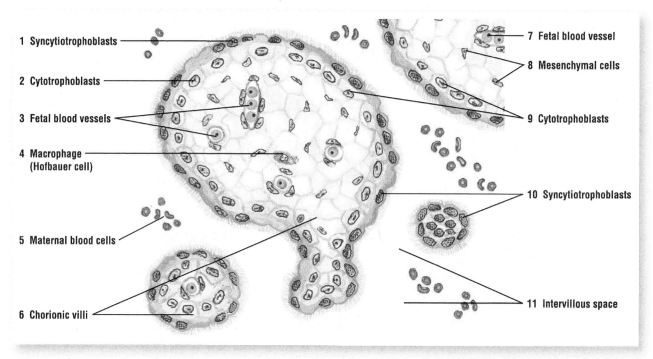

1 Syncytiotrophoblasts
2 Cytotrophoblasts
3 Fetal blood vessels
4 Macrophage (Hofbauer cell)
5 Maternal blood cells
6 Chorionic villi
7 Fetal blood vessel
8 Mesenchymal cells
9 Cytotrophoblasts
10 Syncytiotrophoblasts
11 Intervillous space

FIGURE 21.35 ■ Chorionic villi: placenta during early pregnancy. Stain: hematoxylin and eosin. High magnification.

FIGURE 21.36 | Chorionic Villi: Placenta at Term

The chorionic villi are illustrated from a placenta at term. In contrast to the chorionic villi in the placenta during pregnancy, the chorionic epithelium in the placenta at term is reduced to a thin layer of **syncytiotrophoblasts** (**1**). The connective tissue in the villi is differentiated with more fibers and **fibroblasts** (**4**) and contains large, round **macrophages** (**Hofbauer cells**) (**5**). The villi also contain mature blood cells in the **fetal blood vessels** (**2**) that have increased during pregnancy and the **intervillous space** (**6**) is surrounded by **maternal blood cells** (**3**).

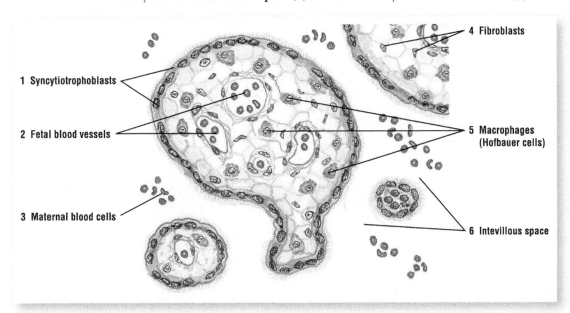

1 Syncytiotrophoblasts
2 Fetal blood vessels
3 Maternal blood cells
4 Fibroblasts
5 Macrophages (Hofbauer cells)
6 Intevillous space

FIGURE 21.36 ■ Chorionic villi: placenta at term. Stain: hematoxylin and eosin. High magnification.

FUNCTIONAL CORRELATIONS 21.8 ■ Placenta

The placenta performs important functions in regulating the **exchange** of substances between the maternal and fetal circulation during pregnancy. One side of the placenta is attached to the uterine wall and the other side to the fetus via the umbilical cord. Maternal blood enters the placenta through blood vessels located in the endometrium and is directed to the **intervillous spaces**, where it bathes the surface of the **chorionic villi** with vessels through which flows the fetal blood. Chorionic villi are separated from the intervillous space by double layers of trophoblast cells (syncytiotrophoblasts and cytotrophoblasts) that form the **placental barrier**. In the intervillous space, metabolic waste products, carbon dioxide, hormones, and water are passed from the fetal circulation to the maternal circulation. Oxygen, nutrients, vitamins, electrolytes, hormones, immunoglobulins (antibodies), metabolites, and other substances pass in the opposite direction. Maternal blood leaves the intervillous spaces through the endometrial veins. The maternal and fetal blood does not mix, and the placental barrier ensures this separation.

The placenta also serves as a temporary—yet major—**endocrine organ** that produces numerous essential hormones for pregnancy. **Placental**

cells (**syncytial trophoblasts**) secrete the hormone **human chorionic gonadotropin** (**hCG**) shortly after the implantation of the fertilized ovum. In humans, hCG appears in urine within 10 days of pregnancy, and its presence can be used to determine **pregnancy** with commercial kits. hCG is similar to luteinizing hormone in structure and function, and it maintains the **corpus luteum** in the maternal ovary during the early stages of pregnancy and stimulates it to continue producing estrogen and progesterone that are essential for maintaining pregnancy. The placenta also secretes **chorionic somatomammotropin**, a glycoprotein hormone that exhibits both **lactogenic** (mammary gland stimulation) and general **growth-promoting** functions.

As pregnancy progresses, the placenta gradually takes over the production of estrogen and progesterone from the corpus luteum to produce sufficient amounts of progesterone to maintain the pregnancy until birth. The placenta also produces **relaxin**, a hormone that softens the cervix and the fibrocartilage in the pubic symphysis to widen the pelvic canal for impending birth and **placental lactogen** that promotes growth and development of the maternal mammary glands.

FIGURE 21.37 | **Inactive Mammary Gland**

The inactive mammary gland is characterized by connective tissue and by a scarcity of the glandular elements. Some cyclic changes in the mammary gland may be seen during the menstrual cycles.

A glandular **lobule (1)** consists of small tubules or **intralobular ducts (4, 7)** lined with a cuboidal or a low columnar epithelium. At the base of the epithelium are the contractile **myoepithelial cells (6)**. The larger **interlobular ducts (5)** surround the lobules (1) and the intralobular ducts (4, 7).

The intralobular ducts (4, 7) are surrounded by loose **intralobular connective tissue (3, 8)** that contains fibroblasts, lymphocytes, plasma cells, and eosinophils. Surrounding the lobules (1) is a dense **interlobular connective tissue (2, 10)** containing blood vessels, a **venule and arteriole (9)**.

The mammary gland consists of 15 to 25 lobes, each of which is an individual compound tubuloalveolar gland. Each lobe is separated by dense interlobular connective tissue. A lactiferous duct independently emerges from each lobe at the surface of the nipple.

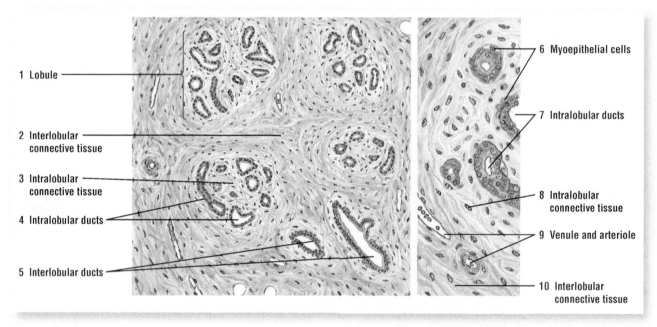

FIGURE 21.37 ■ Inactive mammary gland. Stain: hematoxylin and eosin. *Left,* medium magnification; *right,* high magnification.

FIGURE 21.38 | Mammary Gland: Micrograph of Inactive Mammary Gland

An inactive, or immature, mammary gland consists of undeveloped glandular ducts and dense irregular connective tissue. The **interlobular connective tissue** (4) is located between the glandular **lobules** (3) and the **intralobular connective tissue** (7) between the **intralobular ducts** (1). A larger **interlobular duct** (6) is located outside the lobules (3). Surrounding the intralobular (1) and interlobular (6) ducts are the contractile **myoepithelial cells** (2, 5).

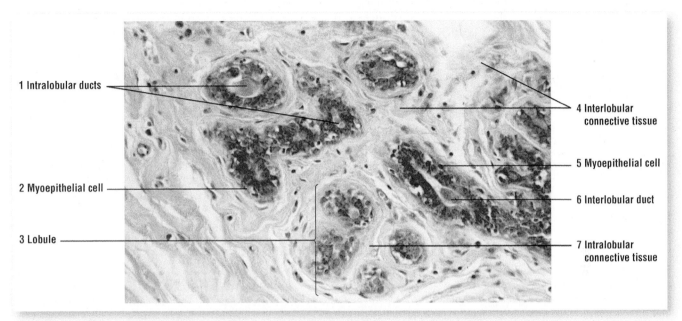

1 Intralobular ducts

2 Myoepithelial cell

3 Lobule

4 Interlobular connective tissue

5 Myoepithelial cell

6 Interlobular duct

7 Intralobular connective tissue

FIGURE 21.38 ■ Mammary gland: micrograph of an inactive mammary gland. Stain: hematoxylin and eosin. ×102.

FIGURE 21.39 | Mammary Gland During Proliferation and Early Pregnancy

For milk secretion (lactation), the mammary gland undergoes structural changes. During the first half of the pregnancy, the intralobular ducts undergo proliferation and form terminal buds that differentiate into **alveoli** (2, 7). At this stage, most of the alveoli are empty, and it is difficult

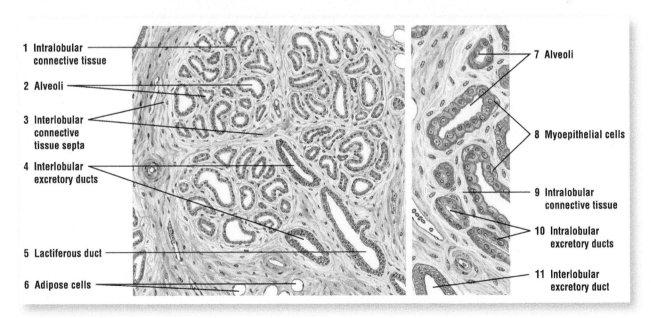

1 Intralobular connective tissue

2 Alveoli

3 Interlobular connective tissue septa

4 Interlobular excretory ducts

5 Lactiferous duct

6 Adipose cells

7 Alveoli

8 Myoepithelial cells

9 Intralobular connective tissue

10 Intralobular excretory ducts

11 Interlobular excretory duct

FIGURE 21.39 ■ Mammary gland during proliferation and early pregnancy. Stain: hematoxylin and eosin. *Left*, medium magnification; *right*, high magnification.

to distinguish between the **small intralobular excretory ducts** (**10**) and the alveoli (2, 7). The intralobular excretory ducts (**10**) appear more regular with a more distinct epithelial lining. The intralobular excretory ducts (**10**) and the alveoli (2, 7) are lined with two layers of cells, the luminal epithelium and a basal layer of flattened **myoepithelial cells** (**8**).

A loose **intralobular connective tissue** (**1**, **9**) surrounds the alveoli (2, 7) and the ducts (**10**); a denser connective tissue with **adipose cells** (**6**) surrounds the individual lobules and forms **interlobular connective tissue septa** (**3**). The **interlobular excretory ducts** (**4**, **11**), lined with taller columnar cells, course in the interlobular connective tissue septa (**3**) to join the larger **lactiferous duct** (**5**) that is lined with a low pseudostratified columnar epithelium. Each lactiferous duct (**5**) collects the secretory product from the lobe and transports it to the nipple.

FIGURE 21.40 | **Mammary Gland During Activation and Early Development**

The activated mammary gland exhibits well-developed secretory **alveoli** (**3**) and branching **intralobular ducts** (**6**) that are lined with a simple cuboidal epithelium and contain secretory products. Both the alveoli (**3**) and the intralobular ducts (**6**) are surrounded by **myoepithelial cells** (**7**). Between the alveoli (**3**) and the intralobular ducts (**6**) are **blood vessels** (**5**). Individual glandular lobules are separated by dense **connective tissue septa** (**4**), whereas the **interlobular connective tissue** (**1**) and the **intralobular connective tissue** (**2**) are thinner and less dense.

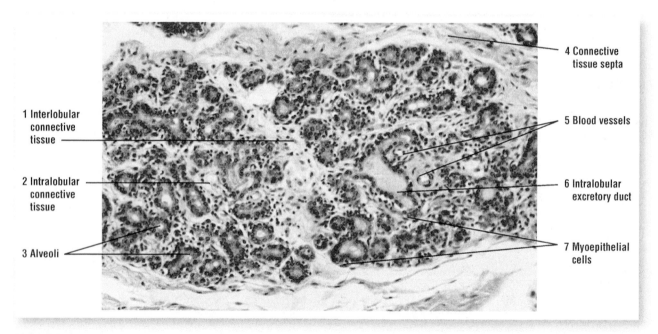

FIGURE 21.40 ■ Mammary gland during activation and early development. Stain: hematoxylin and eosin. ×85.

FIGURE 21.41 | Mammary Gland During Late Pregnancy

A section of a mammary gland with lobules, connective tissue, and excretory ducts is illustrated at lower (*left*) and higher (*right*) magnification. During pregnancy, the glandular epithelium becomes secretory, and the **alveoli** (**2, 8**) and the **ducts** (**1, 7, 13**) enlarge. Some of the alveoli (2) contain a secretory product (2, upper leader). However, the secretion of milk does not begin until after parturition (birth). Because the **intralobular excretory ducts** (1) also contain secretory material, the distinction between alveoli and ducts is difficult.

As pregnancy progresses, the **intralobular connective tissue** (**4, 11**) decreases, whereas the **interlobular connective tissue** (**3, 9**) increases because of the enlargement of the glandular tissue. Surrounding the alveoli are flattened **myoepithelial cells** (**10, 12**), more visible in the higher magnification on the right. Located in the interlobular connective tissue (**3, 9**) are the **interlobular excretory ducts** (**7, 13**), **lactiferous ducts** (**14**) with secretory product in their lumina, various types of **blood vessels** (**5**), and **adipose cells** (**6**).

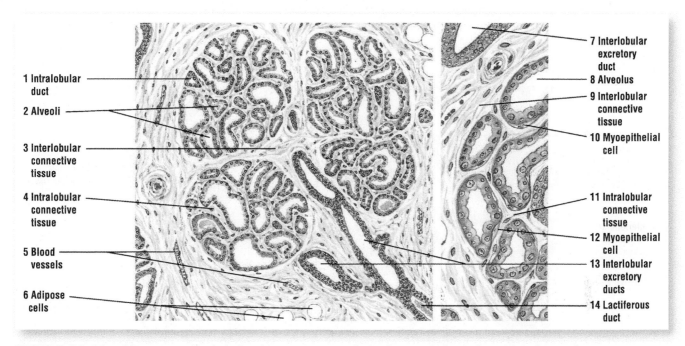

1 Intralobular duct
2 Alveoli
3 Interlobular connective tissue
4 Intralobular connective tissue
5 Blood vessels
6 Adipose cells
7 Interlobular excretory duct
8 Alveolus
9 Interlobular connective tissue
10 Myoepithelial cell
11 Intralobular connective tissue
12 Myoepithelial cell
13 Interlobular excretory ducts
14 Lactiferous duct

FIGURE 21.41 ■ Mammary gland during late pregnancy. Stain: hematoxylin and eosin. *Left*, medium magnification; *right*, high magnification.

FIGURE 21.42 | Mammary Gland During Lactation

This illustration of a mammary gland shows in greater detail the structure of alveoli during lactation at both lower (*left*) and higher (*right*) magnifications.

A lactating mammary gland exhibits distended **alveoli** filled with **secretions** and **vacuoles** (**1, 5, 9**) with some showing irregular **branching** (**1**). Because of increased size of the glandular epithelium (alveoli) and **adipose cells** (**10**), the **interlobular connective tissue** (**3, 7**) is reduced when compared to the inactive gland (Figs. 21.37 and 21.38)

During lactation, not all of the alveoli exhibit secretory activity. The active alveoli (1, 5, 9) are lined with a low epithelium and filled with milk that appears as eosinophilic (pink) material with vacuoles of dissolved fat droplets (1, 5, 9). Some alveoli accumulate secretory product in their cytoplasm, and their apices appear vacuolated, or light staining, because of the removal of fat during tissue preparation. Other alveoli appear **inactive** (**4**) with empty lumina lined with a taller epithelium.

Surrounding the alveoli are the myoepithelial cells (**8**) present between the alveolar cells and the basal lamina. With certain planes of section, the myoepithelial cells (8, upper leader) surround the secretory alveoli in a basket-like fashion. Contraction of the myoepithelial cells expels the milk into the **interlobular excretory ducts** (**2, 6**).

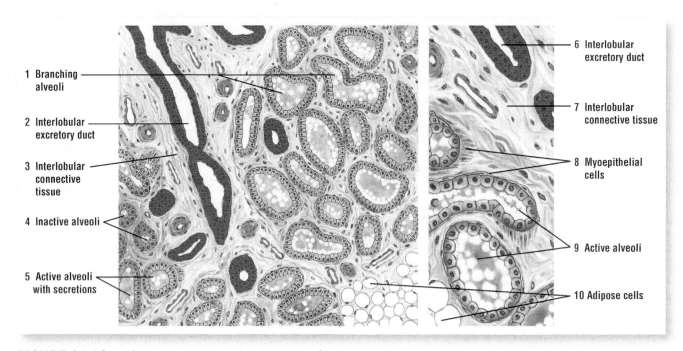

1 Branching alveoli

2 Interlobular excretory duct

3 Interlobular connective tissue

4 Inactive alveoli

5 Active alveoli with secretions

6 Interlobular excretory duct

7 Interlobular connective tissue

8 Myoepithelial cells

9 Active alveoli

10 Adipose cells

FIGURE 21.42 ■ Mammary gland during lactation. Stain: hematoxylin and eosin. *Left*, medium magnification; *right*, high magnification.

FIGURE 21.43 | Lactating Mammary Gland

This photomicrograph illustrates a lobule of a lactating mammary gland that is separated from the adjacent lobule by a layer of **connective tissue** (5). The **alveoli** (2, 3) contain **secretory product** (6) (milk) and are separated by connective tissue septa (5). Some alveoli (3) are single, whereas others are branching alveoli (2). All the alveoli drain into larger excretory ducts that deliver the milk to the lactiferous ducts in the nipple. The mammary glands contain large amounts of **adipose tissue** (1, 4) during lactation.

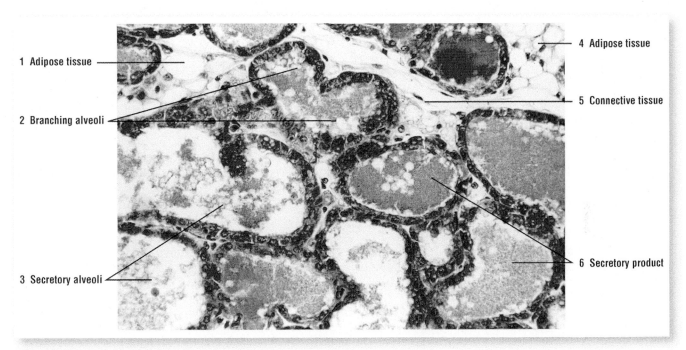

1 Adipose tissue

2 Branching alveoli

3 Secretory alveoli

4 Adipose tissue

5 Connective tissue

6 Secretory product

FIGURE 21.43 ■ Lactating mammary gland. Stain: hematoxylin and eosin. ×75.

FUNCTIONAL CORRELATIONS 21.9 ■ Mammary Glands

Before puberty, the mammary glands are undeveloped and consist of branched **interlobular ducts** that open at the nipple. In males, the mammary glands remain undeveloped. In females, mammary glands enlarge during puberty because of estrogen and progesterone stimulation during menstrual cycles. As a result, adipose and connective tissue accumulate, branching of the ducts increases, and numerous secretory alveoli are formed.

The mammary glands remain inactive until pregnancy. During pregnancy, the mammary glands undergo increased growth because of prolonged stimulation of estrogen and progesterone. As a result, the mammary glands become structurally and functionally mature. Estrogen and progesterone hormones are initially produced by the corpus luteum of the ovary and later by cells in the placenta. In addition, further growth of the mammary glands depends on the pituitary hormone **prolactin**, **placental lactogen**, and **adrenal corticoids**. These hormones stimulate the intralobular ducts of the mammary glands to proliferate, branch, and form numerous **alveoli**. The alveoli then undergo hypertrophy and produce milk during the lactation period. All alveoli become surrounded by contractile **myoepithelial cells**.

After the individual is born (parturition) and pregnancy ends, the mammary gland alveoli initially produce a fluid called **colostrum** rich in proteins, vitamins, minerals, and antibodies (IgA), which provide the newborn with some immunity. Unlike milk, colostrum contains little lipid. Milk is not produced until a few days after parturition. The hormones estrogen and progesterone from the corpus luteum and then placenta suppress milk production by mammary alveoli until their levels decrease.

After parturition and elimination of the placenta, the inhibitory hormones of milk secretion (estrogen and progesterone) are eliminated, and the mammary glands begin actively to secrete milk. As the pituitary hormone **prolactin** activates milk secretion, the production of colostrum ceases. During nursing of the newborn, tactile stimulation of the nipple by the suckling infant promotes further release of prolactin and prolonged milk production. Also, tactile stimulation of the nipple initiates the **milk ejection reflex** that causes the release of the hormone **oxytocin** from the neurohypophysis of the pituitary gland. Oxytocin causes the contraction of myoepithelial cells around the secretory alveoli and excretory ducts in the mammary glands, resulting in milk ejection from the mammary glands toward the nipple.

Decreased nursing and suckling by the infant soon results in the cessation of milk production and eventual regression of the mammary glands to an inactive state.

Chapter 21 Summary

SECTION 2 • Cervix, Vagina, Placenta, and Mammary Glands

CERVIX

- Located between uterus and vagina, with cervical canal passing into uterus
- Undergoes minimal change during menstrual cycle
- Cervical glands exhibit altered secretory activities, depending on menstrual cycle
- During proliferative phase, secretion is watery to allow sperm passage into uterus
- During secretory phase, secretion is viscous, forms a plug, and protects uterus

VAGINA

- Extends from cervix to external genitalia
- Does not have glands, is lined with stratified epithelium, and is lubricated by cervical glands
- Epithelium thickens after estrogenic stimulation but is not shed during menstrual cycles
- Glycogen accumulates during proliferative phase and, after metabolism, becomes acidic
- Vaginal exfoliate cytology (vaginal smear) is closely correlated with the ovarian cycle
- Follicular activity can be determined by predominant cell type in the smear
- Smears of surface epithelium are highly valuable for detecting cervical or vaginal cancers

PLACENTA

- The fetal portion includes the chorionic plate and its villi
- Maternal part includes the decidua basalis layer of endometrium
- Anchoring villi arise from chorionic plate and attach to decidua basalis
- Maternal blood enters intervillous space to bathe villi that contain fetal blood
- Regulates exchange of vital substances between maternal and fetal circulations
- Cells secrete the hormone human chorionic gonadotropin shortly after pregnancy
- Human chorionic gonadotropin appears in urine and is used for pregnancy tests
- Human chorionic gonadotropin stimulates corpus luteum to secrete estrogen and progesterone and other substances
- Takes over function of corpus luteum until birth

MAMMARY GLANDS

- Before puberty, they consist primarily of lactiferous ducts that open at the nipple
- Inactive glands contain connective tissue and ducts, surrounded by myoepithelial cells
- Estrogen and progesterone induce growth in females, forming tubuloalveolar glands
- Development also depends on prolactin, placental lactogen, and adrenal corticoids
- During pregnancy, ducts branch, enlarge, and form terminal buds with alveoli
- Late in pregnancy, alveoli contain some secretory products, but not milk
- At the end of pregnancy, alveolar secretion is colostrum, rich in proteins and antibodies
- During lactation, some alveoli are distended with secretory material containing more fat
- After placenta eliminated, prolactin activates milk secretion
- Suckling of nipple releases oxytocin, causing myoepithelial contraction and milk release

Chapter 21 Review Questions: Section 2

QUESTIONS

In the following multiple choice questions, choose the letter corresponding to the one best answer.

1. The vaginal mucosa is characterized by:

A. cells that produce lactic acid.
B. its surface containing mucous cells for lubrication.
C. its surface being lubricated by cervical glands.
D. its surface being lubricated by submucosal glands.
E. its surface layer being shed during menstrual flow.

2. What produces human chorionic gonadotropin (hCG)?

A. Pituitary gland
B. Endometrium
C. Ovaries
D. Corpus luteum
E. Placental cells (syncytial trophoblasts)

3. What hormone activates milk secretion or lactation?

A. Prolactin
B. Oxytocin
C. Estrogen
D. Progesterone
E. Follicle-stimulating hormone

4. Maternal and fetal blood:

A. mix in the intervillous space.
B. exchange metabolites and nutrients in umbilical veins.
C. are separated by the placental barrier.
D. mix in chorionic villi.
E. mix in the placental barrier.

5. The exchange of nutrients and metabolites for the developing individual occurs in the:

A. placental barrier.
B. umbilical veins.
C. chorionic villi.
D. umbilical arteries.
E. intervillous space.

ANSWERS

1. **Correct Answer: C.** Its surface is lubricated by cervical glands. Although its surface is lined by moist stratified squamous nonkeratinized epithelium, its surface is lubricated by cervical glands.

2. **Correct Answer: E.** Placental cells (syncytial trophoblasts). hCG is produced by the placenta cells and can be detected in urine within about 10 days of pregnancy, and its presence is used to determine pregnancy.

3. **Correct Answer: A.** Prolactin. After the placenta, estrogen, and progesterone are eliminated after parturition, the mammary glands are stimulated by the pituitary hormone prolactin to secrete milk.

4. **Correct Answer: C.** Are separated by the placental barrier. The trophoblast cells form the placental barrier, ensuring that the maternal and fetal blood do not mix.

5. **Correct Answer: E.** Intervillous space. It is in this space that exchange of nutrients and waste products takes place during pregnancy.

ADDITIONAL HISTOLOGIC IMAGES

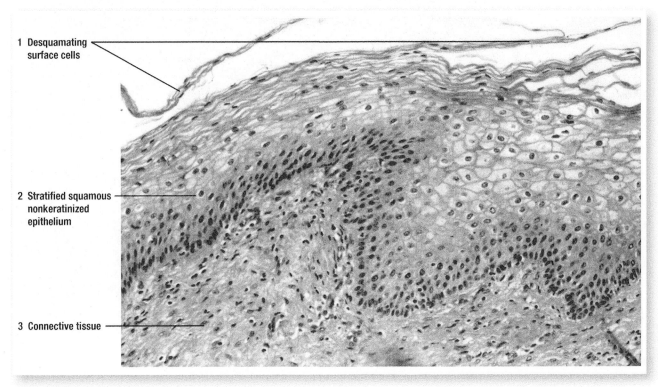

1 Desquamating surface cells

2 Stratified squamous nonkeratinized epithelium

3 Connective tissue

FIGURE 21.44 ■ A section of primate vagina illustrating its epithelium and the underlying connective tissue. Stain: hematoxylin and eosin. ×50.

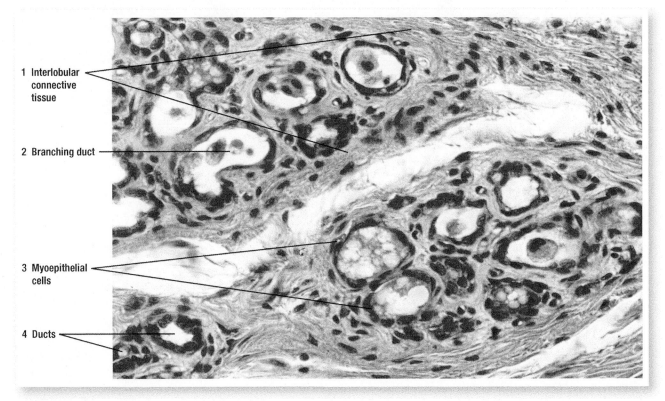

1 Interlobular connective tissue

2 Branching duct

3 Myoepithelial cells

4 Ducts

FIGURE 21.45 ■ A section of an inactive human mammary gland lobule illustrating the ducts and surrounding connective tissue. Stain: hematoxylin and eosin. ×80.

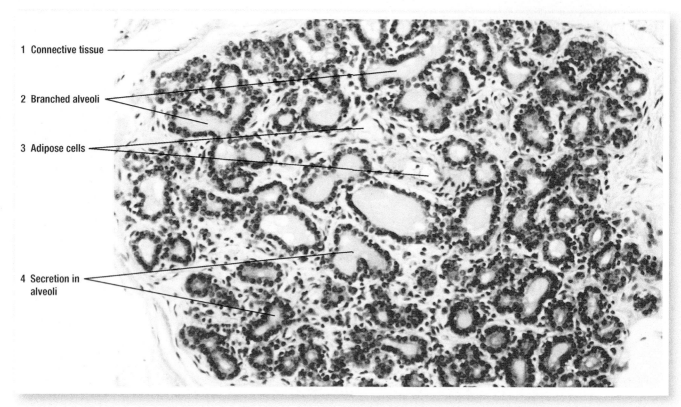

1 Connective tissue

2 Branched alveoli

3 Adipose cells

4 Secretion in alveoli

FIGURE 21.46 ■ A section of a lobule from an active primate mammary gland during pregnancy illustrating the developed alveoli. Stain: hematoxylin and eosin. ×50.

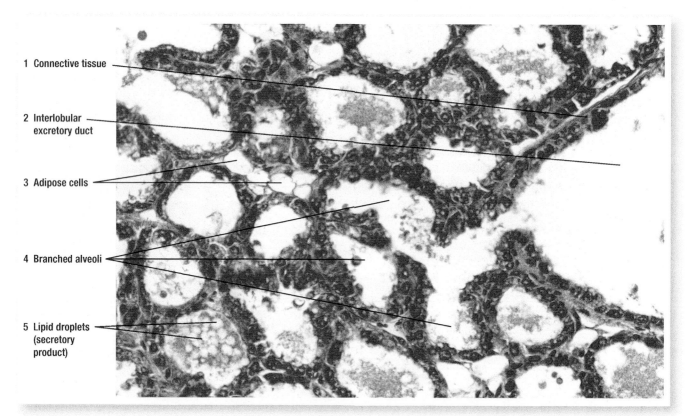

1 Connective tissue

2 Interlobular excretory duct

3 Adipose cells

4 Branched alveoli

5 Lipid droplets (secretory product)

FIGURE 21.47 ■ A section of a lactating rodent mammary gland illustrating alveoli with secretory products and an interlobular excretory duct. Stain: hematoxylin and eosin. ×80.

Organs of Special Senses: Visual Auditory Systems

SECTION 1   Visual System

In the visual system, the eye is a specialized organ for perception of form, light, and color. The eyes are located in cavities within the skull, called **orbits**. Each eye contains a protective cover to maintain its shape, a lens for focusing, photosensitive cells that respond to light stimuli, and cells that process visual information. The visual impulses from the photosensitive cells are conveyed to the brain via the axons that leave the eye in the **optic nerve**.

EYE LAYERS

Each eyeball is surrounded by three layers. The outer fibrous layer consists of cornea and sclera, the middle is the vascular layer, and the inner layer is the sensory retina.

Cornea and Sclera

On the anterior sixth of the eyeball, the fibrous **sclera** is modified into a transparent **cornea**, through which light enters the eye (Fig. 22.1). The posterior five sixths of the sclera is an opaque outer layer of dense connective tissue that extends from the cornea to the optic nerve. The inner layer of the sclera is located adjacent to the **choroid**, which contains connective tissue fibers and cells, including macrophages and melanocytes.

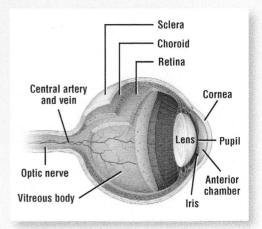

FIGURE 22.1 ■ The internal structures of the eye.

Vascular Layer (Uvea)

Internal to the sclera is the middle or vascular layer (**uvea**) that consists of a densely pigmented layer called the **choroid**, a **ciliary body**, and an **iris**. Choroid is the pigmented dark brown layer with melanocytes that is located between the sclera and the light-sensitive retina. Located in the choroid are blood vessels that nourish the photoreceptor cells in the retina and structures of the eyeball.

Retina

The innermost lining of the posterior chamber of the eye is the **retina** that is in contact with the vascular choroid. The posterior three-quarters of the retina is **photosensitive** and consists of rods, cones, and various **interneurons** that are stimulated by and respond to light (Fig. 22.2). The photosensitive part of the retina terminates in the anterior region of the eye, the **ora serrata**. This **nonphotosensitive** part of the retina continues forward in the eye to line the inner part of the ciliary body and the posterior region of the iris.

EYE CHAMBERS

The eye also contains three chambers.

- The **anterior chamber** is located between the cornea, iris, and lens.
- The **posterior chamber** is situated between the iris, ciliary process, zonular fibers, and lens. The zonular fibers radiate from the ciliary process and insert into the lens capsule, forming the suspensory ligaments of the lens that anchor it in the eyeball.
- The **vitreous chamber** is a larger, posterior space situated behind the lens and zonular fibers and is surrounded by the retina.

Chamber Contents: Aqueous Humor and Vitreous Body

The anterior and posterior chambers of the eye are filled with a clear, watery fluid called the **aqueous humor**. This fluid is continually produced by the epithelial cells of the **ciliary process** located behind the iris in the posterior chamber. Aqueous humor circulates from the posterior chamber to the anterior chamber, where it is drained by veins.

The vitreous chamber is filled with a transparent gelatinous substance called the **vitreous body** containing water with soluble proteins. The fluid component of the vitreous body is called the **vitreous humor**.

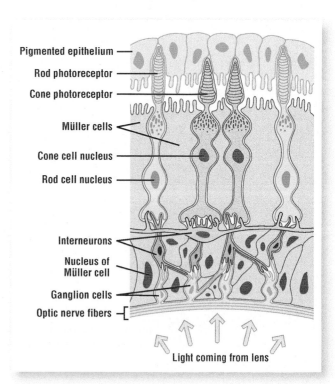

Pigmented epithelium
Rod photoreceptor
Cone photoreceptor
Müller cells
Cone cell nucleus
Rod cell nucleus
Interneurons
Nucleus of Müller cell
Ganglion cells
Optic nerve fibers
Light coming from lens

FIGURE 22.2 ■ The cells that constitute the photosensitive retina.

PHOTOSENSITIVE PARTS OF EYE

The photosensitive retina contains cell types that are organized into distinct cell layers. The light-sensitive layer contains cells called **rods** and **cones** that are stimulated by light rays that pass through the lens (see Fig. 22.2). Leaving the retina are **afferent** (sensory) **axons** (nerve fibers) that conduct light impulses from the retina via the **optic nerve** to the brain for visual interpretation.

The posterior region of the eye also contains a yellowish pigmented spot called the **macula lutea**. In the center of the macula lutea is a depression called the fovea that is devoid of photoreceptive rods and blood vessels. Instead, the fovea contains a dense concentration of photosensitive cones.

the**Point®** Supplemental micrographic images are available at **www.thePoint.com/Eroschenko13e** under Organs of the Special Senses.

FIGURE 22.3 | Eyelid (Sagittal Section)

The exterior layer of the eyelid is composed of thin skin (left side). The **epidermis** (**4**) consists of stratified squamous epithelium with papillae. In the **dermis** (**6**) are **hair follicles** (**1, 3**) with **sebaceous glands** (**3**) and **sweat glands** (**5**).

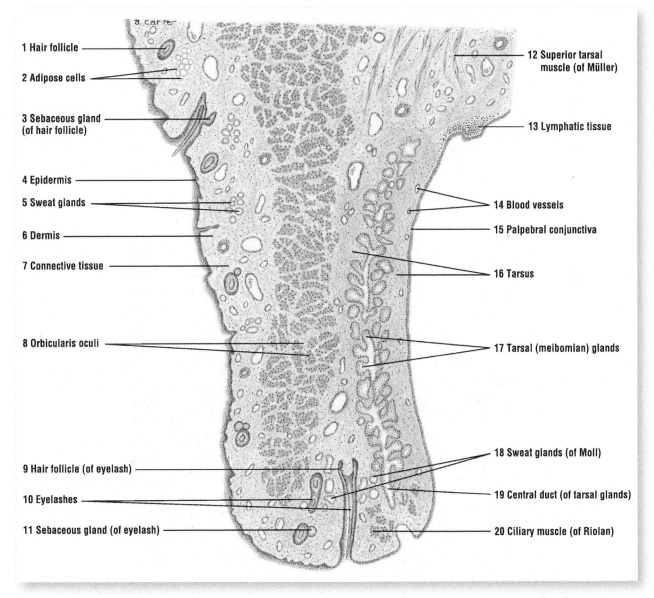

1 Hair follicle
2 Adipose cells
3 Sebaceous gland (of hair follicle)
4 Epidermis
5 Sweat glands
6 Dermis
7 Connective tissue
8 Orbicularis oculi
9 Hair follicle (of eyelash)
10 Eyelashes
11 Sebaceous gland (of eyelash)
12 Superior tarsal muscle (of Müller)
13 Lymphatic tissue
14 Blood vessels
15 Palpebral conjunctiva
16 Tarsus
17 Tarsal (meibomian) glands
18 Sweat glands (of Moll)
19 Central duct (of tarsal glands)
20 Ciliary muscle (of Riolan)

FIGURE 22.3 ■ Eyelid (sagittal section). Stain: hematoxylin and eosin. Low magnification.

The interior layer of the eyelid is a mucous membrane called the **palpebral conjunctiva** (**15**) lined by low stratified columnar epithelium with a few goblet cells. Palpebral conjunctiva is adjacent to the eyeball. The stratified squamous epithelium (4) of the thin skin continues over the margin of the eyelid and then merges into the stratified columnar of the palpebral conjunctiva (15).

The thin lamina propria of the palpebral conjunctiva (15) contains both elastic and collagen fibers. Inferior to the lamina propria is a plate of dense, collagenous connective tissue called the **tarsus** (**16**), which contains specialized sebaceous glands called the **tarsal** (**meibomian**) **glands** (**17**). The secretory acini of the tarsal glands (17) open into a **central duct** (**19**) that runs parallel to the palpebral conjunctiva (15) and opens at the margin of the eyelid.

The free end of the eyelid contains **eyelashes** (**10**) that arise from large, long hair follicles (9). Associated with the eyelashes (10) are small **sebaceous glands** (**11**). Between the hair follicles (9) of the eyelashes (10) are large **sweat glands** (**of Moll**) (**18**).

The eyelid contains three sets of muscles: the palpebral portion of the skeletal muscle, called the **orbicularis oculi** (**8**); the skeletal **ciliary muscle** (**of Riolan**) (**20**) in the region of the hair follicles (9), the eyelashes (10), and the tarsal glands (17); and smooth muscle called the superior **tarsal muscle** (**of Muller**) (**12**) in the upper eyelid.

The connective **tissue** (**7**) of the eyelid contains **adipose cells** (**2**), **blood vessels** (**14**), and **lymphatic tissue** (**13**).

FIGURE 22.4 | Lacrimal Gland

The lacrimal gland consists of several lobes separated into lobules by the **connective tissue** (**2**) septa with **nerves** (**4**), **adipose cells** (**6**), and **blood vessels** (**9**). The lacrimal gland is a serous compound gland that resembles the salivary glands in lobular structure and **tubuloalveolar acini** (**8**). The **myoepithelial cells** (**1, 5**) surround the individual secretory acini (8).

A small **intralobular excretory duct** (**7**), lined with a simple cuboidal or columnar epithelium, is located between the tubuloalveolar acini (8). The larger **interlobular excretory duct** (**3**) is lined with two layers of low columnar cells or pseudostratified epithelium.

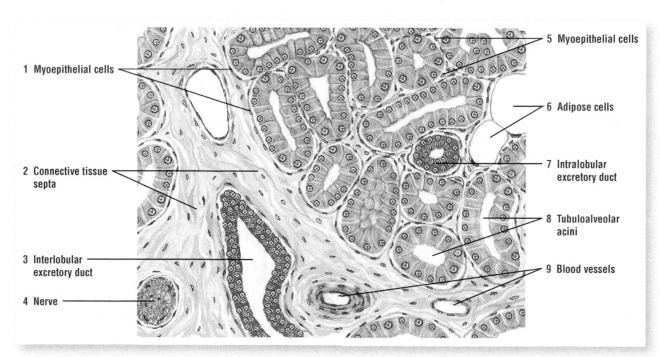

FIGURE 22.4 ■ Lacrimal gland. Stain: hematoxylin and eosin. Medium magnification.

FIGURE 22.5 | Cornea (Transverse Section)

The cornea is a thick, transparent, nonvascular structure of the eye. The anterior surface is covered with a stratified **squamous corneal epithelium** (**1**) that is nonkeratinized with five or more cell layers. The basal cell layer is columnar and rests on a thin basement membrane supported by a thick, homogeneous **anterior limiting (Bowman) membrane** (**4**). The underlying **corneal stroma (substantia propria)** (**2**) forms the body of the cornea. It consists of parallel bundles of **collagen fibers** (**5**) and layers of flat **fibroblasts** (**6**).

The **posterior limiting (Descemet) membrane** (**7**) is also a thick basement membrane that is located at the posterior portion of the corneal stroma (**2**). The posterior surface of the cornea that faces the anterior chamber of the eye is covered with a simple squamous epithelium called the **posterior epithelium** (**3**), which is also the corneal endothelium. These cells are in direct contact with the aqueous humor of the anterior chamber of the eye.

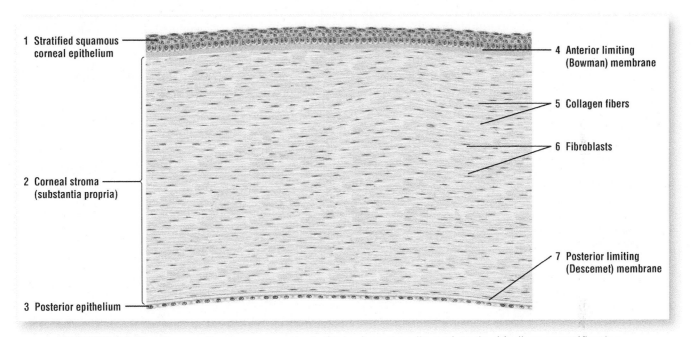

1 Stratified squamous corneal epithelium

2 Corneal stroma (substantia propria)

3 Posterior epithelium

4 Anterior limiting (Bowman) membrane

5 Collagen fibers

6 Fibroblasts

7 Posterior limiting (Descemet) membrane

FIGURE 22.5 ■ Cornea (transverse section). Stain: hematoxylin and eosin. Medium magnification.

FIGURE 22.6 | Whole Eye (Sagittal Section)

The eyeball is surrounded by three layers: an outer, tough fibrous connective tissue layer composed of the **sclera** (**18**) and **cornea** (**1**); a middle layer or uvea composed of the vascular, pigmented **choroid** (**7**), the **ciliary body** (**consisting of ciliary processes and ciliary muscle**) (**4, 14, 15**), and the **iris** (**13**); and the innermost layer composed of the photosensitive **retina** (**8**).

The sclera (18) is a white, opaque, tough connective tissue composed of dense collagen fibers that maintain the rigidity of the eyeball and appears as the "white" of the eye. The junction between the cornea and sclera occurs at the transition area called the **limbus** (**12**), located in the anterior region of the eye. In the posterior region of the eye, where the **optic nerve** (**10**) emerges from the ocular capsule, is the transition between the sclera (18) of the eyeball and the connective tissue **dura mater** (**23**) of the central nervous system.

The choroid (7) and the ciliary body (4, 14, 15) are adjacent to the sclera (18). In a sagittal section, the ciliary body (4, 14, 15) appears triangular and is composed of the smooth **ciliary muscle** (**14**) and the **ciliary processes** (**4, 15**). The fibers in the ciliary muscle (14) exhibit longitudinal, circular, and radial arrangements. The folded and vascular extensions of the ciliary body constitute the ciliary processes (4, 15) that attach to the equator of the **lens** (**16**) by the suspensory ligament or **zonular fibers** (**5**) of the lens. Contraction of the ciliary muscle (14) reduces the tension on the zonular fibers (5) and allows the lens (16) to assume a convex shape.

The **iris** (**13**) partially covers the lens and is the colored portion of the eye. The circular and radial smooth muscle fibers form an opening in the iris called the **pupil** (**11**).

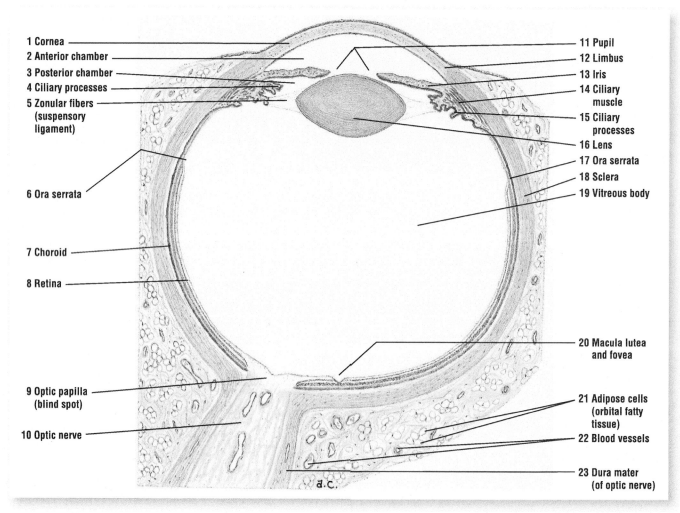

1 Cornea
2 Anterior chamber
3 Posterior chamber
4 Ciliary processes
5 Zonular fibers (suspensory ligament)
6 Ora serrata
7 Choroid
8 Retina
9 Optic papilla (blind spot)
10 Optic nerve
11 Pupil
12 Limbus
13 Iris
14 Ciliary muscle
15 Ciliary processes
16 Lens
17 Ora serrata
18 Sclera
19 Vitreous body
20 Macula lutea and fovea
21 Adipose cells (orbital fatty tissue)
22 Blood vessels
23 Dura mater (of optic nerve)

FIGURE 22.6 ■ Whole eye (sagittal section). Stain: hematoxylin and eosin. Low magnification.

The interior of the eye in front of the lens is subdivided into the **anterior chamber** (**2**) located between the iris (13) and the cornea (1) and the **posterior chamber** (**3**) located between the iris (13) and the lens (16). Both the anterior (2) and posterior (3) chambers are filled with a watery fluid called the aqueous humor. The posterior compartment located behind the lens is the **vitreous body** (**19**) and is filled with a gelatinous material, the transparent vitreous humor.

Posterior to the ciliary body (4, 14, 15) is the **ora serrata** (**6, 17**), a sharp, anteriormost boundary of the photosensitive retina (8). The retina (8) consists of numerous cell layers, one of which contains the light-sensitive cells—the rods and cones. Anterior to the ora serrata (6, 17) lies the nonphotosensitive retina that continues forward in the eyeball to form the inner lining of the ciliary body (4, 14, 15) and posterior part of the iris (13). The histology of the retina is presented in greater detail in Figures 22.8 and 22.9.

In the posterior wall of the eye is the **macula lutea** (**20**) and the **optic papilla** (**9**) or the optic disk. The macula lutea (20) is a small, yellow-pigmented spot, as seen through an ophthalmoscope, with a shallow central depression called the **fovea** (**20**), an area of greatest visual acuity in the eye. The center of the fovea (20) is devoid of rod cells and blood vessels. Instead, it contains a high concentration of cone cells.

The optic papilla (9) is the region where the **optic nerve** (**10**) leaves the eyeball. The optic papilla (9) lacks the light-sensitive rods and the cones and constitutes the "blind spot" of the eye.

The outer sclera (18) is adjacent to the orbital tissue and contains loose connective tissue, **adipose cells** (**21**) of the orbital fatty tissue, nerve fibers, **blood vessels** (**22**), lymphatics, and glands.

FIGURE 22.7 | **Posterior Eyeball: Sclera, Choroid, Optic Papilla, Optic Nerve, Retina, and Fovea (Panoramic View)**

This higher-magnification illustration shows a section of the retina in the posterior region of the eyeball. Visible are the pigmented **choroid** (**7**) with its blood vessels and the connective tissue layer **sclera** (**8**). A shallow depression in the retina is the **fovea** (**5**), which primarily consists of the light-sensitive **cones** (**6**). The rest of the retina contains the **rods** and **cones** (**3**), the different cell and fiber layers of the retina, and **fibers** of the **optic nerve** (**1**) that converge posteriorly in the eyeball to form the **optic papilla** (**2**) and the **optic nerve** (**4**), which exits the eyeball.

The specific cell and fiber layers that constitute the rest of the photosensitive retina are illustrated and described at a higher magnification in Figures 22.8 and 22.9.

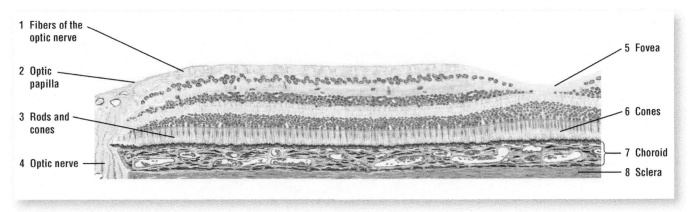

1 Fibers of the optic nerve
2 Optic papilla
3 Rods and cones
4 Optic nerve
5 Fovea
6 Cones
7 Choroid
8 Sclera

FIGURE 22.7 ■ Posterior eyeball: sclera, choroid, optic papilla, optic nerve, retina, and fovea (panoramic view). Stain: hematoxylin and eosin. Medium magnification.

FIGURE 22.8 | Layers of Choroid and Retina (Detail)

The inner layer of the connective tissue **sclera** (**10**) is adjacent to the choroid, which is subdivided into several layers: the **suprachoroid lamina with melanocytes** (**11**), the **vascular layer** (**1**), the **choriocapillaris layer** (**12**), and the transparent limiting membrane or glassy (Bruch) membrane.

The suprachoroid lamina (**11**) consists of fine collagen fibers, a network of elastic fibers, fibroblasts, and melanocytes. The vascular layer (**1**) of the choroid contains medium-sized and large **blood vessels** (**1**). In the connective tissue between the blood vessels (**1**) are **melanocytes** (**2**) that impart a dark color to this layer. The choriocapillaris layer (**12**) contains capillaries with large lumina. The innermost layer of the choroid, the glassy (Bruch) membrane, lies adjacent to the **pigment epithelium cells** (**3**) of the retina and separates the choroid and retina (see Fig. 22.9).

The outermost layer of the retina contains the pigment epithelium cells (**3**) whose basement membrane forms the innermost layer of the glassy (Bruch) membrane of the choroid. The pigment cells (**3**) of the retina contain melanin (pigment) granules in their cytoplasm.

Adjacent to the pigment epithelium cells (**3**) is a photosensitive layer of slender **rods** (**4**) and thicker **cones** (**5**). These cells are situated next to the **outer limiting membrane** (**6**) that is formed by the processes of supportive neuroglial cells called Muller cells.

The outer **nuclear layer** (**13**) contains the **nuclei of rods** (**4, 7**) and **cones** (**5, 7**) and the outer processes of Muller cells. In the **outer plexiform layer** (**14**) are the axons of rods and cones (4, 5)

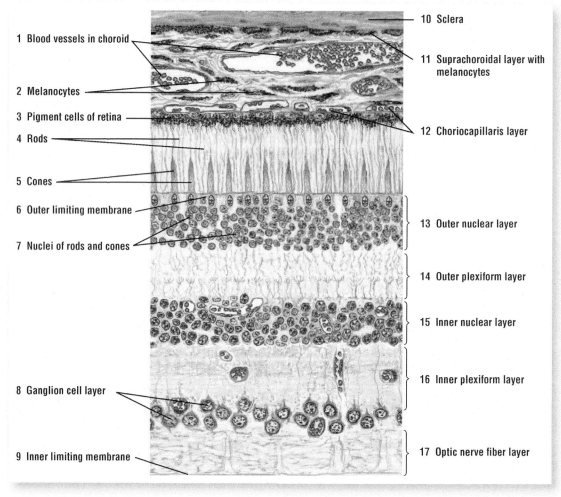

FIGURE 22.8 ■ Layers of the choroid and retina (detail). Stain: hematoxylin and eosin. High magnification.

that synapse with the dendrites of bipolar cells and horizontal cells that connect the rods (4) and cones (5) to the **ganglion cell layer** (8). The **inner nuclear layer** (15) contains the nuclei of bipolar, horizontal, amacrine, and neuroglial Muller cells. The horizontal and amacrine cells are association cells. In the **inner plexiform layer** (16), the axons of bipolar cells synapse with the dendrites of the ganglion (8) and amacrine cells.

The ganglion cell layer (8) contains the cell bodies of ganglion cells and neuroglial cells. The dendrites from the ganglion cells synapse in the inner plexiform layer (16).

The optic **nerve fiber layer** (17) contains the axons of the ganglion cells (8) and the inner fibers of Muller cells. Axons of ganglion cells (8) converge toward the optic disk and form the optic nerve fiber layer (17). The terminations of the inner fibers of Muller cells expand to form the **inner limiting membrane** (9) of the retina.

Blood vessels of the retina course in the optic nerve fiber layer (17) and penetrate the inner nuclear layer (15).

FIGURE 22.9 | **Eye: Layers of Retina and Choroid (Detail)**

This high-magnification photomicrograph illustrates the photosensitive retina. The **choroid** (1) is a vascular outer layer with loose connective tissue and melanocytes that is situated adjacent to the outermost retinal layer—the single-cell, **pigment epithelium** (2) layer. The light-sensitive **rods and cones** (3) form the next layer, which is separated from the dense **outer nuclear layer** (4) by a thin **outer limiting membrane** (5). Deep to the outer nuclear layer (4) is a clear area of synaptic connections, the **outer plexiform layer** (6).

The dense layer of cell bodies of the integrating neurons forms the **inner nuclear layer** (7), which is adjacent to the clear **inner plexiform layer** (8) in whose layer the axons of the integrating neurons form synaptic connections with axons of the neurons that form the optic tract. The cell bodies of the optic tract neurons form the **ganglion cell layer** (9), and their afferent axons form the light-staining **optic nerve fiber layer** (10). The innermost layer of the retina is the inner **limiting membrane** (11), which separates the retina from the vitreous body of the eyeball.

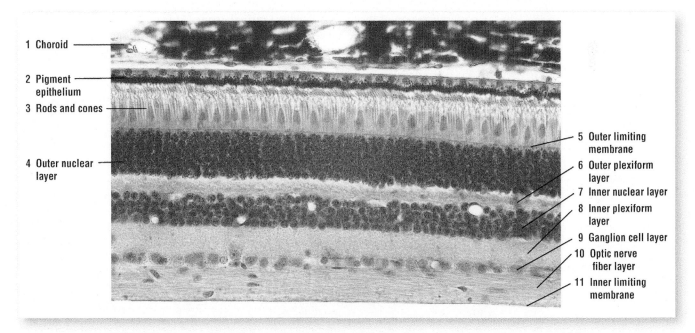

1 Choroid
2 Pigment epithelium
3 Rods and cones
4 Outer nuclear layer
5 Outer limiting membrane
6 Outer plexiform layer
7 Inner nuclear layer
8 Inner plexiform layer
9 Ganglion cell layer
10 Optic nerve fiber layer
11 Inner limiting membrane

FIGURE 22.9 ■ Eye: layers of retina and choroid. Stain: Masson trichrome. ×100.

FIGURE 22.10 | Section of Posterior Eyeball Showing Retina with Fovea Depression

At the posterior region of the eyeball, there is a shallow depression, or an indentation called the **fovea**. Here, the retina does not exhibit any blood vessels, the retinal layers are reduced, and almost all photoreceptor cells are cones. On each side of the depression are visible more expanded retinal layers. The dense-staining **ganglion cells** (**1**), the **inner nuclear layer** (**2**), the **outer nuclear layer** (**3**), and the **pigment epithelium** (**8**) adjacent to **choroid** (**4**) layer are visible. Similarly, the **inner plexiform layer** (**5**), **outer plexiform layer** (**6**), and the photoreceptors **rods and cones** (**7**) adjacent to the pigment epithelium (**8**) are also visible. Surrounding the periphery of the eyeball is the **sclera** (**9**).

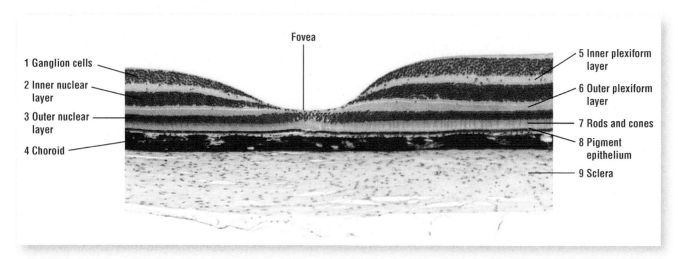

FIGURE 22.10 ■ A section of posterior eyeball showing the retina with a fovea depression. Stain: hematoxylin and eosin. ×17.

FIGURE 22.11 | Optic Papilla (Optic Disk), Optic Nerve, and Section of Retina in Posterior Region of Eyeball

In the posterior region of the eyeball is where **retinal axons** (**5**) from the ganglion cells of the retina converge to form an **optic nerve** that penetrates the connective tissue **sclera** (**3**) and leaves the eyeball. Where the optic nerve leaves the eyeball is the **optic disk** (**optic papilla**), which is

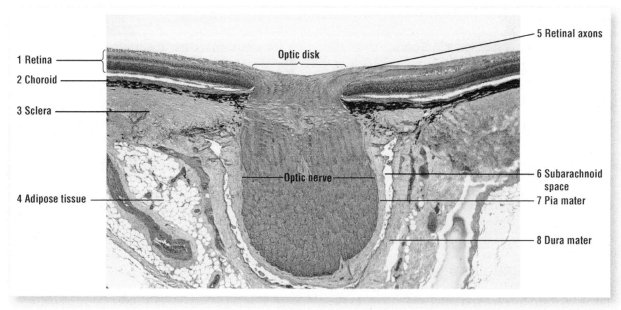

FIGURE 22.11 ■ Optic papilla (optic disk), optic nerve, and a section of retina in the posterior region of the eyeball. Stain: hematoxylin and eosin. ×10.5.

completely insensitive to light because of the absences of the photoreceptor cells and is, therefore, the blind spot in the eye. After leaving the eyeball, the optic nerve in the eye orbit of the skull is surrounded by the meninges of the brain, the **pia mater** (7), a **subarachnoid space** (6), and a thick **dura mater** (8). This low-magnification micrograph also shows different dark-staining cellular and light-staining layers of the **retina** (1) and the adjacent, dense-staining **choroid** (2). Surrounding the exterior of the eyeball are the cells of the **adipose tissue** (4).

FIGURE 22.12 | Section of Posterior Retina with Yellow Pigment of Macula Lutea

With special stains, it is possible to see the yellow area of the macula lutea in the posterior region of the retina. The macula lutea is a small yellow area that surrounds the retinal depression (fovea) and is closely located to the optic disk in the posterior region of the eyeball. This micrograph image shows the yellow color of the macula lutea that is due to the accumulated **yellow pigment** (**xanthophyll**) (7) in the ganglion cells from the fovea. The **ganglion cell layer** (2) and the **retinal axons** (1) are displaced laterally off the fovea so that the light can pass unimpeded to the sensitive cone cells in the center of the fovea. With this stain are also visible the ganglion cell layer (2), the **inner plexiform layer** (8), the **inner nuclear layer** (3), the **outer plexiform layer** (9), the **outer nuclear layer** (4), and the photoreceptors cells—the **rods and cones** (10). Barely visible is the **pigment epithelium** (5) layer that is adjacent to the dense-staining **choroid** (6). Surrounding the retina is the connective tissue **sclera** (11).

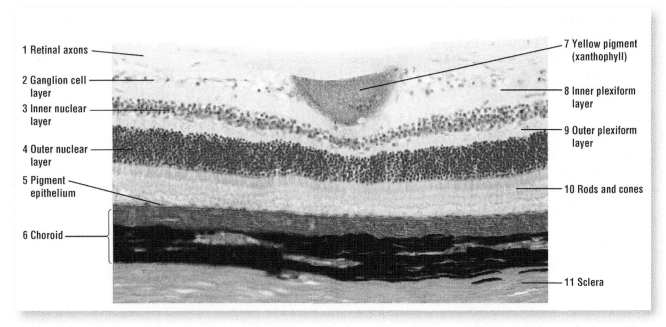

FIGURE 22.12 ■ A section of the posterior retina with the yellow pigment of the macula lutea. Stain: gold and yellow. ×100.

SECRETIONS (TEARS)

Each eyeball is covered on its anterior surface with thin **eyelids** and fine hairs, **eyelashes**, located on the margins of the eyelids. Eyelids and eyelashes protect the eyes from foreign objects and excessive light. Situated above each eye is a secretory **lacrimal gland** that continually produces **lacrimal secretions** or **tears**. Blinking spreads the lacrimal secretion across the outer surface of the eyeball and the inner surface of the eyelid. The lacrimal secretion contains numerous proteins (tear albumins, lactoferrin), mucus, salts, and the antibacterial enzyme **lysozyme**. Lacrimal secretions clean, protect, moisten, and lubricate the surface of the eye (conjunctiva and cornea).

The **tarsal glands** produce an oily secretion that forms a surface layer on the tear film that prevents the evaporation of the tear layer and lubricates the ocular surface. The **sweat glands** (**of Moll**) produce and empty their secretions into the follicles of the eyelashes.

AQUEOUS HUMOR

Aqueous humor is produced by the ciliary epithelium of the **ciliary process** in the eye. This watery fluid flows from the posterior chambers through the pupil into the anterior chamber of the eye between the cornea and lens. Aqueous humor maintains the intraocular pressure, bathes the nonvascular **cornea** and **lens**, and also supplies them with nutrients and oxygen. The fluid is continuously reabsorbed in the angle between the cornea and iris into the canal of Schlemm and the veins of sclera.

VITREOUS BODY

The vitreous chamber of the eye is located behind the lens and contains a gelatinous substance called the **vitreous body**, a transparent colorless gel that consists mainly of water. In addition, the vitreous body contains small amounts of hyaluronic acid, very thin collagen fibers, glycosaminoglycans, and some proteins. The vitreous body transmits incoming light, is nonrefractive, maintains the intraocular pressure and shape of the eyeball, and supports the retina against shock and vibration.

RETINA

The photosensitive retina contains photoreceptive **rods** and **cones**, **bipolar cells**, and **ganglion cells** distributed in different layers. The rods and cones are receptor neurons essential for vision. They synapse with the bipolar cells, which then connect the receptor neurons with the ganglion cells. The afferent axons that leave the ganglion cells converge posteriorly in the eye at the **optic papilla** (optic disk) and leave the eye as the **optic nerve**. The optic papilla, also called the **blind spot**, lacks photoreceptor cells and only contains axons.

Because the rods and cones are situated adjacent to the **choroid layer** of the retina, light rays must first pass through the ganglion and bipolar cell layers to reach and activate the photosensitive rods and cones. The **retinal pigmented epithelial layer** of the choroid absorbs light rays and prevents reflection through the retina that would result in glare. In addition, these epithelial cells phagocytose worn-out outer components of both rods and cones, which are continually shed in renewal processes. The retinal pigment epithelial layer also stores vitamin A, a rhodopsin precursor that initiates visual stimulation. Retinal pigmented epithelial cells utilize vitamin A to form visual pigment molecules for both rods and cones. Cells of the pigment epithelium also form a protective **blood–retina barrier** that isolates the retinal photoreceptive cells and limits the movement of ions, cells, and other substances between the retinal capillaries and the retinal tissue.

RODS AND CONES

The rods are highly sensitive to light and function best in dim or **low light** (at dusk or at night). In the dark, a visual pigment **rhodopsin** is synthesized and accumulates in the rod cells. When rhodopsin interacts with light, it initiates the visual stimulus. In contrast, the cones are less numerous and less sensitive to low light, but respond best to **bright light**. Cones are also essential for visual acuity and **color vision** and contain the visual pigment **iodopsin** that responds maximally to red, green, or blue colors that induce a visual response. Absorption and interaction of light rays with the pigments in rods and cones cause transformations in the pigment molecules. This action excites the rods and/or cones and produces a nerve impulse for vision.

At the posterior region of the eye is a shallow depression in the retina called the **fovea** where its center contains only the **cone cells**, and the blood vessels do not pass over these photosensitive cells. The visual axis of the eye directly passes through the fovea, and the light rays fall directly on and stimulate the tightly packed cones in the center of fovea. As a result, the fovea produces the greatest **visual acuity** and the sharpest **color discrimination**. Immediately adjacent to and surrounding the fovea is the **macula lutea**, a small area that appears yellow in the retina. The yellow color of the macula is due to the presence and accumulation of the yellow pigment **xanthophyll** in the laterally located ganglion cells.

Chapter 22 Summary

SECTION 1 • Visual System

- Eyes are located in protective orbits in the skull
- Visual images are conveyed from eye to brain via optic nerves

EYE LAYERS

- Sclera is the outer layer of eye and is composed of dense connective tissue
- Internal to sclera is the middle or vascular layer uvea that nourishes the retina and the eyeball
- Uvea consists of pigmented choroid, ciliary body, and iris
- Retina is the innermost lining of eye; posterior three-quarters of retina is photosensitive
- Retina terminates anteriorly at ora serrata, which is a non-photosensitive part of retina

WHOLE EYE

- Sclera maintains the rigidity of the eyeball and is the white of the eye
- Anteriorly, sclera is modified into transparent cornea through which light enters eye
- Choroid and ciliary body are adjacent to sclera
- Ciliary processes from ciliary body attach lens by suspensory ligament or zonular fibers
- Iris partially covers the lens and is the colored part of the eye
- Radial smooth muscle forms an opening in the iris, called the pupil

EYE CHAMBERS

- Anterior chamber located between cornea, iris, and lens
- Posterior chamber is a small space between iris, ciliary process, zonular fibers, and lens
- Vitreous chamber is a large posterior space behind lens and zonular fibers, surrounded by retina

Photosensitive Parts of Eye

- Rods and cones in the retina are sensitive to light
- Afferent axons leave retina and conduct impulses from eye to brain for interpretation

Secretions (Tears)

- Each eyeball is covered with an eyelid, which contains sebaceous glands and sweat glands (of Moll)
- Above each eyeball is the lacrimal gland, which produces lacrimal secretions or tears
- Myoepithelial cells surround secretory acini in lacrimal gland
- Tears contain mucus, salts, and antibacterial enzyme lysozyme
- Sebaceous (tarsal) gland secretions form an oily layer on the surface of tear film that prevents evaporation and lubricates ocular surface

Chamber Contents: Aqueous Humor and Vitreous Body

- Produced by ciliary epithelium of the eye and fills both the anterior and posterior chambers
- Bathes nonvascular cornea and lens; supplies them with nutrients and oxygen
- Fluid flows from posterior to anterior chamber via the pupil
- Fluid resorbed in angle between cornea and iris into canal of Schlemm and scleral veins

Vitreous Body

- Vitreous chamber located behind lens and contains transparent gelatinous substance called vitreous body
- Consists mainly of water and water-soluble proteins
- Transmits incoming light, is nonrefractive, and contributes to intraocular pressure of eyeball
- Holds retina in place against pigmented layer of the eyeball
- Supports retina against shock and vibration

Retina

- Contains three types of neurons distributed in different layers
- Rods and cones are receptor neurons essential for vision that synapse with bipolar cells
- Bipolar cells connect to ganglion cells, from which axons converge posteriorly at optic papilla
- Area of optic papilla contains only axons of optic nerve and is the blind spot
- Light rays pass through all cell layers to activate rods and cones

- Pigmented layer of choroid next to retina absorbs light and prevents reflection
- Cells of pigmented layer form blood–retina barrier to isolated photoreceptive cells

Choroid

- Divided into suprachoroid lamina, vascular layer, and choriocapillaris layer
- Suprachoroid layer contains connective tissue fibers and numerous melanocytes
- Vascular layer contains numerous blood vessels and melanocytes
- Choriocapillaris layer contains capillaries with large lumina
- Innermost layer of choroid is glassy membrane and lies adjacent to pigment cells
- Pigment cells separate choroid from retina and perform important functions
- Pigment cells are phagocytic, store vitamin A, and form visual pigments for rods and cones

Rods and Cones

- Rods are highly sensitive to light, function in low light, and synthesize visual pigment rhodopsin
- Cones are sensitive to bright light, essential for visual acuity and color vision
- Cones are most sensitive to red, green, or blue color spectrums and contain visual pigment iodopsin
- Interaction of light with visual pigments transforms their molecules and excites rods and cones
- Pigment xanthophyll accumulates in ganglion cells of macula lutea
- Fovea is in the center of macula lutea and devoid of rods and blood vessels
- Fovea contains a high concentration of the photosensitive cones
- Fovea produces greatest visual acuity and sharpest color discrimination
- Blood vessels do not pass over fovea region in the retina

Chapter 22 Review Questions: Section 1

QUESTIONS

In the following multiple choice questions, choose the letter corresponding to the one best answer.

1. The aqueous humor of the eye:

A. fills the posterior chamber of the eye.
B. covers the lens to maintain moisture.
C. is produced by the cells in the ciliary process.
D. is a gelatinous substance of vitreous chamber.
E. is produced by the tear glands.

2. Where is the antibacterial enzyme lysozyme produced?

A. In the anterior chamber of the eye
B. In vitreous humor
C. In lacrimal secretions
D. In the posterior chamber of the eye
E. In the aqueous humor

3. What does the blind spot in the eye represent?

A. Optic papilla of the optic nerve
B. Nonphotosensitive part of the retina
C. Macula lutea of the retina
D. Fovea of the retina
E. Choroid layer

4. What is rhodopsin?

A. It is a yellow pigment in the choroid.
B. It is a dark pigment in the choroid.
C. It is a visual pigment in the cones.
D. It is a visual pigment in the rods.
E. It is a high concentration of rods.

5. What is found in the fovea?

A. A high concentration of cones
B. A blind spot
C. The macula lutea
D. A high concentration of rods
E. Xanthophyll pigment

ANSWERS

1. **Correct Answer: C.** Is produced by the cells of in the ciliary process. Both anterior and posterior chambers are filled by the aqueous humor produced by the ciliary process located behind the iris in the posterior chamber.

2. **Correct Answer: C.** In lacrimal secretions. The lacrimal gland in the eyelids produces the tears or lacrimal secretions that contain the enzyme lysozyme.

3. **Correct Answer: A.** Optic papilla of the optic nerve. This is the area where the optic nerve leaves the eyeball. There are no photosensitive cells present in the optic papilla.

4. **Correct Answer: D.** It is a visual pigment in the rods. When this pigment interacts with light, it initiates a visual stimulus.

5. **Correct Answer: C.** Macula lutea. This structure surrounds the fovea and contains yellow pigment.

SECTION 2 Auditory System

The **auditory system** consists of the external ear, the middle ear, and the inner ear. The ear is a specialized sensory organ that contains structures responsible for hearing, balance, and maintenance of equilibrium.

EXTERNAL EAR

The auricle, or **pinna**, of the **external ear** gathers sound waves from the environment and directs them through the **external auditory canal** to the eardrum or **tympanic membrane**, from which the sound is directed to the middle ear (Fig. 22.13).

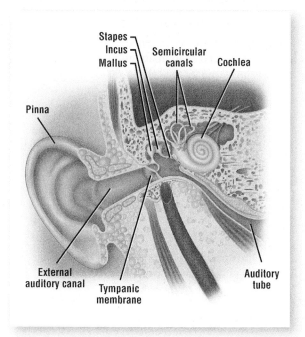

FIGURE 22.13 ■ The internal structures of the ear.

MIDDLE EAR

The **middle ear** is a small, air-filled cavity called the **tympanic cavity**. It is located in and protected by the temporal bone of the skull. The **tympanic membrane** separates the external auditory canal from the middle ear. Located in the middle ear are the **auditory ossicles** consisting of the **stapes**, **incus**, and **malleus** that are attached to the tympanic membrane and to the cochlea of the inner ear; also in the middle ear is the **auditory (eustachian) tube**. The sound waves vibrate the tympanic membrane and are then transmitted through the auditory ossicle bones to the inner ear. The cavity of the middle ear also communicates with the nasopharynx region of the head via the auditory tube. The presence of the auditory tube allows for the equalization of air pressure on both sides of the tympanic membrane during swallowing or blowing the nose.

INNER EAR

The inner ear lies deep in the temporal bone of the skull and consists of small, communicating cavities and canals. These cavities, the **semicircular canals**, **vestibule**, and **cochlea**, are collectively called the **osseous**, or **bony**, **labyrinth**. All sections of the bony labyrinth are filled with perilymph, a fluid rich in sodium and similar in composition to the cerebrospinal fluid (CSF) of the central nervous system. Located within the bony labyrinth is the **membranous labyrinth** that consists of interconnected, thin-walled compartments filled with fluid called **endolymph**.

Cochlea

The organ specialized for receiving and transmitting sound (hearing) is found in the inner ear in the structure called the cochlea (Fig. 22.14). It is a spiral bony canal that resembles a snail's shell that makes three turns on itself around a central bony pillar called the **modiolus**.

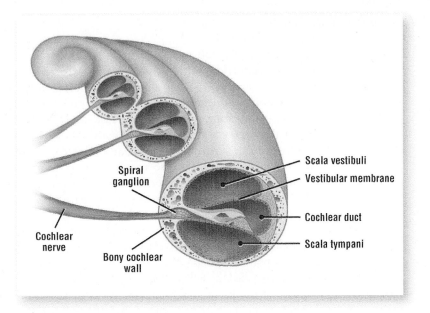

FIGURE 22.14 ■ The cochlea.

Interiorly, the cochlea is partitioned into **vestibular duct** (**scala vestibuli**), **tympanic duct** (**scala tympani**), and **cochlear duct** (**scala media**). Located within the cochlear duct on the **basilar membrane** are specialized receptor cells that detect sound; this is the hearing **organ of Corti** (Fig. 22.15). This organ consists of numerous auditory receptor cells, or **hair cells**, and supporting cells that respond to different sound frequencies. The hair cells contain long, stiff **stereocilia** and project into the fluid-filled cochlear duct. The auditory stimuli (sounds) are carried away from the receptor hair cells via afferent axons of the **cochlear nerve** to the brain for interpretation. A **tectorial membrane** overlies the organ of Corti.

Vestibular Apparatus

The organ of vestibular functions, the **vestibular apparatus**, is responsible for **balance** and **equilibrium**. It is found in the **utricle**, **saccule**, and three **semicircular canals**.

the**Point®**   Supplemental micrographic images are available at **www.thePoint.com/Eroschenko13e** under Organs of the Special Senses.

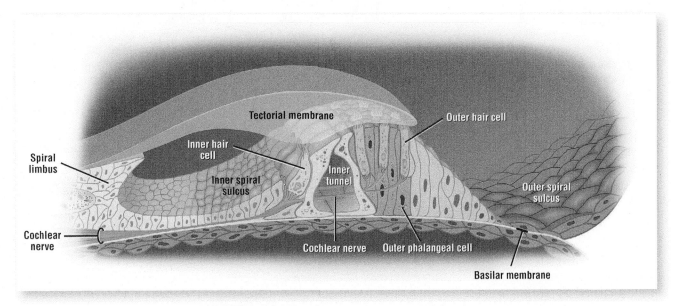

FIGURE 22.15 ■ The hearing organ of Corti.

FIGURE 22.16 | Inner Ear: Cochlea (Vertical Section)

This low-magnification image illustrates the labyrinthine characteristics of the inner ear. The **osseous**, or **bony**, **labyrinth** of the **cochlea** (**14**, **16**) spirals around a central axis of a spongy bone called the **modiolus** (**15**) that contains the **spiral ganglia** (**7**) composed of bipolar afferent (sensory) neurons. The dendrites from the **bipolar neurons** (**7**) extend to and innervate the hair cells located in the hearing **organ of Corti** (**12**). The axons from these afferent neurons join and form the **cochlear nerve** (**13**) that is located in the modiolus (**15**).

The osseous labyrinth (**14**, **16**) is divided into the **osseous** (**bony**) **spiral lamina** (**6**) and the **basilar membrane** (**9**). The osseous spiral lamina (**6**) projects from the modiolus (**15**) about halfway into the lumen of the cochlear canal. The basilar membrane (**9**) continues from the osseous spiral lamina (**6**) to the **spiral ligament** (**11**), a thickening of the connective tissue periosteum on the **outer bony wall** of the **cochlear canal** (**8**).

The cochlear canal (**8**) is subdivided into the lower **tympanic duct** (**scala tympani**) (**4**) and the upper **vestibular duct** (**scala vestibuli**) (**2**). The separate tympanic duct (**4**) and vestibular duct (**2**) continue in a spiral course to the apex of the cochlea, where they communicate through an opening called the **helicotrema** (**1**).

The **vestibular** (Reissner) **membrane** (**5**) separates the vestibular duct (**2**) from the **cochlear duct** (**scala media**) (**3**) and forms the roof of the cochlear duct (**3**). The vestibular membrane (**5**) attaches to the spiral ligament (**11**) in the outer bony wall of the cochlear canal (**8**). The sensory cells for sound detection are located in the organ of Corti (**12**), which rests on the basilar membrane (**9**) of the cochlear duct (**3**). A **tectorial membrane** (**10**) overlies the cells in the organ of Corti (**12**) (see also Figs. 22.17 through 22.19).

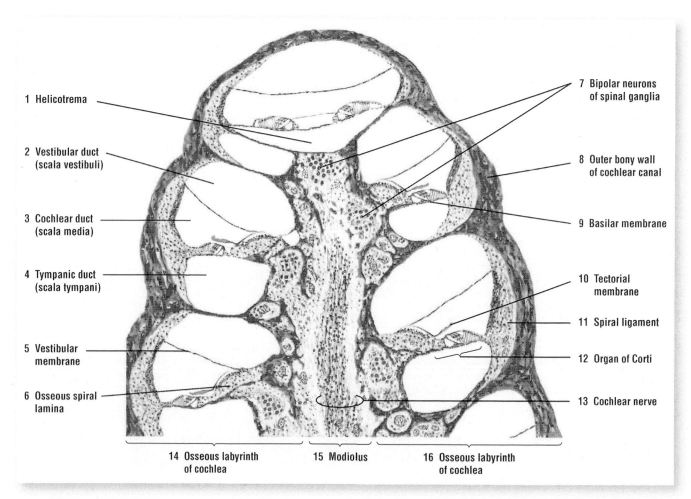

1 Helicotrema

2 Vestibular duct (scala vestibuli)

3 Cochlear duct (scala media)

4 Tympanic duct (scala tympani)

5 Vestibular membrane

6 Osseous spiral lamina

7 Bipolar neurons of spinal ganglia

8 Outer bony wall of cochlear canal

9 Basilar membrane

10 Tectorial membrane

11 Spiral ligament

12 Organ of Corti

13 Cochlear nerve

14 Osseous labyrinth of cochlea

15 Modiolus

16 Osseous labyrinth of cochlea

FIGURE 22.16 ■ Inner ear: cochlea (vertical section). Stain: hematoxylin and eosin. Low magnification.

FIGURE 22.17 | Inner Ear: Cochlear Duct (Scala Media) and Hearing Organ of Corti

This illustration shows in more detail the **cochlear duct (scala media)** (**9**), the hearing **organ of Corti** (**13**), and its associated cells at a higher magnification.

The outer wall of the cochlear duct (9) is formed by a vascular area called the **stria vascularis** (**15**). The stratified epithelium covering the stria vascularis (15) contains a rich intraepithelial capillary network formed from the blood vessels that supply the connective tissue in the **spiral ligament** (**17**). The spiral ligament (17) contains collagen fibers, pigmented fibroblasts, and numerous blood vessels.

The roof of the cochlear duct (9) is formed by a thin **vestibular (Reissner) membrane** (**6**) that separates the cochlear duct (9) from the **vestibular duct (scala vestibuli)** (**7**). The vestibular membrane (6) extends from the spiral ligament (17) in the outer wall of the cochlear duct (9) located at the upper extent of the stria vascularis (15) to the thickened periosteum of the **osseous spiral lamina** (**2**) near the **spiral limbus** (**1**).

The spiral limbus (1) is a thickened mass of periosteal connective tissue of the osseous spiral lamina (2) that extends into and forms the floor of the cochlear duct (9). The spiral limbus (1) is covered by an **epithelium** (**5**) that appears columnar and is supported by a lateral extension of the osseous spiral lamina (2). The lateral extracellular extension of the spiral limbus epithelium (5) beyond the spiral limbus (1) forms the **tectorial membrane** (**10**) that overlies the **inner spiral tunnel** (**8**) and a portion of the organ of Corti (13).

The **basilar membrane** (**16**) is a vascularized connective tissue that forms the lower wall of the cochlear duct (9). The organ of Corti (13) rests on the fibers of the basilar membrane (16) and consists of the sensory **outer hair cells** (**11**), supporting cells, associated inner spiral tunnel (8), and an **inner tunnel** (**12**).

The afferent fibers of **the cochlear nerve** (**4**) from the bipolar cells located in the **spiral ganglion** (**3**) course through the osseous spiral lamina (2) and synapse with outer hair cells (11) in the organ of Corti (13).

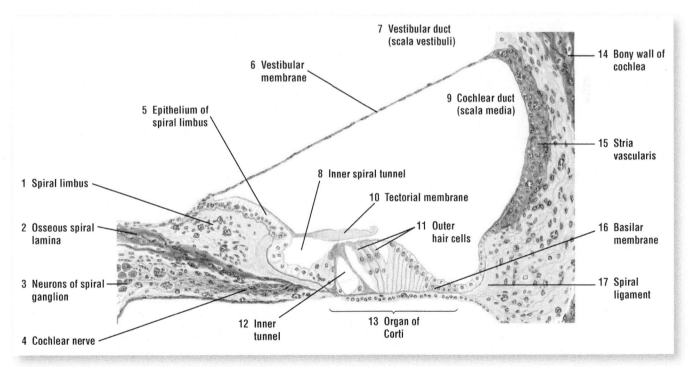

FIGURE 22.17 ■ Inner ear: cochlear duct (scala media) and the hearing organ of Corti. Stain: hematoxylin and eosin. Medium magnification.

FIGURE 22.18 | Inner Ear: Cochlear Duct and Organ of Corti

This higher-magnification photomicrograph illustrates the inner ear with the cochlear canal and the hearing **organ of Corti** (**8**) in the **bony cochlea** (**1, 9**). The cochlear canal is subdivided into the **vestibular duct** (**scala vestibuli**) (**10**), **cochlear duct** (**scala media**) (**3**), and **tympanic duct** (**scala tympani**) (**14**). A thin, **vestibular membrane** (**2**) separates the cochlear duct (3) from the vestibular duct (scala vestibuli) (10). A thicker **basilar membrane** (**7**) separates the cochlear duct (3) from the tympanic duct (scala tympani) (14).

The basilar membrane (7) extends from the connective tissue **spiral ligament** (**6**) to a thickened **spiral limbus** (**11**). The basilar membrane (7) supports the organ of Corti (8) with its sensory **hair cells** (**5**) and supportive cells. Extending from the spiral limbus (11) is the **tectorial membrane** (**4**) that covers a portion of the organ of Corti (8) and the outer hair cells (5). The sensory bipolar **spiral ganglion cells** (**13**) are located in the bony cochlea (1, 9). The afferent axons from the spiral ganglion cells (13) pass through the **osseous spiral lamina** (**12**) to the organ of Corti (8) where their dendrites synapse with its hair cells (5).

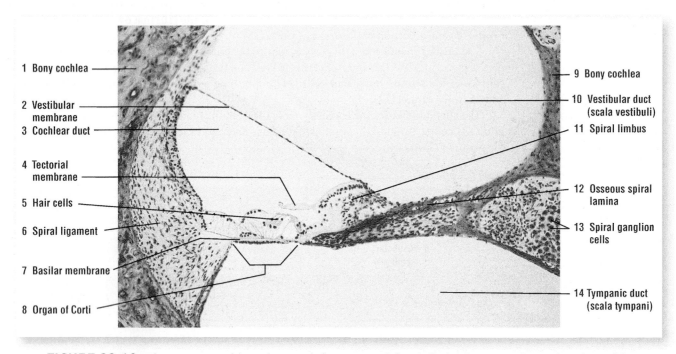

1 Bony cochlea

2 Vestibular membrane
3 Cochlear duct

4 Tectorial membrane

5 Hair cells

6 Spiral ligament

7 Basilar membrane

8 Organ of Corti

9 Bony cochlea

10 Vestibular duct (scala vestibuli)

11 Spiral limbus

12 Osseous spiral lamina

13 Spiral ganglion cells

14 Tympanic duct (scala tympani)

FIGURE 22.18 ■ Inner ear: cochlear duct and the organ of Corti. Stain: hematoxylin and eosin. ×30.

FIGURE 22.19 | Inner Ear: Organ of Corti in Cochlear Duct

This micrograph enlarges the image in Figure 22.18 and shows greater detail of the cochlea and the surrounding cells in the inner ear. The micrograph focuses primarily on the **cochlear duct** (**2**) and the cells and structures in the **organ of Corti** (**14**) situated on the **basilar membrane** (**6**). Visible in the organ of Corti (**14**) are the **outer hair cells** (**12**), the **inner tunnel** (**13**), and the **outer tunnel** (**5**) that separates the cells. Superior to the outer hair cells (**12**) is the **tectorial membrane** (**4**), with the **inner spiral tunnel** (**11**) located inferior to the tectorial membrane (**4**). The thin **vestibular membrane** (**8**) separates the vestibular duct (scala vestibuli) (**1**) from the cochlear duct (**2**). Facing the cochlear duct (**2**) is the vascularized epithelium of **stria vascularis** (**3**) that overlies the connective tissue **spiral ligament** (**7**). The vestibular membrane (**8**) attaches to the **spiral limbus** (**9**) under which are found the axons of the **cochlear nerve** (**10**).

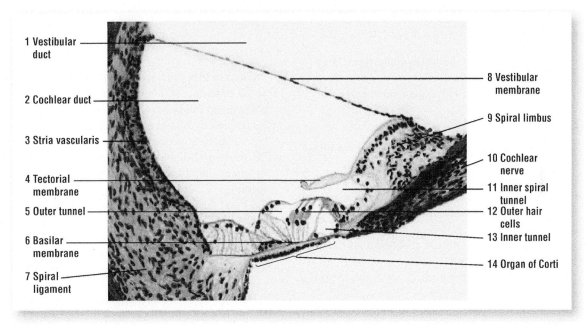

1 Vestibular duct
2 Cochlear duct
3 Stria vascularis
4 Tectorial membrane
5 Outer tunnel
6 Basilar membrane
7 Spiral ligament

8 Vestibular membrane
9 Spiral limbus
10 Cochlear nerve
11 Inner spiral tunnel
12 Outer hair cells
13 Inner tunnel
14 Organ of Corti

FIGURE 22.19 ■ Inner ear: organ of Corti in the cochlear duct. Stain: hematoxylin and eosin. ×50.

FUNCTIONAL CORRELATIONS 22.2 ■ Inner Ear

COCHLEA

The cochlea of the inner ear contains the auditory **organ of Corti**. Sound waves that enter the ear and pass through the **external auditory canal** create mechanical vibrations in the **tympanic membrane** that activate the three bony **ossicles** (stapes, incus, and malleus) in the middle ear. These vibrations are transmitted across the air-filled **middle ear**, or **tympanic cavity**, to the fluid-filled **inner ear**. The sounds vibrate the **basilar membrane** on which are located the sensitive receptor cells for hearing, the hair cells of the organ of Corti that function as **mechano-electrical transducers**. The vibrations of the basilar membrane because of sound, shearing, or bending motion between the hairs (stereocilia) in the hair cells and the overlying **tectorial membrane** activate the release of neurotransmitters from the basal synapse of **hair cells** to the afferent axons. The deflections of the stereocilia on the hair cells convert this mechanical displacement into **nerve impulses**, resulting in transmitting the auditory information to the brain.

Impulses for sound pass along the afferent axons of bipolar **ganglion cells** located in the **spiral ganglia** of the inner ear. The axons from the spiral ganglia form the **auditory** (**cochlear**) **nerve**, which carries the auditory stimuli from the cells in the organ of Corti to the brain for sound interpretation.

VESTIBULAR APPARATUS

The vestibular apparatus consists of the **utricle**, **saccule**, and **semicircular canals**. These sensitive organs respond to linear or angular accelerations or movements of the head. Sensory inputs from the vestibular apparatus initiate the very complex neural pathways that activate specific skeletal muscles that correct balance and equilibrium and restore the body to its normal position.

Chapter 22 Summary

SECTION 2 • Auditory System

- Ear is specialized for hearing, balance, and maintenance of equilibrium

EXTERNAL EAR

- Auricle, or pinna, gathers sound waves and directs them through external auditory canal
- Sound waves reach eardrum or tympanic membrane

MIDDLE EAR

- Contains a small, air-filled cavity called tympanic cavity in temporal bone of the skull
- Tympanic membrane separates external auditory canal from middle ear
- Contains three very small bones, the auditory ossicles: stapes, incus, and malleus
- Contains auditory (eustachian) tube that communicates with nasopharynx
- Auditory tube equalizes air pressure on both sides of tympanic membrane

INNER EAR

- Lies deep in the temporal bone of the skull
- Consists of semicircular canals, vestibule, and cochlea, which is called bony labyrinth

- In bony labyrinth is the membranous labyrinth, a series of compartments filled with fluid
- All sections of bony labyrinth filled with fluid perilymph
- Membranous labyrinth filled with fluid endolymph

Cochlea

- Located in inner ear; receives and transmits sound
- Spiral canal that makes three turns around central bony pillar called modiolus
- Embedded in modiolus is the spiral ganglion composed of bipolar afferent neurons
- Interiorly partitioned into vestibular duct (scala vestibuli), tympanic duct (scala tympani), and cochlear duct (scala media)
- Cochlear duct contains receptor or hair cells in the hearing organ of Corti
- Sound waves vibrate tympanic membrane, which activates the bony ossicles in the middle ear
- Bony ossicles transmit vibrations to inner ear and vibrate basilar membrane
- Organ of Corti is located on basilar membrane; vibrations stimulate hair cells in the organ
- Hair cells (stereocilia displacement) in the organ of Corti convert mechanical vibrations into nerve impulses
- Impulses pass along afferent nerves in spiral ganglia of inner ear to cochlear nerve and brain

Chapter 22 Review Questions: Section 2

QUESTIONS

In the following multiple choice questions, choose the letter corresponding to the one best answer.

1. **The tympanic membrane in the ear separates what structures?**

   A. Auditory ossicles
   B. External auditory canal from the middle ear
   C. Middle ear from the auditory (eustachian) tube
   D. Middle ear from the inner ear
   E. Middle ear from the nasopharynx

2. **The main function of the auditory (eustachian) tube is:**

   A. to conduct sound toward the tympanic membrane.
   B. to reinforce the bony ossicles in the auditory tube.
   C. to direct sounds away from the tympanic membrane.
   D. to equalize pressure on both sides of the tympanic membrane.
   E. nothing.

3. **The bony labyrinth of the ear is filled with:**

   A. perilymph.
   B. air.
   C. hair cells.
   D. endolymph.
   E. bony ossicles.

4. **The organ of Corti is located in(on) the:**

   A. tectorial membrane.
   B. vestibular duct.
   C. basilar membrane.
   D. tympanic membrane.
   E. cochlear duct.

5. **What is the role of the tectorial membrane in sound detection?**

   A. Its vibrations transmit sound from the external ear to the middle ear.
   B. It activates the bony ossicles for sound transmission.
   C. Its interaction with stereocilia in hair cells activates sound transmission.
   D. The hearing organ is attached to its membrane.
   E. It equalizes the sound waves between the external and internal ear.

ANSWERS

1. **Correct Answer: B.** The tympanic membrane in the ear separates the external auditory canal from the middle ear.

2. **Correct Answer: D.** To equalize pressure on both sides of tympanic membrane. This function is utilized during swallowing, blowing the nose, or other pressure alterations that affect the ear.

3. **Correct Answer: A.** Perilymph. This fluid is similar to the cerebrospinal fluid of the central nervous system.

4. **Correct Answer: C.** Basilar membrane. The sounds vibrate the basilar membrane that activates the hair cells (stereocilia) in the organ of Corti and sends nerve impulses for interpretation of sound.

5. **Correct Answer: C.** Its interaction with stereocilia in hair cells activates sound transmission. This activation causes release of neurotransmitters and results in transmission of auditory signals to the brain.

ADDITIONAL HISTOLOGIC IMAGES

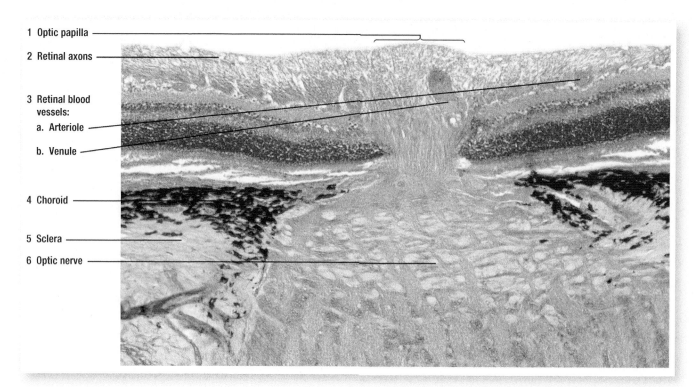

1 Optic papilla

2 Retinal axons

3 Retinal blood vessels:
   a. Arteriole
   b. Venule

4 Choroid

5 Sclera

6 Optic nerve

FIGURE 22.20 ■ A posterior region of primate eyeball illustrating the optic nerve as it leaves the eyeball at the optic papilla. Stain: hematoxylin and eosin. ×25.

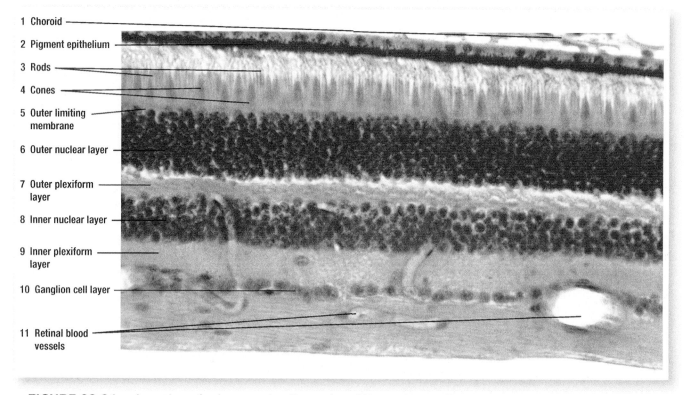

1 Choroid

2 Pigment epithelium

3 Rods

4 Cones

5 Outer limiting membrane

6 Outer nuclear layer

7 Outer plexiform layer

8 Inner nuclear layer

9 Inner plexiform layer

10 Ganglion cell layer

11 Retinal blood vessels

FIGURE 22.21 ■ A section of primate retina illustrating different layers. Stain: hematoxylin and eosin. ×205.

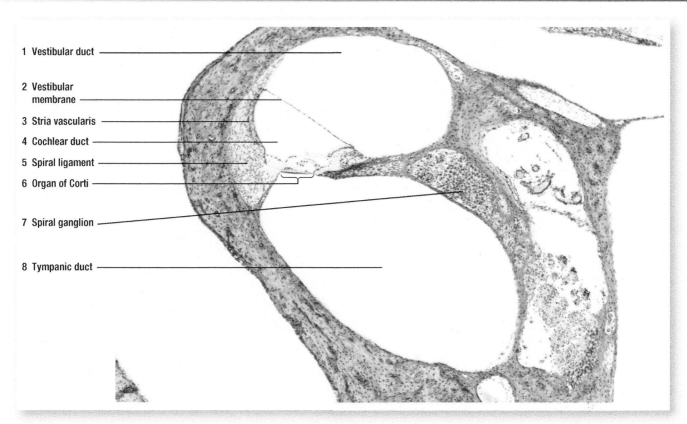

1 Vestibular duct

2 Vestibular membrane

3 Stria vascularis

4 Cochlear duct

5 Spiral ligament

6 Organ of Corti

7 Spiral ganglion

8 Tympanic duct

FIGURE 22.22 ■ A section of primate cochlea illustrating the ducts, their contents, and the surrounding structures. Stain: hematoxylin and eosin. ×13.

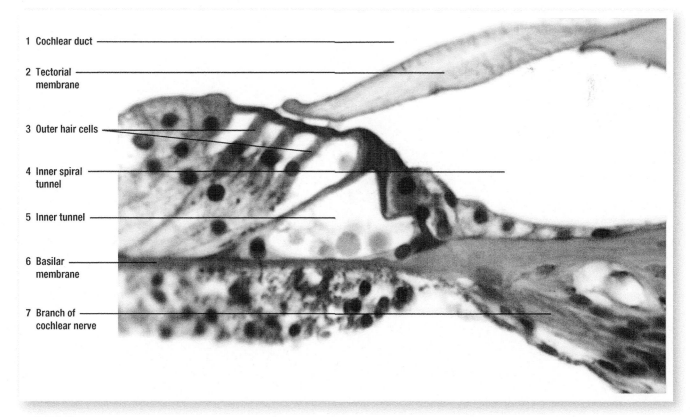

1 Cochlear duct

2 Tectorial membrane

3 Outer hair cells

4 Inner spiral tunnel

5 Inner tunnel

6 Basilar membrane

7 Branch of cochlear nerve

FIGURE 22.23 ■ High magnification of the organ of Corti in a primate. Stain: hematoxylin and eosin. ×320.

INDEX